Keshria Peter

D0202907

FIFTH EDITION

Introduction to Audiologic Rehabilitation

RONALD L. SCHOW

Idaho State University

MICHAEL A. NERBONNE

Central Michigan University

Website Design

Jeff E. Brockett

www.isu.edu/csed/rehab

Boston   New York   San Francisco
Mexico City   Montreal   Toronto   London   Madrid   Munich   Paris
Hong Kong   Singapore   Tokyo   Cape Town   Sydney

Executive Editor and Publisher: Stephen D. Dragin
Editorial Assistant: Katie Heimsoth
Production Supervisor: Joe Sweeney
Editorial–Production Service: Walsh & Associates, Inc.
Composition and Prepress Buyer: Linda Cox
Manufacturing Buyer: Linda Morris
Cover Administrator: Kristine Mose-Libon
Electronic Composition: Omegatype Typography, Inc.

For related titles and support materials, visit our online catalog at
www.ablongman.com.

Library of Congress Cataloging-in-Publication Data

Introduction to audiologic rehabilitation / [edited by] Ronald L. Schow, Michael A.
    Nerbonne. — 5th ed.
        p.   cm.
    Includes bibliographical references and index.
    ISBN 0-205-48292-9
    1. Deaf—Rehabilitation.   2. Audiology.   I. Schow, Ronald L.   II. Nerbonne, Michael A.

RF297.I57   2007
617.8'03—dc22

2006048386

Printed in the United States of America

10   9   8   7   15   14   13   12   11

To our grandchildren—Wyatt, Garrett, McKay, Carter, Shay, Mari, Hayden, Tate, Sadie, Halle, Tyson, Lucas, and others yet unnamed

■ CONTENTS

v

2 Hearing Aids and Assistive Devices 31

H. Gustav Mueller
Earl E. Johnson
Anne S. Carter

7 Psychosocial Aspects of Hearing Impairment and Counseling Basics   245

Kris English

10 Audiologic Rehabilitation for Adults and Elderly Adults: Assessment and Management   367
Kathy Pichora-Fuller
Ronald L. Schow

PART THREE: Implementing Audiologic Rehabilitation: Case Studies   435

11 Case Studies: Children   437

Mary Pat Moeller

12 Case Studies: Adults and Elderly Adults   467

Michael A. Nerbonne
Jeff E. Brockett
Alice E. Holmes

■ PREFACE

As with previous editions of *Introduction to Audiologic Rehabilitation,* our initial steps in generating a new edition centered around gathering feedback from two invaluable sources, our students in the audiologic rehabilitation courses we each continue to teach regularly and numerous colleagues throughout the country and abroad who have relied on our text when teaching their students. Collectively, their input once again has been helpful in providing direction to us as we focused on the changes and additions to be made. Included in their suggestions for this new edition was strong endorsement of the general philosophic approach taken in previous editions as well as support for the basic chapter framework that we have used. Accordingly, the fifth edition has the same organization, and most authors have been retained from the previous edition. We truly are grateful for their loyalty and the expertise they bring.

In terms of changes in the new edition, probably most notable are the extensive modifications and expansion associated with Chapters 2 and 3. In particular, cochlear implants continue to have an ever-expanding impact on our rehabilitation work, and tinnitus and vestibular rehabilitation likewise have increased in scope. Other areas receiving increased attention as they impact audiologic rehabilitation include early intervention programs for infants, short-term rehabilitation in association with hearing aid fittings, and the use of technology in facilitating the rehabilitation of infants and school-age youngsters with hearing loss.

As in the past, this text is mostly designed with the undergraduate in mind, but the utility of the CORE/CARE model makes it useful to graduate students who need a practical guide for how to do this work on a day-to-day basis while making sure they have a systematic approach.

Audiology is now uniformly a doctoral entry level profession. This means the fundamentals covered in diagnostic audiology and in this rehabilitation text will ultimately have a larger structure of knowledge and skill that audiologists will position on a strong foundation. We suggest the rehabilitation fundamentals here are still sound and provide good grounding. For those who use this text from related fields such as speech/language pathology and education of the deaf, we believe you likewise will continue to find the basic material found in this edition to be practical and useful.

We would like to thank the following reviewers for their time and input: Sarah K. Augerman, University of Minnesota; Bopanna B. Ballachanda, University of

New Mexico; Brett E. Kemker, Louisiana Tech University; Frances Miranda, California State University, Northridge; Lynn Norwood, Baylor Unviersity; and Linda I. Rosa-Lugo, University of Central Florida. We also thank those who helped with indexing the book, including Carma Madsen, Judy M. Jones, Andrew Nixon, Jess Stich, and Jackie Stokes.

We are grateful for the support provided by Allyn and Bacon. Thanks to their encouragement, this text will now have an instructor's manual as well as an accompanying website (www.isu.edu/csed/rehab). Watch for the mouse icon, which indicates additional online resources. We hope instructors will find the manual helpful, and students will benefit from the web material, and we encourage you all to take the time to make full use of these additional resources.

Ronald L. Schow
Michael A. Nerbonne

■ CONTRIBUTORS

JEFF E. BROCKETT, ED.D.
Assistant Professor and Director of Audiology
Department of Communication Sciences and Disorders, and Education of the Deaf
Idaho State University
Pocatello, ID 83209

ANNE S. CARTER, PH.D.
Assistant Professor
Department of Communication Sciences and Disorders
University of South Florida
Tampa, FL 33620

DEBORAH S. CULBERTSON, PH.D.
Clinical Associate Professor of Audiology
Department of Communication Sciences and Disorders
East Carolina University
Greenville, NC 27858

KRIS ENGLISH, PH.D.
Associate Professor
Department of Communication Sciences and Disorders
University of Pittsburgh
Pittsburgh, PA 15260

NICHOLAS M. HIPSKIND, PH.D.
Professor Emeritus of Audiology
Department of Speech and Hearing Sciences
Indiana University
Bloomington, IN 47401

ALICE E. HOLMES, PH.D.
Professor of Audiology
Department of Communicative Disorders
University of Florida Health Science Center
Gainesville, FL 32610

EARL E. JOHNSON, M.S.
Research Audiologist/Ph.D. Student
Department of Hearing and Speech Sciences
Vanderbilt University Medical Center
Nashville, TN 37235

MARY PAT MOELLER, PH.D.
Director: Center for Childhood Deafness
Boys Town National Research Hospital
Omaha, NE 68131

H. GUSTAV MUELLER, PH.D
Professor of Audiology
Department of Hearing and Speech Sciences
Vanderbilt University Medical Center
Nashville, TN 37235

MICHAEL A. NERBONNE, PH.D.
Professor of Audiology
Department of Communication Disorders
Central Michigan University
Mt. Pleasant, MI 48859

KATHY PICHORA-FULLER, PH.D.
Associate Professor
Department of Psychology
University of Toronto at Mississauga
Mississauga, Ontario, Canada L5L 1C6

GARY P. RODRIGUEZ, PH.D.
Manatee Hearing and Speech Center
Balance Center of West Florida
701 Manatee Ave. West
Bradenton, FL 34205

RONALD L. SCHOW, PH.D.
Professor of Audiology
Department of Communication Sciences and Disorders, and Education of the Deaf
Idaho State University
Pocatello, ID 83209

MARY M. WHITAKER, AU.D.
Clinical Associate Professor
Department of Communication Sciences and Disorders, and Education of the Deaf
Idaho State University
Pocatello, ID 83209

Fundamentals of Audiologic Rehabilitation

CHAPTER 1

Overview of Audiologic Rehabilitation

Ronald L. Schow
Michael A. Nerbonne

CONTENTS

INTRODUCTION

Most of us have had occasion to converse with someone who has a hearing problem. Unless the person had received proper help for the hearing difficulties, it probably was a frustrating experience for both parties. When the person with hearing loss is a family member or close friend, we become aware that the emotional and social ramifications of this communication barrier can be substantial as well.

Providing help to address all these hearing problems is the focus of this book. Help is possible, but often not utilized. This chapter gives an overview of this process, which is crucial for the welfare of persons who suffer from hearing impairment and, in turn, for those who communicate with them.

Definitions and Synonyms

Simply stated, we may define *audiologic habilitation/rehabilitation* as those professional interactive processes actively involving the client that are designed to help a person with hearing loss. These include services and procedures for limiting the negative effects of and compensating for the hearing impairment. They specifically involve facilitating adequate well-being and receptive and expressive communication (ASHA, 2001; WHO, 2001). A key consideration in this rehabilitation process involves assisting the person with hearing impairment to attain full potential by using personal resources to overcome interpersonal, psychosocial, educational, and vocational difficulties resulting from the hearing loss. Two kinds of important services that are closely related but distinct from the audiologic habilitation/rehabilitation process are *medical intervention* and *education of the deaf.*

Several terms have been used to describe this helping process. *Audiologic habilitation* refers to remedial efforts with children having a hearing loss at birth, since technically it is not possible to restore (rehabilitate) something that has never existed. *Audiologic rehabilitation,* then, refers to efforts designed to restore a lost state or function. In the interest of simplicity, the terms *habilitation* and *rehabilitation* are used interchangeably in this text, technicalities notwithstanding. Variations of the *audiologic rehabilitation* term include *auditory and aural rehabilitation, hearing rehabilitation,* and *rehabilitative audiology.* Terms used to refer to rehabilitative efforts with the very young child include *parent advising/counseling/tutoring* and *pediatric auditory habilitation. Educational* (or *school*) *audiology* is sometimes used to refer to auditory rehabilitative efforts performed in the school setting.

> Audiologic habilitation is sometimes used to refer to those efforts to assist children with hearing loss, since we cannot rehabilitate something that was never there in the first place. Nevertheless, for simplicity's sake, audiologic rehabilitation (AR) is used throughout this text.

Providers of Audiologic Rehabilitation

Audiologic rehabilitation (AR), then, is referred to by different names and is performed in a number of different settings. All aspects of assisting the client in the audiologic rehabilitation process are not performed by one person. In fact, professionals from several different disciplines are often involved, including educators, psychologists, social workers, and rehabilitation counselors. Nevertheless, the audiologist in particular, and in some circumstances the speech–language pathologist or the educator of the deaf, will assume a major AR role. These professionals provide overall coordination of the process or act as advocates for the person with impaired hearing. Audiologic rehabilitation is not something we *do* to a person following a strict "doctor-knows-best" medical model. It is a process designed to counsel and work with persons who are deaf and hard of hearing so that they can actualize their own resources in order to meet their unique life situations. This text has been written with the hope of orienting and preparing such "counselors" or "advocates for the hearing-impaired" so that they can be effective in a problem-solving process.

Education Needs of Providers

There is a newly established professional degree, the Doctorate in Audiology (Au.D.), that now is the minimum educational requirement for those beginning work as audiologists. Along with other professional bodies, the Academy of Rehabilitative Audiology (ARA) adopted a position statement that emphasizes the need for Au.D. students to be well prepared in audiologic rehabilitation. The ARA provides a list of relevant content areas in AR that should be incorporated into any Au.D. program to ensure adequate preparation in this all-important area of audiology. This statement and other documents along similar lines are available on a resource website that goes with this text (see ARA, ASHA, and AAA statements on competencies for AR).

Regardless of academic background, those from the different professions mentioned in the previous section who successfully perform AR must, like competent audiologists, possess an understanding of and familiarity with several areas of knowledge. These include (1) characteristics of hearing impairment, (2) effect of hearing loss on persons, and (3) the previously noted competencies needed for providing audiologic rehabilitation. For purposes of the present treatment, it is assumed that other coursework or study has brought the reader familiarity with the various forms of hearing impairment, as well as procedures used in the measurement of hearing loss. These procedures, referred to as *diagnostic audiology*, serve as a preliminary step toward rehabilitative audiology. The task at hand, then, is to review briefly some characteristics of hearing loss, to explore the major consequences of hearing impairment, and finally to discuss the methods and competencies needed to help with this condition.

■ HEARING LOSS CHARACTERISTICS

Important characteristics of hearing loss as they relate to audiologic rehabilitation include (1) degree and configuration of impairment, (2) time of onset, (3) type of loss, and (4) auditory speech recognition ability.

Degree of Hearing Impairment and Configuration

One major aspect of hearing impairment or loss is the person's hearing sensitivity or degree of loss (see Table 1.1). The amount of loss will vary across the frequency range, leading to different configurations or shapes of hearing loss, including the most common patterns of flat, sloping, and precipitous. (Practice in degree and configuration interpretation is provided on the website.) The category of hearing impairment includes both the hard of hearing and the deaf. Persons with limited amounts of hearing loss are referred to as being *hard of hearing*. Those with an extensive loss of hearing are considered deaf. Generally, when hearing losses, measured by pure-tone average (PTA) or speech recognition threshold (SRT), are poorer than 80 to 90 dB HL, a person is considered to be *audiometrically deaf*. However, deafness can also be described functionally as the inability to use hearing to any meaningful extent for the ordinary purposes of life, especially for verbal

TABLE 1.1		
Degree of Hearing Impairment Descriptions, Based on Pure-Tone Findings		
DEGREES OF HEARING IMPAIRMENT	PTA IN dB BASED ON 0.5, 1, 2 K^a Hz^b	
	Children	Adults
Slight to Mild	21–40	26–40
Mild to Moderate	— 41–55	—
Moderate	— 56–70	—
Severe	— 71–90	—
Profound	— 91 plus	—

[a]K = 1000.

[b]The three frequencies of 0.5, 1, and 2KHz are used for interpreting audiograms and comparing to SRTs. Higher frequencies, including 3KHz and 4KHz, should be considered in hearing aid fitting decisions and compensation cases.

communication. This latter way of defining deafness is independent of the findings from audiometric test results.

The prevalence of hearing impairment may be considered for all persons combined and for children and adults separately. In the United States the prevalence of hearing impairment is estimated to be from 14 to 40 million, depending on whether conservative or liberal figures are used (Goldstein, 1984; Schow, Mercaldo, & Smedley, 1996). These estimates vary depending on the definition of loss; the loss may be self-defined or involve different decibel fence levels, some as low as 15 dB HL, but most are higher, commonly 20 to 25 dB HL. Authorities have suggested that a different definition of loss should be applied for children, because in a younger person the consequences are greater for the same amount of loss. The prevalence of loss also varies depending on whether the conventional pure-tone average (500, 1000, 2000 Hz) is used or whether some additional upper frequencies (like 3000 and 4000 Hz) are included. In this book we recommend that different pure tone average fences be used for children and adults at the "slight-to-mild" degree of loss level, although the degree designation is similar at most levels. In addition, we recommend that either 3000 or 4000 Hz be used in evaluating loss, although the usual three-frequency pure-tone average will typically be used in analyzing audiograms. Table 1.1 indicates that a hearing loss is found in children at a lower (better) decibel level than in adults; this is consistent with ASHA screening levels for school-children that define normal hearing up to and including 20 dB HL (ASHA, 1997). A reasonable estimate from recent prevalence studies would be that at least 10 percent of the population has permanent, significant impairment of hearing (30 million in the United States). Approximately one-third of 1 percent of the total U.S. population is deaf (about 1 million). Thus, the remaining 29 million are in the hard-of-hearing group (Schow et al., 1996).

Children form a subpopulation of the total group of 30 million individuals with impaired hearing. It is estimated that about 3 million U.S. children are deaf and

A reasonable estimate is that 10 percent of the population have hearing loss. In the United States this would be about 30 million persons, but this includes only the most serious problems and not minor hearing difficulties.

Audiometric Patterns of Hearing Loss Using Degree and Configuration

In rehabilitating adults, audiologists may use degree and configuration of loss to group those who are hard of hearing, thus focusing on the most common audiometric patterns. While a focus on the audiogram alone involves a simplification of the many variables discussed in this chapter, it nevertheless allows us to group persons in a useful way for treatment. A recent approach to hearing aid fitting proposed that nine common audiometric categories of flat, sloping, and precipitous configurations constitute the great bulk of all those who are usually fit with hearing aids (McCandless, Sjursen, & Preeves, 2000). The data summarized here categorize loss, similar to this approach, and show a large sample of adult hearing losses (based on the better ear) involving more than 1,200 persons. This sample shows eight exclusive groups of hearing loss: two flat (N=286), two sloping (N=248), two precipitous (N=304), and two groups with loss only at 4000 Hz (N=362). The two 4K loss groups are seldom fit with hearing aids. These eight categories constitute the entire range of hearing losses usually encountered by an average audiologist, but only six show the classic flat, sloping, or precipitous patterns that are usually amplified. For these six, when we look at the configuration (shape) of the loss between 1000 and the average of 2000 and 4000 Hz, almost equal-sized groups show a flat pattern, a sloping pattern, and a precipitous pattern (see Figure 1.1).

Flat 1 = 248*	Sloping 1 = 199*	Precipitous 1 = 250*	Total *N* = 838*
Flat 2 = 38*	Sloping 2 = 49*	Precipitous 2 = 54*	(*6 categories)

See Figure 1.1 and the resource website where the reader may enter better ear thresholds on any client for 1000, 2000, and 4000 Hz to categorize the loss into an exclusive audiometric pattern.

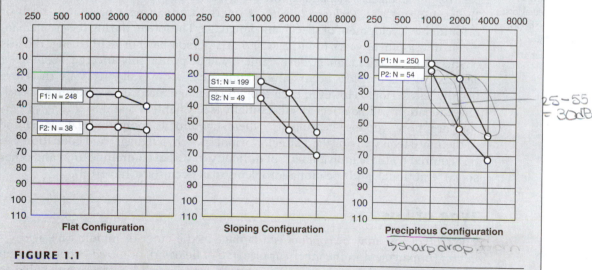

Flat Configuration   **Sloping Configuration**   **Precipitous Configuration**

FIGURE 1.1

Six categories showing flat, sloping, and precipitous hearing configurations on 838 ears tested at health fairs.

Source: Brockett & Schow (2001).

hard of hearing, and even more fit in this category if high-frequency and conductive losses are included (Shepard, Davis, Gorga, & Stelmachowicz, 1981; see Chapter 9). Of these 3 million (2 million in school; 1 million younger), about 50,000 of school age are deaf (American Annals of the Deaf, 2005). As with children, most adults with impaired hearing are considered to be hard of hearing, and only a small minority are deaf (Schow et al., 1996).

Degree (sensitivity), however, is only one of several important dimensions of a hearing loss. Even though it is often the first measure available and provides useful evidence of the impact of the loss, there are exceptions to this generalization. Some children with a profound impairment of 90 dB HL outperform, in language and academic areas, average children who have a loss of only 70 dB HL.

Table 1.2 contains a description of deafness and hard of hearing categories in terms of typical hearing aspects, use of hearing, use of vision, language development, use of language, speech, and educational needs. Prevalence estimates are also shown.

Time of Onset

Cochlear implant recipients are increasingly avoiding the full effects from various kinds of deafness and are an exception to the rule that sensorineural losses cannot be helped medically.

Most hard of hearing youngsters are thought to have hearing loss beginning early in life, but mild losses may not be detected, so prevalence data on young children are scarce and somewhat uncertain (Lundeen, 1991). With youngsters who are deaf or have more severe impairment, the time when a hearing loss is acquired will determine, in part, the extent to which normal speech and language will be present. Severe hearing loss (deafness) may be divided into three categories (*prelingual, postlingual, deafened*) depending on the person's age when the loss occurs (see Tables 1.2 and 1.3). *Prelingual deafness* refers to impairment present at birth or prior to the development of speech and language. The longer during the crucial language development years (up to age 5) that a person has normal hearing, the less chance there is that language development will be profoundly affected. *Postlingual deafness* means that loss occurs after about age 5; its overall effects are therefore usually less serious. However, even though language may be less affected, speech and education will be affected substantially (see Chapters 6 and 8). *Deafened* persons are those who lose hearing after their schooling is completed (i.e., sometime in their late teen years or thereafter). Normal speech, language, and education can be acquired by these individuals, but difficulty in verbal communication and other social, emotional, and vocational problems may occur (see Table 1.3).

Type of Loss

The type of loss may be *conductive* (damage in the outer or middle ear), *sensorineural* (impairment in the inner ear or nerve of hearing), or *mixed* (a combination of conductive and sensorineural). Generally, conductive losses are amenable to medical intervention, whereas sensorineural losses are primarily aided through audiologic rehabilitation. Those with severe and profound sensorineural loss may obtain a cochlear implant (see Chapter 3). Other less common types of loss are possible as well, such as *functional* (nonorganic) problems and *central auditory processing* (CAP or AP) *disorders* (which arise from the processing centers throughout the auditory system, but chiefly in the brainstem or the brain). In the latter type

TABLE 1.2

Categories and Characteristics of Hearing Impairment

Characteristic	Hard of Hearing (29,000,000)[a]	CATEGORY OF DEAFNESS Prelingual (115,000)[a]	CATEGORY OF DEAFNESS Postlingual (230,000)[a]	CATEGORY OF DEAFNESS Deafened (655,000)[a]
Hearing impairment	*Sensitivity:* mild, moderate, or severe; *Recognition:* fair to good (70–90%)	*Sensitivity:* severe or profound degree of loss; *Recognition:* fair to poor		
Use (level) of hearing	Functional speech understanding (lead sense)	Functional signal warning and environmental awareness (hearing minimized)		
Use of vision	Increased dependence		Increased dependence	
Language and speech development	Dependent on rehabilitation measures (e.g., amplification)	Dependent on amplification and early intervention	Dependent on amplification and school rehabilitation	Normal
Use of language	May be affected	Almost always affected	May be affected	Usually not affected
Use of speech	May be affected	Always affected	Usually affected	May be affected
Educational needs	Some special education	Considerable special education	Some special education	Education complete

[a]United States prevalence data for these categories, based on Schow et al. (1996) and Davis (1994), incidence figures and current U.S. census (www.factfindercensus.gov) accessed April 10, 2006.

TABLE 1.3

Definitions of Hearing Impairment

Persons with hearing impairment have been historically divided into the following groups. In general, these are accurate, but early implantation of a cochlear implant and successful audiologic rehabilitation can alter outcomes.

Prelingually deaf persons were either born without hearing (congenitally deaf) or lost hearing before the development of speech and language: 3–5 years (adventitiously deaf). Both speech and language are affected to varying degrees. Some prelingually deaf persons communicate primarily through fingerspelling and signs, but others may primarily communicate via speech, particularly with early successful cochlear implantation.

Postlingually deaf persons are those who became profoundly deaf after the age of 5–10 years but had normal hearing long enough to establish fairly well developed speech and language patterns. While speech generally is affected (more for the 5- than for the 10-year-old), communication may be through speech, signs, fingerspelling, and writing. With successful cochlear implantation, speech may be quite understandable.

Deafened refers to those people who suffer hearing loss after completing their education, generally in their late teens or early twenties and upward. Such people usually have fairly comprehensible, nearly normal speech and language. They face problems of adjustment because of the late onset of their hearing loss.

Hard of hearing persons may have been born thus or subsequently experienced a partial loss of hearing. While they have acquired speech normally through hearing and communicate by speaking, speech may be affected to some extent; for example, the voice may be too soft or too loud. They understand others by speechreading, by using a hearing aid, or by asking the speaker to raise his or her voice or enunciate more distinctly.

Source: Adapted from Moores (1996) and Vernon & Andrews (1990).

of loss the symptoms may be very subtle. In cases of sensorineural loss, auditory speech recognition or hearing clarity is usually affected. This is also the case in difficult listening situations for those with AP problems.

Auditory Speech Recognition Ability

Auditory speech recognition or identification ability (clarity of hearing) is another important dimension of hearing loss. The terms *speech recognition, speech identification,* and *speech discrimination* will be used interchangeably throughout this text, and all are included under the general category of speech perception or comprehension (see Chapter 4). *Speech discrimination* has been used for many years to describe clarity of hearing as measured in typical word intelligibility tests, but *speech recognition* and *identification* have now replaced *discrimination,* since they more precisely describe what is being measured. *Discrimination* technically implies only the ability involved in a same–different judgment, whereas *recognition* and *identification* indicate an ability to repeat or identify the stimulus. *Recognition* is commonly used by diagnostic audiologists, but *identification* meshes nicely with the nomenclature of audiologic rehabilitation procedures as discussed further in Chapter 4. All these terms will at times be used due to historical precedents and evolving nomenclature.

The speech recognition ability in an individual who is hard of hearing typically is better than in a person who is deaf. Persons who are deaf are generally considered unable to comprehend conversational speech with hearing alone, whereas those who are hard of hearing can use their hearing to a significant extent for speech perception. However, some minimal auditory recognition may be present in persons who are deaf even if verbal speech reception is limited, since a person may use hearing for signal warning purposes or simply to maintain contact with the auditory environment (see Table 1.2). Nevertheless, auditory recognition ability and degree of loss are somewhat independent.

In a person of advanced age, a mild degree of loss sometimes may be accompanied by very poor speech recognition. This is referred to as *phonemic regression* and is not unusual in hearing losses among elderly persons who evidence some degree of central degeneration. Disparity in degree of loss and speech recognition ability is also possible in young persons with hearing impairment. For example, a child may be considered deaf in terms of sensitivity, but not in terms of auditory recognition or educational placement. Some children with a degree of loss that classifies them as audiometrically deaf (e.g., PTA = 90+ dB) may have unexpectedly good speech recognition. Thus, speech recognition also is an important variable in describing a hearing loss.

> The degree of loss alone is not adequate to define whether a person is deaf or hard of hearing and to determine a rehabilitation plan. Many other factors, including time of onset and clarity of hearing (word recognition), must be considered.

CONSEQUENCES OF HEARING LOSS: ■ PRIMARY AND SECONDARY

Communication Difficulties

The primary and most devastating effect of hearing loss is its impact on verbal (oral) communication. Children with severe to profound hearing loss do not generally develop speech and language normally, because they are not exposed to the sounds of language in daily living. In a lesser degree of loss or if the loss occurs in adult years, the influence on speech and language expression tends to be less severe. Nevertheless, affected individuals still experience varying degrees of difficulty in receiving the auditory speech and environmental stimuli that allow us to communicate and interact with other humans and with our environment. For children, the choice of a communication (educational) system relates directly to this area of concern. If the educational setting and methods are chosen and implemented appropriately, according to the abilities of the child, the negative impact of the loss can be minimized. Secondary consequences and side effects of hearing loss include educational, vocational, psychological, and social implications (see Chapters 5 and 7 for a discussion of communication systems and their psychosocial implications).

Variable Hearing Disorder/Disability

A health condition, such as a hearing disorder, can be described by a newly revised classification system within the World Health Organization (WHO, 2001), which standardizes terminology throughout the world. If hearing is not "functioning" normally, this is a disorder, and three dimensions are involved within this: (1) *impairment* or problems in body structure and function, (2) *activities*, in this case chiefly communication, and (3) *participation* within life situations. Besides these three dimensions, environmental and personal factors influence the disorder. This provides an excellent framework for the provision of audiologic rehabilitation, and these terms have been incorporated into the rehabilitation model discussed later in the chapter. *Activity* (especially communication) *limitations* can be thought of as the primary consequence of hearing loss, whereas *participation restrictions* involve secondary consequences of the loss that affect social, vocational, and other life situations (see Figure 1.2).

A useful method for measuring the activity limitations and participation restrictions is through self-assessment of hearing, wherein persons make personal estimates about their hearing difficulties. This procedure has been applied with both children and adults. Both the person with impaired hearing and significant others can complete questionnaires independently to provide a more complete picture of the communication, psychosocial, and other effects from the loss (see Chapter 10, Schow & Smedley, 1990).

In preparing to deal with the broad consequences of hearing loss, we must recognize that the impact of a hearing disorder will vary considerably depending on a number of personal and environmental factors. Several of the most important personal factors are presented in Table 1.2. Although not included there, other variables are also important. For example, certain basic characteristics of the individual may have considerable impact on the primary consequences in verbal communication and the secondary effects in education, social, emotional, and vocational areas. The presence of other serious disabilities like blindness, physical limitations, or mental retardation will complicate the situation. A person's native

> The earlier WHO term *disability* has been changed to *activity limitation.* This refers to the primary consequence of hearing impairment.

> The earlier WHO term *handicap* has been changed to *participation restriction.* This refers to the secondary consequences of hearing impairment, including restrictions in the social, emotional, educational, and vocational areas.

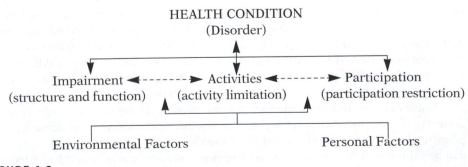

FIGURE 1.2

Model of functioning and disability.
Source: Adapted from WHO (2001), p. 18.

When the eight categories of hearing loss are used, it is possible to develop profiles for *activity limitation* and *participation restriction* for each group using self-report. In this way, expectations for the consequences of hearing loss can be anticipated, and the measurement of rehabilitation success can be compared through the use of outcomes measures. Figure 1.3 shows the eight groupings when activity limitation and participation restriction self-report findings are compared. As can be seen, some configuration categories, such as F2 and S2, tend to produce more activity limitations and participation restrictions than other configuration categories.

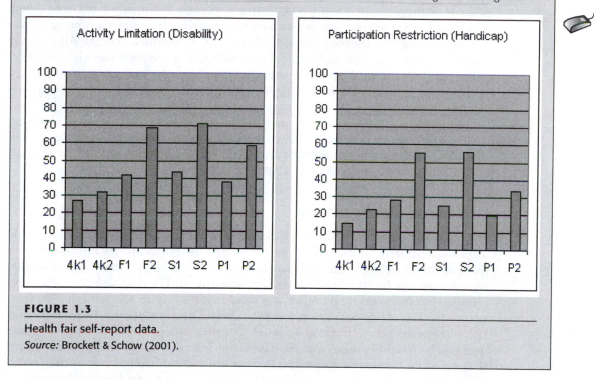

FIGURE 1.3

Health fair self-report data.

Source: Brockett & Schow (2001).

intelligence can also have a tremendous impact in conjunction with a hearing loss. Naturally, basic intelligence will vary from person to person regardless of whether he or she is hearing impaired. However, Vernon (1968) reported on fifty years of research showing that, as a group, persons with hereditary deafness demonstrate a normal range of IQs as measured by performance scales. Whatever the native intellectual ability, it will influence the resultant primary and secondary consequences of hearing loss.

Environmental factors include barriers and facilitators that function with the environment that make things harder or easier for communication to occur.

■ REHABILITATIVE ALTERNATIVES

Little can be done to change basic, innate IQ or native abilities. Nevertheless, a number of AR procedures may have a profound effect on the personal and environmental factors relevant to hearing loss. For example, it is estimated that about 80 percent of Americans who could benefit from hearing aids are not using amplification (Smith, 1991). In addition, there are babies and young children who have hearing loss requiring amplification, but whose losses have not been identified; schoolchildren whose aids are not in good condition; teenagers and young adults who, because of vanity or unfortunate experiences with hearing aids, are not getting the necessary help; adults and elderly individuals who have not acquired hearing aids because of pride or ignorance; and others whose instruments are not properly fitted or oriented to regular hearing aid use. Adults also have been found to be using many poorly functioning hearing aids (Schow, Maxwell, Crookston, & Newman, 1993a). All of these cases represent a need for audiologic rehabilitation. Identifying those who need amplification, persuading them to obtain and use hearing aids or cochlear implants, adjusting them for maximum benefit, and orienting the new user to the instruments are all tasks in the province of AR that may reduce the negative effects of a hearing loss.

Audiologic rehabilitation also includes efforts to improve communication, as well as addressing a variety of other concerns for the hearing impaired person. Before discussing procedures and the current status of audiologic rehabilitation, however, a brief review of the history of AR is in order.

Historical Background

Although audiologic rehabilitative procedures are common today, they have not always been utilized for individuals with hearing loss. For centuries it was assumed that prelingual deafness and the resultant language development delay and inability to learn were inevitable aspects of the impairment. The deaf were thought to be retarded, so for many years no efforts were made to try to teach them. The first known teacher of persons with severe to profound hearing loss was Pedro Ponce de León of Spain, who in the mid- to late 1500s demonstrated that persons who are deaf can be taught to speak and are capable of learning. Other teachers, including Bonet and de Carrion in Spain and Bulwer in England, were active in the 1600s, and their methods gained some prominence. During the 1700s, Pereira (Pereire) introduced education of the deaf to France, and the Abbé de L'Epée founded a school there. Schools were also established by Thomas Braidwood in Great Britain and by Heinicke in Germany. De L'Epée employed fingerspelling and sign language in addition to speechreading, whereas Heinicke and Braidwood stressed oral speech. Beginning in 1813, John Braidwood, a grandson of Thomas Braidwood, tried to establish this oral method in the United States, but he was unsuccessful because of his own ineptness and poor health. Thomas Gallaudet went to England in 1815 to learn the Braidwood oral method, but was refused help because it was feared that he would interfere with John Braidwood's efforts. Consequently, Gallaudet learned de L'Epée's manual method in Paris through contact with Sicard and Laurent Clerc. He returned to the United States and opened his own successful school. (See additional details in Moores, 1996.)

The manual approach to teaching persons who were deaf remained the major force in the United States until the mid-1800s, when speechreading and oral methods were promoted and popularized by Horace Mann, Alexander Graham Bell, and others. The stress on the use of residual hearing had been suggested earlier, but it began to receive strong emphasis with the oral methods used during the 1700s and 1800s. Until electric amplification was developed in the early 1900s, the use of residual hearing required ear trumpets and *ad concham* (speaking directly in the ear) stimulation. More vigorous efforts in the use of hearing followed the introduction of electronic hearing aids in the 1920s (Berger, 1988).

Also in the early 1900s, between 1900 and 1930, several schools of lipreading were started and became quite prominent. Although these institutions were directed principally toward teaching adults with hearing impairment how to speechread, considerable public recognition also was gained for this method of rehabilitating the hearing impaired. (*Speechreading* and *lipreading* will be used interchangeably in this text, although *speechreading* is the more technically accurate term; see Chapter 5 for details.)

BIRTH OF AUDIOLOGY. During World War II, the need to rehabilitate servicemen with impaired hearing resulted in the birth of the audiology profession. The cumulative effect of electronic amplification developments, adult lipreading courses, and the World War II hearing rehabilitation efforts gradually led to the recognition of audiologic rehabilitation as separate from education for persons who are deaf. Eventually, audiologists were recognized as the professionals responsible for providing such services to adults, and soon it was also realized that audiologists could provide crucial help to youngsters who are deaf or hard of hearing.

In the military rehabilitation centers a number of methods were developed to help those with impaired hearing, including procedures for selecting hearing aids. Hearing aid orientation methods requiring up to 3 months of coursework were developed. Considerable emphasis was also placed on speechreading and auditory training.

In the late 1940s and 1950s, as audiology moved into the private sector, the approach to hearing aids changed. Whereas hearing aids were freely dispensed in government facilities, in civilian life people bought amplification exclusively from hearing aid dealers. Methods evolved wherein audiologists would perform tests and recommend hearing aids, but dealers would sell and service the instruments. At that time, the American Speech–Language–Hearing Association (ASHA) maintained that audiologists could not sell hearing aids because this would compromise their professional objectivity. Thus, strict rules were written into the ASHA Code of Ethics, and, except in military facilities, audiologists were excluded from hearing aid sales and follow-up.

In audiologic rehabilitation, audiologists performed preliminary hearing aid work (hearing aid evaluations), but concentrated on providing speechreading and auditory training. These two methods were promoted and used in certain places. For example, speech and hearing centers often set up speechreading and auditory training classes and adult community education programs using these methods. With newer and better hearing aids, however, the magic and motivation of the lipreading schools dissipated, and the ideas worked out in the leisurely three-month military rehabilitation programs were found to be economically unfeasible in the "real world." In one center it was reported that everything had been tried to attract clients for audiologic rehabilitation therapy except "dancing girls" (Alpiner, 1973).

The name *audiology* was first used to describe this new profession in 1946, and Raymond Carhart, who pioneered in the audiologic rehabilitation of World War II servicemen, not only helped name audiology but started the first training program at Northwestern University in 1947.

Because of these setbacks, the 1960s and 1970s were years of examination and reflection for audiologists committed to AR. Such self-examination revealed that the potential clientele for auditory rehabilitation is large and most are not receiving help.

INFANTS. Beginning in the 1960s many audiologists recognized the need for early identification of hearing loss so that management could be initiated during the critical language development years. The incidence of hearing loss in newborns is about 3 per 1,000 children, a higher prevalence than for other disabilities screened routinely in the newborn. Identification methods and programs have evolved to provide early auditory rehabilitation. The advent of cochlear implantation in young children who are deaf has provided another important avenue for management of these youngsters.

CHILDREN. School-age youngsters with hearing impairment were also found to be in need of assistance. Many hard of hearing children are educated in the regular schools, and several studies since the 1960s have indicated that these children are not receiving the specialized support that they need. Even more recent reports indicate that these children are still falling behind, needing special education services, or are being underserved (Blair, Peterson, & Viehweg, 1985; Downs, Whitaker, & Schow, 2003; English & Church, 1999; Flexer, 1992; Matkin, 1984). For example,

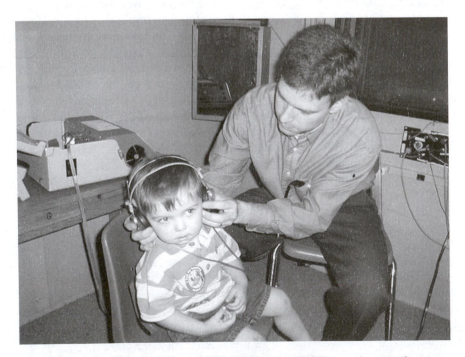

Basic screening is necessary to identify hard of hearing children. Unfortunately, many hard of hearing children are not receiving AR.

Downs et al. (2003) found that in Idaho there were only seven school districts with the services of audiologists. These districts identified and followed five times as many children with hearing loss as compared to seven similar-sized districts without an audiologist. The audiologist-served districts had 2.5 times more hearing aid users and 2.8 times more assistive device users. Unfortunately only one-quarter of the children in the state were in districts with audiologists. Thus, rehabilitation for school-age youngsters is a priority, but there is an acute need for more educational audiologists or highly trained audiologic rehabilitation specialists to serve this population.

ADULTS. Among adults, the needs for hearing rehabilitation are also apparent. Ries's (1994) data revealed that hearing problems are reported by 4 percent of the population from 25 to 34 years of age. This figure rises dramatically with age, so that of those 75 years and older 38 percent of the population report problems. In addition, it is estimated that there are between 5 and 6 million hearing aid users in this country, but conservative estimates suggest that two or three times this many could be using hearing aids. Also, about one-fourth of the aids being used by adults have been shown to be in poor working condition (Schow et al., 1993a).

DIFFICULTIES IN ACCEPTANCE OF AUDIOLOGIC REHABILITATION. When audiologists reflected on the limited acceptance of audiologic rehabilitation, it became apparent that, despite the subject's importance, many in the profession lacked interest. In 1966, the Academy of Rehabilitative Audiology was organized to help audiologists with rehabilitative interests direct their efforts toward reversing these trends. This organization and its members have had an important influence on the emergence of AR as a viable part of audiology.

One reason for the noted neglect of rehabilitation in the past was the hearing aid situation. Primarily because of the success of aggressive sales practices by hearing aid dealers and the ASHA policy that prevented heavy audiologic involvement, 70 to 90 percent of all hearing aids in this country were for many years being sold without active involvement of medical or audiological consultants. Because audiologists did not dispense hearing aids until the 1970s, they were for many years deprived of close contact with clients during the postfitting period. In contrast, the hearing aid dealers were intimately involved in the most crucial rehabilitation process. This situation began to change in the mid- to late 1970s because of relaxation in the ASHA policy prohibiting audiologists from dispensing hearing aids. Finally, due to a Supreme Court decision, ASHA removed these restrictions in 1979. This decision has had a profound effect on AR and the role of the audiologist in working with persons who are deaf and hard of hearing.

Audiologists were not totally free to dispense hearing aids until 1979 because their national association, ASHA, prohibited it.

Current Status

Fortunately, audiologists generally have begun to recognize the opportunities for rehabilitation through early intervention and the provision of services in schools and in neglected adult and geriatric settings. This awareness has been reflected within ASHA, as evidenced in a series of policy statements on rehabilitative audiology issued by special ASHA subcommittees (ASHA, 1992, 1997, 2001). Similar supportive statements on rehabilitation issues have emerged from another major professional organization for audiologists, the American Academy of Audiology (AAA, 1988, 1993, 2000). The Americans with Disabilities Act also created an increased awareness of the need for hearing services (ADA, 1990).

In the past few years, a number of alternative audiologic rehabilitation approaches have been developed, and the profession has gradually moved away from an emphasis on speechreading and auditory training toward a major focus on hearing aid fitting and orientation, with considerable attention to communication patterns and the environment. This change in emphasis has continued and become more widespread, based on recent surveys (Millington, 2001; Schow, Balsara, Smedley, & Whitcomb, 1993b).

A common factor in all new approaches is the recognition that successful hearing aid fitting and orientation and general communication help are the central issues in most audiologic rehabilitation. In most cases now, the focus in AR is on amplification, whereas extensive speechreading and auditory training have become occasional, ancillary procedures. Heavy emphasis on these methods is warranted only in certain instances such as in cochlear implants where auditory training is important.

Recently we have seen the emergence of a new breed of audiologists, more aware of the millions of children and adults in need of audiologic rehabilitation. Results of recent surveys show that approximately 75 to 80 percent of all ASHA audiologists are involved in direct dispensing of hearing aids. According to our most recent survey conducted in 2000, 85 to 92 percent of all audiologists are involved in hearing instrument orientation and rehabilitation counseling. A smaller number (12 to 23 percent) reported being involved in communication rehabilitation, including speechreading and auditory training (Millington, 2001).

PROCEDURES IN AUDIOLOGIC REHABILITATION:
■ **AN AR MODEL—CORE AND CARE**

This section will describe important procedures and elements of audiologic rehabilitation in order to provide a framework for the remainder of this text.

The audiologic rehabilitation model used here emerged in 1980 when the first edition of this text appeared. It has been slightly revised with each new edition of the text, based on the work of Goldstein and Stephens (1981) and other trends in audiology (Stephens, 1996). In its current form it is in harmony with the World Health Organization's (2001) International Classification of Functioning and Disability. The model is intended to encompass all types and degrees of hearing impairment as well as all age groups.

Entry and discharge are considered peripheral to the central aspects of the model. The model consists of two major components: assessment and management. Each component has four divisions and associated subsections. The model is shown in Table 1.4 and Figure 1.4.

TABLE 1.4

Audiologic Rehabilitation Model Used in This Text

	(ENTER THROUGH DIAGNOSTIC–IDENTIFICATION PROCESS)	
Assessment (CORE)	**C**ommunication status: Impairment and activity limitations	Auditory Visual Language Manual Communication self-report Previous rehabilitation Overall
	Overall participation variables	Psychological (emotional) Social Vocational Educational
	Related personal factors	Types I, II, III, IV Personality IQ Age Race Gender
	Environmental factors	Services Systems Barriers Facilitators Acoustic conditions
Management (CARE)	**C**ounseling and psychosocial (modifying personal attitude)	Interpretation Information Counseling and guidance Acceptance Understanding Expectations and goals

	Audibility and impairment	Hearing aid fitting
		Cochlear implants
		Assistive devices
		    Assistive listening
		    Alerting and warning
		    Tactile
		    Communication
		Instruction and orientation

	Remediate communication activity	Tactics to control situation Philosophy based on realistic expectations Personal skill-building
	Environmental/coordination/ participation improvement	Situation improvement Vocational Educational Social Communication partner Community context
	(DISCHARGE)	

Note: This model is based on Goldstein and Stephens (1981), Stephens (1996), and the current WHO (2001) terminology.

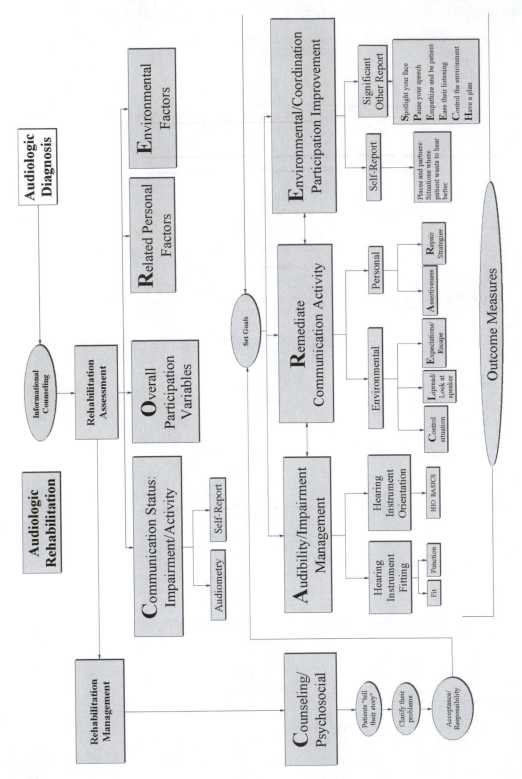

FIGURE 1.4

Model for audiologic rehabilitation.

Source: Schow (2001) and Brockett & Schow (2001).

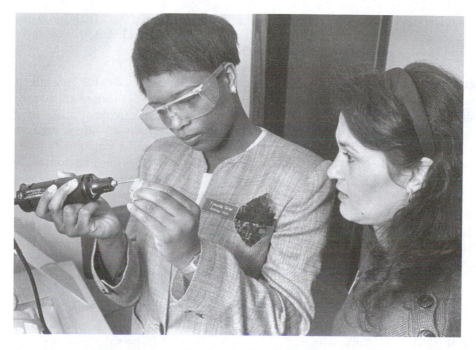

A major aspect of AR involves ensuring that hearing aids are working properly for the patient.

Rehabilitation Assessment Procedures

Following the initial auditory diagnostic tests that indicate the need for audiologic rehabilitation, it is necessary to perform more in-depth workups to determine the feasibility of various forms of audiologic rehabilitation. These assessment procedures should focus on Communication status, Overall participation variables, Related personal factors, and Environmental factors (which are collectively abbreviated as CORE).

The CORE assessment issues help audiologists consider relevant factors that should be evaluated before treatment starts.

COMMUNICATION STATUS. Within the area of *communication* status, which includes impairment and activity, both traditional audiometric tests and questionnaires may be used to assess auditory abilities and self-reported consequences of hearing loss. Visual abilities assessment should include a simple screening and measurement of speechreading abilities. Any evaluation of communication must also consider language, because it is at the heart of verbal communication. If the patient understands a manual–gesture system, this needs to be evaluated, as does any prior treatment. Included in *overall communication* are combined sensory abilities, such as audiovisual and tactile–kinesthetic capacities. Expressive and receptive communication skills should both be considered.

OVERALL PARTICIPATION VARIABLES. Included in this area are participation aspects of hearing loss, including psychological, social, vocational, and educational factors. Social factors such as family and significant others, social class, and lifestyle are to be considered according to the Goldstein and Stephens model. The vocational domain includes position, responsibility, and competence. In addition, the patient's level and form of education must be considered.

RELATED PERSONAL FACTORS. These include the person's attitude, which is considered a crucial aspect of rehabilitation. Goldstein and Stephens (1981) suggested that rehabilitation candidates can be categorized into four types according to attitude. Type I candidates have a strongly positive attitude toward management and are thought to comprise two-thirds to three-quarters of all patients. Most of the remaining candidates fit into Type II: Their expectations are essentially positive, but slight complications are present such as hearing loss that is difficult to fit with amplification. Persons with Type III attitudes are negative about rehabilitation, but show some willingness to cooperate, and those in Type IV reject hearing aids and the rehabilitation process altogether. In the latter two categories, management cannot proceed in the usual fashion until some modification of attitude is achieved. [We consider it important to evaluate attitude prior to rehabilitation.] In the WHO (2001) system, personal factors listed also include age, race, gender, education, personality and character style, aptitude, other health conditions, fitness, lifestyle, habits, upbringing, coping styles (assertiveness), social background, profession, and past and current experiences.

ENVIRONMENTAL FACTORS. These include individual aspects, services, and systems. The individual issues include the physical features of the environment as well as direct personal contacts. The services include social structures and services in the work environment, socially, communication-wise, and transportation-wise. Systems refer to laws, regulations, and rules, both formal and informal. Finally, the acoustic environmental conditions confronted by the hearing-impaired person should be evaluated.

Management Procedures

Once a thorough, rehabilitation-oriented assessment has been completed, management efforts should be initiated. These may take the form of short- or long-term therapy and may involve individual or group sessions. The four aspects of management included here are those detailed in the previous editions of this book. They are also prominently featured in the Goldstein–Stephens model as well as in the WHO (2001) terminology. These include (1) Counseling and psychosocial aspects, (2) Audibility or amplification aspects, (3) Remediation of communication activity, and (4) Environmental coordination/participation improvement (abbreviated as CARE).

CARE defines a management approach that includes four critical components of AR.

Although all four management components are listed sequentially, they may occur simultaneously or in a duplicative and interactive fashion. For example, information about communication is generally introduced early in the counseling phase. However, additional information on how we hear, basics of speech acoustics, visible dimensions of speech, and how to maximize the use of conversational cues may be further emphasized later in the remediation of communication.

COUNSELING/PSYCHOSOCIAL. Counseling/psychosocial includes interpretation of audiologic findings to the client and other significant persons. In addition, pertinent information, counseling, and guidance are needed to help these individuals understand the educational, vocational, psychosocial, and communicative effects of hearing impairment. Considerable understanding and support are necessary in dealing with children who are deaf and hard of hearing, their parents, adults of all ages with hearing impairment, and their families. If the clinician is a good listener, in this process he or she will allow the clients to "tell their own story," and this will in turn help clients to clarify their problems, accept responsibility, and set appropriate goals. This process should bring acceptance and understanding of the conditions along with appropriate expectations for management. It is at this stage that good-attitude (Types I and II) patients must set goals to improve audibility with amplification, whereas clients with poor attitudes (Types III and IV), if not modified toward acceptance and understanding, may not be ready and will resist this type of goal.

AUDIBILITY IMPROVEMENT USING AMPLIFICATION AND ASSISTIVE DEVICES.

AMPLIFICATION FITTING. This phase is sometimes referred to as *hearing aid evaluation,* but it needs to be broader in scope. Here we must consider all forms of amplification, not just hearing aids. For example, cochlear implants, signal warning devices, and other assistive devices like telephone amplifiers should be considered in this phase. In many cases, accurate fitting of these devices will go a considerable way toward resolution of the hearing problem. In most cases, the fitting of hearing devices should be followed by adjustment, modification, and alteration of the basic controls and coupler arrangement until satisfactory amplification is achieved. Effort should be made to ensure that no other amplification arrangements are substantially superior to the ones being used.

HEARING INSTRUMENT ORIENTATION (HIO BASICS). Individuals need to learn about the purpose, function, and maintenance of hearing aids and other assistive devices used by themselves or their child or other family member to avoid misunderstanding and misuse. Amplification units are relatively complex, and this instruction must be given more emphasis than a five-minute explanation or a pamphlet.

> Hearing instrument orientation (HIO), as defined throughout this text, includes basic instruction that should be given to help new hearing aid users. HIO BASICS will be given in Chapter 2.

REMEDIATE COMMUNICATION ACTIVITY. The major impact of hearing loss lies in the area of communication activity. Communication deficits often manifest themselves in educational difficulties for children and in vocational difficulties for adults. In most cases, amplification is considered the most important tool in combating this problem, but some basic communication training and related strategies are recommended for all new amplification users. These involve both environmental and personal adjustments and may provide the basis for more extensive therapy if the client selects goals in this area.

Although a basic overview on communication issues is adequate in most cases of hearing aid fitting, cochlear implants require more extensive skill building wherein the patient learns methods to facilitate communication in conjunction with this new device. Speechreading and improvement of auditory listening strategies are included here, as are related speech and language rehabilitation efforts. Specific communication skills are identified in this phase of therapy and then,

> CLEAR SPEECH is an important new communication strategy as noted in Chapter 4.

through such things as assertiveness training and incorporation of anticipatory and repair strategies, clients may learn to cope better with communication challenges.

ENVIRONMENTAL COORDINATION: PARTICIPATION IMPROVEMENT. Self-reports provide a useful method to help clients select a few situations (places and partners) wherein they would like to improve their hearing and communicating. With the therapist they can identify strategies for improvement. Pre- and post-self-report measures can help determine the success of these efforts. Also in this phase of treatment we include coordination with other sources of help. Disability is not an individual attribute, but rather a collection of conditions, and many of these are created by the social and physical environment. It is a collective responsibility for all elements of society to help make necessary modifications. Although referrals in all areas are not usually necessary, they should be considered. Liaison among client, family, and other agencies is included as are reassessment and modification of the intervention program.

Coordination and teamwork are useful concepts in audiologic rehabilitation. Particularly in the case of the youngster with hearing impairment, many persons may work with or need to work with the child. The parents should be at the center of the rehabilitative process. Also, physicians, social workers, hearing aid dispensers, teachers, school psychologists, and other school personnel need to be coordinated to assist the child and family. For adults, much depends on the particular setting in which the rehabilitation occurs. Sometimes physicians, psychologists, or social workers function in the same clinical setting. In these cases, involvement of another professional may occur naturally and easily. In other situations, the AR therapist can make referrals, when indicated, and encourage the adult to follow up. Sometimes persons are resistant to obtaining medical care or seeing a rehabilitation counselor. Often, parents or adults resist social services, psychiatric assistance, or hearing aid devices. When a client refuses to accept advice, the audiologist must provide whatever insight and help possible, based on the audiologist's background and training, but must respect the rights of the client or the parents. Nevertheless, the audiologic rehabilitation process demands that referrals be made when indicated, and overall coordination within the relevant context is an important dimension that should not be neglected.

Additional clarification and details on this AR model can be found in Goldstein and Stephens (1981) and WHO (2001).

Self-report outcome measures have become a key element to help measure the communication improvement results of AR for different environments and situations (places and partners).

■ SETTINGS FOR AUDIOLOGIC REHABILITATION

Audiologic rehabilitation may be conducted in a variety of settings with children, adults, or the elderly who are either deaf or hard of hearing. A review of these settings may help to demonstrate the many applications of AR (see Table 1.5).

Children

Very young children with hearing impairment and their parents may be recipients of early intervention efforts through home visits or clinic programs. Parent groups are also an important rehabilitation option. As children enter preschool and other school

TABLE 1.5		
Summary of Audiologic Rehabilitation Settings for Children, Adults, and Elderly Persons		
CHILDREN	**ADULTS**	**ELDERLY ADULTS**
Early intervention	University and technical schools	(Most settings listed under Adults)
Preschool	Vocational rehabilitation	Community programs
Parent groups	Military-related facilities	Nursing homes and long-term care facilities
Regular classrooms	ENT clinic–private practice	
School conservation program follow-up	Community, hospital, and university hearing clinics	
School resource rooms	Hearing aid specialists and dispensers	
Residential school classrooms		

settings, audiologic rehabilitation takes on a supportive, coordinative function with teachers of youngsters with impaired hearing managing the classroom learning. Specifically, children in resource rooms, in residential deaf school classrooms, and in regular classrooms can be helped with amplification (both group and individual), communication therapy, and academic subjects. Important help and insights can also be given to the child's parents and teachers, and other professionals may be involved as needed. Hearing conservation follow-up for youngsters who fail traditional school screenings represents another type of rehabilitative work carried out with children.

Adults

Adult AR services are needed for individuals with long-standing hearing loss, as well as for persons who acquire loss during adulthood. Such traumatic or progressive hearing disorders may be brought on by accident, heredity, disease, or noise.

Adults may be served in university or technical school settings, through vocational rehabilitation programs, in military-related facilities, in the office of an ear specialist, or in the private practice of an audiologist. In addition, many adults are served in community, hospital, or university hearing clinics or through hearing aid dealers and dispensers. A variety of rehabilitative services may be provided in all these settings.

Elderly Adults

The vast majority of elderly clients are served through the conventional programs previously described for adults. A substantial proportion of clients seen in these settings for hearing aid evaluations and related services are 65 years of age or older.

The full array of hearing aid and communication rehabilitation services may be provided for the elderly in these clinics, including hearing aid evaluation, orientation, and group and individual therapy. Aside from conventional clinical service, rehabilitation may be provided to the elderly in community screening and rehabilitation programs in well-elderly clinics, retirement apartment houses, senior citizen centers, churches, and a variety of other places where senior citizens congregate. Nursing homes or long-term care facilities also provide opportunities for audiologic rehabilitation since so many residents in these settings have substantial hearing loss and are required to have hearing screening under Medicare law (Bebout, 1991). Nevertheless, rehabilitation personnel should be realistic and anticipate less than 100 percent success with the elderly who are residents in health care facilities (Schow, 1992). Audiologic rehabilitation will be better accepted if it can be applied before persons enter such a facility.

SUMMARY

Audiologic habilitation and rehabilitation involve a variety of assessment and management efforts for the person who is deaf or hard of hearing, coordinated by a professional with audiologic training. Audiology's commitment to this endeavor has waxed and waned during the past sixty-plus years, but recently a resurgence of interest has been spurred by a variety of factors.

A model of rehabilitation has been presented here to provide a framework for assessment and management procedures in audiologic rehabilitation as described in the remaining chapters of this book. Professionals who intend to engage in AR must be familiar with the characteristics of hearing loss reviewed in this chapter if they are to perform effective rehabilitation.

SUMMARY POINTS

- Audiologic rehabilitation (AR) is defined as those professional interactive processes actively involving the client with hearing loss to achieve better communication and minimize the resulting problems. It does not include closely related medical intervention or the teaching of academics to the deaf.
- Audiologists are the chief providers of AR, but speech pathologists and teachers of the deaf also do a great deal of this work. In addition, other professionals such as social workers and rehabilitation counselors may provide key rehabilitative assistance to those with hearing loss.
- AR providers need some background in diagnostic audiology, and they need an understanding of hearing loss and its effect on both children and adults.
- Hearing impairment can be defined in terms of degree of loss, time of onset, type of loss, and word recognition ability. Those with milder forms of hearing loss are called hard of hearing; those with extensive hearing loss who cannot use hearing for the ordinary purposes of life are considered deaf.
- The deaf may be divided into three groups: the prelingually deaf, who are born deaf or acquire it in the first five years of life; the postlingually deaf, who acquire hearing loss after age 5 through the school years; and the deafened, who acquire hearing loss after their education is completed.

- The most serious and primary consequence of hearing impairment is the effect on verbal (oral) communication, referred to as disability. The secondary consequences of hearing impairment may be referred to as a handicap and include social, emotional, educational, and vocational issues. The World Health Organization (WHO) now suggests that communication *activity limitation* be used instead of disability and that we speak of *participation restriction* instead of handicap. In connection with these new terms, WHO also suggests that personal factors and environmental factors are key issues in the provision of AR hearing services. These terms and factors help us properly understand the consequences of hearing impairment and provide the basis for a model of AR.

- Both children and adults are underserved, and many more should receive AR help. Only 20 percent of those who should be using hearing aids obtain them. Even those who have hearing aids can often be shown how to get more effective help from amplification and can benefit from other services to assist them in their communication breakdowns.

- The early history of AR is essentially the history of efforts to help the deaf, beginning in the 1500s. Audiology came into being as a profession in the mid-1940s in connection with World War II, and both audiologic diagnosis and audiologic rehabilitation (AR) are considered key elements within this profession. In recent years, audiologists have become more involved in hearing aid fitting, and new developments such as cochlear implants, assistive listening devices, wider support for disabilities, and the emerging use of outcome measures have helped revitalize AR.

- The model for AR includes assessment and management; rehabilitation assessment includes four elements defined by the acronym CORE. These elements include an assessment of **C**ommunication activity limitations and impairment through audiometry and self-report; **O**verall participation variables, including psychological, social, educational, and vocational factors; **Re**lated personal factors; and **E**nvironmental factors.

- Management includes four elements also, and these are summarized by the acronym CARE. These elements include **C**ounseling, which includes an effort to help clients accept the hearing loss and set reasonable goals; **A**udibility improvement by using hearing aids and assistive devices; **R**emediation of communication; and **E**nvironmental coordination and participation goals.

- Children receive AR services in a variety of settings, including early intervention and school programs. Adults and elderly adults are usually served in settings that dispense hearing aids; these include private practice, medical or ENT offices, hearing aid specialists, military or VA service centers, and community hearing clinics.

- The first eight chapters in this book are organized to provide an overview of the fundamentals in AR, including hearing aids (Chapter 2), cochlear implants and vestibular/tinnitus rehabilitation (Chapter 3), auditory and visual stimuli (Chapters 4 and 5), speech and language issues (Chapter 6), psychosocial issues (Chapter 7), and school AR services (Chapter 8). Two chapters provide comprehensive explanations to illuminate AR for children (Chapter 9) and for adults (Chapter 10). Finally, two case study chapters illustrate how this work is done with children (Chapter 11) and with adults (Chapter 12).

RECOMMENDED READING

Alpiner, J. G., & McCarthy, P A. (2000). *Rehabilitative audiology: Children and adults* (3rd ed.). Baltimore: Williams & Wilkins.

DeConde Johnson, C., Benson, P. V., & Seaton, J. B. (1997). *Educational audiology handbook.* San Diego: Singular.

Gagne, J. P., & Jennings, M. B. (2000). Audiological rehabilitation intervention services for adults with acquired hearing impairment. In M. Valente, H. Hosford-Dunn, & R. Roesser (Eds.), *Audiology treatment.* New York: Thieme Medical Publishers.

Tye Murray, N. (2004). *Foundations of aural rehabilitation* (2nd ed.). Clifton Park, NY: Delmar Learning.

RECOMMENDED WEBSITES

World Health Organization International Classification of functioning, disability, and health:
www.who.int/icidh/

American Academy of Audiology:
www.audiology.org/professional/positions/

American Speech-Language-Hearing Association:
www.asha.org

REFERENCES

Alpiner, J. G. (1973). The hearing aid in rehabilitation planning for adults. *Journal of the Academy of Rehabilitative Audiology, 6,* 55–57.

American Academy of Audiology (AAA). (1988). Early identification of hearing loss in infants and children. *Audiology Today, 2,* 8–9.

American Academy of Audiology (AAA). (1993). Audiology: Scope of practice. *Audiology Today, 5*(1).

American Academy of Audiology (AAA). (2000). *Principles and guidelines for early hearing detection and intervention programs.* Year 2000 position statement from the Joint Committee on Infant Hearing. Accessed April 15, 2006, from www.audiology.org/professional/positions/

American Annals of the Deaf. (2005). Annual survey of hearing-impaired children and youth. *American Annals of the Deaf, 150*(2), 77.

American Speech–Language–Hearing Association (ASHA). (1992). Spotlight on special interest division 7: Audiologic Rehabilitation. *Asha, 34,*18.

American Speech–Language–Hearing Association (ASHA). (1997). *Guidelines for audiologic screening.* Rockville, MD.

American Speech–Language–Hearing Association (ASHA). (2001). Knowledge and skills required for the practice of audiologic/aural rehabilitation. *ASHA Desk Reference Volume 4,* pp. 393–404.

Americans with Disabilities Act (ADA). (1990). (Public Law 101-336), 42 USC Sec. 12101. Equal opportunity for the disabled. Washington, DC.

Bebout, J. M. (1991). Long term care facilities: A new window of opportunity opens for hearing health care services. *Hearing Journal, 44*(11), 11–17.

Berger, K. W. (1988). History and development of hearing aids. In M. C. Pollack (Ed.), *Amplification for the hearing-impaired* (3rd ed.; pp. 1–20). New York: Grune & Stratton.

Blair, J. C., Peterson, M., & Viehweg, S. H. (1985). The effects of mild hearing loss on academic performance among school-age children. *The Volta Review, 87,* 87–94.

Brockett, J., & Schow, R. L. (2001). Web site profiles common hearing loss patterns and outcome measures. *Hearing Journal,* 54(8), 20.

Davis, A. (1994). *Public health perspectives in audiology.* 22nd International Congress of Audiology. Halifax, NS, Canada.

Downs, S. K., Whitaker, M., & Schow, R. (2003). *Audiological services in school districts that do and do not have an audiologist.* Educational Audiology Summer Conference, St. Louis.

English, K., & Church, G. (1999). Unilateral hearing loss in children: An update for the 1990s. *Language, Speech and Hearing Services in Schools, 30,* 26–30.

Flexer, C. (1992). FM classroom public address systems. In M. Ross (Ed.), *FM auditory training systems: Characteristics, selection and use.* Parkton, MD: York Press.

Goldstein, D. P. (1984). Hearing impairment, hearing aids, and audiology. *Asha, 25*(9), 24–38.

Goldstein, D. P., & Stephens, S. D. G. (1981). Audiological rehabilitation: Management Model I. *Audiology, 20,* 432–452.

Lundeen, C. (1991). Prevalence of hearing impairment among school children. *Language, Speech and Hearing Services in Schools, 22,* 269–271.

Matkin, N. D. (1984). Wearable amplification. A litany of persisting problems. In J. Jerger (Ed.), *Pediatric audiology: Current trends* (pp. 125–145). San Diego, CA: College Hill Press.

McCandless, G., Sjursen, W., & Preves, D. (2000). Satisfying patient needs with nine fixed acoustical prescription formats. *Hearing Journal, 53*(5), 42–50.

Millington, D. (2001). *Audiologic rehabilitation practices of ASHA audiologists: Survey 2000.* MS Thesis. Idaho State University.

Moores, D. (1996). *Educating the deaf—psychology, principles, practices* (4th ed.). Boston: Houghton Mifflin.

Ries, P. W. (1994). *Prevalence and characteristics of persons with hearing trouble: United States.* National Center for Health Statistics, *Vital Stat, 24,* 188.

Schow, R. L. (1992). Hearing assessment and treatment in nursing homes. *Hearing Instruments, 43*(7), 7–11.

Schow, R. L. (2001). A standardized AR battery for dispensers. *Hearing Journal, 54*(8), 10–20.

Schow, R. L., Balsara, N. R., Smedley, T. C., & Whitcomb, C. J. (1993b). *American Journal of Audiology, 2*(3), 28–37.

Schow, R. L., Maxwell, S., Crookston, G., & Newman, M. (1993a). How well do adults take care of their hearing instruments? *Hearing Instruments, 44*(3), 16–20.

Schow, R. L., Mercaldo, D., & Smedley, T. C. (1996). *The Idaho hearing survey.* Pocatello, ID: Idaho State University Press.

Schow, R. L., & Smedley, T. C. (1990). (Special Issue) Self assessment of hearing. *Ear and Hearing, 11*(5) (Suppl.), 1–65.

Shepard, N., Davis, J., Gorga, M., & Stelmachowicz, P. (1981). Characteristics of hearing impaired children in the public schools: Part 1—Demographic data. *Journal of Speech and Hearing Disorders, 46,* 123–129.

Smith, M. (1991). The role of age and ageism in the "80% barrier." *Asha, 33*(11), 36–37.

Stephens, D. (1996). Hearing rehabilitation in a psychosocial framework. *Scandinavian Audiolgy, 25* (Suppl 43), 57–66.

Vernon, M. (1968). Fifty years of research on the intelligence of the deaf and hard-of-hearing. A survey of literature and disscussion of implications. *Journal of Rehabilitation of the Deaf, 1,* 1–11.

Vernon, M., & Andrews, J. (1990). *The psychology of deafness.* White Plains, NY: Longman Press.

World Health Organization (WHO). (2001). International classification of functioning, disability and health. Geneva: World Health Organization.

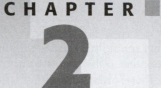

CHAPTER 2

Hearing Aids and Assistive Devices

H. Gustav Mueller
Earl E. Johnson
Anne S. Carter

CONTENTS

INTRODUCTION

In nearly all cases, audiologic rehabilitation involves working with individuals who can benefit from the use of hearing aids or other assistive listening devices. While all forms of auditory rehabilitation are important, reliance on visual and situational cues is inversely related to the quality of the hearing aid fitting. A critical first step for most patients, therefore, is to provide amplification that makes speech and environmental sounds of various inputs audible, optimizes intelligibility and sound quality, and assures that loud inputs are not uncomfortable or distorted. This might sound like a fairly straightforward task; however, hearing aids are sometimes fitted in a haphazard manner, without careful consideration of these underlying principles. Getting the most appropriate hearing aids on a patient, and adjusting them precisely for that patient's listening needs, can facilitate significantly many of the other aspects of auditory rehabilitation.

Twenty years ago many master's degree training programs in audiology covered the study of hearing aids in a single three-credit course. Today, as audiology has moved to a four-year Au.D. degree, two or three courses are devoted solely to the selection and fitting of hearing aids. Why the change? The selection, fitting, and verification of hearing aids has become increasingly complex, and dispensing hearing aids has become an integral part of the scope of practice of audiology. To do it right, extensive training is necessary.

In recent years, several factors have had a significant impact on the way we select and fit hearing aids, which indirectly has influenced the amount of training required for proficiency. As you are reading this chapter, it is important to keep these issues in mind, as they are shaping the way that we do our job.

Programmable: A hearing aid, either digital or analog, that is programmed digitally using a PC or remote control device.

Digital: A hearing aid that uses digital processing of the signal.

Probe-mic measures: Using a tiny silicone tube placed near the tympanic membrane, which is attached to a miniature microphone, the gain and output of the hearing aid are assessed in the patient's ear.

- *Advanced circuit design.* Each year new hearing aid circuits are introduced that provide a variety of new signal processing algorithms. Today, some hearing aids have twenty or more separate channels of signal processing, each one requiring patient-specific adjustments of several processing features. Additionally, special features such as digital noise reduction, directional microphone technology, etc., must be considered and programmed accordingly.
- *Digital/programmable hearing aids.* Essentially all hearing aids are now programmable, and the majority of these hearing aids are digital. These instruments are programmed through the use of a personal computer, and the audiologist must be familiar with the fitting software and the thousands of fitting options in order to obtain the optimum fit for the patient.
- *Probe-microphone measurements.* The ability to measure reliably the output of hearing aids at the patient's tympanic membrane allows for the use of precise verification protocols. Additionally, the performance of many other hearing aid features can be evaluated and quantified. The equipment is available today that allows us to do all our testing and fitting in ear canal sound pressure level (SPL).
- *Computerization.* Hearing aid specifications, prescriptive fitting methods, automated testing procedures, hearing aid selection algorithms, and self-assessment inventories are now all available from computer software. Combine this with digital/programmable hearing aids and PC-based probe-microphone measurements and the personal computer becomes the workstation for audiometric testing, hearing aid selection, adjustment, fitting, and validation.
- *Delivery system.* Thirty years ago it was considered unethical for audiologists to sell hearing aids for profit. Today, the majority of hearing aids are dispensed by audiologists, and the percentage increases annually. Dispensing hearing aids

is a business; understanding the business part of fitting hearing aids is essential for any audiologist in private practice.

- *Internet.* Prospective hearing aid users now use the Internet to learn about hearing aids at manufacturers' websites, have their hearing aid questions answered through audiology discussion groups, and in some cases, even purchase their hearing aids online. Educated consumers often have high expectations.

In this chapter, we will cover a wide range of information about hearing aids, beginning with a simple description of how they work, how they are tested, and eventually leading to the latest details concerning automated fitting procedures and modern digital instruments. We will also discuss some other important assistive listening and rehabilitative devices used, with or as an alternative to hearing aids.

■ HEARING AIDS

A successful hearing aid fitting, which should lead to a happy hearing aid user, is dependent upon the audiologist's understanding of hearing aid technology and how to apply this technology to different types of hearing losses, loudness growth functions, and listening needs.

To get things started, the following is a simplified description of what makes a hearing aid work. Later in this chapter we'll provide a more detailed description of some of these components.

Basic Components

The purpose of a hearing aid is to amplify, or make sounds louder, and to accomplish this with respect to the input signal and the patient's hearing loss configuration. There are certain basic components, common to all types of hearing aids (see block diagrams in Figure 2.1). Here's a step-by-step walk through of how things work:

1. Sound waves enter the hearing aid through the *microphone.*
2. The *microphone* converts the sound waves into an electrical signal.
3. The *amplifier* increases the strength of the electrical signal.
4. A smaller loudspeaker called a *receiver* functions to convert the amplified signals back into sound waves.
5. The amplified sound is channeled from the *receiver* directly to the ear canal. For hearing aids that fit behind the ear, the receiver sends the amplified sound into a clear plastic tube attached to a custom-made earmold. For those hearing aids that fit into the ear, the amplified sound is channeled into the ear canal by a small piece of tubing within the shell of the instrument.
6. The *battery* provides electrical energy to power the hearing aid and enable the amplification process to occur.

The typical hearing aid of today has many other features. As we go on in this chapter, you will see that there are variations of each one of these basic components. It is these variations, along with other controls and features, that allow us to customize each hearing aid for the individual patient.

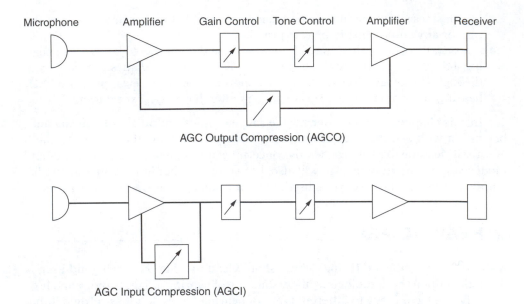

FIGURE 2.1

Block diagram illustrating basic components of output compression and input compression hearing aids.
Source: Olsen (1986).

Controls and Features

In addition to the basic components that we've just discussed, many hearing aids include additional controls or circuits. The following is a listing of the most common of these features:

1. *On-off switch.* Allows the user to turn the hearing aid off when not in use. In some hearing aids, this switch also activates the telecoil (see below). Generally, the "M" position indicates that the microphone is on, "O" turns the aid off, and the "T" (if present) activates the telecoil. For most custom instruments, the on-off switch (if present) usually is part of the volume control wheel.

2. *Telecoil.* A special circuit designed to enhance use of the hearing aid with the telephone. A telecoil switch may be incorporated into a toggle on-off switch or exist as a separate control. Electromagnetic signals are picked up by the telecoil from the receiver of the telephone (leakage), amplified, and transduced to acoustic energy before entering the ear. Thus, the telecoil takes the place of the hearing aid microphone as the input component of the hearing aid system. While proven beneficial for many users, there is substantial variability in the performance of the telecoil within each individual hearing aid, particularly custom instruments, due to size and placement restrictions, making it necessary to carefully evaluate performance characteristics of each device. Telecoils are not available on some smaller custom hearing aids due to space limitations. Often, hearing aids with multiple

Individuals with mild-to-moderate hearing loss often can do quite well on the telephone using the hearing aid in traditional microphone mode.

memories will devote one memory to the telecoil. In these instances, it can be accessed through a programming button on the hearing aid, or by the use of a remote control device.

3. *Volume control.* The volume of the hearing aid can be controlled by a toggle switch, a rotating wheel, or through a remote control device. This allows the user to select a preferred listening level for a specific listening situation. As mentioned earlier, in some smaller hearing aids, the volume control also acts as an on-off switch.

Many instruments do not employ a manual volume control. In some cases this is based on the notion that the hearing aid is programmed to *automatically* adjust the volume for different input signals (by using input-controlled compression in multiple channels). Additionally, for the very small completely-in-the-canal instruments, there usually is no volume control (other than remote control) due to space limitations.

4. *Control of frequency-specific gain.* Using a digitally controlled programmable system, the audiologist makes adjustments for each patient so that there is greater or lesser amplification in certain frequency regions. For example, a patient's hearing loss may involve only the frequencies above 2000 Hz. The hearing aid is then adjusted so that it will not amplify substantially any frequencies below 2000 Hz. Conversely, a patient with an upward sloping hearing loss might need some reduction of amplification in the higher frequencies. Today's digital hearing aids have precise gain control in ten to twenty frequency bands, allowing for appropriate adjustment of the frequency response for any type of hearing loss configuration.

5. *Compression.* Essentially all hearing aids use some form of automatic gain control (AGC), commonly referred to as compression, to limit maximum output.

Compression can be used for controlling the input (AGCi) or controlling the output (AGCo), and usually is used for both. AGCo allows the audiologist to control the maximum output of the hearing aid; the purpose of this adjustment is to assure that loud sounds are not uncomfortably loud to the user. Modern hearing aids often have two circuits for output limiting: one prior to the amplifier (to prevent overload) and one after the amplifier (to prevent listener discomfort). AGCo monitors the output of the hearing *after* the amplifier.

As the name suggests, AGCi monitors the input, or the signal *before* it is amplified. In this case the compression parameters are adjusted so that incoming signals, when amplified, are placed within the patient's dynamic range. For both types of compression, precise adjustments of parameters (e.g., kneepoints and/or ratios) can be made by the audiologist at the time of the fitting to tailor the compression activation to the loudness growth function of the individual patient. These are illustrated in Figure 2.1.

In summary, compression is used to accomplish two fitting goals: repackaging "the world" so that it fits into the patient's residual dynamic range (AGCi) and limiting the output just below the patient's LDL without introducing distortion (usually AGCo).

6. *Directional microphone technology:* A desirable option, available for many hearing aids, is the use of a directional microphone. Directional amplification can be obtained using a single directional microphone, or by using two or three

Even though research has shown that when the hearing aids are programmed correctly, many patients do not *need* a volume control, it is *desired* by most patients, especially if they are previous users of hearing aids equipped with volume controls.

At one time it was common to use peak clipping as a method to limit the maximum output. This circuitry can introduce distortion when peak clipping occurs, and therefore most hearing aids today use compression technology for output limiting.

Most of today's hearing aids have more than one compression circuit, often both input-controlled *and* output-controlled, operating independently in several channels.

Most patients fitted with directional microphone amplification also desire omnidirectional (equal amplification from all directions) for some listening situations. Most directional hearing aids are equipped with a button that allows the patient to switch to omnidirectional when needed, or the hearing aid does this automatically—more on this later.

omnidirectional microphones that have been electronically designed to produce a directional effect. Using directional amplification, the patient can improve the signal-to-noise (S/N) ratio of a listening situation by assuring that the desired speech signal is arriving from directly in front of him or her—the surrounding noise signal will then receive less amplification, improving the S/N ratio by as much as 6 dB or more for some listening environments. Nearly all patients will benefit from directional hearing aids for some listening situations (see Mueller & Ricketts [2000] for review).

As we stated earlier, all types of hearing aids include the microphone, amplifier, receiver, and power source, and most have highly adjustable compression and the option of directional microphone technology. It should be noted that the basic features described thus far are not the only options available. We will discuss the more specialized features of modern digital hearing instruments later in this chapter.

Some of the optional controls and circuitry must be selected depending on the needs of the user. As an example, for the patient who wants a very small hearing aid and seldom uses the telephone, it might not be necessary to include a telecoil in the hearing aid. Similarly, directional technology is not available for all hearing aids due to space limitations. If a patient will only wear very small hearing aids, it may be necessary to sacrifice the directional features in order to assure that the hearing aids are used. Thus, in selecting the appropriate device for a patient, we must consider the type of hearing loss, as well as the special needs of the user. This information will then guide the audiologist in choosing the most appropriate style of hearing aid, so let's talk about hearing aid styles next.

Hearing Aid Styles

There are currently six primary styles of hearing aids available. These include (1) body aid, (2) eyeglass aid, (3) behind-the-ear (BTE) aid, (4) in-the-ear (ITE) aid, (5) in-the-canal (ITC) aid, and (6) completely-in-the-canal (CIC) aid. Why so many choices? Over the years various hearing aid styles have been developed to reflect changing technology (miniaturization) and to meet the hearing needs and cosmetic desires of listeners with hearing impairments.

The earliest nonelectric hearing aid styles were made out of animal horns or other materials to form an ear-trumpet-style device. However, during the twentieth century, the hearing aid market was comprised of mostly electronic hearing aids powered by batteries using analog technology that became smaller and more efficient throughout the century. The electronic components (e.g., capacitors, resistors, transistors) utilized in these hearing aids were contained within various shell casing sizes referred to as the hearing aid style. In 1996, the first 100 percent digital hearing aid was introduced to the hearing aid market, and today, over 90 percent of the U.S. hearing aid market consists of digital products. However, for the most part, digital platform technology is still contained within the same hearing aid styles that analog technology was available in during the 1990s. Figure 2.2 provides an illustration of the four most common hearing aid styles. Each of the shown hearing aid styles as well as some additional styles will be discussed individually regarding current market share. In addition, issues related to each hearing aid style will be highlighted to give you a better idea of the need for different styles of hearing aids and

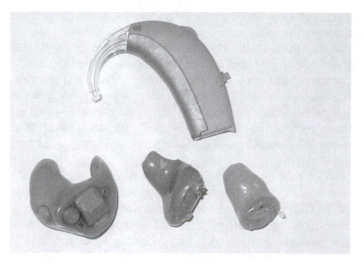

FIGURE 2.2

Four most common styles of hearing aids. The BTE is on top, while the ITE, ITC, and CIC are below.

the reasons why each style may or may not be selected for a particular patient. We will first describe two hearing aids styles that are not shown in Figure 2.2.

BODY AID. Given that the body aid was the style of the 1920s, it may come as a surprise to learn that this type of hearing aid is still manufactured. Over the years body aids sometimes have been utilized because of their larger controls, which can be helpful for elderly patients who have dexterity and vision problems. While body aids do not represent much of the current hearing aid market in the United States or Europe (less than 1%), they have found a place in many developing countries. Because of their larger size and standard construction, they can be manufactured less expensively. Additionally, they are popular in countries where hearing aid batteries are a rarer commodity and can be very expensive relative to earned salaries. Body aids utilize larger, cheaper batteries such as the AA size, whereas other styles of hearing aids use less commonly available battery sizes. Some body aids even utilize alternative energy sources such as solar cells. Fully charged, some solar-powered body aids can last up to two weeks without recharging. However, users are generally advised to charge them one hour each day during midday direct sunlight. An example of a solar-powered body-worn hearing aid may be found at www.comcareinternational.org.

EYEGLASS HEARING AID. The eyeglass/hearing aid combination device has almost disappeared from the global hearing aid market, but still yet is mentioned under available hearing aid styles because it was an innovative concept in its day during the 1960s. Conceptually, the combination eyeglass and hearing aid unit sounds like a good idea. In practice, however, there are several drawbacks. For example, in cases where the hearing aid or the eyeglasses component needed to be modified in some way or needed a service repair, the entire device had to be mailed back to the manufacturer, and the patient would be without both. This, as well as other issues, has resulted in the eyeglass style not being utilized today except in rare instances.

In contrast to the less prevalent devices mentioned above, the following section will review the four basic styles of hearing aids that generally are available from all the major hearing aid manufacturers. Recall that the style of a hearing aid relates to the cosmetic design of the device, not the level of technology in the device. So, when hearing aid manufacturers introduce a new product every other year or so, the technology of that particular model will be compact enough to fit into even the smallest style of hearing aids, although some advanced features, such as directional microphones and user controls, may not be able to be included on smaller styles due to limited space on the faceplate of the hearing aid.

BTE. The behind-the-ear (BTE) hearing aid is worn over the pinna and is typically coupled to tubing with an earmold that directs the amplified sound to the tympanic membrane. In some cases, the BTE may only be connected to tubing that is inserted directly in the ear canal for a more open fitting. The BTE is generally less expensive than comparable custom-made hearing aids incorporating similar levels of technology. The BTE aid requires no special modifications to the shell case and can thus be completely manufactured in advance of a placed order from a hearing aid dispenser. Many hearing aid dispensers actually keep a stock supply of BTE aids in their offices for same-day fittings with a temporary earmold. In contrast, the circuitry for custom-made products must be inserted and attached to the hearing aid shell casing that is made from an ear impression unique to each patient. The fabrication of the hearing aid shell casing and wiring of electronic components is performed at a manufacturer's product assembly plant prior to shipping.

Sales of hearing aids in the United States are reported to the Hearing Instrument Association (HIA), and statistics for different styles are published. According to a recent HIA survey, the BTE model is about 25 percent of the hearing aid market. It should be noted that in spite of the fact that BTEs have became smaller and more cosmetically appealing in the past few years, BTE hearing aids still seem to carry a negative connotation associated with their size.

However, BTEs are still the favored and most appropriate choice for fitting children. With a BTE fitting, only the earmold needs to be replaced as the child grows. This is much less costly than recasing a custom-made hearing aid. In addition, because BTEs are the most powerful hearing aid style in terms of gain and output, they remain the premiere choice for fitting severe-to-profound hearing losses. BTEs are also often selected because of their compatibility with a large variety of assistive listening devices. The larger sizes of BTEs allow for use of a larger battery, in turn giving the hearing aid a longer operating life before a battery change is necessitated. This is important, as it can be quite difficult for elderly individuals with limited manual dexterity and visual impairments to change a battery. In addition, larger user controls may be placed on the BTE-style hearing aid, making them easier to see and manipulate.

In recent years a modification of the traditional BTE has been introduced (see Figure 2.3). This new product has a small case that fits discreetly behind the ear. It also utilizes a smaller tubing size,

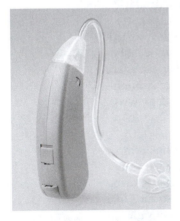

FIGURE 2.3

"Open fitting" BTE hearing aid.

Courtesy of Siemens Hearing Instruments, Inc.

which is then transmitted to an "open fitting" within the ear canal. In general, this style of BTE instruments employs advanced feedback control systems. Limited research has shown that this new BTE style can provide adequate gain while minimizing the negative aspects of the occlusion effect (one's own voice sounding hollow).

ITE. The in-the-ear (ITE) hearing aid resides in the concha portion of the pinna, with the receiver portion extending into the ear canal. The ITE style became commercially available in the 1960s. The HIA reports that the ITE-style hearing aid accounts for about 40 percent of annual sales. Currently, there are three variants of the ITE style: full shell, low profile, and half shell. The full shell ITE fills the entire concha portion of the outer ear. The low profile ITE fills the inner portion of the concha from top to bottom, but does not protrude outwards as much as the full shell ITE. The half shell ITE style fills only the lower half of the concha. The full-concha ITE usually is used when more gain and output is required, although not producing as much gain as can be obtained with the BTE style. In general, the ITE and smaller styles are easier to insert and remove in comparison to the BTE. Additionally, ITEs and smaller styles are less susceptible to wind noise, which can be quite annoying when hearing aids are worn outside.

ITC. The in-the-canal (ITC) hearing aid only partially fills the lower approximate one-quarter of the concha. The HIA reports that the ITC style accounts for approximately 20 percent of annual sales. Currently, it is also the smallest style of hearing aid that can contain directional microphone technology, because a directional microphone needs port spacing of several millimeters on the faceplate to function effectively. Because it represents a compromise between amplification power and size, the ITC hearing aid may be appropriate for patients who have cosmetic concerns with hearing aids, less severe hearing losses, and/or moderate loss of dexterity.

CIC. As its name implies, the completely-in-the-canal (CIC) hearing aid is completely contained within the ear canal; this style accounts for approximately 15 percent of annual sales. The low percentage of total sales for the CIC is somewhat surprising, as most patients typically ask for the smallest hearing aid possible. One explanation for this may be that audiologists are counseling patients away from this smallest of the hearing aid styles toward larger styles that have many advantages over the CIC.

CICs may not offer the gain/output appropriate for patients with moderate to more severe hearing losses. Another disadvantage of the CIC is its lack of a directional microphone, which is usually advantageous for improving understanding performance in the presence of background noise. CICs also require more frequent repair than other hearing aid styles. The electronics contained within the CIC shell are more susceptible to perspiration and cerumen, as the CIC is placed deeper in the ear canal of the patient. Moreover, while a volume control is not desired by all patients (or audiologists, for that matter), the faceplate of the CIC is oftentimes too small to accommodate one when it is wanted or needed. Kochkin (2003) showed that 78 percent of all hearing aid consumers want a volume control, and 33 percent of those consumers without a volume control on their present hearing aid would like to have one.

Finally, it's important to mention the ITD hearing aid. Many newer students to the field of audiology may be unfamiliar with this abbreviation, but according to several MarkeTrak surveys of hearing aid owners, as many as 15 percent of this group are very familiar with this type of hearing aid, which stands for "in-the-drawer." Note that this is not truly a style of hearing aid but instead a clever use of abbreviations to categorize over 1 million *purchased hearing aids* in the United States that are not worn by patients. For a number of different reasons, many hearing aid owners do not wear the hearing aids that they invested so much money in just months or years before. The five most cited reasons for dissatisfaction with hearing aids leading to ITD aids are poor perceived benefit, inability to hear in background noise, poor fit/comfort, negative side effects of hearing aids, and price/cost of repairs (Kochkin, 2002). We obviously still have a lot of work to do.

SUMMARY. For many patients, either the BTE, ITE, ITC, or CIC hearing aid style may be fit successfully to candidates with mild-to-moderate hearing losses. However, it will continue to be necessary to select the appropriate style based on the audiologic needs of the wearer, as well as his or her expectations and preferences. For example, it will be nearly impossible to satisfy a hearing aid wearer with a BTE if he or she is opposed to the larger device from the outset of the selection/fitting process for cosmetic reasons. However, the advantages and disadvantages of all hearing aid styles should be presented to the hearing aid candidate so that an informed decision can be made. Matching the right hearing aid style to the patient is an important first step in the hearing aid fitting procedure, although it is not always an easy task. Sometimes a little trial and error must be applied. There will be some cases in which more specialized types of hearing aid fittings may be more appropriate.

■ SPECIALIZED FITTING OPTIONS

CROS/BICROS

CROS-style hearing aids are now available with both digital processing and directional microphone technology.

For the individual who has an unaidable hearing loss in one ear and normal hearing or an aidable hearing loss in the other ear, Contralateral Routing of Signal (CROS) or Bilateral Contralateral Routing of Signal (BICROS) amplification may be the most appropriate hearing aid arrangement. A CROS hearing aid is used when there is good hearing in one ear and the opposite ear cannot benefit from amplification. This device has a microphone on the side of the poor ear and its receiver directed to the normal ear, so the good ear can receive sound from the opposite side of the head. We have made the person a "two-sided" listener, but importantly, *not* a "two-eared" listener.

Somewhat different from the CROS fitting, BICROS hearing aids are used in cases where one ear is unaidable but there is some degree of aidable hearing loss in the other. This device has two microphones, one near the better ear and the other near the poorer ear. The acoustic signals from both sides are delivered to a single amplifier and receiver, and the output is then directed into the best ear.

For both CROS and BICROS, the transmission of sound can be either via hardwire or FM. In the *hardwire* system, the signal is carried from one side of the head to the other by wires concealed within the eyeglass frame or by a tube or cord around the back of the neck, as in the ITE and BTE styles. If an *FM system* is utilized, signals are transferred across the head by an FM transmitter and picked up by an FM receiver positioned near the better ear. The signal is then converted back to acoustic energy and presented to the better ear.

There also is a fitting arrangement referred to as a *transcranial CROS*. In this case, a powerful hearing aid is fitted to the unaidable ear (BTEs, ITEs, and CICs all have been used), with the hope that sound crosses over to the normal ear via bone conduction. There has been some limited success with this approach, but it requires that the bone conduction thresholds of the good ear are within normal limits.

A final method of accomplishing the patient benefit desired from a CROS fitting is to use an implantable hearing aid. This fitting option will be discussed in the next section.

Bone Conduction Hearing Aids

Conventional hearing aids usually are designed to utilize an air conduction receiver, and thus far, we have described the various styles of air conduction hearing aids that deliver the acoustic output in the ear canal. Some individuals with hearing loss, however, are unable to use conventional air conduction devices. They may have congenital atresia (missing or incomplete ear canals), chronic infection of the middle or outer ear that is made worse when a hearing aid or earmold is worn, or significant middle ear structure damage, making it difficult to obtain the necessary gain. In these cases, bone-conduction hearing aids are a practical solution.

TRADITIONAL BONE-CONDUCTION DEVICES. In traditional bone-conduction devices, amplified sound is delivered through a vibrator placed behind the ear and over the mastoid bone. These devices are most commonly integrated into body- or eyeglass-style hearing aids. In the body aid, a vibrating device is held against the mastoid process by a metal headband. In the eyeglass hearing aid, the vibrator is mounted into the stem of the eyeglass that extends behind the ear. Sound is picked up by the microphone and amplified, causing the bone conduction device to vibrate, which in turn sets the skull into vibration, resulting in the transmission of sound to the cochlea. These traditional bone conduction devices have a number of drawbacks and are rarely used today.

Implantable Hearing Aids

BAHA. BAHA is short for bone anchored hearing aid. It is a device that is implanted surgically behind the ear in the mastoid area. This surgical placement might be expected because this is also where the bone vibrator is placed for bone conduction audiometry. Additionally, the BAHA is most often used for conductive and mixed hearing losses. Use of the BAHA has been most strongly advocated for those patients where traditional hearing aids are unsatisfactory. The most ideal patients for BAHAs are those with congenital atresias or longstanding middle ear dysfunction (Chasin, 2002). The BAHA has also been used for the medical management of single-sided deafness as a transcranial device. Speech understanding performance and perceptual benefit measures obtained on patients wearing both a BAHA and a CROS aid system have shown the BAHA to provide significant improvement over a conventional CROS aid system (Wazen et al., 2003). However, longer follow-up research is still needed to determine if these improvements outweigh the risk of an implantation surgery, surgery cost, and device maintenance (Niparko, Cox, & Lustig, 2003).

Currently, the BAHA style is only manufactured by one company, Entific Medical Systems (see www.entific.com), and it is conveniently named BAHA®. The device has been FDA approved for individuals over the age of 5 years with conductive and mixed losses. Chasin (2002) reported that since 1977 over 9,000 people had been fit worldwide with the BAHA®. Figure 2.4A shows a percutaneous abutment that has been surgically placed in the mastoid bone, and Figure 2.4B shows an ear-worn BAHA® that has been snapped onto the abutment. Coupling of this device to the mastoid bone allows sound to be transmitted to the cochlea via vibration of the mastoid bone. Management of patient care for individuals with a BAHA® is most often a collaborative effort between both the surgeon and the audiologist.

MEI. MEI is an abbreviation for another type of implantable hearing aid known as the middle ear implant. The MEI may be used for both conductive and/or sensorineural hearing losses. However, it is most often used to treat sensorineural hearing losses. Two methods of transduction for MEIs are piezoelectric and electromagnetic.

Piezoelectric implementation of MEIs involves an external microphone placed by the ear that transduces sound to an implanted middle ear crystal. The crystal

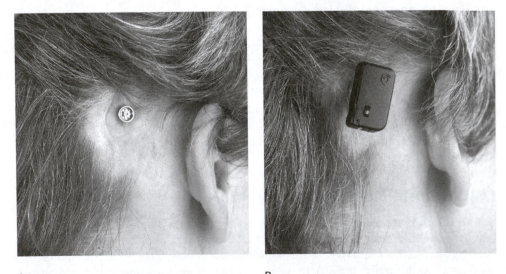

A   B

FIGURE 2.4

The BAHA® percutaneous abutment is shown on the left with the BAHA® device attached to the abutment on the right.

Courtesy of Entific Medical Systems.

bends in response to stimulation from sound transduction. This bending of the crystal then causes the ossicular chain in the middle ear space to vibrate, and sound transmission continues on to the cochlea. A major advantage of the piezoelectric implementation over the electromagnetic implementation is smaller components, allowing for a more discreet completely implantable device.

Because of its larger size the electromagnetic implementation of MEIs is only partially implantable. Most of these implants have an external coil connected to a microphone and an amplifier. An implanted magnet located at or near the incuostapedial joint of the ossicular chain oscillates as electromagnetic field waves move past the magnet, thus electromagnetic energy is converted to mechanical energy, and the sound propagates along the auditory pathway to the oval window of the cochlea.

Three useful websites related to middle ear implants include www.symphonix .com, www.medel.com, and www.otologics.com.

CI. A cochlear implant (CI) is a biomedical device that bypasses the middle ear, the traveling fluid wave in the scala media of the cochlea, and sensory cells on the basilar membrane to electrically stimulate neurons of the cochleovestibular (VIIIth) nerve. The purpose of a CI is to provide improvement beyond that offered by conventional amplification to people with severe-to-profound hearing loss. Most individuals with even severe-to-profound hearing loss have some functional auditory nerve fibers that can be stimulated in this way. Much like hearing aids, CIs aim to provide the detection and correct identification of environmental and speech sounds. A simulation of CIs may be found on the Internet at www.utdallas.edu/~loizou/cimplants/cdemos.htm. A comprehensive discussion of CIs may be found in Chapter 3.

■ THE EARMOLD

The earmold serves a variety of important functions. As you may recall, the earmold couples the hearing aid to the user's ear via a tube, as in the case of the BTE and eyeglass-style hearing aids (or a wire cord and external receiver, as in the body-style hearing aid). Figure 2.5 shows samples of many of the earmold styles that are available. As such, the earmold provides support for the BTE hearing aid, and most important, it directs and modifies the amplified sound that reaches the ear canal.

As with custom hearing aids, custom earmolds come in various styles, ranging from large models that fill the entire concha of the outer ear to models in which only a small piece of tubing extends into the ear canal. In general, the greater the hearing loss, the larger the earmold needed.

Once the earmold is coupled to the hearing aid, the properties of the sound reaching the user's ear are changed. The acoustic properties of the earmold itself and the length and diameter of the connecting tube play an important part in the final acoustical characteristics of the hearing aid system.

> While this section is geared toward earmolds, it is important to remember that many of the same principles and techniques applied to earmolds also can be used with custom hearing aid shells.

Acoustic Effects of Earmolds and Hearing Aid Shells

The most important characteristic of the earmold or hearing aid shell is that each can be modified to alter the amplified signal delivered to the user's ear. As we'll

BTE AND EYEGLASS TUBE TYPE

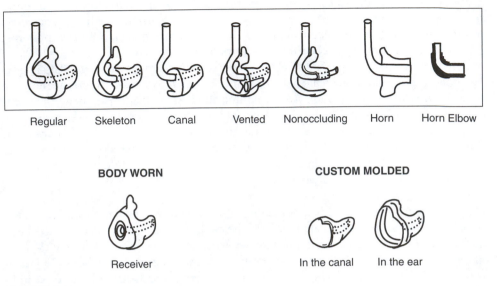

| Regular | Skeleton | Canal | Vented | Nonoccluding | Horn | Horn Elbow |

BODY WORN

Receiver

CUSTOM MOLDED

In the canal   In the ear

FIGURE 2.5

Basic types of earmolds.
Source: Stabb & Lybarger (1994).

discuss later, it is important that the real-ear frequency response is tailored for each patient. By utilizing the following techniques, the audiologist can modify one or more portions of the frequency response of the hearing aid in order to deliver the acoustic signal more appropriately.

LOW-FREQUENCY MODIFICATION

THE VENT. The most common modification is called a vent, which is a small hole drilled into the canal portion of the earmold or shell. The vent is usually parallel to the sound bore, although in some instances a diagonal vent is used. Earmolds (and custom hearing aids) are vented for three primary reasons:

- To allow unwanted amplified low frequencies to escape from the ear canal
- To release pressure to avoid a "plugged ear" sensation
- To allow the normal input of unamplified sound

"Select-A-Vent" is a common term used to identify the small plastic plugs of various vent diameters.

Vents can be drilled to various diameters, depending on the results desired. The diameter of a vent may vary from a small pressure equalization vent to an "open earmold" where the vent has been enlarged until nothing remains but the outermost portion of the earmold. In general, the larger the vent size, the more low-frequency attenuation (reduction). In recent years, there has been an increase in "open fittings." In this case, a special nonoccluding earmold with a small tube is used. An example of this is shown in Figure 2.3. Variable vents are also available that use small plastic plugs or different sizes of tubing that can totally occlude an existing vent or provide smaller openings of various diameters.

MID-FREQUENCY MODIFICATION

THE DAMPER. Acoustic dampers are placed within the tubing or earhook of BTE-style hearing aids and in the receiver tubing of custom instruments. They are small inserts that act as resistors, altering the acoustic dimensions of the hearing aid system. In general, dampers will smooth out peaks of the frequency response and reduce the overall output. Metal pellets, mesh screens, cotton, and lamb's wool have all been used for this purpose. Without the use of dampers, some hearing aids produce a strong output peak in the mid-frequency range, typically near 1500 Hz, that can cause discomfort to the user. The effects of acoustic dampers on the hearing aid response depend on the value of the acoustic resistance of the dampers. Higher ohm values (acoustic resistance) cause more flattening of peaks and reduction in overall output.

HIGH-FREQUENCY MODIFICATION

THE ACOUSTIC HORN. An acoustic horn is produced by progressively increasing the internal diameter (e.g., 2 mm to 3 mm to 4 mm) of the earmold tubing or custom shell sound bore. The effect is an enhancement of high-frequency gain, especially in the important 3000 to 4000 Hz region. Not all ear canals are large enough to accommodate 4 mm diameter tubing, and the use of a 3 mm diameter horn is more common.

> The acoustic horn approach cannot be used effectively with custom instruments.

Even with high-end digital technology, there are cases when the adjusted programmed gain and output does not meet desired targets. Through the use of venting and horning (and sometimes the use of dampers), it is possible to shape the hearing aid's frequency response to a variety of different desired gain characteristics. It is important to remember that any modification to the hearing aid–earmold system can change the output delivered in the ear canal, and many of these alterations cannot be predicted from 2 cc coupler measurements. We recommend measuring real-ear output (using probe-microphone measurements), therefore, whenever alterations in the earmold or hearing aid shell are made.

Ear Impressions

While professionals bring their own style and tools to the making of an ear impression, each professional must follow certain steps to ensure that an accurate representation of the concha and ear canal is obtained while protecting the patient from possible discomfort or even injury. Most professional malpractice suits in the field of audiology arise from ear impressions that have caused injury to a patient. An improper ear impression can cause swelling or irritation of the ear canal, as well as bleeding. In the worst cases, it can actually rupture the tympanic membrane. Ear impression material can sometimes be inserted past the narrowest part of the ear canal where it can harden and become unable to be removed easily from the ear canal. In this circumstance, a physician or other medical professional must cut and remove small portions of the hardened material from the ear canal until the remaining material can be pulled back through the narrow portion of the ear canal.

It is necessary that the ear impression is precise, as this will be used to fabricate the earmold or shell of the hearing aid. A poor fit can easily lead to hearing aid rejection. The first step in making an ear impression is to perform otoscopy. Otoscopy must be performed to determine if the ear canal is clear or mostly clear of cerumen.

Next, an otolight is used to place an eardam just beyond the second bend of the ear canal. The light ensures that the ear canal is clearly visible so that placement of the eardam is precise. Eardams may consist of materials such as a cotton block, sponge, or foam plug. The purpose of the eardam is to help ensure that the impression material does not come into contact with the tympanic membrane. Otoscopy is then performed again to reaffirm proper placement of the eardam. The impression material is then opened from its packaging. Ear impression material consists of two parts: a base and a catalyst. These parts are mixed and inserted into a syringe. The mixture is injected into the ear canal starting at the eardam moving outward in a swirling motion until all crevasses in the concha and helix are filled. The material is given time to harden, usually about 5 minutes, before removal. Once sufficiently hardened, the pinna is lifted up and back to help loosen the impression. The impression is then pulled out of the ear with a slight forward and downward rotation and inspected for deficiencies or flaws. If not satisfactory, it may need to be remade. The ear canal is finally reinspected once more to ensure that the eardam as well as all impression material has been removed along with no injury to the ear canal or tympanic membrane. Finally, the impression is then sent to an earmold laboratory or hearing aid manufacturer for fabrication of the final product.

Recently, ear impression scanning equipment has come into use and is causing a shift in the ear impression to earmold or custom hearing aid shell process. The equipment uses a three-dimensional scanner to create a digital image of the ear impression with extreme accuracy. It is expected that many practice sites will begin scanning ears in their own office and ordering earmolds and custom shells electronically via submission of an electronic order and image file of the ear's structure.

■ BATTERIES

There are five common hearing aid battery sizes. The battery sizes in descending order of size are the 675, 13, 312, 10, and 5. Notice that the numbers do not follow a convenient descending pattern that reflects the size of the battery. The size 13 battery is indeed larger than the size 312 battery. Typically, larger batteries are found in larger hearing aids, such as the BTE and ITE styles, and smaller batteries are for ITC and CIC styles. However, there are exceptions; in an effort to maintain a small case design, some BTE style hearing aids designed for fitting mild-to-moderate high-frequency hearing losses utilize a small size 10 battery.

Nearly all hearing aid batteries are now zinc-air. Zinc-air means that the batteries are comprised of zinc but are activated by air once a protective tab is removed from the positive terminal of the battery. In the past hearing aid batteries have been made of mercury and silver oxide. The mercury batteries were shown to have toxic environmental effects when decomposing, and the silver oxide batteries became cost-prohibitive to produce as the cost of silver per ounce increased in the 1970s.

Table 2.1 shows the nominal voltage and storage capacity of current for different sizes of hearing aid batteries.

The operating life of a battery is typically expressed in hours. However, this may also be expressed in days. The typical conversion rate from hours to days is 16 to 1. However, this conversion rate may be changed to reflect the actual hour usage per

TABLE 2.1

Voltage and Current Capacity Hours for Different Battery Sizes

BATTERY TYPE	NOMINAL VOLTAGE	CAPACITY (MILLIAMP HOURS)
Zinc-Air 5	1.3V	50–60 mAh
Zinc-Air 10	1.3V	50–60 mAh
Zinc-Air 312	1.3V	100–120 mAh
Zinc-Air 13	1.3V	170–230 mAh
Zinc-Air 675	1.3V	400–550 mAh

Source: Adapted from Mueller & Hall (1998).

day for any given hearing aid user. In order to determine the expected operating life of a hearing aid battery, the current drain on the battery from the specific hearing aid's processing must be known. Current drain will vary systematically in accordance to gain needed for meeting prescriptive targets for the hearing loss and other hearing aid specialty features employed such as a noise reduction system or feedback reduction system. Current drain can be determined utilizing most hearing aid test systems and is always reported in the product specifications of hearing aid products.

An example is as follows: Assume that the measured current drain on a size 13 battery from a specific hearing aid is .79 mA per hour. Then, referencing the chart in Table 2.1, it can be determined that a size 13 battery has an average storage capacity of 200 mAh (midpoint of 170 and 230). The 200-hour storage capacity is then divided by .79. This yields an expected battery life of approximately 253 hours or 16 days (assuming 16 hours of use per day). If the patient used the hearing aid for only 8 hours a day, then the days of battery life would double.

■ ELECTROACOUSTIC PROPERTIES

The electroacoustic performance characteristics of hearing aids are defined in several standards. One of these standards is referred to as the American National Standards Institute (ANSI) S3.22, which is maintained by volunteer hearing professionals, scientists, and engineers. The standard has been revised numerous times since it was introduced in 1977, the most recent being 2003.

All manufactured or repaired hearing aids must operate within the specifications of this standard. Electroacoustic evaluations of a hearing aid should always accompany a new or repaired hearing aid when it arrives from the manufacturer, but it is quite simple to actually perform your own electroacoustic analysis with a hearing aid test system in your practice setting. Examples of two hearing aid analyzers from one manufacturer are shown in Figure 2.6.

An electroacoustic analysis should take only a few minutes. It is an integral part of the hearing aid fitting protocol and a quantifiable method of documenting hearing aid performance. Prior to the initial hearing aid fitting, testing is conducted to

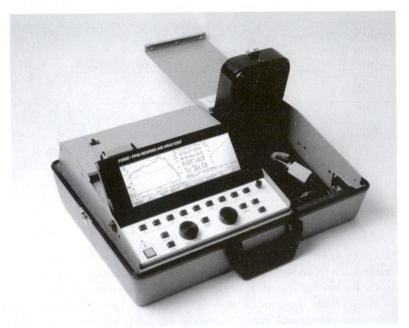

Fonix FP40: Portable Hearing Aid Analyzer

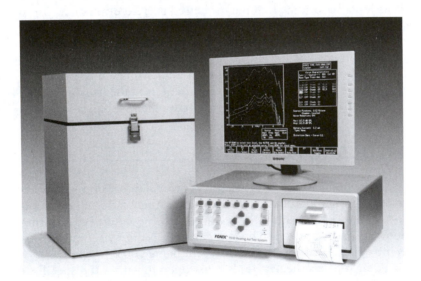

Fonix 7000: Hearing Aid Test Analyzer

FIGURE 2.6

Hearing aid analyzers.

Courtesy of Frye Electronics.

Terms Related to Electroacoustic Analysis

Output Sound Pressure Level (OSPL90): Represents the maximum output level in dB SPL the hearing aid is able to produce with an input of 90 dB SPL.

High Frequency Average (HFA) OSPL90: The average output for a 90 dB SPL input at 1000, 1600, and 2500 Hz (or at three special-purpose average frequencies in certain situations).

High Frequency Average Full-On Gain (HFA FOG): Average difference between the output SPL in a 2 cc coupler and the input SPL set to the hearing aid's full-on position at 1000, 1600, and 2500 Hz (or at three special-purpose average frequencies in certain situations).

High Frequency Average Reference-Test Gain (HFA RTG): Average difference between the output SPL in a 2 cc coupler and the input SPL in a 2 cc coupler at 1000, 1600, 2500 Hz (or at three special-purpose average frequencies in certain situations), with the hearing aid set to its RTG position. The RTG position is described as HFA OSPL90 – 77 dB.

Frequency Range: The useful range of frequencies that fall within a lower and upper designated frequency. The useful range is defined as the frequencies that have greater output SPL values than the HFA output response level – 20 dB at the hearing aid's RTG position.

Total Harmonic Distortion (THD): Unwanted signals created by the hearing aid that occur at integer multiples of an input sine wave. It is most often reported at test frequencies of 500, 800, and 1600 Hz. For each test frequency, the power of all distortion products is summed and expressed relative to the power of the wanted output signal in a percentage value.

Equivalent Input Noise (EIN): The internal noise generated by microphones and amplifiers in the hearing aid.

More detailed definitions and definitions for other electroacoustic characteristics may be found in the ANSI S3.22 1996 or 2003 standard.

---

assure that the instrument is performing according to specifications. Following hearing aid use, testing is conducted to assure that the desired performance is maintained.

The electroacoustic analysis is performed within a hearing aid test box; a reference microphone monitors the level of the input signal while another microphone measures the output from the hearing aid in a 2 cc coupler. A 2 cc coupler is a standardized coupler used across the hearing aid industry with a volume of 2 cubic centimeters; it may either be an HA-1 or HA-2 style. With an HA-1 coupler, the receiver of the hearing aid is placed into a large opening; putty material is then placed around the case of the hearing aid to seal off the opening. An HA-2 coupler can accept both a body aid button-type receiver and a BTE aid with the use of an additional snap-on piece with standard earmold tubing.

■ THE SELECTION AND FITTING OF HEARING AIDS

To this point in this chapter, we have provided some general information concerning how hearing aids are constructed, how they work, the variety of styles that are available, and how we can measure their performance on a standard coupler. Now comes the hard part: fitting and adjusting the sophisticated technology to the dyanamic characteristics and listening needs of the patient. We have outlined a five-step protocol for selecting and fitting hearing aids. While it is tempting to grab a couple of hearing aids out of a box and go directly to Step 4, you will find that the key to successful fittings is directly related to the time and thought that is expended during Steps 1, 2, and 3.

Step 1: Selecting the Hearing Aid Candidate

Several issues must be considered when an individual is selected as a hearing aid candidate. Three of the most important factors are degree of hearing loss, amount of communication difficulty, and motivation to use hearing aids. Quite frequently, these three factors interrelate, and it is difficult to make a fitting decision based on information from only one or two of these categories.

DEGREE OF HEARING LOSS. Usually the first step in determining hearing aid candidacy is to examine the pure-tone thresholds. If the patient has a profound hearing loss (with accompanying poor word recognition), it might be that the hearing impairment is too severe to be helped with conventional hearing aids. It is then appropriate to consider the alternative amplification devices that we discuss elsewhere in the chapter.

A more common decision that needs to be made is to determine if the hearing loss is severe enough to warrant amplification. There are no strict rules for this determination, but most audiologists agree that if hearing is normal or near-normal (thresholds of 25 dB or better) for 4000 Hz and below, it is unlikely that hearing aids will be beneficial. As hearing loss starts to affect the higher speech frequencies of 3000 and 4000 Hz, which is the typical pattern, the patient will need to be considered for amplification. Many successful hearing aid users today have normal or near-normal hearing through the frequencies of 1500 to 2000 Hz.

One method to assess the effects of the pure-tone impairment is to calculate an Audibility Index, or AI. An AI is the percent of average speech that is audible to the patient. The chart shown in Figure 2.7, developed by Mueller and Killion (1990), can be used for this purpose. Simply plot the audiogram on the chart and count the dots that are not audible (above the threshold line). Subtract this from 100 percent and you have the Audibility Index. Anyone with an audibility index below 85 percent could probably benefit from hearing aids, *but* only if the criteria of the next two categories are met.

DEGREE OF COMMUNICATION DISABILITY. A patient can have a significant hearing loss based on pure-tone findings, yet might not believe that he or she has a hearing disability (or at least a hearing disability that needs to be treated). This can be influenced by the patient's lifestyle, occupation, and the amount of time spent communicating with others. In some cases, it is denial, or simply a lack of awareness of the problem—"I can hear fine, it's just that my family members mumble."

A standardized self-assessment tool (also referred to as self-report) is an excellent way to survey each individual's communication problems. While much of the same information could be gleaned from an extensive case history, a standard questionnaire is a more reliable and efficient method of collecting this information.

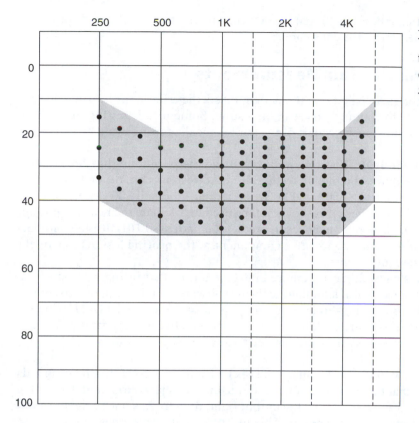

FIGURE 2.7

The count-the-dot audiogram form for calculation of the Audibility Index (Articulation Index), or AI.
Source: Mueller & Killion (1990).

There are several self-assessment questionnaires available, some specific to communication, some related to personality traits and expectations, others related to social and emotional issues (see Chapter 10 for a review). Several useful websites for information on computerized self-assessment tools include

> www.ausp.memphis.edu/harl
>
> www.ihr.gla.ac.uk
>
> www.isu.edu/csed/rehab

Hearing aid outcome measures that are designed to measure handicap, benefit, or satisfaction also can be used to measure expectations and unaided communication difficulties.

MOTIVATION TO USE HEARING AIDS. A final area concerning hearing aid candidacy is related to the motivation of the patient to use hearing aids. A person might have a significant hearing loss, admit that he or she has communication problems, yet not be willing to use hearing aids. Logic suggests that these patients probably won't be happy hearing aid users, and it is tempting to simply tell them "Come back when you're ready." There is some evidence to suggest, however, that if we somehow can get these people to start using hearing aids, they might become successful hearing aid users—sort of a "Try it, you'll like it" approach.

Certainly, as with other health care providers, it is our responsibility to firmly tell the patient what we believe is the best treatment for him or her. Given that no one *really* wants to use hearing aids, a lukewarm recommendation is often viewed as no recommendation by the patient. Obviously, the final decision to purchase hearing aids lies in the patient's hands.

Step 2: Preselection Measurements

Once it has been established that the patient meets the criteria for hearing aid candidacy, it is time to conduct preselection testing. Some of this testing might have been conducted previously as part of the audiologic diagnostic evaluation.

PURE-TONE THRESHOLDS. You might already have the pure-tone thresholds available from the auditory diagnostic testing. If not, thresholds are needed for all frequencies of interest (e.g., 250 to 6000 Hz, including 1500 and 3000 Hz). For most prescriptive methods, these thresholds will be used to calculate the hearing aid gain requirements and in some instances to predict the patient's LDLs. It is also important to know if there is a conductive component to the hearing loss, as this might alter your gain requirements.

These thresholds either are entered into the automated fitting software for a given product or used with stand-alone fitting software and then applied to a given product. It also is common to use an umbrella software, termed *NOAH*, which is then linked to the software of different manufacturers. In this way, patient data can be stored in a central location and applied to any hearing instrument.

LOUDNESS DISCOMFORT LEVEL (LDL). One of the leading reasons that hearing aids are rejected is that the maximum output of the aid was placed too high. Obtaining the data that will assist in getting the output right, therefore, is one of the most important preselection measurements. This measurement, sometimes referred to as *uncomfortable level (UCL)* or *threshold of discomfort (TD)* rather than LDL, is conducted using pure tones (or very narrow bands of noise) at two or three key frequencies (e.g., 500 Hz, 1500 Hz, and 3000 Hz). We recommend using the chart shown in Table 2.2; a rating of "loud, but OK" is the value used for specifying the hearing aid's maximum output (see Mueller & Hornsby, 2002, for a review).

SPEECH-IN-NOISE TESTING. Often, success with hearing aids depends on the patient's ability to understand speech in background noise. It is difficult to predict a patient's speech-in-noise understanding based on his or her pure-tone thresholds, as many factors can influence the results, including central auditory processing difficulties. For this reason, many audiologists conduct prefitting speech-in-noise testing using insert earphones to obtain a general impression of how the patient might perform in background noise using hearing aids. A common test to use for this purpose is the QuickSIN (www.etymotic.com).

Step 3: Hearing Aid Selection

There are several important aspects of the hearing aid selection procedure, ranging from the style of the hearing aid to the type of signal processing, to whether the hearing aid should be analog or digital, to whether the hearing aid should be re-

TABLE 2.2
Categories of Loudness

Uncomfortably loud (7)

Loud, but OK (6)

Comfortable, but slightly loud (5)

Comfortable (4)

Comfortable, but slightly soft (3)

Soft (2)

Very soft (1)

Source: Cox, R. M. (1995). Using loudness data for hearing aid selection: The IHAFF Approach. *The Hearing Journal 48*(2), 39–44.

mote controlled. Many of these decisions require input from the patient, since a mistake in any one area potentially could lead to hearing aid rejection.

HEARING AID STYLE. Earlier in this chapter we summarized the pros and cons of different hearing aid styles. Using the information obtained from the preselection testing, it is now time to find the best style for your patient. In addition to the audiometric information available and necessary features for the patient (e.g., telecoil, directional microphone), you must also consider such aspects as the patient's dexterity, the pinna and ear canal geography, and the need for a cosmetically acceptable product. Financial resources cannot be overlooked, as some styles (e.g., CIC) tend to be more expensive than others.

GAIN AND FREQUENCY RESPONSE. Hearing aids are programmable and can be adjusted to fit a wide range of hearing losses. However, it is still necessary for manufacturers to have products of two or three different power categories. That is, when a patient has a severe-to-profound loss, a more powerful hearing aid must be ordered than if the patient had a mild-to-moderate hearing loss.

The desired gain and output of the hearing aid usually are selected using a validated prescriptive fitting method. Through research it has been determined that theoretical formulae can be applied using the patient's thresholds and/or LDLs. These gain and output targets can be expressed in either 2 cc coupler or in ear canal gain or SPL values. While these prescriptive targets may not be the ideal fitting for all patients, it has been shown that they will optimize the fitting for the average patient. The following are two fitting methods that are currently used:

- National Acoustic Laboratories' Nonlinear method v.1 (NAL-NL1) (see www.NAL.gov.AU)
- Desired Sensation Level method v.4.1 (DSL4.1) (see www.DSL@nca.uwo.ca)

In general, most audiologists use the NAL method with adults and the DSL method with children, although there is considerable overlap. These prescriptive methods not only provide desired targets for gain and output, but also provide guidance for selecting compression parameters. An example is shown in Figure 2.8. Some hearing aid manufacturers have developed their own prescriptive approaches, which are implemented in their fitting software. None of these methods, however, have the supporting research of the NAL or the DSL.

Hearing aids are available with a wide range of signal processing features. At one time, digital processing was considered a special feature. Today, nearly all hearing aids utilize digital processing, so this is no longer considered to be special. However, the type and number of digital processing algorithms vary significantly from product to product. For this chapter, we'll divide the products into two categories: basic features and advanced features. Some of the basic features were briefly discussed earlier, and additional basic features are listed below.

MULTIPLE CHANNELS. Signals are processed separately in several different channels throughout the frequency range of speech. This allows for gain and compression to

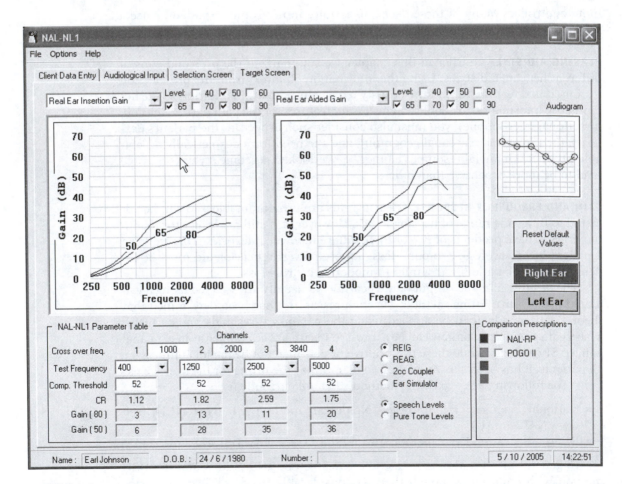

FIGURE 2.8

NAL-NL1 software recommendations for prescriptive targets.

be applied more precisely in accordance with the patient's hearing loss and dynamic range.

MULTIPLE MEMORIES. Many hearing aids have two or three memories. Each memory can be programmed with different fitting parameters for different listening conditions. Possible choices might be listening in background noise, on the telephone, or listening to music. In some models a memory is used for the directional microphone feature. The different memories can be accessed by a remote device or by a button on the hearing aid.

COMPRESSION. Another basic feature is compression. One type of compression is WDRC (AGCi), which is used to remap inputs from very soft to loud into the patient's residual dynamic range. The WDRC designator suggests that the hearing aid has a low kneepoint (e.g., around 40 dB SPL or lower). The design is based on the philosophy that speech should always, or nearly always, be in compression. A second type of compression is limiting compression (AGCo) which is used to maintain high inputs below the patient's LDL. Many products employ both of these compression features.

> Dynamic range: The difference between a listener's Loudness Discomfort Level (LDL) and threshold for that signal (either pure tones or speech).

EXPANSION. Another feature that often is combined with WDRC compression is audio expansion. Expansion compresses signals below the kneepoint and is used to minimize annoyance from amplified microphone noise and low-level environmental sounds. Expansion often allows the patient to use the gain necessary to make soft speech audible without the negative side effects of excessive amplification of ambient noise.

DIRECTIONAL TECHNOLOGY. Even the "entry-level" hearing aids, space permitting, employ directional microphone technology.

The use of directional microphone technology is the most effective method to improve the signal-to-noise ratio. Directional hearing aids improve the signal-to-noise ratio based on spatial location, not spectral content. That is, if a patient is able to position himself so that he is facing the primary talker, and the background noise is surrounding or from behind the patient, directional hearing aids will provide a significant improvement in SNR when compared to omnidirectional amplification. The degree of improvement depends on several variables (e.g., distance from primary talker, reverberation of room, azimuth of noise sources), but in general, research has shown that a 3 to 6 dB improvement in the SNR can be expected. For some patients, in some listening situations, this SNR advantage can improve speech understanding by 50 percent or more. It's likely that nearly all patients will obtain some benefit in some listening conditions.

> Most directional hearing aids today do not utilize directional microphones *per se*, but employ omnidirectional microphones and utilize electronic phase cancellation techniques to accomplish the desired directional effect.

There are other important features available with today's digital products. The following are some of the algorithms associated with the more "advanced" hearing aid products.

- *Automatic digital noise reduction.* The incoming signal is analyzed in several different channels, and if the signal is determined to be noise, an automatic gain reduction occurs in that channel. Typically, the speech versus noise decision is based on the modulations of the signal. Other types of noise reduction use a filtering approach. While noise reduction has not shown to improve the signal-to-noise ratio significantly, it does seem to improve listening comfort and reduce listener fatigue (see Mueller & Ricketts, 2005, for review).

■ *Adaptive feedback reduction.* Acoustic feedback is a problem for many hearing aid users, and it can lead to hearing aid rejection. The acoustic feedback is perceived by users and sometimes those around them as a squeal or a whistle. In today's instruments, when transient acoustic feedback occurs (such as when a telephone receiver is placed at the ear) the hearing aid automatically identifies the frequency and employs a frequency-specific temporary gain reduction to eliminate or reduce the feedback. This can be accomplished by using phase cancellation or by introducing a narrow notch filter. Adaptive feedback cancellation has two possible patient benefits: First, if the patient isn't bothered by annoying feedback, she will be more apt to use a higher gain setting, which will result in greater audibility of soft speech sounds. Secondly, an effective feedback suppression system allows for the use of a more open fitting—this can help reduce or eliminate the occlusion effect.

■ *Directional microphone control.* Directional hearing aids can be automatic and/or adaptive. Automatic means that the hearing aid will automatically switch back and forth between omnidirectional and directional depending on the listening situation. This is considered a desirable feature because research has shown that many hearing aid users fail to switch to the directional setting when they are in background noise. Adaptive means that while in the directional mode, the hearing aid will automatically change the strength and pattern of the directional amplification based on the intensity, spectrum, and azimuth of the noise source.

■ *Linked hearing aids.* Hearing aids are now available that "talk to each other." Through radio frequency transmission, the hearing aids (a bilateral fitting) share information. This has some direct patient benefit in that the patient only has to change gain on one hearing aid and the gain of the other hearing aid will automatically change the same amount. The same result is present for changing listening programs. Additionally, the sound classification system is linked, which means that automatic switching of both hearing aids occurs in parallel.

> Data logging is a feature available in some digital hearing aids that produces a record of information related to the listening environments a hearing aid user has been in, as well as the extent to which the user has utilized options like a directional microphone. This information can be helpful to the clinician in resolving fitting issues with some patients.

BILATERAL FITTINGS. Like shoes, gloves, and eyeglasses, hearing aids are usually fitted in pairs. It was once thought that a single hearing aid was satisfactory for someone with an aidable hearing impairment in both ears, but fortunately few professionals continue to hold this outdated belief. There are many advantages of a binaural fitting over a monaural one, and binaural is nearly always the fitting of choice. Some of the advantages include increased gain, improved localization, better sound quality, and improved speech understanding in background noise (see Mueller & Hall, 1998, for a complete review of the benefits of binaural fittings).

OTHER CONSIDERATIONS. We have discussed many of the most important features of hearing aid selection. Some other decisions that might need to be made include the need for a telecoil, direct audio input, or other special circuits. It is important to review all the features that we mentioned earlier in this chapter to assure that everything has been considered when the hearing aids are ordered.

Step 4: Verification

As mentioned in the preceding section, hearing aids typically are programmed for the patient according to a validated prescriptive fitting method. Once you have selected the prescriptive method that you believe is best, which might be different for different patients, the gain and output must then be verified.

The first verification procedure is to measure the performance of the hearing aids in the 2 cc coupler, as discussed earlier in this chapter. The gain, frequency response, OSPL90, and distortion of the hearing aid is checked to assure that it matches specifications and is consistent with the electroacoustic characteristics that are desired.

The most important verification procedures are conducted when the patient is wearing the hearing aids. In general, there are four different methods used to verify if the hearing aids being fitted have the correct gain, frequency response, and signal processing characteristics. Some audiologists might use different methods for different patients or combine methods for a single patient. The most essential of these measures is probe-microphone assessment, but we will discuss three other complementary measures first.

INFORMAL RATING OF SPEECH QUALITY AND INTELLIGIBILITY. "So, how does that sound?" This is perhaps the most popular question posed to a new hearing aid user. While this question is commonly asked, opinions vary concerning how much emphasis should be placed on the patient's answer. Can a patient reliably select what is best for him or her? Can he or she hear the difference between small but important changes in the frequency response? Is the frequency response that *sounds the best* necessarily the one that will result in the *best understanding of speech*? Probably not. It is, of course, always important to listen to the comments from the patient, but we believe that this should be used only as an adjunct to more structured verification protocols.

SPEECH RECOGNITION OR INTELLIGIBILITY TESTING. Because the patient usually sought amplification because of difficulty understanding speech, it seems logical that the verification procedure should measure his or her ability to understand aided speech. A speech testing approach can be used fairly successfully to compare *unaided* to *aided*; however, it is difficult to use speech testing for selecting the best frequency response or signal processing strategy. So, clinical speech testing can be used successfully to determine if hearing aids are better than no hearing aids, but usually not for determining which hearing aid adjustments are the best.

If aided speech testing is used, we suggest using tests that employ sentences in background noise. Two tests that work well for assessing hearing aid performance are

- Hearing In Noise Test (HINT): Available from Maico (www.maico-diagnostics.com)
- Quick Speech-in-Noise (QuickSIN) test: Available from the developer, Mead Killion, Ph.D. (www.etymotic.com)

LOUDNESS SCALING. If part of your fitting goal is to restore normal loudness perceptions, then some type of aided loudness verification is warranted. This can be

A self-assessment tool, the Profile of Aided Loudness (PAL), can be used to determine if the patient has normal aided loudness perceptions of everyday sounds in the real world.

conducted using frequency-specific signals, but usually connected-speech testing is adequate. An example protocol would be as follows (using the chart shown in Table 2.2):

- Present connected speech at 45 dB SPL. A 2 rating is desired, 1 or 3 rating is acceptable.
- Present connected speech at 65 dB SPL. A 4 rating is desired, 3 or 5 rating is acceptable.
- Present connected speech at 85 dB SPL. A 6 rating is desired, 5 rating is acceptable.

When a desired or acceptable rating is not obtained, make adjustments to gain, compression, and/or output and repeat the protocol.

Probe-microphone assessment often is referred to as "real ear" testing, or real ear measures (REM).

PROBE-MICROPHONE MEASUREMENTS. The most reliable method to verify the performance of hearing aids, and the preferred method described in published protocols, is to measure the output of the hearing aid at the tympanic membrane of the hearing aid user. This is accomplished by placing a small silicone tube in the ear canal that is attached to a measurement microphone. A loudspeaker is used to present a variety of test signals (e.g., noise, shaped speech, real speech), and the output from the hearing aid in the user's ear is analyzed using computerized equipment. Given the complexity of modern hearing aids, it usually is desirable to use real speech (either recorded or live voice) as the input signal. The results are displayed on a monitor and can be printed for the patient's file. Figure 2.9 shows two different popular probe-microphone systems.

There are few reasons *not* to use probe-microphone measurements as part of the verification procedure. Although there is an initial outlay of funds to purchase this equipment, the long-term payoff is well worth the investment. In addition to verification of gain and frequency response, this equipment has a variety of other uses in the evaluation of hearing aids and assistive listening devices. Using probe-microphone measurements, the real-ear gain of the hearing aid can be compared to the gain and output specified by a validated prescriptive fitting protocol. Additionally, varied inputs can be presented to the hearing aid to evaluate the effects of different automatic signal processing strategies. The hearing aid's directional microphone, noise reduction, telephone coil, and other special features also can be reliably assessed using this equipment.

Step 5: Postfitting Counseling, Orientation, and Outcome Measures

Even the best hearing aid, with the best circuitry adjusted precisely for the patient's hearing loss, can be a failed fitting if appropriate counseling and follow-up is not conducted.

POSTFITTING COUNSELING AND HEARING INSTRUMENT ORIENTATION (HIO). After the verification procedure is completed, it's time to sit down with the patient and walk through the use and care of the instruments. This is not something that can be rushed through. If possible, include significant others who spend time with the

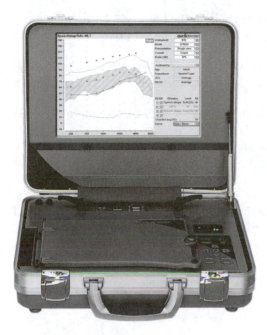

Audioscan RM500 SL   Audioscan VERIFIT

FIGURE 2.9

Examples of probe microphone systems.
Courtesy of Etymotic Design.

hearing aid user. It is good to have a handout that includes all the information that you will be presenting verbally (the user guide furnished by the manufacturer will have some of the information). Here is a basic list of things that you will want to discuss at the time of the hearing aid orientation. The acronym to help you remember the nine topics of this list is **HIO BASICS** (Hearing Instrument Orientation BASICS) (Schow, 2001).

1. **H** = Hearing expectations: Unfortunately, hearing aids do not work just like eyeglasses. Everything will not be perfectly clear once they are put in place. Additionally, adjustment to amplification requires days, weeks, and even months for some patients. The patient needs to know this.
2. **I** = Instrument operation: The patient should be able to turn the hearing aid on and off, change programs (if necessary), adjust volume, activate telecoil (if present), demonstrate use of hearing aid on telephone, discuss assistive telephone listening devices.
3. **O** = Occlusion effect: Have the patient talk with the hearing aids in his or her ears, *but turned off*—see if an occlusion effect is present. If so, and if it is bothersome, conduct treatments for reducing the occlusion effect (e.g., increase venting, lengthen canal) or explain why you can't make it go away (assuming that you can't).
4. **B** = Batteries: Discuss different battery types and sizes, what batteries the patient uses, how to obtain batteries, how long a battery lasts, and what to do with

those funny sticky tabs (don't put them back on the battery!). Have the patient demonstrate proficiency in opening and closing the battery door, inserting and removing the battery.

5. A = Acoustic feedback: Demonstrate what acoustic feedback, or squealing, sounds like (if the patient can hear it), what causes it, when it is OK, and when it is not OK.

6. S = System troubleshooting: Provide the patient with a troubleshooting chart to assess basic problems (see Table 2.3).

7. I = Insertion and removal: Demonstrate insertion and removal on an artificial ear, then have the patient practice in front of mirror. The patient should be able to do this before leaving the office.

8. C = Cleaning and maintenance: Show patient where wax accumulates in receiver tubing, demonstrate wax cleaning tool, show how the hearing aid itself can be wiped clean. Talk about taking battery out when storing the instrument, using of a dry-aid kit if moisture is a problem, keeping the instrument away from water, excessive heat, and hair spray, avoiding dropping hearing aid on hard surface, and other potential hazards.

TABLE 2.3

Troubleshooting of Common Problems with Hearing Aids

PROBLEM	CAUSE	POSSIBLE SOLUTION
Instrument has no sound or sound is weak	Battery polarity reversed	Make sure battery is inserted correctly
	Low or dead battery	Replace with fresh battery
	Instrument not turned on	Rotate volume control
	Clogged wax guard	Clean wax guard
	Volume turned down	Turn up volume control
Instrument whistles	Improper seating in ear	Reinsert the instrument until it fits securely
	Volume control too high	Turn down volume control
	Clogged wax guard	Clean wax guard
	Excessive wax in the ears	Consult your hearing health care professional
Sound is distorted or intermittent	Low battery	Replace battery
	Battery compartment is not completely closed	Gently close the battery compartment
Buzzing sound	Low battery	Replace battery
Swelling or discharge in ear		Check with your physician

9. S = Service, warranty, and repairs: Explain warranty and repair policies, give patient warranty card, explain how repairs are handled in your office (do you allow walk-ins?).

A thorough orientation also will include material on tips for effective communication. This will include discussion of listening styles (passive, aggressive, assertive), material on family communication dynamics (spouse, family members), information on using repair and anticipatory strategies, and the effective use of vision. In short, there are personal and environmental adjustments that the hearing aid user should try to utilize to complement the audibility improvements derived from amplification. Chapters 4 and 10 will provide more information regarding these topics, notably SPEECH and CLEAR in Chapter 10.

FOLLOW-UP VISITS AND OUTCOME MEASURES. On follow-up visits, it is useful to recheck some of the verification procedures that were conducted at the time of the fitting. Some general postfitting verification procedures might be the following:

- Present average-level speech to the patient (e.g., 65 dB SPL). Determine if the programmed gain continues to be appropriate.
- With the volume control wheel set for speech at MCL, present loud speech (e.g., 85 dB SPL) to assure that it is not uncomfortably loud (you can use the chart shown in Table 2.2. If loud speech is only judged as being at 5, it might be appropriate to reduce compression or raise the output to provide the patient with more headroom.
- Many manufacturers have "Fitting Assistant Modules" in their software that will help make adjustments for other specific problems that the patient might report.

This is also a good time to repeat the self-assessment questionnaires that you gave the patient before the hearing aids were fitted in order to derive additional outcome measures regarding benefit. The patient can now respond to the questions relative to his or her performance with hearing aids, including use, benefit, and satisfaction measures. At this time it is also appropriate to consider providing additional audiologic rehabilitation in addition to hearing aids, which is designed to further facilitate communication for the patient. Both short- and long-term forms of AR are discussed in detail in the chapters to follow.

Several things to consider during your postfitting testing, adjustments, and counseling are:

Acclimatization. Some research has suggested that it takes several weeks or even several months for the brain to adjust to a new acoustic input; that is, the new speech spectrum delivered by the hearing aid. It is possible, therefore, that maximum performance, or improvement in performance from a previous hearing aid, will not occur until acclimatization is complete.

Acclimatization can occur for a variety of hearing aid related factors: hearing new environmental sounds, soft speech, or a different speech spectrum.

Unaided ear effect. It is common to fit a person bilaterally who has been a long-time monaural hearing aid user. Research has suggested that for a person who has previously been aided monaurally, the ear that has not been aided for a period of time possibly will show a decline in performance for understanding speech. Can this decline be reversed? Possibly. Hence, speech understanding for this previously unaided ear, after some hearing aid use, might be better than predicted based on standard testing prior to the fitting of the hearing aids. More evidence in this area is needed, but this may be a compelling reason for fitting hearing aids bilaterally whenever possible.

■ CONSIDERATIONS FOR THE PEDIATRIC PATIENT

In many respects, fitting hearing aids to infants and young children is the same as for adults; the goals of maximizing intelligibility and quality, making soft speech audible, average speech comfortable, and loud speech loud, but not too loud are equally important for this population. But children are not simply little adults—there are some additional factors that must be considered and some procedural variations as well (see Bentler [2000] for review; see the American Academy of Audiology pediatric fitting protocol).

Prefitting Testing

For infants and young children it often is not possible to obtain precise pure-tone thresholds or loudness growth functions. However, in many cases, pure-tone thresholds for different frequency regions can be estimated from auditory electrophysiologic testing. Methods are available to estimate loudness discomfort levels for children based only on threshold data. Because precise threshold and loudness data often are not available, two factors are important: (1) The child should be reevaluated frequently so that changes in the fitting can be made as additional audiometric information becomes available, and (2) the child should be fitted with hearing aids that are highly adjustable so that alterations in the gain or output can be made easily.

Fitting Considerations

When fitting infants and children, it is important to use probe-microphone measures to assess the increased output of the hearing aid due to the smaller ear canal residual volume. This measure is termed the real ear coupler difference, or RECD.

As we have discussed previously, different types of assistive listening technology rely on bypassing the hearing aid's microphone, either through direct auditory input (DAI) or through the hearing aid's telecoil. For children who are developing speech and language, this becomes even more critical. This reason alone might dictate the hearing aid style that is selected; for example, the telecoil of an ITE might not provide enough gain and output. As with adults, binaural amplification should be the standard fitting whenever there are two aidable ears.

Prescriptive fitting approaches are available that are specifically designed for children. As mentioned earlier, the most commonly used today is the Desired Sensation Level (DSL) 4.1 method. In particular, this selection procedure takes into account the need to deliver extended high-frequency information to the child, to consider the small residual ear canal volume of the child, and to limit the output to "safe levels." Other methods, such as the NAL-NL1, also have been used successfully with the pediatric population.

Verification of Fitting

Older children can provide self-report information to help in fitting issues, but because the infant or young child cannot provide subjective reports of the hearing aid performance, parents can provide this (see Chapter 9). In addition, objective verification strategies are essential. The prescriptive fitting method can be verified easily using probe-microphone measurements. With even the somewhat uncooperative child, this testing can be reliably conducted with a little patience. On occasion, young children are sedated for the electrophysiology measures; some audiologists also conduct their probe-microphone measurements at this opportune moment.

Probe-microphone measurements will reveal the amount of gain that is present throughout the frequency range. Importantly, this testing will also determine the maximum output that is delivered in the child's ear canal. Because the child's ear canal is much smaller than an adult's, the real-ear output often is 10 to 15 dB higher than shown in the 2 cc coupler. A hearing aid gain/output that is too high can result in discomfort for the child, and possibly the child's obtaining a noise-induced hearing loss. As the child becomes older (e.g., 3 to 4 years of age), it is possible to conduct reliable loudness behavioral testing using specially designed charts (see Mueller & Bright, 1994). Just because a child says that sounds are not uncomfortably loud, however, does not guarantee that the hearing aid output is not damaging the ear—this is why objective ear-canal SPL measurements are essential.

Postfitting Procedures

Extensive parent counseling following the fitting is very important. The parents must know how to adjust and care for the hearing aid. Several practical accessories for children's hearing aids are available; a list of these accessories can be reviewed with the parents.

Follow-up visits for children need to be scheduled more frequently than for adults:

1. The hearing loss needs to be monitored to ensure that it is not progressive, to verify previous findings, and to obtain additional information for hearing aid adjustment.
2. The fit of the hearing aid or earmold in the ear must be monitored. Because of the rapid ear growth of children, an earmold might become loose in a few months, causing acoustic feedback. Periodic remakes or replacements of the earmold or custom shell are common.
3. The electroacoustic characteristics of the hearing aids should be monitored. Children's hearing aids are subject to many bumps and bruises; it is important to ensure that the hearing aid maintains its appropriate gain and frequency response and that excessive distortion is not present.
4. Parent counseling and training regarding hearing aid use and other aspects of their children's AR programs should be ongoing.

■ ASSISTIVE DEVICES

Although hearing aids are designed to assist individuals with hearing impairment in almost all listening environments, some patients, because of their age, degree of hearing loss, or other factors, may not derive significant benefit from hearing aids.

Thus, there is a need for other assistive devices (ADs). ADs used by individuals with deafness and impaired hearing to improve communication are called assistive listening devices (ALDs), while other ADs are used for alerting and signaling of environmental events. It is probably a bit optimistic and unrealistic to think that all facilities in the world or even the United States are readily equipped with ADs at this time, so those individuals with hearing impairments often carry their own individual ADs with them. However, U.S. legislation, specifically the Rehabilitation Act of 1973 and the Americans with Disabilities Act of 1990, has mandated that all facilities and programs receiving federal money can be accessed and used by all people with disabilities, including hearing impairments. Thus, ADs of some type should be available on request at many locations (i.e., schools, colleges, universities, hospitals, nursing homes, police and fire departments, libraries, museums, movie or theater facilities, parks). A request may be filed under the Freedom of Information Act to determine the facilities and programs that receive federal funds in your living community.

Assistive Listening Devices and Other Communication Devices

There are four main types of assistive listening devices (ALDs) for the hearing impaired. These types include hardwire, induction loop, infrared, and Frequency Modulation (FM) systems. ALDs may either be for personal use or for an entire group. It has been shown that even many normal hearing individuals can benefit from assistive listening devices (Crandell & Smaldino, 1996; Crandell et al., 1995).

HARDWIRE SYSTEMS. As the name implies, a hardwire system employs direct wiring from the microphone to the amplifier and receiver. A microphone is first placed near the desired speaker of interest. A wire then routes to a direct audio input (DAI) of a hearing aid or some type of receiver box attached to an earphone headset to deliver the sound to the listener. An example of a hardwire system without an earphone headset is shown in Figure 2.10. Most systems in this category are for personal use only.

BENEFITS

Inexpensive
Lightweight and portable

LIMITATIONS

Limited by length of wires between components
May have reduced sound quality in comparison to other ALDs

INDUCTION LOOP AMPLIFICATION (ILA) SYSTEM. This system involves wiring that is looped around the perimeter of a room typically near the ceiling or under the carpet. Again, a microphone is placed near the listener and the sound source is sent via either a wired connection or a FM signal to a receiver that converts the signal into electrical energy. The electric current is

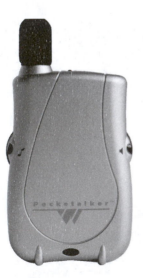

FIGURE 2.10

Pocket Talker™ system without earphones.
Courtesy of Williams Sound.

then carried around the room via the wire loop that surrounds the room. The electric current creates a magnetic field that can be detected by a hearing aid telecoil or other type of telecoil receiver. The induction loop system can be used by anyone in the room wearing a telecoil receiver unit. The induction loop system is demonstrated in Figure 2.11 below. The telecoil is then able to convert the magnetic field into an acoustic signal that is amplified for the person. The hearing aid telecoil is discussed later in more detail in the section on communication with the use of a telephone.

BENEFITS

- Does not require a hardwired connection to the listener
- Will work with existing telecoil in a listener's hearing aid
- Relatively inexpensive

LIMITATIONS

- Wire loop must be installed in the room
- Not a portable system
- Affected by orientation of hearing aid telecoil
- Increasing distance from wire loop will decrease signal strength
- Multiple induction loops installed within the same building are not always isolated from one another

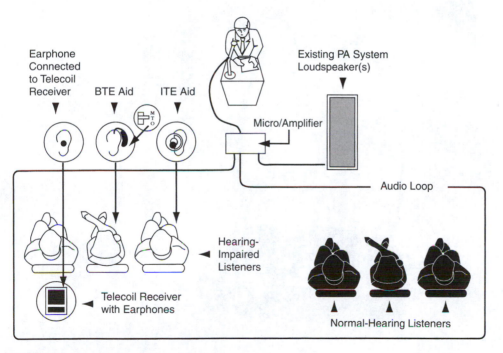

FIGURE 2.11

Room-sized induction loop system in which listeners with hearing impairment are using telecoil circuits to better understand the speaker.

Source: Reprinted with permission from Compton, C. (1991). *Assistive devices: Doorways to independence.* Annapolis, MD: Van Comp Associates.

INFRARED SYSTEMS. With an infrared system, a microphone is again placed near the speaker of interest. The microphone converts the acoustic signal into electrical energy, which is then converted into an infrared light by a transmitter. The infrared light must be directed in a clear line of sight toward an infrared light receiver. The receiver unit then converts the light signal back to an electrical signal, which may be amplified. The signal is once more converted, this time into an acoustic signal. These systems are most often used at theatrical or musical productions because the infrared light will not extend beyond the audience listening area. These productions can and have been pirated when induction loops or FM systems are used. Infrared systems are worn usually worn by a single person, but multiple infrared units may be installed in any given room or auditorium. An infrared unit is shown in Figure 2.12 below.

BENEFITS

- Inexpensive
- Wireless transmission
- Will not extend outside a designated listening area
- Can be used in adjacent rooms without interference

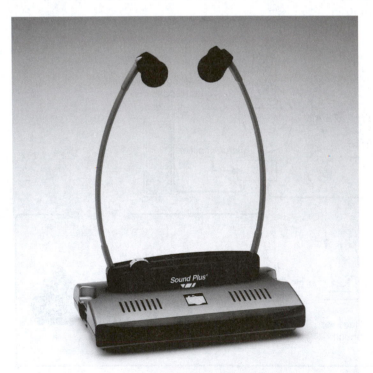

FIGURE 2.12

Infrared device.
Courtesy of Williams Sound.

LIMITATIONS

- Requires a direct line of sight
- Will not work outdoors in direct sunlight
- Person confined to a certain area for listening

FM SYSTEMS. Frequency Modulation (FM) systems operate under regulations imposed by the Federal Communications Commission (FCC). An FM system for individuals with hearing impairments can, in a sense, be thought of as a miniature radio station. Traditional radios found in most cars or homes have a tuner that receives FM signals between approximately 87.9 MHz and 107.9 MHz that have been broadcasted over relatively long distances (usually several miles). In contrast, FM systems for individuals with hearing impairments operate at different bandwidths that have been allocated specifically for the hearing impaired and can only broadcast short distances (several hundred feet). FM systems have traditionally operated between 72 and 75.9 MHz and have recently been allocated additional bandwidth from 216 to 217 MHz. However, much like a radio station, FM systems can transmit acoustic signals from the sender to the receiver with excellent fidelity.

The personal FM system receiver is either worn by or placed close to the listener. The speaker/talker wears a microphone and the transmitting unit. The FM signal is then transmitted to the receiving device. Two examples of individual use FM systems are illustrated in Figure 2.13. Methods of connecting the FM receiver to the listener are shown in Figure 2.14. Another example of a personal FM system receiver not shown in the figures is a "lunchbox"-size electronic speaker placed on the student's desk in a classroom setting. These speakers are usually covered with a colorful, well-designed fabric in order to appeal to a young child.

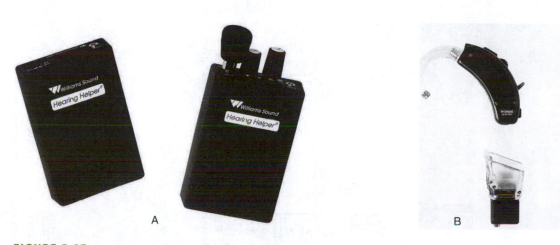

A   B

FIGURE 2.13

Two examples of FM: (A) Personal FM transmitter and receiver (Courtesy of Williams Sound).
(B) BTE hearing aid with FM receiver boot (Courtesy of Williams Sound).

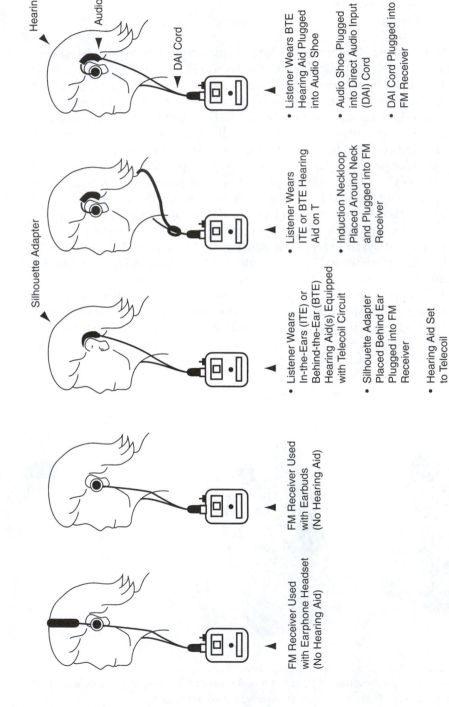

FM Receiver Used with Earphone Headset (No Hearing Aid)

FM Receiver Used with Earbuds (No Hearing Aid)

- Listener Wears In-the-Ears (ITE) or Behind-the-Ear (BTE) Hearing Aid(s) Equipped with Telecoil Circuit

- Silhouette Adapter Placed Behind Ear Plugged into FM Receiver

- Hearing Aid Set to Telecoil

- Listener Wears ITE or BTE Hearing Aid on T

- Induction Neckloop Placed Around Neck and Plugged into FM Receiver

- Listener Wears BTE Hearing Aid Plugged into Audio Shoe

- Audio Shoe Plugged into Direct Audio Input (DAI) Cord

- DAI Cord Plugged into FM Receiver

FIGURE 2.14

Methods of sound pickup from an FM receiver.

Source: Reprinted with permission from Compton, C. (1991). *Assistive devices: Doorways to independence.* Annapolis, MD: Van Comp Associates.

BENEFITS

- Portable
- Wireless transmission
- Easy to operate
- Can be used indoors and outdoors
- Can be used simultaneously in adjacent rooms
- Electromagnetic interference is not a problem
- Does not require that receiver be in direct line of sight with receiver
- Great sound quality

LIMITATIONS

- Radio interference possible

Soundfield FM systems, for group use, utilize multiple electronic speakers placed strategically throughout the room to provide all listeners with a better signal-to-noise ratio. These speakers in effect place the all listeners closer to the speaker/talker of interest. One major disadvantage of a soundfield FM system is the lack of portability in comparison to a personal FM system. However, a soundfield FM system can greatly improve the speech understanding performance of even normal-hearing individuals in the audience group.

TELEVISION. As evidenced by the category name, this device aims to increase an individual's ability to understand television audio. This type of device is connected to the audio output on the television. It may use a direct wired connection, induction loop, or FM system to transfer audio to the listener, but more commonly, an infrared light connection from the transmitter placed near the television to the receiver is used. Figure 2.15 shows different ways an infrared device can be integrated with receiver units worn by the listener. In addition to improving understanding of the television with this device, other individuals with normal hearing who watch television alongside the individual with hearing impairment can now listen to the television at more normal levels. Another common infrared device for use with the television is shown in Figure 2.12.

Closed captioning is another option for those individuals with hearing impairments. Closed captioning displays typed subtitles on the screen delayed a bit from the audio signal, but the individual can comprehend the program by simply reading the subtitles. It is now required that all televisions 13 inches or greater in size have closed-captioning capability as mandated by the Television Decoder Circuitry Act of 1990, which took effect July 1, 1993.

TELEPHONE AND CELL PHONE. Assistive listening devices are vital for individuals with hearing impairment to communicate by means of a phone. As phone conversations are only auditory-only, it requires a much better signal-to-noise ratio for equivalent understanding of the same conversation in a face-to-face conversation, which includes many visual cues. These devices may range from a separate amplifier that is connected between the telephone and the headset or an entire telephone with internal volume adjustments designed for the hearing impaired as shown

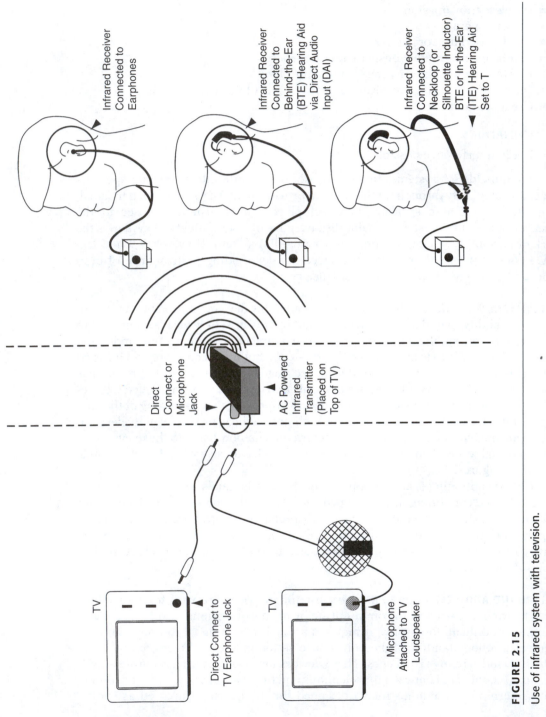

FIGURE 2.15

Use of infrared system with television.

Source: Reprinted with permission from Compton, C. (1991). *Assistive devices: Doorways to Independence.* Annapolis, MD: Van Comp Associates.

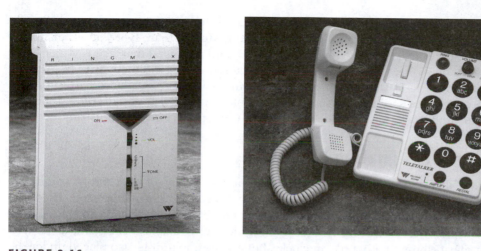

FIGURE 2.16

Assistive devices for use of the telephone.
Courtesy of Williams Sound.

respectively in Figure 2.16A and B. In addition, these phones may utilize flashing lights to signal that the phone is ringing and needs to be answered.

The most common device used to integrate a telephone with a hearing aid is the telecoil, often shortened to *t-coil*. The t-coil is a small coil of wire that creates voltage when an alternating magnetic field flows through it (Dillon, 2001). All LAN phones produce a small magnetic field around them when in use. A magnetic field is produced by electrical current that has the same wavelength as the audio signal. Therefore, when the telephone is placed near the ear, hearing aids with an "auto t-coil" will switch to the t-coil mode automatically when a magnetic field of sufficient strength is detected. The voltage created by the t-coil is then processed by the hearing aid and presented to the hearing aid user as an acoustic signal with proper frequency and output shaping for the person's hearing loss. Many hearing aids will not switch to t-coil mode automatically and still require the wearer to manually change the hearing aid program by activating a program selector control prior to using the telephone. The use of a t-coil eliminates problems of acoustic feedback when trying to use a telephone.

Cell phones also utilize volume adjustments and, of course, ear buds that allow for the audio output to be routed directly into the ear canal. Cell phones may also utilize the hearing aid t-coil feature. A recent change in the Hearing Aid Compatibility Act (HAC Act) requires that all manufacturers of cell phones increase the percentage of their products that are compatible with existing hearing aid t-coil technology. If a cell phone is not hearing aid compatible from the manufacturer, the cell phone can still be used with an additional induction neck loop. The neck loop is placed around the neck and connects to the audio output of the cell phone. The neck loop then converts the signal into a magnetic field that is picked up by the t-coil in the hearing aid.

For those individuals with more severe-to-profound hearing loss who are still unable to communicate with an amplified telephone or telecoil, a teletype device may be used. This device is referred to as a text telephone (TT) or a telephone device

Automatic t-coils are now available in hearing aid styles as small as the ITC.

for the deaf (TDD). TDDs are computerized systems that allow the user to directly call another person having similar equipment. Messages are typed and transmitted to the other individual's telephone and TDD, and the typed message is visually displayed on a screen. Calls from a TDD user can be placed indirectly with individuals not having a TDD through a relay system (www.fcc.gov/cgb/dro/trs.html). The process of transcribing the spoken words into text and vice versa is often called *relaying* and is a service provided by the U.S. General Services Administration.

Alerting/Signaling Devices

These devices signal the hearing impaired or deaf person of happenings around his or her environment that would be heard by those with normal hearing. These devices either vibrate, flash lights, or further amplify sound. The alarm clock is one example of the vibrating type of alerting device. It displays time and is set in a similar fashion to other alarm clocks, but a vibrating unit is also placed under the pillow inside the pillow case as to shake the person awake at the appropriate time. Flashing light units may be connected to lamps, smaller LED lights, or other lights in the home to signify the ringing of a doorbell, telephone, or even a baby crying.

Bluetooth technology (a short-range wireless communication system) is revolutionizing the way the public responds to hearing aids and telephones.

Last, an example of an alerting device that further amplifies sound is a fire/smoke alarm detector. These fire/smoke alarms may also include a strobe light. Interestingly, most of these fire/smoke alarm devices only output an "audible" 90 dB tone centered around 3100 Hz at a distance of 10 feet from the alarm (Ross & Mulvaney, 2005). This is precisely the frequency region where most hearing-impaired listeners have hearing loss, and those with deafness will have thresholds worse than 90 dB in the 3000 Hz region. So, it is certainly debatable whether the tone will be audible, and it certainly may not be loud enough to wake someone from a sleeping state. Therefore, Hearing Loss Association of America (SHHH) has recommended that the output of audible alarms be concentrated in the low frequencies (sweeping between 200 and 600 Hz) at an intensity level between 85 dB minimum and 120 dB maximum, exceeding prevailing sound level in the room by at least 15 dB (Ross & Mulvaney, 2005).

In addition, more recent devices have incorporated radio transmission in alerting devices that will directly send a message to a pager-like unit that will vibrate and display a message describing the currently transpiring event. Numerous alerting devices and variants of the abovementioned assistive devices may be found by searching the Internet and by contacting alerting device manufacturing companies, as well as organizations for persons with hearing impairment.

CONCLUDING REMARKS

Hopefully, after reading about the above amplification options that are available to those individuals with hearing impairments, it is apparent that there is not a shortage of choices in amplification devices. In fact, due to advancements in electronics and computer technology, most of these amplification devices are capable of reproducing amplified sounds and speech for individuals with hearing impairments with considerably higher fidelity and output levels than ever before. However, according to the MarkeTrak VI survey (Kochkin, 2001), only 22 percent of those individuals with a hearing loss that could receive benefit from amplification devices actually seek out and receive professional services. Thus, audiologists have the formidable task of informing the general population about amplification products and services and dispelling many of the misconceptions regarding amplification that currently exist today.

SUMMARY POINTS

- The basic components of a hearing aid are the microphone, the amplifier, the receiver, and the battery. Behind-the-ear (BTE) instruments also require an earmold to channel the sound into the ear canal.
- The majority of today's hearing aids are programmable, meaning that the method in which the hearing aid processes sound can be adjusted and tailored for the patient using computer software.
- Hearing aid circuits can be either analog or digital. Digital processing, introduced in 1995, is rapidly becoming the standard. Two key components, the microphone and the receiver, however, are the same for both digital and analog technology.
- Hearing aid compression can be input controlled (before the amplifier) or output controlled (after the amplifier). Most modern hearing aids have both input and output compression onboard the digital chip.
- Hearing aid compression can be used to prevent loud sounds from being too loud and uncomfortable (usually accomplished with output compression), or can be used to "repackage" the wide intensity range of speech into the patient's reduced dynamic range (accomplished using input compression).
- A popular category of compression is termed wide-dynamic range compression (WDRC). It is available in all the current digital products and is especially useful for providing audibility of soft speech.
- Common hearing aid styles include the behind-the-ear (BTE), in-the-ear (ITE), in-the-canal (ITC), and completely-in-canal (CIC). Essentially the same technology can be obtained in each. Of the four styles, the ITC and CIC are appealing to many, primarily because of cosmetic advantages. However, the ITE is the most frequently used at the present time.
- BTE hearing aids require coupling to an earmold. Earmolds can be modified through venting (low frequencies), the use of damping (mid-frequencies) or through the use of horn tubing (high frequencies).
- Hearing aids are assessed, both at the manufacturer and in the clinic, using 2 cc coupler measures. These results are used to determine if the hearing aid meets a set of preestablished specifications. These results *do not* assure that the hearing aid is appropriate for a given patient.
- Whenever possible, it is recommended that individuals with hearing loss in both ears be fitted with binaural amplification. Some of the advantages include increased gain, improved localization, better sound quality, and improved speech understanding in noise.

- Verification of the hearing aid fitting can include the following: informal patient judgments of quality and intelligibility, measures of speech understanding, loudness scaling, probe-microphone measurements, and self-report measures (daily use time and satisfaction/benefit). When prescriptive fitting procedures are used, probe-microphone measures are the preferred method for determining if desired gain and output values have been achieved.
- After the fitting, it's important to remember HIO BASICS: Hearing expectations, Instrument operation, Occlusion effect, Batteries, Acoustic feedback, System troubleshooting, Cleaning and maintenance, and Service, warranty, and repairs.
- When fitting hearing aids to infants and children, it's important to remember that because of their small ear canals, the output of the hearing aid will be greater than with adults. Probe-microphone measures can be used to determine this difference value.
- In addition to hearing aids, many individuals can benefit from assistive devices, which can be used for special listening situations (e.g., an amplifier for the telephone, an FM or infrared device for listening to the TV), or other applications (e.g., alarms and other alerting devices).

RECOMMENDED READING

Bentler, R. A. (2000). Amplification for the hearing-impaired child. In J. G. Alpiner & P. A. McCarthy (Eds.), *Rehabilitative Audiology* (pp. 106–139). New York: Lippincott Williams & Wilkins.

Chasin, M. (1997). Current trends in implantable hearing aids. *Trends in Amplification, 2*(3), 84–107.

Dillon, H. (2001). *Hearing aids.* Sydney: Boomerang Press.

Mueller, H. G., & Hall, J. W. (1998). *Audiologists' desk reference, Volume II.* San Diego: Singular Publishing Group.

Mueller, H. G., Hawkins, D. B., & Northern, J. L. (1992). *Probe microphone measurements.* San Diego: Singular Publishing Group.

Palmer, C. V., & Mueller, H. G. (2000). Hearing aid selection and assessment. In J. G. Alpiner & P. A. McCarthy (Eds.), *Rehabilitative audiology* (pp. 332–376). New York: Lippincott Williams & Wilkins.

Ross, M. (1994). *Communication access for persons with hearing loss.* Baltimore: York Press.

Tyler, R. S., & Schum, D. J. (1995). *Assistive devices for persons with hearing impairment.* Boston: Allyn & Bacon.

Valente, M., Hosford-Dunn, H., & Roeser, R. (Eds.). (2000). *Audiology: Treatment.* New York: Thieme.

RECOMMENDED WEBSITES

www.entific.com
www.symphonix.com

www.medel.com

www.otologics.com

www.utdallas.edu/loizou/cimplants.cdemos.htm

www.ausp.memphis.edu/harl

www.ihr.gla.as.uk

www.isu.edu/csed/rehab

www.NAL.gov.AU

www.DSL@nca.uwo.ca

www.phonicear.com

www.tvears.com

www.williamsound.com

www.shhh.org

www.harcmercantile.com

REFERENCES

American National Standards Institute (ANSI). (1996). *ANSI S3.22-1996-Specification of hearing aid characteristics*. Melville, NY: Acoustical Society of America.

Bentler, R. A. (2000). Amplification for the hearing-impaired child. In J. G. Alpiner & P. A. McCarthy (Eds.), *Rehabilitative audiology* (pp. 106–139). New York: Lippincott Williams & Wilkins.

Chasin, M. (2002). Bone anchored and middle ear implant hearing aids. *Trends in Amplification, 6*(2), 33–38.

Compton, C. L. (1991). *Assistive devices: Doorways to independence*. Washington, DC: Assistive Device Center, Gallaudet University.

Cox, R. M. (1995). Using loudness data for hearing aid selection: The IHAFF approach. *The Hearing Journal, 48*(2), 10, 39–44.

Crandell, C., & Smaldino, J. (1996). Soundfield amplification in the classroom: Applied and theoretical issues. In F. Bess, J. Gravel, & A. Tharpe (Eds.), *Amplification for children with auditory deficits* (pp. 229–250). Nashville: Bill Wilkerson Center Press.

Crandell, C., Smaldino, J., & Flexer, C. (1995). *Soundfield FM amplification: Theory and practical applications*. San Diego, CA: Singular Publishing Group.

Dillon, H. (2001). *Hearing aids*. Sydney: Boomerang Press.

Kochkin, S. (2001). The VA and direct mail sparks growth in hearing aid market. *Hearing Review, 8*(12), 16–24, 63–65.

Kochkin, S. (2002). Consumers rate improvements sought in hearing instruments. *Hearing Review, 9*(11), 18–22.

Kochkin, S. (2003). Isolating the impact of the volume control on patient satisfaction. *Hearing Review, 10*(1), 26–35.

Mueller, H. G. (2000). What's the digital difference when it comes to patient benefit? *The Hearing Journal, 53*(3), 23–32.

Mueller, H. G., & Bright, K. E. (1994). Selection and verification of maximum output. In M. Valente (Ed.), *Strategies for selecting and verifying hearing aid fittings* (pp. 38–63). New York: Thieme.

Mueller H. G., & Hall, J. W. (1998). *Audiologists' desk reference, Volume II.* San Diego, CA: Singular Publishing Group.

Mueller, H. G., & Hornsby, B. (2002). Selection, verification and validation of maximum output. In M. Valente (Ed.), *Strategies for selecting and verifying hearing aid fittings* (2nd ed.). New York: Thieme.

Mueller, H. G., & Killion, M. C. (1990). An easy method for calculating the articulation index. *The Hearing Journal, 43*(9), 14–17.

Mueller, H. G., & Ricketts, T. A. (2000). Update on directional microphone hearing aids. *The Hearing Journal, 53*(5), 10–17.

Mueller H. G., & Ricketts, T. A. (2005). Digital noise reduction: Much ado about something? *The Hearing Journal, 58*(1), 10–17.

Niparko, J., Cox, K., & Lustig, L. (2003). Comparison of the Bone Anchored Hearing Aid Implantable Hearing Device with Contralateral Routing of Offside Signal Amplification in the rehabilitation of unilateral deafness. *Otology & Neurotology, 24*(1), 73–78.

Olsen, W. (1986). Physical characteristics of hearing aids. In W. Hodgson (Ed.), *Hearing Aid Assessment and Use in Audiologic Habilitation* (3rd ed.). Baltimore: Williams & Wilkins.

Ross, M. (1994). *Communication access for persons with hearing loss.* Baltimore: York Press.

Ross, M., & Mulvany, D. (2005). *Smoke alarms: What consumers should know.* Pennsylvania Self Help for Hard of Hearing People. Accessed June 15, 2005, from http://www.pa-shhh.org/ross/ross61.html.

Schow, R. L. (2001). A standardized AR battery for dispensers is proposed. *The Hearing Journal, 54*(8): 10–20.

Stabb, W., & Lybarger, S. (1994). Characteristics and use of hearing aids. In J. Katz (Ed.), *Handbook of Clinical Audiology* (4th ed.). Baltimore: Williams & Wilkins.

Wazen, J. J., Spitzer, J. B., Ghossaini, S. N., Fayad, J. N., Niparko, J. K., Cox, K. M., Brackmann, D. E., & Soli, D.S. (2003). Transcranial contralateral stimulation in unilateral deafness. *Otolaryngology—Head and Neck Surgery, 124*(3), 248–254.

Cochlear Implants and Vestibular/Tinnitus Rehabilitation

Alice E. Holmes
Gary P. Rodriguez

CONTENTS

INTRODUCTION

New breakthroughs in audiology now allow us to assist persons in ways never thought of thirty years ago. Persons with profound sensorineural loss now have the potential to receive sound information through the use of cochlear implants. Treatment plans are now available for dizzy patients and tinnitus sufferers. This chapter will provide an overview of these new advances in audiology.

Most persons who are diagnosed with a sensorineural hearing loss are fit with hearing aids and can receive varying amounts of benefit from these devices.

Unfortunately, for some individuals with severe-to-profound hearing loss, these traditional amplification devices may offer only limited or no help, even with extensive experience and audiologic rehabilitation. Even the most powerful amplifiers are unable to provide meaningful information for environmental sound awareness or speech perception for persons with little or no residual hearing. Cochlear implant technology has offered many of these individuals an alternative means to receive some important information from their impaired auditory systems.

Cochlear implant: Device that electrically stimulates the auditory nerve of patients with severe-to-profound hearing loss to provide them with sound and speech information.

A cochlear implant is a device that electrically stimulates the auditory nerve of patients with severe-to-profound hearing loss to provide them with sound and speech information. It is not an amplifier that increases the level of the acoustic signal, but a surgically implanted device that bypasses the peripheral auditory system to directly simulate the auditory nerve. The cochlear implant does not restore normal hearing. Cochlear implant recipients vary in the amount of benefit that they receive from the device. Some individuals are provided with auditory awareness, detection of environmental sounds, and improvement in their speechreading abilities while other patients are able to achieve open set speech perception without visual cues. Many individuals are able to conduct conversations over the telephone.

■ COCHLEAR IMPLANTS

How Does a Cochlear Implant Work?

Open set speech perception tests: Listener has an unlimited number of response possibilities.

A number of cochlear implant systems are available worldwide. Each has its own unique characteristics, advantages, and disadvantages, but all operate using the same basic principles. All cochlear implant systems commonly in use consist of an externally worn headset connected to a speech processor, with a battery source and a surgically implanted internal receiver stimulator attached to the electrode array that is placed in the cochlea.

Figure 3.1 shows one of the commercially available cochlear implant systems with an ear-level speech processor. The behind-the-ear device (1) consists of a microphone, speech processor, and transmitter coil. The transmitter coil has a magnet that adheres to the head over the skin where the receiver stimulator is placed. The microphone picks up the sound wave, converts it into an electrical signal, and sends it to the speech processor. The speech processor codes the information using a device-specific strategy and sends it to the external transmitter coil. The coil sends the information through the skin via FM radio waves to an internal receiver (2), which in turn sends the information to the implanted electrodes (3) that stimulate the available auditory nerve fibers (4). The auditory nerve then sends the information to the brain so that the person can perceive sound stimulation. This all occurs in a matter of microseconds.

Closed set speech perception tests: Listener is given a choice of multiple responses.

History of Cochlear Implants

In 1972, the first wearable cochlear implant was implanted in an adult at the House Ear Institute. The House/3M device consisted of a single electrode implanted in the basal end of the cochlea with a ground electrode placed in the eustachian tube. This

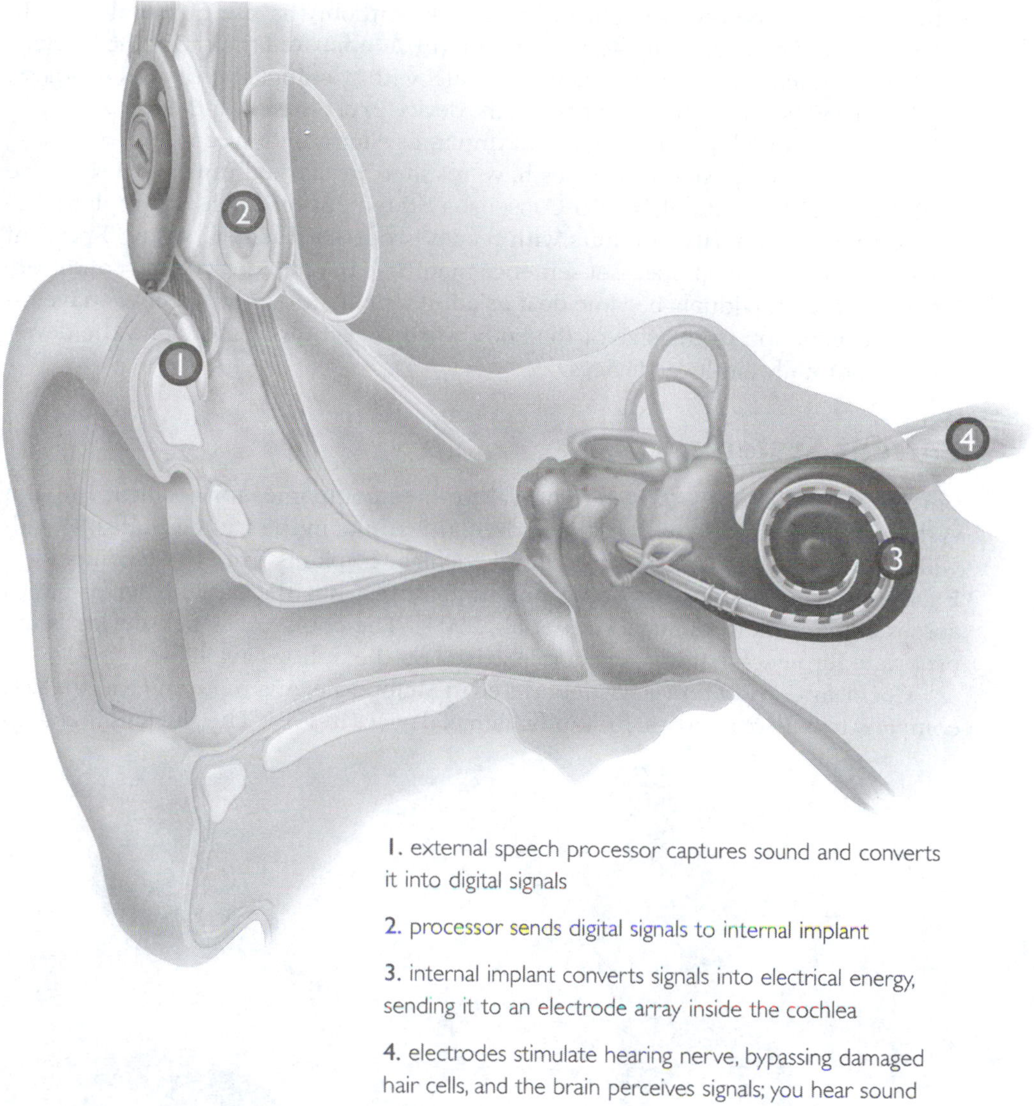

1. external speech processor captures sound and converts it into digital signals

2. processor sends digital signals to internal implant

3. internal implant converts signals into electrical energy, sending it to an electrode array inside the cochlea

4. electrodes stimulate hearing nerve, bypassing damaged hair cells, and the brain perceives signals; you hear sound

FIGURE 3.1

Components of a cochlear implant system and how it works.
Courtesy of Cochlear Ltd.

device was capable of providing the patient with information on the presence or absence of sound, durational cues, and intensity cues. Even with this limited information, many individuals had improved speechreading abilities and were able to learn to identify many environmental sounds with training. Over 1,000 persons received this commercially available device. In 1980 the device became available for use in children over the age of 2 years (Wilson, 2000).

Multielectrode devices came into wide use in the 1980s. With these systems, limited frequency cues became available to the patients, and many patients were achieving some open-set speech understanding without the use of visual cues. In 1985, the U.S. Food and Drug Administration (FDA) approved the use of the Nucleus 22-Channel Cochlear Implant System for adults with postlingual profound deafness. In 1990, the FDA also approved the use of the device in children over the age of 2 years.

Continued development of cochlear implant systems and the speech processing strategies over the past two decades have resulted in marked improvements. The 1995 National Institute of Health Consensus Statement on Cochlear Implants reported that the majority of adults with recent processors achieve over 80 percent correct on high-context open-set sentence materials in an auditory-only condition. Most of these individuals became deaf as adults. Cosmetic improvements have included a reduction in the size of the body-worn speech processors and the development of totally ear-level devices.

Current Systems

Currently, the FDA has granted approval to three companies for cochlear implant systems for general use with both children and adults in the United States. World-wide over 100,000 persons have received cochlear implants from these companies. Each of the companies has some unique features, but the patient performance across companies is similar (Firzt et al., 2004). The choice of which device is appropriate for which patient is generally based on the options available.

Cochlear Corporation is headquartered in Melbourne, Australia, and was the first company to receive approval for multichannel devices in 1985. The Nucleus Freedom

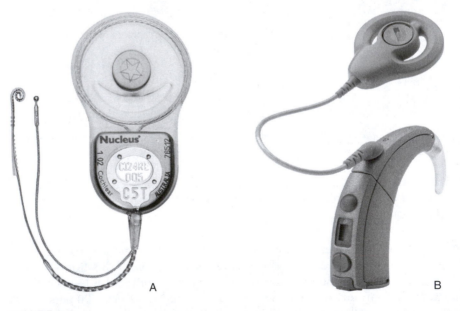

A   B

FIGURE 3.2

Nucleus New Freedom cochlear implant system: (A) cochlear implant, (B) speech processor and coil.

Photos courtesy of Cochlear Corporation, Englewood, CO.

System (Figure 3.2) was launched from Cochlear Corporation in April 2005. It has the option of four programs using various processing and noise reduction strategies. The external device is the first "splash- and sweatproof" digital speech processor.

The HiResolution™ Bionic Ear System from Advanced Bionics (Figure 3.3) was developed in and is manufactured in the United States. It has the fastest processing speed and has a rechargeable battery for the ear-level device.

The third device approved for use in the United States was developed and is manufactured by Med El Corporation in Austria. The implant for its most recent

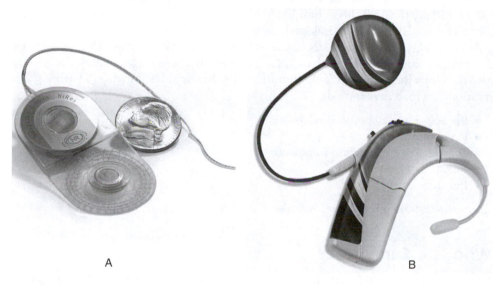

A   B

FIGURE 3.3

Advanced Bionics HiResolution cochlear implant system: (A) cochlear implant (B) speech processor and coil.

Photos courtesy of Advanced Bionics, Sylmar, CA.

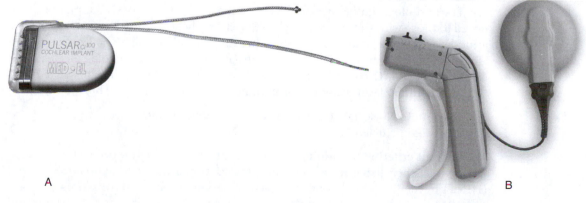

A   B

FIGURE 3.4

MED-EL Pulsar cochlear implant system: (A) cochlear implant (B) speech processor and coil.

Photos courtesy of MED-EL Corporation, Durham, NC.

system, the Pulsar (Figure 3.4), is in a ceramic case that allows for low-level Magnetic Resonating Imaging (MRI). The other companies require surgical removal of the internal magnet prior to an MRI. For persons who know they may need multiple MRIs, this is often the implant of choice.

The Cochlear Implant Team

A multidisciplinary team is necessary for a successful cochlear implant program. These team members should be involved in the entire process from the evaluation for candidacy through the re/habilitation process. The team must include both an otolaryngologist and an audiologist, who serve as the team leaders. The otolaryngologist makes the medical decisions and performs the surgery. The audiologist determines audiologic candidacy and programs the speech processor. He or she also develops the audiologic rehabilitation plan in conjunction with the other team members, which may include

- Speech–language pathologists
- Psychologists
- Teachers of the hearing impaired
- Social workers
- Parents

Communication among team members is vital to success of the cochlear implant.

Who Is a Candidate?

Not everyone is a candidate for a cochlear implant. Candidacy evaluations generally consist of a number of evaluations with several team members. With the improved outcomes, the criteria for implantation have vastly expanded since the 1980s when only adults with profound postlingual hearing impairments were eligible. Currently, the FDA has approved the use of cochlear implants in persons over the age of 12 months.

The audiologic guidelines are based on the performance of CI recipients as opposed to those with similar hearing losses wearing hearing aids. Patients must have a moderate-to-profound sensorineural hearing loss bilaterally. The Committee on Hearing and Equilibrium of the American Academy of Otolaryngology—Head and Neck Surgery (AAO-HNS; Luxford, 2001) recommends testing in quiet at a 70 dB SPL presentation level using the Minimum Speech Test Battery. This includes

- Hearing In Noise Test (HINT): Two 10-sentence lists in quiet
- Consonant-Nucleus-Consonant Test (CNC): One 50-word list

The current criterion for adults is ≤50 percent speech recognition in the ear to be implanted when listening at normal conversational levels to sentence material (HINT) in the best-aided conditions. The opposite ear must have scores ≤60 percent. Medicare has stricter guidelines for payment requiring speech recognition scores of 40 percent or less. Currently, there are clinical trials on elders using more lenient criteria. These criteria with technology are changing rapidly, and it is im-

TABLE 3.1

Candidacy Guidelines

	AGE GROUP		
	ADULTS (≥18 YEARS OF AGE)	YOUNG CHILDREN (12 MONTHS TO 3 YEARS)	OLDER CHILDREN (3 TO 18 YEARS)
Hearing Loss	Moderate-to-profound in the low frequencies; severe-to-profound in the mid to high frequencies (≥70 dB HL)	Profound (≥90 dB HL)	Severe-to-profound in the low frequencies (>70 dB HL); profound in the mid to high frequencies (≥90 dB HL)
Aided Speech Recognition @ 70 dB HL	≤50 percent aided speech recognition on recorded sentence material in the ear to be implanted ≤60 percent aided speech recognition on recorded sentence material in the unimplanted ear	Lack of development in simple auditory skills over a three- to six-month period	≤30 percent best-aided word score
Communication/ Education	Desire to be a part of the hearing world	Therapy program that emphasizes the development of auditory skills	Educational/therapy program that emphasizes the development of auditory skills
Medical	No medical contraindications	No medical contraindications	No medical contraindications
Other	Highly motivated parents Patient has appropriate expectations	Highly motivated patient Parents have appropriate expectations	Highly motivated parents and child Parents and child have appropriate expectations

portant for professionals to remain current. As systems and performance with the devices improve, the criteria are expanded.

For children, the audiologic criteria include a bilateral severe-to-profound sensorineural hearing loss with limited benefit from traditional amplification. For a young child, this is often difficult to determine and is defined as little to no progress in auditory development with appropriate amplification and audiologic habilitation. In older children, the criterion is ≤30 percent word recognition at normal conversational levels in the best-aided condition.

Formal evaluations should include standard audiometric unaided test batteries, otoacoustic emissions, aided speech perception testing, and aided speechreading evaluations. Speech and language evaluations should be completed on all children and all adults with prelingual hearing loss. Otologic–medical evaluations are done

CT scan: Computerized tomography scans of the temporal bone provide information on the surgical anatomy of the cochlea.

by the physician. CT scans or MRIs are necessary to determine if the device can be implanted.

In addition to the audiometric guidelines for sensorineural hearing loss listed above, several other criteria are required prior to a person's receiving a cochlear implant. There should be no medical contraindications, such as the absence of the VIII nerve. The person must be free of active middle ear infections and be able to undergo surgery and anesthesia.

Patients and their families also should be counseled on the costs of cochlear implantation, and insurance reimbursement information needs to be provided. The cost of the cochlear implant system, surgery, and rehabilitative program ranges from $60,000 to $80,000. Most major insurance carriers (e.g., Blue Cross/Blue Shield), Medicare, and, in some states, Medicaid cover the procedure. Vocational rehabilitation services in some states also will pay for the cochlear implant. Several studies on the cost–utility of the procedures have shown the cochlear implant to be a cost-effective procedure that often results in less expensive educational training for the recipient and more employability.

CANDIDACY FOR ADULTS. Adults must have had at least a three- to six-month trial period with appropriate amplification and show limited benefit from the hearing aids as defined by less than 50 percent auditory-only speech recognition performance with open-set sentences. Individuals must have a strong support system and be motivated to undergo the rehabilitative process of speech processor programming and audiologic rehabilitation. They must have realistic expectations. Honest counseling about the range of benefits that people receive is necessary. The limitations of the device need to be covered. Potential candidates need to be told that not everyone is able to use the telephone even after training. Some individuals may only receive enhancement of their speechreading abilities and awareness of environmental sounds. It is helpful to have them contact other patients who have the cochlear implant. Caution should be taken not to have them talk only to the highest functioning users, as this often leads to unrealistic expectations. The team leaders may make the appropriate referrals for further evaluations to other team members such as the psychologist if it is suspected that there may be problems with the patient's or family members' expectations.

Individuals must also want to be part of the hearing world. Adults with prelingual hearing loss have poorer prognoses for success with a cochlear implant. Although speechreading abilities may be improved in these individuals, very few have achieved any open-set speech perception without visual cues. This is particularly true in those individuals who lack oral communication skills. Referrals for psychological and speech–language pathology consultations are often necessary in this population.

CANDIDACY FOR CHILDREN. Candidacy for children is sometimes very difficult to determine and should be done by the entire team of professionals mentioned above. Children must have at least a six-month trial period with appropriate and consistent binaural hearing aid use and must be receiving auditory training during that period (see Chapter 4). Hearing loss from some etiologies, such as meningitis, can

> ### Case 3.1. SK
>
> SK was an 89-year-old who had had a bilateral profound hearing loss for approximately two years. He relied on his wife for all communications. He was implanted in our facility and received good benefit from his cochlear implant as measured by a 92 percent score on the HINT in quiet. At the time of his initial evaluation, his wife had been diagnosed with Alzheimer's disease. About one year after he received his implant, his wife's condition had declined enough that their roles were reversed, and he became her caregiver. Due in part to the benefits derived from the implant, both were able to remain in their home together and neither had to be institutionalized. There is no upper age limit for cochlear implantation. As long as the person meets all other criteria, he or she is a candidate. The issue is quality of life, not longevity.

cause ossification of the cochlea soon after onset. In these cases, the hearing trial may be decreased to two or three months. Limited benefit from amplification in young children is defined as lack of development in simple auditory skills over a three- to six-month period. In older children, when speech perception tests can be completed, limited benefit is defined as scores of less than 30 percent with open-set material.

The earliest recommended age for implantation is 12 months. The prognosis for development of speech and language is better with early intervention and implantation (Robbins et al., 2004). In some cases of definitive diagnosis of profound hearing loss, the surgery can be done earlier (Colletti et al., 2005). The key issue is appropriate diagnosis. It is very difficult to accurately predict an audiogram and amplification potential benefit from objective measures, such as auditory brainstem response (ABR) testing, or from behavioral testing. Implanting a very young child should only be considered after a comprehensive audiological evaluation by a skilled pediatric audiologist.

Motivation and expectations of the family must be assessed, and they must be counseled to have appropriate expectations. Both the psychologist and the social worker on the team are helpful in assessing the family situation and assisting with compliance after the child receives the implant. Many families hope that the cochlear implant will correct the child's hearing. They must be told that the implant is not a cure and will not give the child normal hearing. As with adult recipients, these children's parents should be given the opportunity to talk with other families who have gone through the process with their child. They need to understand that intensive therapy will be a very important part of the child's audiologic and communication development. It is important to have all members of the team, including the teacher of the hearing impaired and the speech–language pathologist, active in the process. They can provide much of the support needed in training the child and family members.

The communication mode that the child uses does not determine candidacy, but the child's educational program must emphasize the development of auditory skills. Children trained in an auditory–verbal or auditory–visual mode of communication do progress more rapidly with their implants. Children placed in total communication programs do receive benefit from the implant if audition and speech are also encouraged along with signing (Meyer, Svirsky, Kirk, & Miyamoto, 1998).

Teenagers pose an additional challenge when determining candidacy. Well-meaning relatives and friends who want the child to be part of the hearing world make the referrals. If the teen has some oral speech and language skills and wants the implant for him- or herself, then he or she may be a candidate. However, many of the teenagers themselves have no desire or motivation to get a cochlear implant. In addition, the plasticity of the auditory system appears to decline rapidly after about 6 years of age. Therefore, congenitally deafened teens have poorer prognoses for success with an implant, much like that of prelingual adults. They also may have made the choice to enter the Deaf community and have no interest in hearing.

The Nottingham Children's Implant Profile (NChIP; Nikolopoulos, Archbold, & Gregory, 2005) is a good tool for summarizing the evaluation process for children. Ten items are scored by the implant team as "no concern (0), mild-to-moderate concern (1), or great concern (2)." Items cover the children's demographic details (chronological age and duration of deafness), medical and radiological conditions, the outcomes of audiological assessments, language and speech abilities, multiple handicaps or disabilities, family structure and support, educational environment, the availability of support services, expectations of the family and deaf child, cognitive abilities, and learning style. Patients with a high NChIP score are not deemed appropriate candidates for a cochlear implant.

Deaf Culture and Cochlear Implants

The Deaf community defines Deafness with a capital "D" as a culture rather than a disability. It is characterized by having its own language, American Sign Language (ASL). Some individuals within the Deaf community have expressed strong opinions against the use of cochlear implants, especially in children. They resent anyone who is trying to "fix a Deaf child." They have likened cochlear implants to foot binding in ancient China by trying to shape the child into actively using hearing. Many of their feelings stem from years of professionals forcing oral programming for all children with hearing loss and their own frustrations with traditional hearing aids.

Over the past fifteen years, the National Association of the Deaf (NAD) has softened its criticisms of cochlear implants. In 1990 the organization came out in strong opposition to the FDA approval of cochlear implants in children, stating that the research being conducted on children had no regard for the child's quality of life as a deaf adult. In their 2000 Position Statement on Cochlear Implants, the NAD recognized the technology of cochlear implants as a tool for use with some forms of communication. They asserted that the parents have the right to choose the cochlear implant but emphasized that parents must be given all the options, including the option of sign language and the choice to be part of the Deaf world instead of the hearing world. They continue to assert that young prelingually deafened children do not have the auditory foundation to learn spoken language easily, and therefore cochlear implants in these children may have less than favorable results. This is in direct conflict with data by Miyamoto et al. (1993) and Waltzman and Cohen (1998) that demonstrated that children implanted at a young age received significant speech perception benefits.

Implant teams must make parents aware of the Deaf Culture issues. The parents do need to make informed decisions with knowledge of all options. Implant teams should be cognizant of the Deaf Culture issues and be prepared to address them when counseling parents. It is also important to provide information to Deaf clubs on the current status of cochlear implants and the possible benefits and limitations of the devices.

Treatment Plans for Cochlear Implant Recipients

Once the evaluation and patient counseling have been completed and the decision has been made to proceed with the cochlear implant, the implant team may suggest that the patient go through some pretraining. With adults and older children the pretraining may include speechreading therapy and training in the use of communication strategies for communication breakdowns (Chapters 4, 5, and 10). For children the pretraining may include conditioning for play audiometry using tactile or visual stimulation, which then will allow for more accurate assessment of hearing sensitivity with and without the implant.

SURGERY. The cochlear implant surgery is completed under general anesthesia. Typically, the surgeon makes an incision behind the ear and drills a small area in the mastoid bone for the placement of the receiver stimulator and the insertion of the electrode array. The electrode array is then threaded through the mastoid and the middle ear cavity and then inserted in the scala-tympani of the cochlea through the round window. Insertion depths can range up to 30 mm depending on the implant system being used. The operation normally ranges from one to three hours and often is done on an outpatient basis.

After surgical placement of the internal receiver/stimulator and the electrode array, the patient must wait approximately three to six weeks before the external headset and speech processor can be fit. This waiting period allows for healing of the incision area prior to placing the magnet on the sensitive surface where the external transmitter is placed.

HOOK-UP. The initial fitting and programming of the cochlear implant, commonly called the hook-up, usually takes 1½ to 2 hours. During the hook-up or fitting of the headset and speech processor, the audiologist must program the speech processor using a specific manufacturer-designed diagnostic programming system interfaced with a personal computer.

All the current generation implants have the capability of testing the integrity of the internal device by using a technique called telemetry (Abbas & Brown, 2000). Electrode voltages and impedances can be measured when current is supplied through the system. In this manner the audiologist can check the internal device prior to programming the system. If any of the electrodes are found to be out of compliance with standard values, they will not be programmed for use. In some implant centers, telemetry is also completed by the audiologist in the operating room at the time of surgery to ensure proper device functioning before surgical closure.

In order to create the program, or MAP, for the speech processor, the audiologist must determine the electrical dynamic range for each electrode used (Figure 3.5).

MAP: Cochlear implant program that encodes the acoustic signal and translates it into electrical stimulation levels based on the measured T and C levels.

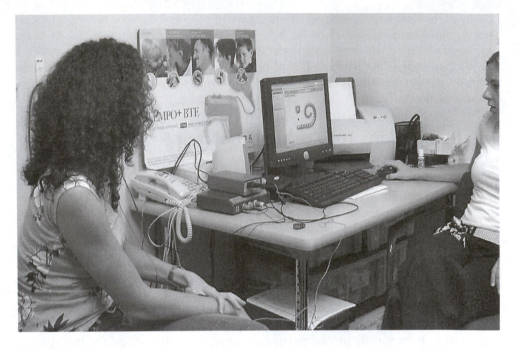

FIGURE 3.5

Programming an adult patient.

The programming system delivers an electrical current through the cochlear implant system to each electrode in order to obtain the electrical threshold (C-level) and maximal level of current that is comfortably loud (C- or M-level) measures. T-level or minimum stimulation level is the softest electrical current that produces an auditory sensation by the patient 100 percent of the time. The C- or M-level is the loudest level that can be listened to comfortably for a long period of time. The speech processor is then programmed or "mapped" using one of the several encoding strategies so that the electrical current delivered to the implant will be within this measured dynamic range between T- and C-levels. Obviously, T- and C-levels are much easier to obtain on adults and older children with postlingual hearing loss. Techniques for testing the T-levels in young children are similar to testing pure tone hearing thresholds, ranging from observational testing to conditioned play audiometry. Using a team approach with two audiologists is very helpful when programming or mapping the cochlear implants of young children. Obtaining the C-levels in children is a challenging task, with the audiologist often relying totally on behavioral observation. Neural Response Telemetry (NRT; Cochlear Corp.) or Neural Response Imaging (NRI; Advanced Bionics) are objective techniques that can be used to estimate the dynamic ranges in young children or difficult-to-test patients. NRT and NRI offer a means of testing the compound action potential of the nerve using two of the electrodes in the array as recording electrodes and two as stimulating electrodes. No additional equipment is necessary. From these measures, T- and C-levels can be estimated (Abbas & Brown, 2000). With children, au-

Neural response telemetry (NRT): Allows the implant system to function as a miniature evoked potential system by sampling and recording action potentials generated by electrical stimulation.

diologists will often evaluate only a limited number of electrodes spaced throughout the electrode array during the initial hook-up and either estimate the levels for the other electrodes or only include the tested electrodes in the initial program.

After T- and C- levels are established and the MAP is created, the microphone is then activated so that the patient is able to hear speech and sounds in the environment. The initial reaction to speech varies among patients. Most adults describe speech as sounding mechanical and cartoonlike. Children often react with tears. This is understandable, considering that they may have no concept of what sound and hearing are and may find the stimulation frightening. Often they are hearing their own voice, including their crying, for the first time. As they are calmed down, they often realize that when they stopped crying, the stimulation stopped. This can be the first step to auditory awareness.

Most current generation systems have multiple memories that allow the audiologist to save more than one MAP in the speech processors. This is very helpful to the audiologist since, due to acclimatization to sound, the initial T- and C-levels are often not the final values. Higher current values can be used to make alternative MAPs, which can be saved into the processor's multiple memories so that patients have the option of increasing the power between clinic visits.

> Acclimatization to sound: Adaptation to sound stimulation that changes the measured T- and C-levels allowing the individual to tolerate higher levels.

The patient and family should also be instructed on the daily care and maintenance of the system. They must know how to place the processor and coil on the head, change batteries, manipulate the controls, and troubleshoot the unit. Parents need to be shown how to check the system prior to putting it on the child. Spare cords or cable should be supplied. Suggestions on wearing the units using belts, harnesses, or clips should be given. Accessories should be explained and demonstrated. Warnings on the dangers of electrostatic discharge (ESD) should be given, as well as any other safety factors. Static electricity can corrupt stored programs or, in rare cases, cause damage to the internal unit when the external device is being worn. Parents are told to remove the device when their child plays on plastic slides or on other static-generating materials. Warranty and loss and damage insurance information should be covered.

> Electrostatic discharge (ESD): Occurs when static electricity (accumulation of electrical charge) transfers between two objects charged to different levels.

The patients or the parents of young users are asked to keep a diary or log of their listening experiences. They are asked to record both positive and negative experiences. Significant others are also asked to keep a record of their observations when they are with the implant user. This helps in reprogramming the units on subsequent visits and also in developing the most appropriate treatment plans.

FOLLOW-UP PROGRAMMING AND THERAPY. The second programming session is usually performed within one week of the initial hook-up. Review of the patient diary and experiences with the implant are helpful in determining if the programs provided sufficient power for sound awareness and detection or if any sounds were uncomfortably loud, indicating that the C-levels were set too high. During this visit, the T- and C-values are reevaluated, and new MAPs are placed in the processor.

During this session, an initial screening of the patient's abilities should be completed. Table 3.2 contains examples of tests commonly used for patients with cochlear implants. Children should be tested using various auditory training screening materials that are age-appropriate. These results will help guide the treatment plan. Auditory training programs developed for aided children with hearing loss can be

TABLE 3.2	

Examples of Tests Commonly Used for Patients with Cochlear Implants

AGE GROUP	TESTS
Preschool	Early Listening Function (ELF; Anderson, 2003b)
	Early Speech Perception Test (Moogs & Geers, 1990)
	Infant Toddler Meaningful Auditory Integration Scale (IT-MAIS; Zimmerman-Phillips, Robbins, & Osberger, 2001)
	Meaningful Auditory Integration Scale (MAIS; Robbins, Renshaw, & Berry, 1991)
School Age	Children's Hearing in Noise Test (C-HINT; Nilsson, Soli, Gelnett, 1996)
	Children's Home Inventory for Listening Difficulties (CHILD; Anderson et al., 2003a)
	Craig Lip-reading Inventory (Craig, 1992)
	Lexical Neighborhood Test (LNT; Kirk, Pisoni, & Osberger, 1995)
	Multisyllabic Lexical Neighborhood Test (MLNT; Kirk et al., 1995)
	NU-Chips (Elliott & Katz, 1980)
	Phonetically Balanced Kindergarten Test (PBK; Haskins, 1949)
Adults	CID Everyday Sentence Test (Davis & Silverman, 1970)
	Consonant Nucleus Consonant Test (CNC; Peterson & Lehiste, 1962)
	CUNY Sentence Test (Boothroyd, Hanin, & Hnath, 1985)
	Hearing in Noise Test (HINT; Nilsson, Soli, & Sullivan, 1994)
	Minimal Auditory Test Battery (MAC; Owens, Kessler, Tellen, & Shubert, 1981)
	NU-6 Monosyllabic Word Test (Tillman & Carhart, 1966)

used with cochlear implant users as well. Excellent reviews of screening devices and suggestions for treatment plans can be found in Nevins and Chute (1996) and Estabrooks (1998).

For adults, several programmed therapy plans have been developed for implant users. These include screening tests to help the clinician in determining the starting point in the plans (Cochlear Corporation, 1998; Wayner & Abrahamson, 1998). Auditory training methods such as speech tracking are extremely helpful in both treatment and monitoring progress with the device. Software programs, such as Sound and Beyond® and Earobics®, are available for both children and adults and can be used both in the clinic and at home.

The amount and length of therapy with the cochlear implant depend on the patient. In many cases, the implant user will receive device programming and monitoring at the cochlear implant center and other audiologic re/habilitation and speech–language therapy through their schools or local audiologists and therapists. A coordinated effort on the part of all professionals and parents is very important in developing and implementing the treatment plans. Face-to-face meetings, teleconferencing, written reports, and email are all means of maintaining contact with all parties involved. Parent-maintained notebooks that all professionals may use are also excellent. By having the parent in charge of a notebook that has records and

Speech tracking: A therapeutic procedure in which subjects are presented with prose and asked to repeat verbatim what they hear (De Filippo & Scott, 1978).

communications to be shared by professionals, the parent can be empowered to be part of the process. Teachers and therapists who are not familiar with implants need to be provided with literature on cochlear implants and given instructions on how to check and troubleshoot the devices. They need to understand that the cochlear implant is designed to give the child more auditory information. They can still use similar teaching techniques with these children as they used prior to the implant, but they need to raise their expectations concerning what the child can accomplish using audition. The habilitation programming discussions in Chapter 9 can easily be adapted for cochlear implant users. In working with a young child who is learning to listen through a cochlear implant, the focus should be on listening. The child's world needs to have rich, repetitive spoken language. Information needs to be given auditorially first, and then visual cues can be incorporated. Parents need to be involved, because they are the true teachers and therapists for their children.

Programming follow-ups for adult patients with postlingual hearing loss usually consist of approximately six visits in the first two months of use, then at three months, six months, and annually thereafter. For young children the programming schedule suggested is weekly visits for two months, then at six months, nine months, and every six months thereafter. These schedules can be modified to include more or less visits depending on the person's adaptation to the implant, auditory responsiveness, and ease of programming.

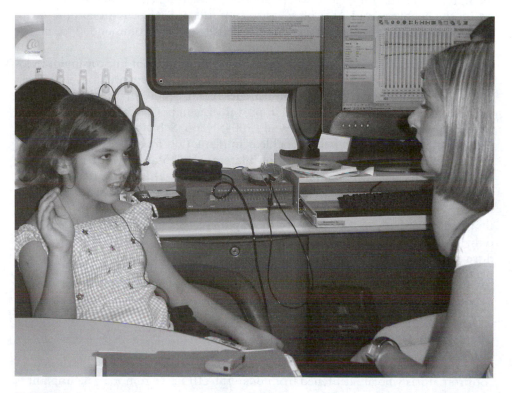

FIGURE 3.6

Therapy with a child cochlear implant user.

Variables Affecting Performance

As stated previously, patient performance varies greatly among cochlear implant users. Many users are able to achieve open-set speech recognition even in the presence of background noise whereas some patients receive only improvement in their speechreading abilities and awareness of environmental sounds. Age of onset, length of deafness, age of implantation, length of implant use, etiology of the hearing loss, nerve survival, mode of communication, cochlear implant technology, surgical issues, audiologic re/habilitation methods, and motivation are examples of variables that affect success with the implant. Some of these are known factors, such as age of onset and length of deafness. Studies have shown that the shorter the length of severe-to-profound hearing loss and better the preimplant discrimination score, the better the prognosis for benefit from the cochlear implant (Rubenstein, Parkenson, Tyler, & Gantz, 1999). Others are unknown quantities, such as the amount of nerve survival, both prior to and following surgical insertion of the electrode array. Patients, parents, and significant others need to be made aware of the many variables that can affect performance.

Nerve survival: The amount of VIII nerve fibers that are available for stimulation.

BILATERAL HEARING WITH COCHLEAR IMPLANTS. Recent studies have shown that some of the benefits of binaural hearing, such as localization and improved hearing noise, can be accomplished when the patient wears a hearing aid in the ear opposite the cochlear implant (Ching et al., 2001, 2004; Seeber, Baumann, & Fastl, 2004). Currently, a hearing aid trial in the opposite ear is recommended for all patients receiving unilateral cochlear implants.

Bilateral cochlear implantation has also shown significant improvement in localization and hearing in noise in adults (van Hoesel, 2004; van Hoesel & Tyler, 2003). The binaural benefits in children are less clear. Studies have indicated some children get limited localization and improvements in noise while others show no clear binaural advantage (Litovsky et al., 2004; Nopp, Schleich, & D'Haese, 2004). The possible benefits of bilateral cochlear implantation must be weighed against the possible disadvantages. The cost of bilateral implantation will be $40,000 to $60,000 greater than with a unilateral cochlear implant. This cost is not only monetary: Surgical risks are also increased. In addition, one must consider the possibility that some future device may be developed that could only be used in an ear that had never had an implant. With the rapid changes in technology, if the child only has the implant in one ear, the other ear would be available so the new procedure could be performed. When reviewing the options for a young child whose expected lifespan is 70 to 75 years, the importance of keeping one ear open for future options needs to be considered.

Auditory Brainstem Implant

An auditory brainstem implant (ABI) has been developed for individuals with neurofibromatosis who are deafened from bilateral VIII nerve tumors. The implant is placed on the cochlear nucleus of the brainstem during the surgery to remove the tumor. To date, over 100 patients have received the ABI, and in early November 2000, the Nucleus 24 ABI was approved by the USFDA for use in cases of neurofi-

> ### Case 3.2. May
>
> May was identified through newborn screening in the hospital two days after birth. She was fit with hearing aids bilaterally at 8 weeks of age, and her parents started with her in a total communication therapy program that emphasized auditory training. At 13 months she was showing little to no progress in her speech/auditory development, and she was evaluated for a cochlear implant. At 15 months she was implanted. She continued using total communication, but speech and audition were emphasized in her therapy at home and by her family. May is now 9 years old and is in a regular classroom performing well educationally. She rarely uses sign language unless with her Deaf friends. Her speech and language development is at the level of her normal hearing peers. She is active in Girl Scouts and sports at her school. The cochlear implant has given her a chance to function as a well-adjusted happy young lady in the hearing world.

bromatosis for patients over the age of 12 years (Cochlear Corporation, 2000). Results with this implant are similar to early generation multielectrode implants and show promise to those who have not been able to benefit from cochlear implants because they lack functioning VIII nerves.

Future Trends in Cochlear Implants

Advances in cochlear implants are occurring rapidly in design, programming techniques, coding strategies, and determining candidacy. Both internal and external devices are becoming smaller. The introduction of behind-the-ear speech processors has provided cosmetic advantages that are particularly attractive to adolescent and young adult users.

Acoustical/electrical stimulation is currently being investigated (Gantz, Turner, Gfeller, & Lowder, 2005). Many individuals have usable hearing in the low- to mid-frequency range but have no hearing in higher frequencies. These people with "dead regions" of the cochlea receive little to no high-frequency information from hearing aids. With electrical/acoustic stimulation, the cochlear implant electrode array is placed only in basal portion of the cochlea and programmed for high-frequency sounds. At the same time the low- to mid-frequencies are amplified using standard hearing aid technology. This cochlear implant/hearing aid combination could help many individuals who currently do not qualify for cochlear implants, but are dissatisfied with their hearing aids because the higher pitches cannot be amplified.

■ VESTIBULAR EVALUATION AND REHABILITATION

The evaluation and treatment of vestibular disorders can be extremely challenging and rewarding. Often the precise etiology cannot be fully identified by conventional testing, yet the symptoms can be life changing for the patient. Putting together the puzzle requires an interdisciplinary approach involving physicians,

Vestibular rehabilitation: Treatment techniques to aid in the recovery from vestibular weakness or dizziness.

physical therapists, and audiologists, along with other specialists in various fields of study. For instance, there are many balance centers throughout the country for evaluation and rehabilitation that are jointly operated by audiologists and physical therapists. These facilities receive many patient referrals from general physicians and ear specialists in the area.

About half the people in the United States will experience some form of balance or dizziness problem in their lifetimes (AAA, 2005). Between 5 and 8 million physician consults per year are due to dizziness (Desmond, 2000). This estimate increases with age with one study reporting that 65 percent of individuals over 60 experience dizziness or loss of balance (Hobeika, 1999).

Although balance and dizziness disorders are frequently considered an inner ear problem, in reality complex interactions between several systems are required to maintain our stability. The somatosensory and visual systems, along with the vestibular portion of the inner ear, all work together to obtain an accurate picture of our environment and position in space. This information is then analyzed by the brainstem, cerebellum, and cortex to initiate reflexive and voluntary motor responses (Figure 3.7).

Somatosensory input is obtained from the legs, hips, ankles, and feet, which transmit specific information depending on the surface we are standing on. Dif-

FIGURE 3.7

Sensory input contributing to balance are the visual, somatosensory, and vestibular systems.
Courtesy of NeuroCom® International, Inc.

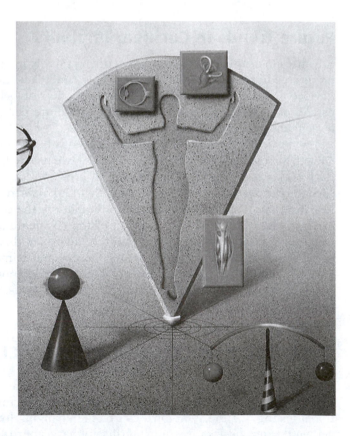

ferent signals are sent to the brain if we are standing in our dining room, walking the beach in soft sand, or rocking on a boat. Under normal circumstances somatosensory input provides a major role in balance maintenance.

For example, if we stand on a ladder to change a light bulb in an overhead fixture, most of us can accomplish this task without any problem. However, if we need to change a different light bulb located over our bed, using the mattress to stand on, the task becomes more difficult. The mattress moves and gives while we are reaching over our head, compromising input from the lower half of our body. This requires greater concentration and more time and could even be a bit fatiguing because we are using additional resources, both mental and physical, to replace the bulb. If the surface becomes even more unstable, greater reliance is required from the visual system.

Vision is another key component to balance function. Visual input is compared and contrasted with other systems to determine how we perceive the world around us. When a discrepancy occurs, this can result in sensory conflict within the central nervous system, impairing our ability to maintain our equilibrium. When somataosensory input is compromised, the visual system becomes the dominant player in the sensory integration hierarchy. If further deterioration occurs to both visual and somatosensory input, we are forced to rely more heavily on inner ear function (Nashner, 1993).

The inner ear has two divisions: the cochlea, which is responsible for hearing, and the vestibular portion, comprised of the semicircular canals and vestibule (Figure 3.8). The semicircular canals are fluid-filled structures and respond to head motion. These sensors are linked with the visual system in the brainstem. Different cranial nerves and processing centers control the muscles of each eye and work in a complementary manner with the inner ear structures. Three canals in each ear allow us to sense head movement in various directions. This type of sensory integration is crucial for keeping our eyes focused on targets of interest (Baloh & Honrubia, 2001).

This relationship is easy to demonstrate by focusing on your finger out in front of you at arm's length. If you move your head from the center position to the right, the fluid in the horizontal semicircular canal moves to the left, stimulating sensory structures in both ears. One side increases its neural response while the other decreases. This alerts your brain of the direction and speed of that head movement. Simultaneously, your eyes move in an equal and opposite direction so that the object can remain in focus. A similar response will occur in the opposite direction, or if you move your head up and down instead of left to right. This is just one example of how vestibular and visual systems work together. Other reflexive eye movements occur depending on the nature and speed of the visual target.

The enlarged portion in the middle of the inner ear is the vestibule. These structures have sensory organs that are most sensitive to linear acceleration—for example, moving straight forward in a car from a stop sign or up and down in an elevator. The sensory structures in the vestibule seem to be more closely involved with postural control. Together with other motor responses, the vestibular reflexes help maintain ocular stability and postural control and produce appropriate muscle activity to maintain equilibrium (Honrubia & Hoffman, 1993).

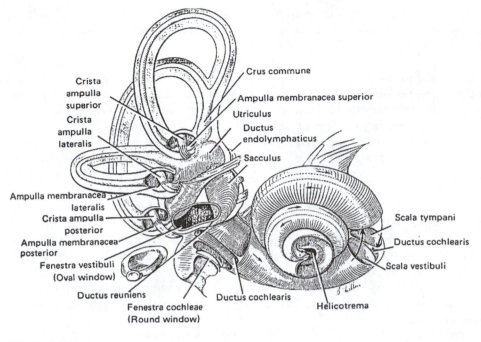

FIGURE 3.8

Anatomy of the inner ear including the cochlea (hearing) and vestibular portion (balance).

Source: Used with permission from *Some Pathological Conditions of the Ear, Nose and Throat: An Atlas.* Courtesy Abbott Laboratories, Abbott Park, Illinois.

As outlined in Figure 3.9, balance control is a multifaceted process. In addition to accurate sensory input, appropriate motor output is vital for maintaining balance. These actions need to be analyzed and readjusted in our constantly changing environment within fractions of a second. Simultaneously, the brain needs to select which input is correct and ignored or minimize aberrant information to determine body position. Selected body movements are the result of reflexive, learned, and volitional response patterns. These require quick changes in muscle groups to adjust to new experiences (Nashner, 1993).

Causes of Balance Problems

One of the main causes of disequilibrium is medicine. Frequently, medications create unwanted side effects or interact with other prescriptions. Careful monitoring of pharmaceutical products should be coordinated by all physicians. Damage to visual, vestibular, and proprioception systems may also impair one's abilities to process sensory input. Cataracts, vestibular neuritis, or peripheral neuropathy can all have a deleterious effect on balance function. Insults to the central nervous system created by strokes, tumors, or poor circulatory function can lead to balance difficulties. Systemic problems in the cardiovascular, respiratory, or endocrine system can result in chronic dizziness. Neurologic disorders and cranial nerve function can

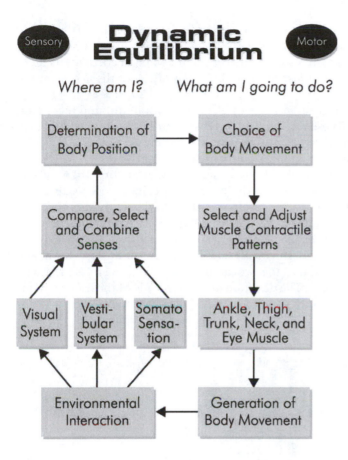

FIGURE 3.9

Sensory and motor components of Dynamic Equilibrium.

Courtesy of NeuroCom® International, Inc.

contribute to balance problems. For this reason we rely on a multidisciplinary approach to balance assessment that begins with a physician.

Medical Evaluation

A thorough exam is completed of the head, neck, and functional balance by an otologist. History is a key component to identifying problems. A review of systems is completed along with cranial nerve examination, functional balance screening, and assessment of vital signs. Determining the characteristics of a balance problem is critical to making the appropriate decisions regarding patient care. Diagnostic evaluations including blood work, imaging studies, and outside referral to other specialists such as neurologists, opthamologists, and orthopedists are made if necessary.

Audiologic and Balance Testing

Since the inner ear is comprised of a hearing and vestibular portion, disease processes that affect one may affect the performance of the other. Therefore, a thorough audiologic evaluation is usually part of a balance workup. Assessment of the vestisbulo-ocular pathways, positioning and positional testing, along with sensory organization testing, is accomplished through videonystagmography (VNG) and computerized dynamic posturography (CDP). Electrophysiologic testing such as auditory brainstem responses may also be incorporated when needed. Many audiologists are involved in the administration and interpretation of these specialized tests.

Videonystagmography utilizes video goggles to closely monitor and record eye movements (Figure 3.10). These recordings are subsequently analyzed with help of a computer to evaluate inner ear structures, sensory and motor function of ocular muscles, and brainstem processing that coordinates these activities.

During the test the patient is asked to look in different directions, follow visual targets, and move his or her head and body in various positions. Recordings are then compared to normative data. The test is also used to detect nystagmus. Nystagmus is an involuntary eye movement resulting from the connections between our eyes, brain, and balance sensors in our ears. It frequently occurs whenever someone is experiencing dizziness. During the caloric portion of the test, warm and cool air or water are introduced into the ear canal. This typically results in nystagmus and a sensation of dizziness. The direction and magnitude of these movements are of diagnostic significance to the audiologist and physician. VNG can help dis-

FIGURE 3.10

Videonystagmography
Photo courtesy of ICS.

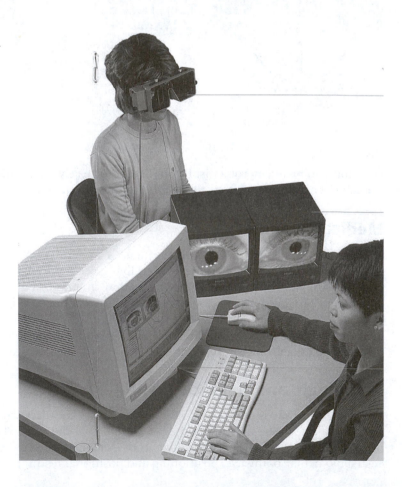

tinguish between problems in the ear, brainstem pathways, or other processing centers in the cerebellum.

Frequently, the precise etiology of chronic balance disturbances is unknown. In older populations, this is especially true. Computerized dynamic posturography (CDP) can be particularly useful under these circumstances. CDP is conducted to test one's ability to maintain balance under various conditions (see Figure 3.11). It utilizes a pressure sensitivity footplate and computer monitoring to measure shifts in body weight and center of gravity under normal and sensory compromised conditions. Because CDP is more of a functional evaluation, results are extremely useful in documenting deficits in balance performance. In many instances, abnormal CDP provides critical objective documentation of a patient's symptoms.

The Sensory Organization Test (SOT) is extremely useful for this purpose. During the evaluation the patient is asked to maintain his or her balance under a variety of conditions (Figure 3.12). Some of the subtests allow visual, somatosensory, and vestibular input to be used normally, while others purposefully disrupt visual input with a moving visual field or somatosensory input by induced movement of the platform surface. Certain conditions are completed with eyes open, others with eyes closed. Analysis is then completed using age-corrected normative data. These findings help document patients' balance problems, assist in development of a rehabilitation program, and confirm progress gained from individualized management protocols (Black, Angel, Pesznecker, & Gianna, 2000).

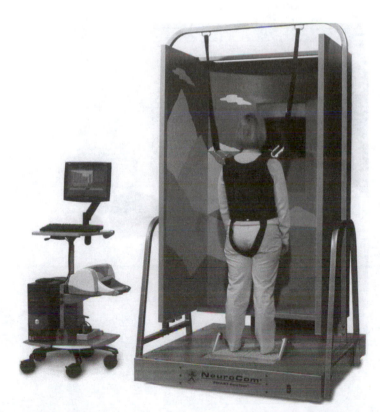

FIGURE 3.11

Computerized Dynamic Posturography.
Photo courtesy of NeuroCom® International, Inc.

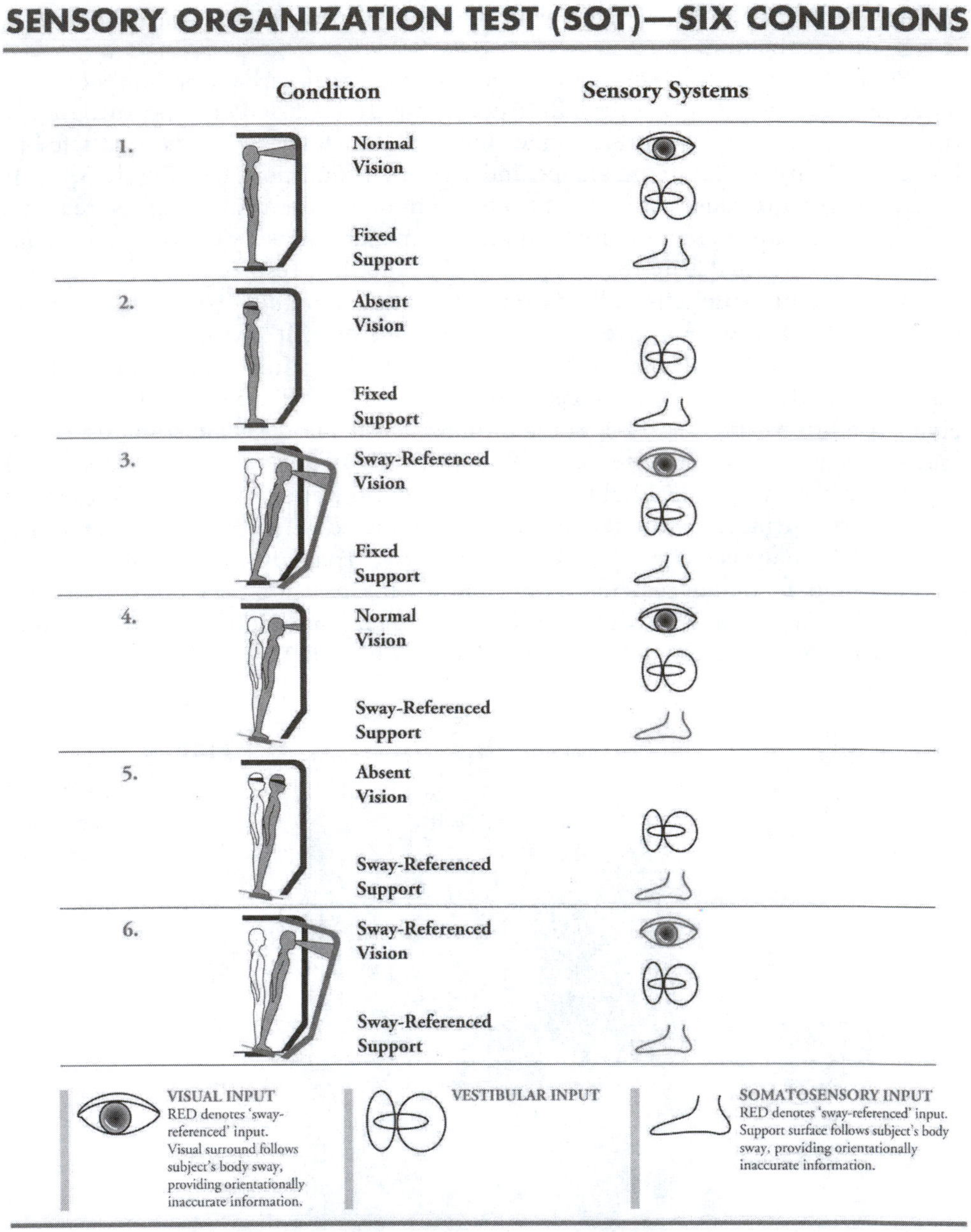

SENSORY ORGANIZATION TEST (SOT)—SIX CONDITIONS

	Condition	Sensory Systems
1.	Normal Vision / Fixed Support	
2.	Absent Vision / Fixed Support	
3.	Sway-Referenced Vision / Fixed Support	
4.	Normal Vision / Sway-Referenced Support	
5.	Absent Vision / Sway-Referenced Support	
6.	Sway-Referenced Vision / Sway-Referenced Support	

VISUAL INPUT
RED denotes 'sway-referenced' input.
Visual surround follows subject's body sway, providing orientationally inaccurate information.

VESTIBULAR INPUT

SOMATOSENSORY INPUT
RED denotes 'sway-referenced' input.
Support surface follows subject's body sway, providing orientationally inaccurate information.

FIGURE 3.12

Conditions of the Sensory Organization Test.

Courtesy of NeuroCom® International, Inc.

Vestibular Rehabilitation

An increasing number of audiologists are involved in vestibular rehabilitation. More frequently, physical therapists do this work, or there is a collaborative effort between these paraprofessionals. Since much of vestibular rehabilitation (VR) is a symptom-driven process, history information is obtained from a treatment perspective rather than a strict medical site-of-lesion model. Symptoms are scrutinized in detail regarding onset, duration, activity, environment, frequency of occurrence, and severity of dizziness. Physical data is collected including posture, range of motion, strength, and sensation. Visual/vestibular movements are checked along with static balance, gait, and positional testing. Administration of the Dizziness Handicap Inventory (Jacobsen & Newman, 1990) is completed to explore the impact that dizziness has in the lives of our patients. This scale was designed to investigate the physical, emotional, and functional problems related to dizziness and is very useful to document patient improvement before and after treatment.

REHABILITATION CANDIDATES. Patients who respond well to VR typically report chronic conditions of motion-provoked dizziness or generalized disequilibrium. Individuals with abnormal postural control or gait problems are also good candidates. In addition, people who have demonstrated difficulties integrating visual, vestibular, or somatosensory input as confirmed by CDP or during clinical evaluations can benefit from VR (Smith-Wheelock, Shepard, & Telian, 1991). In contrast, people experiencing progressive medical pathologies that involve balance centers or severe disability may not realize the same level of improvement (Shepard & Telian, 1995). Fluctuating or spontaneous episodes of dizziness may not be stable long enough to provide time for reorganization of sensory and motor processes. Conditions of severe disability may not have adequate residual function of sensory or motor output to complete many of the protocols required in VR.

> About 20% of all dizziness and 50% of dizziness in older persons is caused by benign paroxysmal positional vertigo (BPPV).

Vestibular therapy works due to the exquisite ability of the central nervous system to change depending on need or condition. Goebel (1993) points out, "If not for this capacity to alter the motor output to different stimuli, the highly integrated balance system could not adapt to the myriad of novel situations which occur in everyday life" (p. 655). Because of this ability, we can develop changes in muscle response (adaptation) and reduce the action of reflexive responses with repeated stimulation (habituation), which are crucial to the principles underlying vestibular rehabilitation (Goebel, 1993).

TREATMENT. Most of us would avoid movements or activities that make us feel bad. If you become dizzy whenever you move to the right, you would probably avoid that movement or at least do it very slowly. Over time you might slow down enough that you develop a sedentary lifestyle. Vestibular therapy encourages patients to do the opposite of what may come naturally. Inactivity is substituted with safe activity. Movements that make you feel "funny" are programmatically initiated. Patients are counseled that "they will probably feel worse before they feel better," but most do get better. Typically, they are asked to withdraw from "dizziness medication," which may only serve to sedate the brain and delay recovery. These issues must be well understood by the patient and family prior to the initiation of therapy so they will

> Canalith repositioning, which involves simple head movements, is successful in treating about 80% of cases with BPPV.

Case 3.3. ES

ES was a 66-year-old female referred with a one-year history of general disequilibrium and dizziness. Her symptoms were exacerbated with quick movements, and she had some difficulty walking due to back and hip pain. She used glasses for reading and admitted she had a bit of a hearing loss. She took care of her 93-year-old mother and enjoyed gardening. She had heavy reliance on medications to control her dizziness. She stated "I had to take three pills to make it to this appointment and am going to take two when I get home." She had experienced one fall and maintained lights throughout her house all night long because she is afraid of falling. She only went to church and the doctor's office for socialization. She was frustrated because she could not maintain her household chores and take care of her mother without assistance. She also wanted to return to tending her garden.

Although videonystagmogarphy revealed no significant deficits, CDP and evaluation with the physical therapist and an audiologist indicated that she was an appropriate candidate for vestibular rehabilitation. Her Dizziness Handicap Inventory score was 34, consistent with a mild degree of impairment. She was originally given some vestibulo-ocular exercises with head movement in several plains, timed stance tasks under eyes open and eyes closed conditions on a stable surface, and walking while focusing on a visual target. These were to be completed three times a day. General conditioning was also encouraged. She was asked to discontinue her "dizzy medication."

Following the first week of therapy, her muscles were sore and actually felt a bit worse at times. She was compliant completing her at-home exercises even though she experienced some nausea and increased dizziness. She saw some improvement in her ability to complete therapeutic exercises during the second week of treatment, although consistently waited until her daughter arrived home to do her "homework." During her third week of vestibular rehabilitation she reduced her "dizzy medicine" and continued to see improvement in her balance. Exercises were modified and difficulty increased as therapy progressed. After a month, she required no medication to treat her symptoms and only became dizzy and slightly nauseous riding in a car. Following six weeks of home exercises and clinic visits, she reported no significant balance or dizziness problems. She stated, "I feel so good, I almost can't remember feeling bad." Her DHI score dropped by 28 points and CDP overall score improved 15 percent. She reported a decrease in her symptoms by 90 percent. She returned to house duties and caring for her mother, and has happily returned to pulling weeds. At follow-up one month after discharge from therapy, she was "Doing real good."

know what to expect and be properly motivated. Counseling, education, and compliance with at-home exercises are crucial to the success of the program.

The goals of VR are to improve balance and gait by retraining muscle response to varying conditions. The exercises completed in the clinic and at home must reflect normal daily activities in a wide variety of contexts to be integrated into new learned behavior (Herdman, 1989). Typically, the patient is shown the precise protocol and completes the exercises in the clinic. Written instructions are provided along with specific details of each movement. This generates confidence in the individual, which allows him or her to continue therapy at home. If habituation exercises are incorporated into the rehabilitative plan, care must be taken to ensure safety, especially in the home setting (Smith-Wheelock et al., 1991). It is usually evident at the next visit who has been doing his or her "homework" and who has not!

Developing an individualized therapy program that gradually becomes more challenging over the course of treatment is typically implemented. Rehabilitative protocols can incorporate head movement while focusing on a visual target. This helps facilitate coordination between vestibular and ocular pathways. The task can be altered to include a busy background behind the target. Exercises can be modified to include walking while maintaining focus on a target and utilizing different rates of head movement in both the horizontal and vertical plane. Further difficulty can be introduced by standing on a cushion or walking on an unstable surface. As they progress, specific exercise protocols are developed to challenge the patient.

This type of individualized program has proven extremely successful. Retrospective studies have shown that 85 percent of those enrolled in a custom-designed VR program see improvement in their condition. Approximately 30 percent reported complete recovery (Smith-Wheelock et al., 1991). Improvements can be seen in several weeks, with the typical program lasting two months or so. In addition, these protocols seem appropriate regardless of age or gender (Shepard & Telian, 1995). Older populations typically require longer rehabilitation programs and closer monitoring but experience similar gains in function as younger patients (Shepard et al., 1993).

This course of treatment and recovery represents relatively typical results utilizing individualized vestibular rehabilitation protocols. Highly motivated and compliant patients realize a return to normal activities with perseverance and dedication. Many require continued home routines and generalized conditioning to maintain the gains achieved during therapy.

■ TINNITUS EVALUATION AND REHABILITATION

Tinnitus can range from a minor annoyance to a debilitating condition with a wide range of associated symptoms. It can result in sleep disorders, depression, anxiety, and other medical problems. Depending on the definition, the incidence of tinnitus can vary from approximately 10 percent to over 30 percent in various populations (Davis & Rafaie, 2000; Newell et al., 2001). Patients frequently describe their tinnitus as a ringing, hissing, or buzzing sound in their ears or head. These sounds can be intermittent or continuous and are frequently high-pitched in nature, although they can manifest themselves in a vast array of auditory experiences. While hearing loss and age have been correlated with the experience of tinnitus (Newell et al., 2001), not all elderly people with hearing loss encounter this problem. According to the American Academy of Audiology, over 40 million people suffer from tinnitus in the United States alone (AAA, 2001). Although many individuals experience tinnitus at one time or another, only about 20 percent of these cases are considered clinically significant.

Tinnitus: A ringing or buzzing sound in the ear that is not caused by external sound simulation.

Causes of Tinnitus

The precise etiology of tinnitus is unknown. However, it can arise from problems throughout the auditory system, and can be very different across individuals.

Recent literature suggests that the cochlea and subcortical and cortical levels of the brain may be involved in the generation or lack of control of neural activity that contributes to the perception of tinnitus (Jastreboff, 2000; Salvi, Lockwood, & Burkard, 2000). These mechanisms are extremely complex, and we are just beginning to discover some of the mysteries of this process.

Sound is not just passively transmitted from the ear to the cortex like a telephone line. Important processing centers are present throughout the central auditory pathways. These signals are analyzed and modulated throughout the system. There are also connections between auditory and nonauditory centers of the central nervous system (Jastreboff, 2000). Interactions between auditory messages and portions of the brain that are involved with emotion and metabolic function can create real and challenging problems for the person suffering from tinnitus. This may explain why some individuals feel their tinnitus is only a minor annoyance, and others seem to be completely debilitated and obsessed by the sound.

Clinically significant tinnitus is most likely initiated from problems in the peripheral auditory system (Ruth & Hamill-Ruth, 2001). Auditory insults such as noise exposure, Ménière's disease, acoustic neuroma, and presbycusis (hearing loss due to the aging process) have all been associated with tinnitus. Certain medications can also influence or damage inner ear structures that may predispose someone to tinnitus. These changes in inner ear function typically result in alteration of neural activity, which may disrupt processing at various levels of the central nervous system (Jastreboff, 2000; Tyler & Bergan, 2001).

Evaluation

Although audiologists play a central role in the evaluation and treatment of tinnitus, a team approach seems more productive for severe cases. A thorough medical examination by an otolaryngologist is preferred to rule out any significant medical or pharmacologic issues that could be causing the tinnitus. Many patients experience emotional and psychological problems as a result of or in addition to their tinnitus. Depression and anxiety about their condition often requires health care specialists that have appropriate training in these matters. This makes a psychologist or psychiatrist an invaluable member of the treatment team (Sweetow, 2003).

Tinnitus assessment typically begins with a comprehensive audiologic evaluation. In addition to speech and pure-tone threshold testing, quantification of the tinnitus is often completed. This generally includes methods to match the pitch or frequency of the sound, its loudness, and at what levels it can be "masked" or covered up by another sound. Loudness discomfort levels are also obtained for a variety of stimuli. Otoacoustic emission studies used to evaluate inner ear function are also part of the tinnitus workup.

An important facet of the tinnitus evaluation includes exploring the impact it has on someone's life. Currently there are a variety of history forms and self-report questionnaires that are used to help quantify these symptoms. The Tinnitus Handicap Inventory (Newman, Jacobson, & Spitzer, 1996), Tinnitus Reaction Questionnaire (Wilson, Henry, Bowen, & Haralambous, 1991) and Tinnitus Severity Scale (Sweetow & Levy, 1990) are some popular questionnaires frequently administered. These tools have been extremely useful at describing the distress, loss of sleep, and emotional impact of tinnitus. In addition, they can be used to validate the course of treatment utilized in patients suffering from this problem.

Treatment

Education is a critical component of tinnitus treatment and recovery. Once serious causative conditions have been ruled out, the realization that this condition does not involve a serious medical illness is invaluable to the patient. Explanation of auditory anatomy and physiology and possible causes of their tinnitus assists patients in gradually gaining control of this situation. This insight then motivates them to develop strategies to better deal with this challenge.

Currently, there is no universal cure that can be used to successfully treat all forms of tinnitus. While medical, surgical, and pharmacological possibilities exist, most treatments still lack complete success in the recovery from tinnitus. In fact, most of the currently available protocols used to help patients suffering from tinnitus are nonmedical in nature.

Hearing loss is frequently present when an individual experiences tinnitus. For this reason, hearing aids probably are the most common and most effective tool used to help the person suffering from this problem. The amplification from the hearing aid can in some people interfere with the perception of the tinnitus and helps it become less noticeable. Under these circumstances, hearing aids can not only help the patient improve his or her communication abilities, but may have a positive effect on the tinnitus as well. Unfortunately, this is not always the case. The tinnitus does not always respond to conventional amplification. For some, the tinnitus and the sounds being amplified are very different from one another. Under these circumstances, noise generators or ear level masking devices can be used to help ameliorate the problem.

Noise generators can include a variety of devices to help decrease the awareness of ongoing tinnitus. Noise generators are not necessarily implemented to completely cover up the tinnitus, just to make it less intrusive. Counseling and other behavioral methods can then be used more effectively in the management of tinnitus. Noise generators can be as simple as a radio tuned to a station that diverts attention from the tinnitus to flowing water, soothing music, or specifically tuned devices that cover up or mask the offending sound.

Dr. Jack Vernon and his colleagues at the Oregon Hearing Research Center have been pioneers in the evaluation and treatment of tinnitus (Vernon, 1998; Vernon & Meikle, 2000). They have developed protocols and conducted research for the use of tinnitus maskers, hearing aids, and combination devices. With proper evaluation, the masking signal is adjusted to meet the person's individual needs. Most ear level devices look similar to hearing aids. Open or nonoccluding systems that do not completely plug up the canal are generally recommended for a more natural sound and feel. Combination devices can generate a specifically tuned sound to mask the tinnitus and provide amplification for the hearing loss encountered in many tinnitus patients. In this way, *habituation* to the tinnitus can occur slowly over time.

One of the key principles in tinnitus treatment is to avoid total quiet and develop a rich auditory environment (Henry, Schechter, Nagler, & Fausti, 2002). This

Habituation can be defined as "a disappearance in reaction induced by a stimulus" (Jastreboff, 2000). This phenomenon is present in many sensory systems and allows for adaptive changes to occur in the central nervous system. This plasticity facilitates modifications of neural processing and analysis within the brain.

practice helps patients reduce the intrusion tinnitus has in their lives on a daily basis. One analogy frequently described is that of a candle burning in a room (Henry, Jastreboff, Schechter, & Zaugg, 2003). If that candle is glowing in the corner on a dark and moonless night, its presence is almost magnified by the environment. In contrast, if that same candle is burning in the brightness of a sunny afternoon, its brilliance is reduced and may even go unnoticed. This is similar to one strategy used in tinnitus management.

Jastreboff coined the term "Tinnitus Habituation Therapy," which has received widespread acceptance as "Tinnitus Retraining Therapy," or "TRT." This treatment is based on the Neurophysiologic Model of Tinnitus (Jastreboff, 2000). This model proposes that disruption of cochlear function results in changes in neural activity coming from the ear. These changes can produce abnormal signal processing within the central nervous system at subcortical levels. If negative thoughts are attached to the tinnitus, they can be manifested by clinically significant tinnitus. This association occurs due to interconnections between auditory and nonauditory portions of the brain, specifically the limbic system, which modulates emotional behavior, and the autonomic nervous system, which regulates processes such as heart rate, breathing, and other bodily functions. These connections can result in extremely negative emotions and significant physiologic changes in the individual. The objective of this treatment is to condition the patient not to respond to the tinnitus in an emotional way. Protocols are designed to make the tinnitus an unimportant sound that is in the background of consciousness (Henry et al., 2002; Jastreboff, 2000), similar to the air conditioner of your car that you notice when you first turn it on, then it gradually fades away into the background and goes unnoticed. TRT is accomplished through directive counseling and sound therapy.

Directive counseling is used to educate and condition the patient not to view the tinnitus in a threatening manner. Information is delivered and coping strategies are developed to help make this transition occur. Sound therapy facilitates the process of habituation by providing low-level background sounds to make the tinnitus less noticeable. Noise generators and combination units are used to accomplish this task. It should be noted that TRT is a long-term proposition. Since changes within the central nervous system are required for success, patients must be committed to their treatment. Time demands are also significant for the service provider. Patients are informed that TRT may take several months to produce noticeable improvement and up to two years for habituation to be complete.

Although tinnitus remains one of the most challenging conditions to treat by hearing health care professionals, progress continues to be made. Modifications to TRT and other intervention strategies have been used with promising success (Henry et al., 2002; Sweetow, 2000; Tyler & Bergan, 2001). New technologies are allowing closer inspection of the mechanisms involved in tinnitus production (Kaltenbach, 2000; Salvi et al., 2000). The American Tinnitus Association (ATA) is a valuable resource for professionals and patients dealing with tinnitus. They support funding for research and provide information to tinnitus sufferers and the professionals who treat patients (American Tinnitus Association, 2005). In addition, ATA publishes *Tinnitus Today*, a quarterly journal, and maintains an up-to-date website on tinnitus. Through these efforts continued progress is being made on behalf of those who suffer from this problem.

SUMMARY POINTS

- The scope of audiologic rehabilitation has increased dramatically in the past two decades. Clinicians must keep current on new technologies and techniques to aid their patients in all types of disorders that involve either the auditory or vestibular portions of the ear.
- Cochlear implants offer an alternative for sound stimulation to individuals who receive limited benefits from traditional amplification.
- Careful evaluation by a team of professionals is needed to determine candidacy for cochlear implantation and to develop the appropriate treatment plans for these individuals. Audiologic re/habilitation is an integral part of the cochlear implant process, including speech processor programming and training. With training, the cochlear implant can improve the quality of life for persons with severe-to-profound hearing loss.
- Patients with balance problems or complaining of tinnitus no longer must be told there are no successful treatment plans available. Research in vestibular and tinnitus rehabilitation promises hope to the many individuals suffering from vertigo and tinnitus. New advances in these areas have helped many patients resume active and productive lives.

RECOMMENDED READING

COCHLEAR IMPLANTS

Biderman, B., & Thomas, W. (1998). *Wired for sound: A journey into hearing.* Ontario, Canada: Trifolium Books.

Clark, G. (2003). *Cochlear implants: Fundamentals and applications.* New York: Springer-Verlag.

Cullington, H. E. (Ed.). (2003). *Cochlear implants: Objective measures.* Philadelphia: Taylor & Francis.

Estabrooks, W. (1998). *Cochlear implants for kids.* Washington, DC: Alexander Graham Bell Association for the Deaf.

Farley, C. (2002). *Bridge to sound with a "bionic" ear.* Wayzata, MN: Periscope Press.

Nevins, M. E., & Chute, P. M. (1996). *Children with cochlear implants in educational settings.* San Diego, CA: Singular Publishing Group.

Niparko, J. K. (2000). *Cochlear implants: Principles and practices.* Philadelphia: Lippincott Williams & Wilkins.

Parker, J. A. (Ed.). (2004). *The official patient's sourcebook on cochlear implants.* San Diego, CA: Health Publications.

Romoff, A. (2002). *Hear again: Back to life with a cochlear implant.* New York: Sterling Publishing Co.

Waltzman, S. B., & Cohen, N. L. (2000). *Cochlear implants.* New York: Thieme.

Wayner, D. S., & Abrahamson, J. E. (1998). *Learning to hear again with a cochlear implant: An audiologic rehabilitation curriculum guide.* Austin, TX: Hear Again.

Wayner, D. S., Abrahamson, J., & Casterton, J. (1998). *Better communication and cochlear implants.* Austin, TX: Hear Again.

Zeng, F. G., & Popper, A. N. (2004). *Cochlear implants.* New York: Springer-Verlag.

VESTIBULAR REHABILITION

Herdman, S. J. (2000). *Vestibular rehabilitation. Contemporary Perspectives in Rehabilitation* series. Philadelphia: F. A. Davis.

Jacobson, G. P., Newman, C. W., & Kartush, J. M. (Eds). (1993). *Handbook of balance function testing.* St. Louis: Mosby-Yearbook.

Shepard, N. T., & Telian, S. A. (1996). *Practical management of the balance disorder patient.* San Diego, CA: Singular Publishing Group.

TINNITUS

Tyler, R. S. (2000). *Tinnitus handbook.* San Diego, CA: Singular.

Vernon, J. A. (1998). *Tinnitus treatment and relief.* Boston: Allyn and Bacon.

RECOMMENDED WEBSITES

COCHLEAR IMPLANTS

Nucleus Cochlear Implant Systems:
http://www.cochlear.com.html

Advanced Bionics Cochlear Implant Systems:
http://www.cochlearimplant.com/index.html

Med EL Cochlear Implant Systems:
http://www.medel.com/intro.html

National Association of the Deaf (NAD):
http://www.nad.org/infocenter/newsroom/papers/CochlearImplants.html

Cochlear Implants in Adults and Children, National Institutes of Health, Consensus Development Conference Statement, May 15–17, 1995:
http://consensus.nih.gov/cons/100/100_statement.htm

AAA Position Statement on Cochlear Implants in Children:
http://www.audiology.org/professional/positions/cochlear.php

VESTIBULAR REHABILITATION

American Academy of Audiology:
http://www.audiology.org

Vestibular Disorders Association:
http://vestibular.org

Neurocom International, Inc:
http://www.onbalance.com

TINNITUS

American Tinnitus Association:
http://www.tinnitus@ata.org

American Academy of Audiology:
http://www.audiology.org

REFERENCES

Abbas, P. J., & Brown, C. J. (2000). Electrophysiology and device telemetry. In S. B. Waltzman & N. L. Cohen (Eds.), *Cochlear implants.* New York: Thieme.

American Academy of Audiology. (2001, March/April). American Academy of Audiology position statement on audiologic guidelines for the diagnosis and management of tinnitus patients. *Audiology Today, 13,* 2.

American Academy of Audiology (AAA). (2005). Position statement on the audiologist's role in the diagnosis and treatment of vestibular disorders. *Audiology Today, 17.*

American Tinnitus Association. (2005). About ATA. *American Tinnitus Association.* Accessed 2005 from http://www.ata.org/about_ata/

Anderson, K. L. (2003a). CHILD—Children's Home Inventory for Listening Difficulties. Accessed 2005 from http://www.phonak.com/diagnostic

Anderson, K. L. (2003b). ELF—Early Listening Function. Accessed 2005 http://www.phonak.com/diagnostic

Baloh, R. W., & Honrubia, V. (2001). *Clinical neurophysiology of the vestibular system. Contemporary neurology series.* New York: Oxford University Press.

Black, F. O., Angel, C. R., Pesznecker, S. C., & Gianna, C. (2000). Outcome analysis of individualized rehabilitation protocols. *American Journal of Otology, 21,* 543–551.

Boothroyd, A., Hanin, L., & Hnath, T. (1985). *A sentence test of speech perception: Reliability, set equivalence and short term learning: Internal report RCI 10.* New York: Speech and Hearing Sciences Research Centre, City University of New York.

Ching, T. Y. C., Incerti, P., & Hill, M. (2004). Binaural benefits for adults who use hearing aids and cochlear implants in opposite ears. *Ear and Hearing, 25,* 9–21.

Ching, T. Y. C., Psarros, C., Hill, M., Dillon, H., & Incerti, P. (2001). Should children who use cochlear implants wear hearing aids in the opposite ear? *Ear and Hearing, 22,* 365–380.

Craig, W. N. (1992). *Craig Lip-reading Inventory: Word Recognition.* Englewood, CO: Resource Point.

Cochlear Corporation. (1998). *Rehabilitation manual.* Englewood, CO: Author.

Cochlear Corporation. (2000). *Nucleus24ABI: The multichannel auditory brainstem implant.* Englewood, CO: Author.

Colletti, V., Carner, M., Miorelli, V., Guida, M., Colletti, I., & Fiorino, F. G. (2005). Cochlear implantation at under 12 months: Report on 10 patients. *Laryngoscope, 115*(3), 445–449.

Davis, A., & Rafaie, E. A. (2000). Epidemiology of tinnitus. In R. S. Tyler (Ed.), *Tinnitus handbook* (pp. 1–23). San Diego, CA: Singular Publishing Group.

Davis, H., & Silverman, R. (1970). *Hearing and deafness.* New York: Holt, Rinehart and Winston.

DeFilippo, C. L., & Scott, B. L. (1978). A method for training and evaluating the reception of ongoing speech. *Journal of the Acoustical Society of America, 63,* 1186–1192.

Desmond, A. L. (2000). Vestibular rehabilitation. In M. Valente, H. Hosford-Dunn, & R. J. Roser (Eds.), *Audiology treatment.* New York: Thieme.

Elliot, L. L., & Katz, D. (1980). Development of a new children's test of speech discrimination (technical manual). St. Louis, MO: Auditec.

Estabrooks, W. (1998). *Cochlear implants for kids.* Washington, DC: Alexander Graham Bell Association for the Deaf.

Firszt, J. B., Holden, L. K., Skinner, M. W., Tobey, E. A., Peterson, A., Gaggl, W., Runge-Samuelson, C. L., & Wackym, P. A. (2004). Recognition of speech presented at soft to loud levels by adult cochlear implant recipients of three cochlear implant systems. *Ear & Hearing, 25*(4), 375–387.

Gantz, B., Turner, C., Gfeller, K., & Lowder, M. W. (2005). Preservation of hearing in cochlear implant surgery: Advantages of combined electrical and acoustical speech processing. *Laryngoscope, 115,* 795–802.

Goebel, J. A. (1993). Plasticity and compensation within the vestibular system. In I. Kaufman Arenberg (Ed.), *Dizziness and balance disorders: An interdisciplinary approach to diagnosis treatment and rehabilitation.* New York: Kugler Publications.

Haskins, H. A. (1949). *A phonetically balanced test of speech discrimination for children.* Masters thesis. Evanston, IL: Northwestern University.

Henry, J. A., Jastreboff, P. J., Schechter, M., & Zaugg, T. (2003). *Tinnitus research therapy: Research perspectives.* Presentation to the American Academy of Audiology, San Antonio, TX.

Henry, J. A., Schechter, M. A., Nagler, S. M., & Fausti, S. A. (2002). Comparison of tinnitus masking and tinnitus retraining therapy. *Journal of American Academy of Audiology, 13,* 559–581.

Herdman, S. J. (1989). Exercise strategies for vestibular disorders. *Ear, Nose and Throat Journal, 68,* 961–964.

Herdman, S. J. (2000). Vestibular rehabilitation. *Contemporary perspectives in rehabilitation.* Philadelphia: F. A. Davis.

Hobeika, C. P. (1999). Equilibrium and balance in the elderly. *Ear, Nose, Throat Journal, 78*(8), 558–562.

Honrubia, V., & Hoffman, L. F. (1993). Practical anatomy and physiology of the vestibular sysytem. In G. P. Jacobson, C. W. Newman, & J. M. Kartush (Eds.), *Handbook of balance function testing.* San Diego, CA: Singular Publishing Group.

Jacobson, G. P., & Newman, C. W. (1990). The development of the dizziness handicap inventory. *Archives of Otolaryngology—Head Neck Surgery, 116,* 424–427.

Jastreboff, P. J. (2000). Tinnitus Habituation Therapy (THT) and Tinnitus Retraining Therapy (TRT). In R. S. Tyler (Ed.), *Tinnitus handbook* (pp. 357–376). San Diego, CA: Singular.

Jastreboff, P. J., & Jastreboff, M. M. (2000). Tinnitus Retraining Therapy (TRT) as a method for treatment of tinnitus and hyperacusis patients. *Journal of the American Academy of Audiology, 11,* 162–177.

Kaltenbach, J. A. (2000). Neurophysiologic mechanisms of tinnitus. *Journal of the American Academy of Audiology, 11,* 125–137.

Kirk, K. I., Pisoni, D. B., & Osberger, M. J. (1995). Lexical effects on spoken word recognition by pediatric cochlear implant users. *Ear & Hearing, 16,* 470–481.

Litovsky, R. Y., Parkinson, A., Arcaroli, J., Peters, R., Lake, J., Johnstone, P., & Gonquang, Y. (2004). Bilateral cochlear implants in adults and children. *Archives of Otolaryngology—Head and Neck Surgery, 130,* 648–655.

Luxford, W. M. (2001). Minimum speech test battery for postlingually deafened adult cochlear implant patients. *Archives of Otolaryngology—Head and Neck Surgery 124*(2), 125–126.

Meyer, T., Svirsky, M., Kirk, K., & Miyamoto, R. (1998). Improvements in speech perception by children with profound prelingual hearing loss: Effects of device, communication mode, and chronological age. *Journal of Speech Hearing Research, 41,* 846–858.

Miyamoto, R., Osberger, M., Robbins, A., Myres, W., & Kessler, K. (1993). Prelingually deafened children's performance with the Nucleus multichannel cochlear implant. *American Journal of Otology, 14,* 437–445.

Moogs, J. S., & Geers, A. E. (1990). *Early Speech Perception Test for Profoundly Hearing-Impaired Children.* St. Louis, MO: Central Institute for the Deaf.

Nashner, L. M. (1993). Practical biomechanics and physiology of balance. In G. P. Jacobson, C. W. Newman, & J. M. Kartush (Eds.), *Handbook of balance function testing.* St. Louis: Mosby-Yearbook.

National Association of the Deaf. (2001, January). NAD Position Statement on Cochlear Implants. NAD Broadcaster.

National Institute of Health (NIH). (1995, May 15–17). *Cochlear Implants in Adults and Children. National Institutes of Health, Consensus Development Conference Statement.*

Nevins, M. E., & Chute, P. M. (1996). *Children with cochlear implants in educational settings.* San Diego, CA: Singular Publishing Group.

Newell, P., Mitchell, P., Sindhussake, D., Golding, M., Wigney, D. Hartley, D., Smith, D., & Birtles, G. (2001). Tinnitus in older people: It is a widespread problem. *Hearing Journal, 54*(11), 14–18.

Newman, C. W., Jacobson, G. P., & Spitzer, J. B. (1996). Development of the tinnitus handicap inventory. *Archives of Otolaryngology—Head and Neck Surgery, 122,* 143–148.

Nikolopoulos, T. P., Archbold, S. M., & Gregory, S. (2005). Young deaf children with hearing aids or cochlear implants: Early assessment package for monitoring progress. *International Journal of Pediatric Otorhinolaryngology, 69*(2), 175–186.

Nilsson, M. J., Soli, S. D., & Gelnett, D. J. (1996). *Development of the Hearing in Noise Test for Children (HINT-C).* Los Angeles: House Ear Institute.

Nilsson, M. J., Soli, S. D., & Sullivan, J. A. (1994). Development of the Hearing in Noise Test for the measurement of speech reception in quiet and in noise. *Journal of the Acoustical Society of America, 95,* 1085–1099.

Nopp, P., Schleich, P., & D'Haese, P. (2004). Sound localization in bilateral users of MED-EL Combi 40/40+ cochlear implants. *Ear and Hearing, 25,* 205–214.

Owens, E., Kessler, D. K., Tellen, C. C., & Shubert, E. D. (1981). Minimal Auditory Test Battery (MAC) battery. *Hearing Aid Journal, 9,* 32.

Peterson, G., & Lehiste, I. (1962). Revised CNC lists for auditory tests. *Journal of Speech and Hearing Disorders, 27,* 62–70.

Robbins, A., Koch, D., Osberger, M., Zimmerman-Phillips, S., & Kishon-Rabin, L. (2004). Effect of age at cochlear implantation on auditory skill development in infants and toddlers. *Archives of Otolaryngology—Head and Neck Surgery, 130,* 570–574.

Robbins, A. M., Renshaw, J. J., & Berry, S. W. (1991). Evaluating meaningful auditory integration in profoundly hearing-impaired children. *American Journal of Otolaryngology, 12* (Suppl.), 144–150.

Rubinstein, J. T., Parkenson, W. S., Tyler, R. S., & Gantz, B. J. (1999). Residual speech recognition and cochlear implant performance: Effects of implantation criteria. *American Journal of Otology, 20,* 445–452.

Ruth, R. A., & Hamill-Ruth, R. (2001). A multidisciplinary approach to management of tinnitus and hyperacusis. *Hearing Journal, 54*(11), 26–32.

Salvi, R. J., Lockwood, A. H., & Burkard, R. F. (2000). Neural plasticity and tinnitus. In R. S. Tyler (Ed.), *Tinnitus handbook.* San Diego, CA: Singular.

Seeber, B. U., Baumann, U., & Fastl, H. (2004). Localization ability with bimodal hearing aids and bilateral cochlear implants. *Journal of Acoustical Society of America, 116*(3), 1698–709.

Shepard, N. T., & Telian, S. A. (1995). Programmatic vestibular rehabilitation. *Archives of Otolaryngology—Head and Neck Surgery, 112,* 173–182.

Shepard, N. T., & Telian, S. A. (1996). *Practical management of the balance disorder patient.* San Diego, CA: Singular Publishing Group.

Shepard, N. T., Telian, S. A., Smith-Wheelock, M., & Raj, A. (1993). Vestibular and balance rehabilitation therapy. *Annals of Otology, Rhinology, & Laryngology, 102*(3), 198–205.

Silverman, S. R., & Hirsh, I. J. (1955). Problems related to the use of speech in clinical audiometry. *Annals of Otology, Rhinology, & Laryngology, 64,* 1234–1244.

Smith-Wheelock, M., Shepard, N. T., & Telian, S. A. (1991). Physical therapy program for vestibular rehabilitation. *American Journal of Otology, 13*(3), 224–225.

Sweetow, R. W. (2000). Cognitive-behavior modification. In R. S. Tyler (Ed.), *Tinnitus handbook* (pp. 297–311). San Diego, CA: Singular Publishing Group.

Sweetow, R. W. (2003). *Tinnitus patient management.* Presentation to the American Academy of Audiology, San Antonio, TX.

Sweetow, R. W., & Levy, M. C. (1990). Tinnitus severity scaling for diagnostic/therapeutic usage. *Hearing Instrument, 41,* 20–21.

Tillman, T. W., & Carhart, R. (1966). An expanded test for speech discrimination utilizing CNC monosyllabic words. Northwestern University test No. 6. Brooks Air Force Base, TX: USAF School of Aerospace Medicine Technical Report.

Tyler, R. S., & Bergan, C. J. (2001). Tinnitus retraining therapy: A modified approach. *Hearing Journal, 54*(11), 36–42.

van Hoesel, R. J. (2004). Exploring the benefits of bilateral cochlear implants. *Audiologic Neurootology, 9*(4), 234–246.

van Hoesel, R. J., & Tyler, R. S. (2003). Speech perception, localization, and lateralization with bilateral cochlear implants. *Journal of Acoustical Society of America, 113*(3), 1617–1630.

Vernon, J. A. (1998). Introduction. In J. A. Vernon (Ed.), *Tinnitus treatment and relief.* Boston: Allyn and Bacon.

Vernon, J. A., & Meikle, M. B. (2000). Tinnitus masking. In R. S. Tyler (Ed.), *Tinnitus handbook.* San Diego, CA: Singular Publishing Group.

Waltzman, S. B., & Cohen, N. L. (1998). Cochlear implantation in children younger than 2 years old. *American Journal of Otology, 19,* 1083–1087.

Wayner, D. S., & Abrahamson, J. E. (1998). *Learning to hear again with a cochlear implant: An audiologic rehabilitation curriculum guide.* Austin, TX: Hear Again.

Wilson, B. S. (2000). Cochlear implant technology. In J. K. Niparko et al. (Eds.), *Cochlear implants: Principles and practices.* Philadelphia: Lippincott, Williams & Wilkins.

Wilson, P. H., Henry, J., Bowen, M., & Haralambous, G. (1991). Tinnitus reaction questionnaire: Psychometric properties of a measure of distress associated with tinnitus. *Journal of Speech Hearing Research, 34,* 197–201.

Zimmerman-Phillips, S., Robbins, A. M., & Osberger, M. J. (2001). *Infant-Toddler Meaningful Integration Scale.* Sylmar, CA: Advanced Bionics Corp.

CHAPTER 4

Auditory Stimuli in Communication

Michael A. Nerbonne
Ronald L. Schow

CONTENTS

■ INTRODUCTION

The importance that communication plays in our lives cannot be overstated. Communication can take a variety of forms and involves one or more of our sensory modalities. The form of communication most often used to express oneself, oral communication, involves utilization of speech. This creates an extraordinary dependence on the sense of hearing in order to receive and perceive accurately the complex network of auditory stimuli that comprise speech. The sense of hearing, therefore, is crucial to the process of oral (verbal) communication.

The onset of a significant auditory impairment in an individual can seriously impede the ability to communicate. Although a hearing loss may trigger other difficulties of a psychosocial, educational, or vocational nature, the inability of the person with hearing impairment to communicate normally serves as a fundamental cause of these other problems. Based on the critical role of audition in communication, audiologic rehabilitation represents an extremely important process whereby an individual's diminished ability to communicate as the result of a hearing loss can, it is hoped, be sharpened and improved. One area of audiologic rehabilitation that has traditionally been included in this process is often referred to as auditory training. This procedure generally involves an attempt to assist the child or adult with a hearing impairment in maximizing the use of whatever degree of residual hearing remains.

This chapter will provide information regarding auditory training with patients with hearing impairment, including objectives and applications, assessment of auditory skills prior to therapy, and exposure to some of the past and present approaches to providing auditory training. Because of the conviction that the professional providing auditory training must be familiar with the basic aspects of oral communication, information is also provided about the oral communication process. This includes the introduction of a communication model, information regarding auditory perception and the acoustics of speech, and a discussion of the possible effects of hearing loss on speech perception.

■ A COMMUNICATION MODEL

Although a portion of the communication that normally takes place between individuals is nonverbal, we remain heavily dependent on our ability to receive and interpret auditory stimuli presented during oral communication. Successful oral communication involves a number of key components that deserve elaboration so that the reader may gain an appreciation of the basic process. All oral communication must originate with a *source* or *speaker* who has both a purpose for engaging in communication and the ability to properly encode and articulate the thought to be conveyed. The actual thought to be expressed is termed the *message*. The message is made up of auditory stimuli organized in meaningful linguistic units. Visual and tactile cues are also provided by the speaker in conjunction with the production of the auditory message. Another critical component of the process is the auditory *feedback* provided to the speaker while producing speech, which then provides an opportunity for any needed adjustments or corrections to occur. The communication situation in which the message is conveyed is referred to as the *environment*. Factors associated with the environment, such as the presence of competing background noise, can drastically alter the amount and quality of the communication that takes place. The final major component of the communication process is the *receiver* or *listener*, who is charged with the responsibility of receiving and properly decoding and interpreting the speaker's intended thought. The listener also provides additional feedback to the speaker about how the message is being received.

These basic components of the oral communication process and their sequence are found in Figure 4.1. All the major components are equally important in ac-

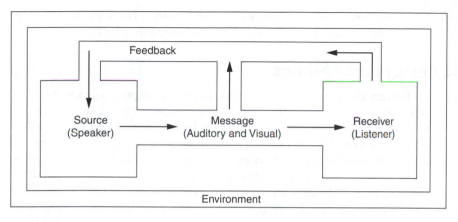

FIGURE 4.1

A simple model of the oral, or verbal, communication process.

complishing the desired end—communication. Disruption or elimination of any one part may result in partial or complete failure of the communication process. Proper application of this communication model is of concern to us throughout the chapter and the entire book.

■ AUDITORY PERCEPTION

Our ability to communicate verbally with others depends to a great extent on the quality of our auditory perception of the various segmental (individual speech sounds) and suprasegmental (rate, rhythm, intonation) elements that comprise speech. The following sections will focus on the basic aspects of auditory perception; the intensity, frequency, and duration components of speech; and transitional cues. The impact of hearing loss on speech perception is also discussed.

Development of Auditory Skills

It is both important and amazing to realize that the unborn infant possesses a functional auditory system that allows the child to begin perceiving auditory stimuli several weeks prior to birth. This is followed by further development and refinement in the neonate's auditory-processing skills in the days and weeks immediately following birth. As a result, the newborn infant not only is capable of detecting auditory stimuli, but also can make gross discriminations between various auditory signals on the basis of frequency and intensity parameters. This process of selective listening is extended to speech stimuli within a few weeks following birth. The rather rapid emergence of auditory skills, as described by Northern and Downs (2002), is crucial for the development of speech processing abilities, as well as the emergence of speech and language in the infant. Without the benefit of a normal-functioning auditory system and extensive exposure to auditory stimuli, however, the development of auditory and speech–language skills may be seriously affected.

Basic Perception Abilities

Detection simply involves knowing that a sound is present, whereas *discrimination* is the ability to distinguish when two separate sounds are different.

Although the human auditory system has sophisticated perceptual capabilities, it is limited, to some extent, in terms of the signals it can process. Optimally, the normal human ear is capable of perceiving auditory signals comprising frequencies ranging from about 20 to 20,000 Hz. Stimuli made up entirely of frequencies below and above these limits cannot be detected. Intensity limits, as shown in Figure 4.2, vary as a function of the frequency of the auditory stimulus. The maximum range of intensity we are capable of processing occurs at 3000 to 4000 Hz and varies from about 0 to approximately 130 to 140 dB SPL. Signals with intensity of less than 0 dB SPL are generally not perceived; in contrast, signals in excess of 130 to 140 dB SPL produce the sensations of feeling and pain rather than hearing.

In addition to the detection of acoustic signals, the human ear is also able to discriminate different stimuli on the basis of only minor differences in their acoustical properties. Our ability to discriminate changes in the frequency, intensity, or duration of a signal is influenced by the magnitude of each of the other factors. Stevens and Davis (1938) estimated that the normal ear is capable of perceiving approximately 340,000 distinguishable tones within the audible range of hearing. This total number was based only on frequency and intensity variations of the stimuli, and it suggests that our auditory system possesses amazing discrimination powers.

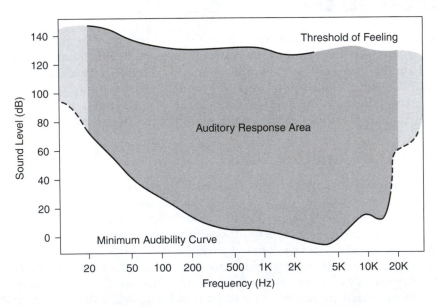

FIGURE 4.2

The auditory response area for persons with normal hearing.

Source: Durrant, J. D., & Lovrinic, J. H. (1995). *Bases of Hearing Science* (3rd ed.). Baltimore: Williams & Wilkins. Reprinted by permission.

Acoustics of Speech

Knowledge about the acoustical properties of speech is important for understanding how speech is perceived. Therefore, basic information relevant to this process will be covered in the following sections.

INTENSITY PARAMETERS OF SPEECH. The normal human ear is capable of processing signals within an intensity range approaching 130 dB; however, the range of intensity normally found in speech is relatively small. The average intensity of speech, when measured at a distance of approximately 1 meter from the speaker, approximates 65 dB SPL. This corresponds to a value of about 45 dB HL when expressed audiometrically. The average shout will approach 85 dB SPL (65 dB HL), and faint speech occurs at about 45 dB SPL (25 dB HL). Thus, a potential range of about 40 dB exists between the average intensities found, with the softest and loudest speech that we are exposed to in common communication situations. Factors such as distance between the speaker and listener can influence the intensity levels for a given communication situation.

Considerable variability also exists in the acoustical energy normally associated with individual speech sounds. Table 4.1 lists the relative phonetic powers of the phonemes, as reported by Fletcher (1953). As illustrated, the most powerful phoneme, /ɔ/, possesses an average of about 680 times as much energy as the weakest phoneme, /θ/, representing an average overall difference in intensity between the two speech sounds of approximately 28 dB. Since a considerable amount of variability also exists in the intensity of individual voices, Fletcher estimated that, collectively, different speakers may produce variations in the intensity of these two phonemes as great as 56 dB. The relative power of vowels, according to Fletcher, is significantly greater than that of consonants, with the weakest vowel, /i/, having more energy than the most powerful consonant. Further, typical male speakers produce speech with an overall intensity that is about 3 dB greater than that of female speakers.

TABLE 4.1

Relative Phonetic Power of Speech Sounds as Produced by an Average Speaker

ɔ	680	l	100	t	15
ɑ	600	ʃ	80	g	15
ʌ	510	ŋ	73	k	13
æ	490	m	52	v	12
ʊ	460	tʃ	42	ð	11
ɛ	350	n	36	b	7
u	310	dʒ	23	d	7
ɪ	260	ʒ	20	p	6
i	220	z	16	f	5
r	210	s	16	θ	1

Source: Fletcher, H. (1953). *Speech and Hearing in Communication.* Princeton, NJ: D. VanNostrand.

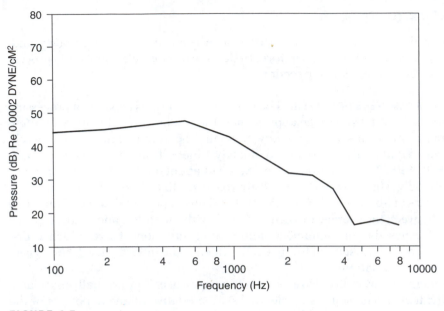

FIGURE 4.3

Long-interval acoustic spectrum of male voices. Measurement made with micro-phone 18 inches from speaker's lips.

Source: Miller, G. A. (1951). *Language and Communication* (p. 87). New York: McGraw-Hill.

FREQUENCY PARAMETERS OF SPEECH. The overall spectrum of speech, as seen in Figure 4.3, is composed of acoustical energy from approximately 50 to 10,000 Hz (Denes & Pinson, 1993). Closer examination of this figure also reveals that the greatest amount of energy found in speech generally is associated with frequencies below 1000 Hz. Above this frequency region, the energy of speech decreases at about a 9 dB/octave rate. The concentration of energy in the lower frequencies can be largely attributed to the fundamental frequency of the adult human voice (males, 130 Hz; females, 260 Hz), and the high intensity and spectral characteristics associated with the production of vowels. As shown in Figure 4.3, the greatest energy for male speech is around 500 Hz. This is due to resonance in the vocal tract rather than just fundamental frequency. It should be noted that the fundamental frequency of children is substantially higher than that of adults, around 400 Hz (Hegde, 1995). As a result, the major energy concentration for this age group occurs higher on the frequency scale than for adults.

A key aspect of speech production and perception is the information associated with the segmental elements of speech. The segmental components consist of the numerous features associated with the individual vowel and consonant phonemes of the language. The vowels in English are composed mainly of low- and mid-frequency energy and, as indicated earlier, contribute most of the acoustic power in speech. Specifically, the frequency spectrum of each vowel contains at least two or three areas of energy concentration that result from the resonances that occur in the vocal tract during phonation. These points of peak amplitude are referred to as *formants,* and their location and pattern on the frequency continuum are unique for each vowel. Figure

Formant refers to a band of frequencies that are resonated, or boosted in energy, by the vocal tract.

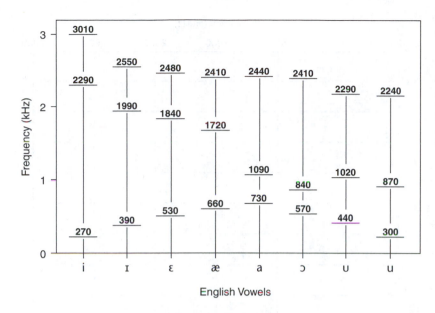

FIGURE 4.4

Mean values of formant frequencies of vowels of American English for adult males.

Source: Peterson, G. E., & Barney, H. L. (1952). Control methods used in the study of the vowels. *Journal of the Acoustical Society of America, 32,* 693–703.

4.4 illustrates the approximate location of the major formants associated with the vowels, as spoken by adult males. Formants provide important acoustic cues for the identification of vowels. However, it is important to note that even though each of the vowels has several formants, we need only hear the first two or three to be able to perceive accurately the vowel spoken (Peterson & Barney, 1952).

The consonants in English display a broader high-frequency spectral composition than do vowels. This is particularly true for those consonants for which voicing is not utilized and whose production involves substantial constriction of the articulators. Although they contain relatively little overall energy, or intensity, when compared with vowels, consonants are extremely important in determining the intelligibility of speech. Consequently, accurate perception of consonants is vital.

Figure 4.5 contains estimates of the combined intensity and frequency values generally associated with the individual speech sounds in English. Specifically, the vertical axis presents the intensity levels in dB HL of the major components of each sound (if a particular sound has more than one major frequency component, each is noted by the same phonetic symbol), while the horizontal axis expresses the general frequency region associated with each speech sound. A close inspection of this figure discloses, as indicated earlier, that the vowels can generally be characterized as having considerable acoustic energy, for the most part confined to the low- and mid-frequency range. On the other hand, the consonants demonstrate decidedly less intensity overall and a much more diffuse frequency distribution as a group. The voiced consonants generally possess a greater amount of low- and mid-frequency energy, while the unvoiced consonants are made up of mid- and high frequencies. All consonants appear in the upper portion of the figure, reflecting their weaker intensity values.

In addition to the spectral properties associated with each of the consonants, it is important to identify the frequency characteristics related to the distinctive features associated with the production of these phonemes. Miller and Nicely's (1955)

FIGURE 4.5

Intensity and frequency distribution of speech sounds in the English language. The values given should be considered only approximations, and are based on data reported by Fletcher (1953) and Ling and Ling (1978). Sounds with more than one major component appear in more than one location in the figure.

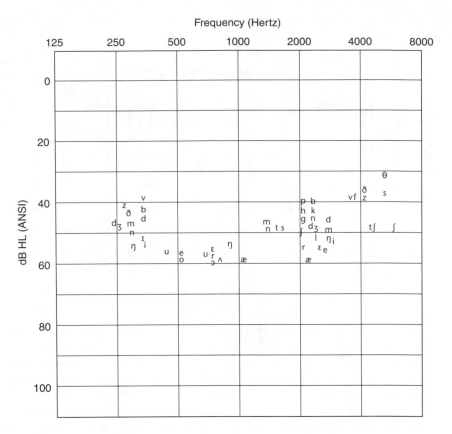

The segmental components of speech are the features associated with the individual speech sounds. The suprasegmental components (rhythm and prosody, pitch, rate) are overall features of speech that are superimposed on phonemes and words.

classification system includes five features: voicing, nasality, affrication, duration, and place of articulation. The voiced–voiceless distinction, as well as cues for nasality and affrication, are primarily carried by low-frequency energy. Information about place of articulation, on the other hand, is contained in the higher frequencies. Table 4.2 categorizes each consonant phoneme by its place and manner of articulation and voicing features.

Another major component of speech is the suprasegmentals. The suprasegmental aspects are those features that are present in speech but are not confined to any single segment or phonemic element. Suprasegmental features, such as intonation, rhythm, stress, and pitch, are superimposed throughout speech as overall features. The suprasegmentals convey important information for speech perception, and this information is conveyed primarily in the low frequencies through acoustic cues associated with the fundamental frequency and other related aspects of speech.

TEMPORAL PARAMETERS OF SPEECH. The duration of individual speech sounds in our language covers a range from about 30 to 300 msec (Fletcher, 1953; Lehiste, 1976). A number of factors can significantly influence the duration of a given phoneme, making the direct comparison of duration among phonemes difficult. However, vowels generally have a longer duration than consonants. Fletcher (1953) considered vowels to have average durations of between 130 and 360 msec, while

---

TABLE 4.2

Categorizing Consonants on the Basis of Manner and Place of Articulation and Voicing

MANNER OF ARTICULATION	PLACE OF ARTICULATION						
	Bilabial	Labiodental	Linguadental	Alveolar	Palatal	Velar	Glottal
Plosives or Stops	p b			t d		k g	
Fricatives		f v	θ ð	s z	ʃ ʒ		h
Affricates					ʧ ʤ		
Nasal	m			n		ŋ	
Liquid				l,r			
Glide	w					j	

Note: Voiceless consonants are listed first, with voiced consonants underneath.

the duration of consonants ranges from 20 to 150 msec. In spite of variations in absolute durational properties, individual phoneme duration does contribute toward speech perception. For instance, Minifie (1973) pointed out that the duration of stop consonants (examples: /p/ and /b/) varies systematically in a vowel-consonant-vowel context, with correct perception of the speech sound depending, to a degree, on the durational property of the phoneme produced.

As we all know, the overall rate of speech differs considerably from speaker to speaker. The research of Goldman-Eisler, as discussed by Lehiste (1970), demonstrates that the average rate of speech used during connected discourse ranges from about 4.4 to 5.9 syllables per second. The normal rate of speech, as expressed in phoneme output, averages about 12 phonemes per second, but can approach 20 phonemes when the speaker is excited (MacKay, 1987). Thus, the articulatory process is swift and capable of producing a flood of speech sounds and words that must be processed as effectively by the receiver, or listener, as they were produced by the speaker. Both of these are challenging tasks!

TRANSITIONAL CUES. The acoustic properties of a given phoneme spoken in isolation are altered significantly when the phoneme is produced with other phonemes in conversational speech. In conversational speech the dynamic movements of the articulators in the production of adjacent phonemes produce acoustical by-products, termed *transitional cues*. These cues make up a large portion of the total speech signal and are very important in the perception of speech, since they contain valuable information related to individual phoneme perception, especially for diphthongs and consonants.

For example, the second and third formants of vowels often contain transitions in frequency produced by the flowing movement of the articulators that signal the

Transitional cues result from the influences of coarticulation of individual speech sounds when combined into words, phrases, and so on.

presence of particular consonants that immediately follow. These formant transitions occur as the vocal resonances shift during articulation of vowels and consonants, which are combined in speech. Likewise, the durational aspects of vowels in connected speech can be altered to convey information regarding the phoneme to follow. For example, a voiced consonant in the final position is often accompanied by increased duration of the vowel immediately before it. The prolonged vowel duration contributes to our perception of voicing in the consonant that follows. This is an example of why formant transitional cues are a vital part of the speech signal and are quite important for speech perception.

Speech Perception and Comprehension

Our discussion has emphasized the segmental and suprasegmental aspects that constitute speech. The organization and production of these crucial elements into a meaningful oral message by the speaker and the accurate reception of this dynamic signal by the listener represent a highly complex, sophisticated process. However, mere reception of the segmented and suprasegmental elements of speech by a listener does not ensure proper perception of the message. Perception of speech implies understanding and comprehension, and the reception of speech by the auditory mechanism is only a first step in its perception.

In its most basic form, the perception of speech may be thought of as involving a number of important components. Among these are the following:

Detection. This basic aspect of auditory perception simply involves being aware of sound. Our ability to detect speech is influenced by our hearing acuity and the intensity level of the speech signal.

Discrimination. Speech discrimination refers to the ability to distinguish among the individual speech stimuli (phonemes, syllables, etc.) of our language.

Identification. The ability to identify or label what one has heard by pointing to, or naming.

Attention. A fundamental ingredient in the perception of speech relates to attending to or focusing on the speaker and the message being conveyed. The degree and quality of the listener's attention will influence how well speech is perceived.

Memory. A key component in speech perception is the ability to retain or store verbal information for relatively brief periods or, in some instances, extended lengths of time. Memory is also fundamental to other components of speech perception and enables us to combine individual speech units for the purpose of deriving meaning from an entire verbal message, rather than from each individual unit of the message.

Closure. The perceived speech elements must be brought together into a meaningful whole. This process, termed closure, helps a person to recognize speech even when some cues are absent, as with hearing loss.

Comprehension. Full perception and understanding of the meaning of an auditory message.

Our task in audiologic rehabilitation should be to take into consideration what is currently known concerning speech perception as we work with individuals with hearing impairments.

Speech Perception and Hearing Loss

Our success in processing speech is closely related to a number of important factors, and some of these will be discussed in the next section.

PHYSICAL PROPERTIES. Information concerning the physical properties of speech is most relevant when considering the relationship between the perception of speech and hearing loss, for the degree of our success in processing speech appears closely related to our ability to receive the coded acoustical information that makes up the signal.

The normal ear is well equipped to receive and process speech in most situations. Since speech is normally presented at average intensity levels of around 45 dB HL, it is well within the sensitivity range of the normal human ear. Also, although we are capable of hearing auditory signals ranging in frequency from about 20 to 20,000 Hz, only a portion of the entire range is required for the reception of speech, since speech contains energy from roughly 50 to 10,000 Hz. Consequently, in most listening conditions, those with normal hearing will have no difficulty in adequately hearing the speech sounds found in oral communication.

The same does not hold true for persons with hearing impairment. No longer are the intensity and frequency ranges of the impaired ear always sufficient to provide total perception of the speech signal. One or both of these stimulus parameters may be limited such that it becomes difficult to hear specific speech sounds adequately for identification purposes. For example, a person with 50 dB thresholds from 2000 to 8000 Hz would have considerable difficulty perceiving the phonemes with spectral compositions that primarily involve those higher frequencies. The information in Figure 4.5 regarding the relative frequency and intensity characteristics of individual speech sounds as spoken at a typical conversation level helps in understanding why this occurs.

While factors such as type of hearing loss and test materials can influence the outcome of investigations concerning hearing loss and the perception of phonemes, some general patterns of speech-perception difficulties have been observed for persons with hearing loss. For instance, most hearing-impaired listeners experience only minimal difficulty in vowel perception (Owens, Benedict, & Schubert, 1971). Specifically, in their research the vowel phonemes /ɛ/ and /o/ were found to have the highest probability of error. Only when the degree of impairment is severe to profound does the perception of vowels become significantly altered (Erber, 1979). Consonant perception, however, presents a far more difficult listening task for those with hearing impairment. Owens (1978) found phonemes such as /s/, /p/, /k/, /d/, and /θ/ to be among the most frequently missed by adults with sensorineural hearing loss. He also found misperceptions to be more frequent for phonemes in the final position of words than in the initial position. The most common errors in consonant phoneme perception occur with the place of articulation feature, followed by manner of articulation. Errors in the perception of nasality and voice among consonants are generally far less frequent.

Owens and his colleagues conducted a series of investigations regarding the perception of consonants. In one such study Owens, Benedict, & Shubert (1972) examined the relationship between the configuration of the audiogram and the specific consonant perceptual errors made by a group of hearing-impaired individuals. The /s/, /ʃ/, /tʃ/, /dʒ/ and the /t/ and /θ/ in the initial position only were found to be difficult for listeners with sloping configurations on the audiogram. The authors noted that these phonemes became increasingly difficult to hear accurately as the steepness of the sloping high-frequency hearing loss increased. Correct recognition of /s/ and the initial /t/ and /θ/ were found to be closely related to hearing sensitivity above 2000 Hz, while perception of /ʃ/, /tʃ/, and /dʒ/ was very dependent on sensitivity between 1000 and 2000 Hz. These findings point out the crucial role which hearing in this frequency region plays in the perception of several consonant phonemes. A similar study by Sher and Owens (1974) with listeners having high-frequency impairments confirmed that individuals with normal hearing to 2000 Hz and a sharp-sloping sensitivity loss for frequencies above that experience difficulty in adequately hearing a number of consonant phonemes. These authors pointed out that information concerning specific phoneme errors is useful in establishing audiologic rehabilitation strategies for persons with hearing losses of this type.

As can be seen, the actual overall degree of difficulty in speech perception imposed on an individual is related to the intensity and frequency features of the hearing loss found on the conventional audiogram. However, difficulty with speech perception can also be influenced by other related variables, which will be discussed elsewhere in this chapter and throughout the text. Therefore, while the audiogram usually is our most useful single predictor of a person's speech perception abilities, other factors to be discussed in the next section must be considered as well.

The redundancy of speech relates to its predictability; the greater the redundancy, the better the odds will be that a listener can guess what was said, even when he or she did not hear the entire message.

REDUNDANCY AND NOISE. The perception of speech is a highly complex process that involves more than the acoustics of speech or the hearing abilities of the listener, even though these are important variables, to be sure. Ultimately, for oral communication to be successful, sufficient information must be present in the message of interest for it to be perceived. The amount of information available for a given communication situation is closely associated with the concepts of redundancy and noise.

Conversational speech generally can be described as being highly redundant. That is, it contains information from a variety of sources that is available for a listener to use in comprehending a message, even though portions of the communication may not have been heard. The degree of redundance in oral communication varies from one expression to the next, so the extent to which a listener can predict what was said will also vary. Basically, the more redundant a message, the more readily it can be perceived by the listener, especially in difficult listening situations. A number of factors present in a given communication situation can influence the amount of redundancy present, and Table 4.3 provides a list of some of these.

Among the many factors associated with the redundancy, or predictability, found in conversational speech for the listener to use for perception are syntactic, semantic, and situational constraints (see Table 4.4). Syntactic, or structural, constraints relate to the predictable manner in which linguistic units are chained to-

TABLE 4.3

A Partial List of Factors That Can Influence the Amount of Redundancy in Speech

Within the speaker	Compliance with the rules of the language
	Use of appropriate articulation, intonation, stress
	Size and appropriateness of the vocabulary used to convey the message
Within the message	Number of syllables, words, etc.
	Amount of context
	Frequency composition of the speech signal
	Intensity of the speech signal
Within the communication environment	Amount of acoustic noise
	Degree of reverberation
	Number of situational cues present that are related to the message
Within the listener	Familiarity with the rules of the language
	Familiarity with the vocabulary of the message
	Knowledge of the topic of conversation
	Hearing abilities

Source: Adapted from Sanders (1971).

TABLE 4.4

Examples of Linguistic Constraints Available to Enhance Speech Perception

Syntactic constraints: Refer to the fact that every language is governed by a set of grammatical rules that specifies the relationship between words used to communicate. For example, adjectives may be used to qualify nouns (as in "the *blue* shoes"); adjectives are not used to qualify verbs (as in "he *blue* ran").

Semantic constraints: Refer to the fact that the words used in a sentence are usually related to each other in a meaningful way. For example, although the sentence "Put the salt on the cloud" is syntactically correct; semantically, it is highly improbable.

Situational constraints: Refer to the fact that language usually takes place within a physical and social context. Generally, the use of language bears some relationship with the context in which it is used. For example, in a stadium, during a football game, it is more likely that the topic of discussion will center around sports-related activities than around religious beliefs and values.

Source: Adapted from Gagne & Jennings (2000).

gether according to the rules associated with acceptable English. The selection and use of phonemes and words in an utterance are strongly influenced by these rules, making it easier for the listener to predict what is to follow after having heard only the initial portion of the sentence. Such syntactic clues can be used in conjunction with another factor related to redundancy, namely semantic constraints, which allow the listener to predict the type of vocabulary and expressions to be used based

TABLE 4.5	
Some Potential Sources of Noise in Oral Communication	
Within the speaker	Poor syntax
	Abnormal articulation
	Improper stress or inflection
Within the communication environment	Abnormal lighting
	Competing or distracting visual stimuli
	Competing or distracting auditory stimuli
	Reverberation
Within the listener	Lack of familiarity with the rules of the language
	Inability to identify the topic of the message
	Poor listening skills

Source: Adapted from Sanders (1971).

on the general semantic content of the expression. When the topic of conversation is food, for example, the listener can expect to hear a rather restricted range of vocabulary peculiar to that particular topic. Use of this small range of words will increase the redundancy of the message, making it easier to predict what is said. Situational constraints also create redundancy. Our conversational partner, the location of the conversation, the time of day it takes place, and other similar factors all influence what we say and how we say it, which also can make conversational speech more predictable. All these types of constraints, along with other factors listed in Table 4.3, collectively produce the redundancy that makes the perception of speech easier for us all.

Noise in oral communication refers to a host of factors that can actually reduce the amount of information present for the listener to use. In this context, "noise" refers to a variety of variables that can be counterproductive to communication, not just competing auditory noise. Table 4.5 provides a partial list of the potential sources of noise associated with oral communication with which the listener must contend. Each of these factors may reduce the amount of information in a spoken message, thus reducing the amount of redundancy, or predictability, which is available for the listener to use in perceiving speech.

Thus, the degree of information available for the listener to use in perceiving a message is influenced in a positive or negative manner by a number of related variables that are part of oral communication. For the listener, particularly one with hearing impairment, the importance of each of these variables to the process of speech perception cannot be overstated.

■ THE AUDITORY TRAINING PROCESS

Traditionally, auditory training has been considered a major component of the audiologic rehabilitation process. Thus, its potential in assisting those with hearing loss has been expressed in major textbooks within the field of audiology, both in the past (Davis & Hardick, 1981; Davis & Silverman, 1960; Oyer, 1966) and recently (Alpiner & McCarthy, 2000; Tye-Murray, 2004).

The intent of the next major section of this chapter is to familiarize the reader with both the traditional and the current forms of auditory training and how they fit into the entire audiologic rehabilitation process.

Definition and Application of Auditory Training

Numerous attempts have been made to define auditory training in the past. Though similar in some respects, these definitions vary considerably according to the orientation of the definer and special considerations dictated by factors associated with hearing loss, such as its degree and time of onset.

Probably the most commonly referred to definition of auditory training is attributed to Carhart (1960), who considered auditory training a process of teaching the child or adult with hearing impairment to take full advantage of available auditory clues. As a result, Carhart recommended an emphasis in therapy on developing an awareness of sound, gross discrimination of nonverbal stimuli, and gross and fine discrimination of speech.

Later, in discussing the use of auditory training with children, Erber (1982) described it as "the creation of special communication conditions in which teachers and audiologists help hearing-impaired children acquire many of the auditory perception abilities that normally hearing children acquire naturally without their intervention" (p. 1). Erber stated further that "Our intent is to help the hearing-impaired child apply his or her impaired auditory sense to the fullest capacity in language communication, regardless of the degree of damage to the auditory system. Usually progress is achieved through careful application of amplification devices and through special teaching techniques" (p. 29).

The hearing abilities that a person with hearing loss has left are often referred to as residual hearing.

When considering auditory training for adults, two general objectives are usually relevant: (1) learning to maximize the use of auditory and other related cues available for the perception of speech and (2) adjustment and orientation to facilitate the optimum use of amplification, including cochlear implants and tactile devices.

Inherent in the various views of auditory training, as well as those of other professionals in audiologic rehabilitation, is the notion that persons with hearing impairment can be trained to maximize the use of whatever amount of hearing they possess. The ultimate aim of auditory training is, therefore, to achieve maximum communication potential by developing the auditory sensory channel to its fullest. In a sense, auditory training is often designed to improve one's listening skills, which will result in improved speech perception. Although the primary goal of auditory training is usually to maximize receptive communication abilities, it is important to point out that achieving this basic goal can result in other important accomplishments as well, including acquisition of more proficient speech and language skills, educational and vocational advancement, and successful psychosocial adjustment. As indicated earlier, if the communication skills of persons with hearing impairment can be improved, other areas of concern, such as educational progress, will be facilitated as well.

Early Efforts in Auditory Training

The earliest efforts in auditory training date back at least to the nineteenth century. Individuals in Europe used auditory training with the hearing impaired throughout the 1800s, with some success noted. Impressed with their accomplishments, Goldstein (1939) introduced a similar approach to auditory training in the United States in the late 1890s and early 1900s. Known as the Acoustic Method, this approach centered around systematic stimulation with individual speech sounds, syllables, words, and sentences to improve speech perception and to aid deaf persons in their own speech production. The Acoustic Method was utilized in a number of facilities throughout the country, including the Central Institute for the Deaf in St. Louis, Missouri, which Goldstein founded. Goldstein exerted a significant influence on the thinking of many professionals over the years regarding the potential of auditory training with persons with hearing impairment.

Until World War II, the primary focus of auditory training was its use with severely/profoundly deaf children in an effort to facilitate speech and language acquisition and increase their educational potential. However, the activities that occurred at VA audiology centers during World War II served to demonstrate on a large scale that adults with mild-to-severe hearing impairments could profit from auditory training as well. Led by Raymond Carhart, personnel in these centers developed and applied auditory training exercises with large numbers of adults, most with noise-induced hearing loss. Carhart (1960) later authored a book chapter that influenced the thinking of audiologists regarding auditory training with children and adults for years to come.

Raymond Carhart made many contributions to the profession of audiology and is considered by many to be the Father of Audiology.

CARHART. Carhart's approach to auditory training for prelingually impaired children was based on his belief that since listening skills are normally learned early in life, the child possessing a serious hearing loss at birth or soon after will not move through the normal developmental stages important in acquiring these skills. Likewise, when a hearing loss occurs in later childhood or in adulthood, some of the person's auditory skills may become impaired even though they were intact prior to the onset of the hearing loss. In each instance, Carhart believed that auditory training was warranted.

CHILDHOOD PROCEDURES. Carhart outlined four major steps or objectives involved in auditory training for children with prelingual deafness:

1. Development of awareness of sound
2. Development of gross discriminations
3. Development of broad discriminations among simple speech patterns
4. Development of finer discriminations for speech

Development of an awareness of auditory stimuli and the significance of sound involves having the child acknowledge the presence of sound and its importance in his or her world. The development of gross discrimination initially involves demonstrating with various noisemakers that sounds differ. Once the child can successfully discriminate grossly different sounds, he or she is exposed to finer types of discrimination tasks that include variation in the frequency, intensity, and durational properties of sound. When the child is able to recognize the presence of sound and can perceive gross differences with nonverbal stimuli, Carhart's approach calls for the introduction of activities directed toward learning gross discrimination for speech signals. The final phase consists of training the child to make fine discriminations of speech stimuli in connected discourse and integrating an increased vocabulary to enable him or her to follow connected speech in a more rapid and accurate fashion. Carhart also felt that the use of vision by the child should be encouraged in most auditory training activities.

ADULT PROCEDURES. Because adults who acquire a hearing loss later in life retain a portion of their original auditory skills, Carhart recommended that auditory training with adults focus on reeducating a skill diminished as a consequence of the hearing impairment. Initially, Carhart felt that it was important to establish "an attitude of critical listening" in the individual. This involves being attentive to the subtle differences among sounds and can involve a considerable amount of analytic drill work on the perception of phonemes that are difficult for the adult with hearing impairment to perceive. Lists of matched syllables and words that contain the troublesome phonemes, such as *she–fee, so–tho, met–let,* or *mash–math,* are read to the individual, who repeats them back. Such training should also include phrases and sentences, with the goal of developing as rapid and precise a recognition of the phonetic elements as is possible within the limitations imposed by the person's hearing loss. Speechreading combined with a person's hearing was also encouraged by Carhart during a portion of the auditory training sessions.

Because we often communicate under less than ideal listening circumstances, Carhart advocated that auditory training sessions for adults be conducted in three commonly encountered situations: (1) relatively intense background noise, (2) the presence of a competing speech signal, and (3) listening on the telephone. This emphasis on practice in speech perception under listening conditions with decreasing amounts of redundancy has been emphasized more recently by Sanders (1993) and numerous other audiologic rehabililationists.

According to Carhart, the use of hearing aids is vital in auditory training, and he recommended that they be utilized as early as possible in the auditory training program. These recommendations were consistent with Carhart's belief that systematic exposure to sound during auditory training was an ideal means of allowing a person to adequately adjust to hearing aids and assist in using them as optimally as possible.

■ CURRENT APPROACHES TO AUDITORY TRAINING

The basic intent of more recent methods of auditory training remains the same, that is, to maximize communication potential by developing to its fullest the auditory channel of the person with hearing impairment. This next section will discuss how this form of audiologic rehabilitation currently is being applied with the hearing impaired.

Candidacy for Auditory Training

In recent times, auditory training therapy has been utilized selectively with certain types of patients, but only occasionally with most others. Its most common use is with children with prelingual sensorineural hearing impairment, especially those with moderate to profound degrees of loss with congenital onset. Another targeted population for auditory training in recent times has been cochlear implant recipients, both children and adults. There is strong evidence that a structured program of listening training enhances the benefits derived from a cochlear implant. Although extensive auditory training typically is not utilized with hard of hearing adults, certain factors, such as exceptionally poor speech perception and/or a severe to profound degree of loss, may result in its application on a selective basis.

Assessment of Auditory Skills

An integral part of a comprehensive auditory training program is the assessment of individual auditory skills. Before, during, and at the conclusion of auditory training the clinician should attempt to evaluate the auditory abilities of the person with hearing impairment. Information of this nature is important for several reasons, including

1. Determining whether auditory training appears warranted.
2. Providing a basis for comparison with post-therapy performance, to assess how much improvement in auditory performance, particularly speech perception, has occurred.
3. Identifying specific areas of auditory perception to concentrate on in future auditory training.

The nature of the auditory testing that takes place will vary considerably depending upon a number of variables, such as the age of the client, his or her language skills, and the type and degree of the hearing loss. The clinician must exercise care in selecting appropriate test materials for the individual patient, particularly with regard to the language levels required for a given test. Actually, when testing speech perception performance via hearing or vision, a number of variables need to be kept in mind that can influence the degree of difficulty of the perceptual task. These include

that affect the degree of difficulty of the perceptual task

■ The nature of the perceptual task (detection, discrimination, identification, comprehension).
■ The use of either an open or closed set (e.g., multiple choice) response format.
■ The degree of context present (e.g., monosyllabics presented in isolation, or sentences).
■ The level of sophistication and the age level of the vocabulary used in the test (instructions and test items).
■ The signal-to-noise ratio present (figure–ground).

Manipulation of any one of these variables can make the test either easier or harder for an individual, and the clinician should be mindful of all this when selecting and administering tests. A variety of tests, both formal and informal, should be available for assessment purposes so that the particular needs of each individual can be met adequately.

EVALUATING CHILDREN. Both the degree and the sophistication of testing appropriate for young children are limited by their physical and cognitive development. Therefore, informal testing and observation are relied upon heavily with this age group. For the infant, the initial goal of assessment for auditory training purposes may not center on speech perception. Rather, an effort may be made to identify the extent to which auditory skills have emerged, such as gross discrimination and localization of a variety of stimuli. Once this information is known, a specific program for developing auditory skills, such as that described in Chapter 9, can be implemented in conjunction with therapy related to development of speech and language.

For older children, more formal, in-depth assessment of overall speech perception abilities generally is possible. Specifically, materials have been developed that require the child to respond in a prescribed manner to individual words or phonemes presented at a comfortable listening level. Some of the commonly used formal tests of this type that have been designed for assessing speech perception in children with hearing impairment include the following:

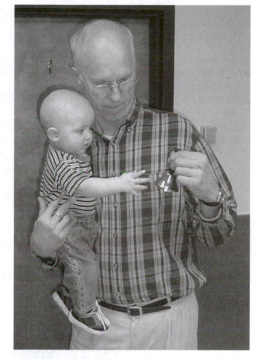

Informal assessment of auditory awareness/localization skills.

1. *Word Intelligibility by Picture Identification (WIPI) (Ross & Lerman, 1970).* The authors of the *WIPI* modified an existing test for children (Myatt & Landes, 1963) to include only vocabulary appropriate for children with hearing impairment. The *WIPI* includes four lists that each contain 25 monosyllabic words. The child provides a picture-pointing response in a closed-set format. According to the authors, the test is suitable for use with children with hearing loss and limited receptive and expressive language abilities.

2. *Northwestern University Children's Perception of Speech (NU-CHIPS) (Katz & Elliott, 1978).* This test consists of 50 monosyllabic nouns that have been scrambled to form four individual lists. Like the *WIPI*, the *NU-CHIPS* uses a response format that requires that the child point to the one picture from several options that best represents the test items. Because of the basic vocabulary included and the nonverbal response format, use of the *NU-CHIPS* with many children with hearing loss appears appropriate.

3. *Six Sound Test by Ling (1976, 1989).* Six isolated phonemes (/m/, /a/, /u/, /i/, /s/, and /ʃ/) are spoken to the child at a normal conversational level. Those with usable residual hearing up to 1000 Hz should be able to detect the vowels. Children with some residual hearing up to 2000 Hz should detect /ʃ/, and those with residual hearing up to 4000 Hz (not worse than 90 dB HL at 4000 Hz) should detect /s/.

Tests use either a closed-set or open-set format. A closed-set format for a test of speech perception involves presenting a test item (e.g., a word) and having the listener choose the correct response from a limited set of options (multiple choice). In an open-set format, the listener can respond with any word he or she feels is correct.

Additional test batteries are designed to assess varied aspects of auditory skills development in children. Examples include the following:

Figure–ground refers to the ability to perceive a target signal that is presented simultaneously with other competing signals.

1. *Test of Auditory Comprehension (TAC), developed through the Audiologic Services of the Los Angeles County Schools (Trammel, 1981).* Designed for children ages 4 to 12 years with moderate to profound hearing losses, the *TAC* is the evaluation part of a comprehensive auditory skills instructional plan. The instrument has 10 subtests that assess several areas of auditory perception, including speech discrimination, memory sequencing, figure–ground discrimination, and story comprehension. Results of TAC subtests are used to establish baseline performance and direction for the companion auditory training curriculum.

2. *Glendonald Auditory Screening Procedure (GASP), developed at the Glendonald Auditory School for the Deaf in Australia (Erber, 1982).* GASP is based on a model of auditory perception described in the next section of this chapter (see Figure 4.6). The basic test battery associated with *GASP* consists of three subtests of speech perception: ① phoneme detection, ② word identification, and ③ sentence comprehension. The *GASP* phoneme detection subtest is similar in format to the *Six Sound Test* developed by Ling (1976, 1989). According to Erber, the results from *GASP* can aid in planning auditory training because the child's performance on the subtests is predictive of other, related auditory tasks.

3. *Developmental Approach to Successful Listening (DASL) Test (Stout & Windle, 1994).* This comprehensive test of auditory skills evaluates numerous aspects

Response Task	Speech Stimulus					
	Speech Elements	Syllables	Words	Phrases	Sentences	Connected Discourse
Detection	1					
Discrimination						
Identification			2			
Comprehension					3	

FIGURE 4.6

An auditory stimulus–response matrix showing the three *GASP* subtests: Phoneme Detection (1), Word Identification (2), and Sentence (Question) Comprehension (3).

Source: Erber, N. (1982). *Auditory training.* Washington, DC: Alexander Graham Bell Association for the Deaf. Reprinted by permission.

of sound awareness, phonetic listening, and auditory comprehension. Children from 3 years of age can be evaluated with the *DASL Test,* and some normative information is available for children with varying degrees of hearing loss.

These tests all attempt to take into account the limitations of hearing-impaired youngsters' receptive vocabulary level and their ability to respond orally. However, the variability observed in the receptive and expressive communication skills of these children makes it unwise to draw any firm generalizations about the specific age range of children for whom any of these tests are suited. Vocabulary age rather than chronological age is a key consideration in selecting the appropriate test to use.

EVALUATING ADULTS. A number of formal tests of speech perception also are available for use with adults. Any of the traditional monosyllabic word lists, such as the *CID W-22s* (Hirsh et al., 1952) or the *Northwestern University Auditory Test No. 6* (Tillman & Carhart, 1966), may be employed to evaluate overall word-recognition abilities.

Other tests allow for more in-depth assessment of the perception of consonants, which can be especially difficult for persons with hearing impairment to perceive accurately. For example, Owens and Schubert (1977) produced a 100-item, multiple-choice consonant perception test called the *California Consonant Test (CCT).* Thirty-six of the test items assess consonant perception in the initial word position, while 64 items test perception in the final position. Each of the 100 items is presented to the listener in a closed-set, multiple-choice format, as shown in Figure 4.7. Research by Schwartz and Surr (1979) demonstrated that, compared to the *NU-6s,* the *CCT* is more sensitive to the speech recognition difficulties experienced by individuals with high-frequency hearing loss. Consequently, the *CCT* is often relied on in assessing the speech recognition abilities of adult patients.

Tests that employ sentence-type stimuli also can be informative. Kalikow, Stevens, and Elliott (1977) developed a test called *Speech Perception in Noise,* or *SPIN.* This test is unique in that it attempts to assess a listener's utilization of both linguistic and situational cues in the perception of speech. Sentence material is

> Word recognition testing typically involves presenting a 25- or 50-word list of monosyllabic words at a comfortable intensity level for the listener. A percent correct score is calculated.

ROBE _____	MAP _____	BAIL _____
RODE _____	MATCH _____	JAIL _____
ROSE _____	MATH _____	DALE _____
ROVE _____	MAT _____	GALE _____
LASS _____	DIES _____	LEAF _____
LAUGH _____	DIED _____	LEASE _____
LATCH _____	DIVE _____	LEACH _____
LASH _____	DINE _____	LEASH _____
FIN _____	PEAK _____	RAISE _____
PIN _____	PEACH _____	RAID _____
KIN _____	PEAT _____	RAGE _____
TIN _____	PEEP _____	RAVE _____

FIGURE 4.7

Examples of multiple-choice test items for the *California Consonant Test.*
Source: Owens & Schubert (1977).

presented against a background of speech babble, with the listener's task being to identify the final word in the sentence. Ten 50-item forms of *SPIN* have been generated, each version containing sentences with either high or low predictability relative to the final word in each sentence. Examples of each are shown in Table 4.6. Bilger, Rzcezkowski, Nuetzel, and Rabinowitz (1979) have revised the forms to make them more equivalent to each other. The SPIN test can provide important information concerning how effectively a given listener makes use of contextual information in the perception of speech, in addition to providing insight regarding how the listener perceives the acoustical properties of speech.

The *Central Institute for the Deaf (CID) Everyday Speech Sentences* (Davis & Silverman, 1978) have been used extensively to evaluate a listener's ability to perceive connected discourse. They consist of ten 10-sentence sets, as shown in Table 4.7. The sentences vary in length and form and possess several characteristics associated with typical conversation.

Results of these tests, as well as others, should provide the clinician with specific information concerning a client's consonant perception in a word and/or sentence context, as well as the ability to comprehend speech in sentence form.

Additional information about speech perception can be gained by introducing competing noise to the test situation and varying the degree of redundancy in the

TABLE 4.6

Examples of Low- and High-Predictability Sentences from the *SPIN* Test

SENTENCE	LEVEL OF PREDICTABILITY
The honey bees swarmed round the *hive*.	High
The girl knows about the *swamp*.	Low
The cushion was filled with *foam*.	High
He had considered the *robe*.	Low

Source: Kalikow, Stevens, & Elliott (1977).

TABLE 4.7

Examples of a 10-Sentence Set of *CID Everyday Speech Sentences*

1. *It's time* to go.
2. If you *don't want these old magazines, throw them out.*
3. *Do* you *want to wash up?*
4. It's a *real dark night so watch your driving.*
5. *I'll carry* the *package* for *you.*
6. Did *you forget* to *shut off* the *water?*
7. *Fishing* in a *mountain stream* is my *idea* of a *good time.*
8. *Fathers spend* more *time* with their *children than* they *used to.*
9. *Be careful not to break your glasses!*
10. *I'm sorry.*

Source: Davis & Silverman (1978).

test material. Also, addition of visual cues via speechreading during test administration in a bisensory perceptual condition can provide useful information regarding a person's overall integrative skills (see Chapters 5 and 10).

Owens, Kessler, Telleen, and Shubert (1985) developed a comprehensive set of tests, the *Minimal Auditory Capabilities (MAC) Battery*, for assessing auditory and visual skills of patients with severe-to-profound hearing impairment. The level of difficulty of the *MAC* is suitable for individuals for whom conventional speech perception tests may be too challenging, such as with persons having profound hearing loss. Included in the *MAC* battery are 14 subtests that evaluate both basic and more complex auditory perception abilities involving a variety of listening tasks with speech. One of the subtests also assesses speechreading skills. The battery is presently being used in the evaluation of cases considered for a cochlear implant. Another assessment battery used for this purpose is the *Iowa Cochlear Implant Battery* (Tyler, Preece, & Lowder, 1983), as is the *HINT (Hearing in Noise Test)*, developed by Nilsson, Sali, and Sullivan (1994).

Bisensory refers to using hearing and vision together.

Methods of Auditory Training

The more current approaches to auditory training vary considerably. According to Blamey and Alcantara (1994), it is possible to categorize them into one of four general categories, based on the fundamental strategy stressed in therapy:

1. *Analytic:* Attempts to break speech into smaller components (phoneme, syllable) and incorporate these separately into auditory training exercises. Examples include exercises that emphasize same–different discrimination of vowel or consonant phonemes in syllables (e.g., /bi–ba/) or words (e.g., /kIp–kIt/) or require the listener to identify a word within a closed-set response format (e.g., run–money–bat).

2. *Synthetic:* Emphasizes a more global approach to speech perception, stressing the use of clues derived from the syntax and context of a spoken message to derive understanding. Training synthetically involves the use of meaningful stimuli (words, phrases, sentences). This might involve practicing sentence perception based on prior information about context (e.g., having lunch, a classroom discussion on government) or having the clinician name a topic and present related words or phrases that the individual must repeat back.

3. *Pragmatic:* Involves training the listener to control communication variables, such as the level of speech, the signal-to-noise ratio, and the context or complexity of the message, in order to obtain the necessary information via audition for understanding to occur. For example, the person with hearing impairment practices how to effectively use conversation repair strategies, like asking questions or requesting that a statement be repeated or clarified, to comprehend a paragraph read by the clinician. A similar activity centers around the use of QUEST?AR (Erber, 1996). Here, the patient is given a series of questions related to a specified topic, such as those listed in Table 4.8. The patient asks the clinician each question. The clinician answers each question, and the patient then must correctly repeat the answer given before moving on

Signal-to-noise ratio refers to comparing the intensity of the signal you wish to hear with all the other auditory signals present in that listening situation.

TABLE 4.8

Topics and Questions from QUEST?AR[a]

Where did you go? museum, restaurant, post office, shopping, camping, doctor, zoo, beach, airport, swimming, mountains, picnic, music lesson, Mars, supermarket, and so forth

Questions:

1. Why did you go there?
2. When did you go?
3. How many people went with you?
4. Who were they? (names)
5. What did you take with you?
6. Where is (the place where you went)?
7. How did you get there?
8. What did you see on the way?
9. What time did you get there?
10. What did you do first?
11. What did you see?
12. How many? What colour? etc.
13. What happened at (the place where you went)?
14. What else did you do?
15. What were other people doing at (the place where you went)?
16. What was the most interesting thing that you saw?
17. What was the most interesting thing that you did?
18. What did you buy?
19. What kind? What flavour? What colour? etc.
20. How much did it cost?
21. Did anything unusual happen? What?
22. How long did you stay?
23. What did you do just before you came home?
24. When did you leave?
25. How did you get home?
26. What happened on the way home?
27. What time did you get home?
28. How did you feel then?
29. When are you going back?
30. Do you think that I should go sometime? Why?

[a]QUESTions for Aural Rehabilitation.
Source: Erber (1996).

to the next question. This conversationlike therapy strategy can be done in an auditory-only or auditory-visual mode.

4. *Eclectic:* Includes training that combines most or all of the strategies previously described.

While the auditory training programs to be described all have analytic, synthetic, or pragmatic tendencies, most would best be described as eclectic, since more than one general strategy for the training of listening skills typically is used with a given child or adult.

ERBER. A flexible and widely used approach to auditory training designed primarily for use with children has been described by Erber (1982). This adaptive method is based on a careful analysis of a child's auditory perceptual abilities through the use of the *GASP* assessment battery (described briefly in the earlier portion of this chapter devoted to assessment). Recall that *GASP*'s approach to evaluating a child's auditory perceptual skills takes into account two major factors: (1) the complexity of the speech stimuli to be perceived (ranging from individual speech elements to connected discourse) and (2) the form of the response required from the child (detection, discrimination, identification, or comprehension). Several levels of stimuli and responses are involved, as shown in Figure 4.6. The *GASP* test battery evaluates only the three stimulus–response combinations indicated in the figure. However, Erber encourages the use of other available test materials to evaluate other stimulus–response combinations from the matrix in Figure 4.6, when appropriate.

Once the child's auditory capabilities are determined, an auditory training program is outlined using the same stimulus–response model as discussed for *GASP* assessment, when establishing goals and beginning points for therapy. Those stimulus–response combinations found not to be processed well during the *GASP* assessment phase logically become the same combinations targeted in auditory training activities that follow. Erber's approach is flexible and highly adaptable to children with a wide variety of auditory abilities, since the stimulus and response combinations range from the simplest (phoneme detection) to the most complex (sentence comprehension) perceptual tasks.

Erber also described three general styles that the clinician may use during auditory training, depending on the communication setting. These styles differ in specificity, rigidity, and direction and are described in Table 4.9. Adaptive procedures, where the child's responses to speech stimuli are used to determine the next activity, can be employed with any of these styles. In attempting to develop a child's auditory abilities, Erber (1982) stated:

> Auditory training need not follow a developmental plan where, for instance, you practice phoneme detection first and attempt comprehension of connected discourse last. Instead, you might use the "conversational approach" during all daily conversation, and apply the "moderately structured approach" as a follow-up to each class activity. During each activity, you will note consistent errors. Later, you might provide brief periods of specific practice with difficult material. In this way, you can incorporate auditory training into conversation and instruction, rather than treat listening as a skill to be developed independently of communication. (p. 105)

Erber's emphasis on integrating the development of auditory skills into all activities with children with hearing impairment is shared by many, including Sanders (1993) and Ling and Ling (1978), who recommend that auditory training "be viewed as a supplement to auditory experience and as an integral part of language and speech training" (p. 113). Thus, therapy directed toward the development of auditory and language skills can and should be done in an integrated, mostly seamless manner.

As mentioned earlier, Erber's levels of perception model (detection, discrimination, identification, and comprehension) is widely used with both children and adults in rehabilitation therapy involving the development and improvement of auditory and visual perceptual skills for speech perception.

TABLE 4.9

Three General Auditory Training Approaches

Natural conversational approach	1. The teacher eliminates visible cues and speaks to the child in as natural a way as possible, while considering the general situational context and ongoing classroom activity. 2. The auditory speech perception tasks may be chosen from any cell in the stimulus–response matrix, for example, sentence comprehension. 3. The teacher adapts to the child's responses by presenting remedial auditory tasks in a systematic manner (modifies stimulus and/or response), derived from any cell in the matrix.
Moderately structured approach	1. The teacher applies a closed-set auditory identification task, but follows this approach activity with some basic speech development procedures and a related comprehension task. Thus, the method retains a degree of flexibility. 2. The teacher selects the nature and content of words and sentences on the basis of recent class activities. 3. A few neighboring cells in the stimulus–response matrix are involved (for example, word and sentence identification and sentence comprehension).
Practice on specific tasks	1. The teacher selects the set of acoustic speech stimuli and also the child's range of responses, prepares relevant materials, and plans the development of the task, all according to the child's specific needs for auditory practice. 2. Attention is directed to a particular listening skill, usually represented by a single cell in the stimulus–response matrix (e.g., phrase discrimination).

Source: Erber, N. (1982). *Auditory Training.* Washington, DC: Alexander Graham Bell Association for the Deaf. Reprinted by permission.

DASL II. Stout and Windle (1994) have developed a sequential, highly structured auditory-training curriculum called the Developmental Approach to Successful Listening II, or DASL II. Like Erber's (1982) approach, the DASL II consists of a hierarchy of listening skills that are worked on in relatively brief, individualized sessions.

The DASL II curriculum can be used with persons of any age, but it mainly has been utilized with preschool and school-age youngsters using either hearing aids or cochlear implants. Three specific areas of auditory skill development are focused on the following:

1. *Sound awareness:* Deals with the development of the basic skills of listening for both environmental and speech sounds. The care/use of hearing aids and cochlear implants is also included.
2. *Phonetic listening:* Includes exposure to fundamental aspects of speech perception such as the duration, intensity, pitch, and rate of speech. The discrimination and identification of vowels and consonants in isolation and in words are included in this area.

3. *Auditory comprehension:* Emphasizes the understanding of spoken language by the child with hearing impairment. Includes a wide range of auditory processing activities from basic discrimination of common words to comprehension of complex verbal messages in unstructured situations.

The authors have developed a placement test that enables the clinician to evaluate the child's auditory skills relative to each of these three main areas. Specific subskills are tested, making it possible to determine the particular listening skills which a child has or has not acquired. As with the *GASP* approach, information from the DASL II placement test enables the clinician to determine the appropriate placement of the child within the auditory skills curriculum. The test's developers provided numerous activity suggestions for the clinician. These address each of the many subskills of the three main areas of listening which make up DASL II. These are organized from the simplest to the most difficult listening task. The following example is a list of subskills related to sound awareness that are included in the DASL II. Similar subskill lists and related activities are provided by the developers for all components of DASL II.

DEVELOPING SOUND AWARENESS SUBSKILLS

1. Responds to the presence of a loud, low-frequency gross environmental sound. (Example: loud banging on a hard surface)
2. Responds to the presence of a loud speech syllable or word.
3. Responds to the presence of a variety of different gross environmental sounds.
4. Indicates when ongoing environmental sounds stop.
5. Indicates when a sustained speech syllable or word stops.
6. Indicates when teacher or parent turns both hearing aids (or processor) on or off.
7. Discriminates between presence of spoken syllable or word and silence.
8. Discriminates between a variety of familiar environmental sounds in a set of two choices.
9. Discriminates between a variety of familiar environmental sounds in a set of three choices.
10. Discriminates between a variety of environmental sounds in a set of four choices.
11. If the student is amplified binaurally, locates the direction of sound on the same plane.
12. If the student is amplified binaurally, locates the direction of sound on different planes.
13. Identifies common environmental sounds.
14. If the student is amplified binaurally, he or she can detect when one aid is on versus when both aids are on in a structured situation.

A team approach is encouraged with DASL II, with the audiologist, speech–language pathologist, classroom teacher, and parents working in a coordinated fashion on relevant subskills. This makes it vital that frequent communication occurs among the team members.

SKI-HI. Clark and Watkins (1985) developed this comprehensive identification and home intervention treatment curriculum for infants with hearing impairment and

Home intervention involves guiding the parents as they carry out important components of an early audiologic rehabilitation program in the home for an infant diagnosed with a hearing loss.

their families, and it is in wide use nationally (see Chapter 9 for more details). One of the major components of SKI-HI's treatment plan is a developmentally based auditory stimulation–training program. It is utilized in conjunction with language–speech stimulation and consists of 4 phases and 11 general skills, which are listed in Table 4.10. Although these phases and skills are organized developmentally, infants may not always move sequentially from one phase or skill on the list to the next higher one in a completely predictable manner. SKI-HI provides an extensive description of activities that the clinician and parent or caregiver may utilize in working on subskills related to each of the specific general skills included in each phase of the auditory training program. The structure and completeness of SKI-HI's auditory training component make it user-friendly for parents under the guidance of clinicians. Table 4.11 provides a summary of an example of listening activities which are part of SKI-HI's comprehensive auditory stimulation program.

TABLE 4.10

The Four Phases and Eleven Skills of the SKI-HI Auditory Program

The approximate time line indicates the estimated amount of time spent by a profoundly deaf infant in each phase. The age of the child upon entry into the program and the amount of hearing loss are among the factors that will affect the time needed to progress through the four phases.

PHASES	SKILLS
Phase I (4–7 months)	1. *Attending:* Child is aware of presence of home and/or speech sounds but may not know meanings; stops, listens, etc.
	2. *Early vocalizing:* Child coos, gurgles, repeats syllables, etc.
Phase II (5–16 months)	3. *Recognizing:* Child knows meaning of home and/or speech sounds but may not be able to locate; smiles when hears Daddy home, etc.
	4. *Locating:* Child turns to, points to, locates sound sources.
	5. *Vocalizing with inflection:* High/low, loud/soft, and/or, up/down
Phase III (9–14 months)	6. *Hearing at distances and levels:* Child locates sounds far away and/or above and below
	7. *Producing some vowels and consonants*
Phase IV (12–18 months)	8. *Environmental discrimination and comprehension:* Child hears differences among and/or understands home sounds
	9. *Vocal discrimination and comprehension:* Child hears differences (a) among vocal sounds, (b) among words, or (c) among phrases and/or understands them
	10. *Speech sound discrimination and comprehension:* Child hears differences among and/or understands distinct speech sounds
	11. *Speech use:* Child imitates and/or uses speech meaningfully

Source: Adapted from Watkins & Clark (1993); Watkins (2004).

TABLE 4.11	

A Lesson in SKI-HI's Auditory Stimulation and Training Program

Recognition of objects and events from sound source (Phase II, Skill 3, Subskill 6)

Parent objective	Parent will provide repeated meaningful opportunities for his or her child to associate environmental and speech sounds with their source.
Child objective	Child will demonstrate recognition of environmental and speech sounds by realizing their source.
Lesson	Review with the parent the sounds and activities that you have been utilizing for previous work on attending. Continue these activities, ensuring that the child is aware of the source of the sound and that the sounds are relevant to the child.
Materials	Naturally occurring environmental sounds and voice.
Activities	1. Ask everyone who comes to visit to knock several times, pause, and knock again. When someone knocks, take your child to the door and say, "listen," etc.
	2. Encourage the child to discover different sounds that toys make by providing him or her play time with several different sound toys.
	3. Stimulate the child to produce sounds by manipulating objects or toys (banging pans, squeezing toy, etc.) and stimulate vocalization by making sounds as you play with the toys.
	4. Imitate the child's actions, such as shaking a rattle, and imitate all vocalizations.
	5. Associate speech with all major movements (e.g., saying "roll" each time you roll the child over and "up" when you pick him or her up).
	6. Stimulate association of particular voices with particular people by having siblings/relatives use voice as they play with the child.

Source: Adapted from Clark & Watkins (1985); Watkins & Clark (1993); Watkins (2004).

SPICE. Moog, Biedenstein, and Davidson (1995) developed the Speech Perception Instructional Curriculum and Evaluation (SPICE) to provide a guide for clinicians in evaluating and developing auditory skills in children with severe-to-profound hearing loss. It contains goals and objectives associated with four levels of speech perception. The first level, *detection,* is intended to establish an awareness and responsiveness to speech. The second and third levels, *suprasegmental* and *vowel and consonant perception,* are worked on in tandem. In the suprasegmental section, children work on differentiating speech based on gross variations in duration, stress, and intonation. In the vowel and consonant section, children begin to make perceptual distinctions among individual word stimuli with similar duration, stress, and intonation features, but with different vowels and consonants. With progress, the child is introduced to the fourth level, *connected speech.* Now the emphasis is

Connected or running speech is natural or conversational speech.

the perception of words in a more natural environment (phrases and sentences). Activities for SPICE are done with combined auditory–visual presentation, as well as auditory-only listening situations. Much of these activities are carried out in short, structured therapy sessions that concentrate on specific listening skills. As the child progresses, the newly acquired skills can be refined further in more natural, informal conversation. Recently, SPICE has been used extensively with children using cochlear implants as an approach to developing listening skills in conjunction with their expanded auditory input.

COCHLEAR IMPLANT MANUFACTURERS. The major cochlear implant manufacturers have made available some excellent supportive programs for developing/improving auditory skills and facilitating the use of cochlear implants for both children and adults. For example, Cochlear Corporation distributes Sound and Beyond, a self-paced interactive software program designed for use by adults at home to practice their listening skills. Another program, designed for teenagers, Nucleus Hear We Go, contains numerous listening activities related to a variety of topics of interest (sports, food, television, etc.). Finally, Listen, Learn, and Talk is a comprehensive program for developing listening skills and language in children from birth to school-age. Information regarding each of these programs can be obtained via www.cochlearamericas.com/Support/41/asp. MED-EL (www.medel.com) has made available a training program titled AUDITRAIN, which is designed to help adult cochlear implant users maximize the use of their hearing through 22 individual lesson plans that contain both analytic and synthetic listening activities. Finally, Advanced Bionics (www.bionicear.com) has developed an extensive videotape series for parents of recently implanted children, as well as members of the cochlear implant team. These films cover a variety of important topics, including detailed information and activities related to auditory skill development.

CONSONANT RECOGNITION TRAINING. This approach to auditory training mainly has been used with adults and relies primarily on an analytic approach to facilitate improved speech perception. In addition to its use in auditory training, consonant recognition training frequently incorporates speechreading into a combined auditory–visual training approach. Walden et al. (1981) originally described consonant recognition training as it was utilized initially at Walter Reed Army Medical Center. Briefly, a large number of training exercises were developed with each exercise concentrating on a select number of consonants presented in a syllable context. The listener's task is to make same–different judgments between syllable pairs and to identify the nonsense syllables presented individually. The position of the consonants within the syllable is varied between exercises. The person with hearing impairment receives immediate feedback regarding the correctness of his or her response. This general procedure allows for intense drill to occur for a select number of consonants during a relatively short therapy session.

Walden and others presented data to support the efficacy of this approach to auditory training. They noted an 11.6 percent average improvement in consonant recognition. More impressively, a 28.2 percent average improvement was found in perception of sentences presented in a combined auditory–visual mode. A follow-up study (Montgomery, Walden, Schwartz, & Prosek, 1984) utilized a similar training protocol for consonant recognition that combined work on speechreading and auditory training. Using sentence material to assess performance, they noted a substantial improvement in speech recognition for adults with hearing impairment.

Another investigation (Rubenstein & Boothroyd, 1987) also examined the effectiveness of consonant recognition training as part of a larger study comparing analytic and synthetic therapy approaches to improving speech perception. Rubenstein and Boothroyd found that consonant recognition training did produce modest improvement in speech perception for a group of adults with hearing impairment, but the amount of improvement observed was not any greater than was achieved with a synthetic approach to auditory training. However, the results from Kricos and Holmes (1996) did not support the efficacy of consonant recognition training with older adults.

More research needs to be focused on the relative merits of consonant-recognition training as it is used in attempting to improve auditory perception. Also needed is further clarification of the basic roles played by auditory and visual speech perception, both individually and when utilized in a combined manner, in the processing of speech by persons with hearing impairment (Gagne, 1994; Walden & Grant, 1993). In the meantime, interest in using consonant-recognition training continues, and its use has been extended in recent years to include computer-based programming as well (Lansing & Bienvenue, 1994; Tye-Murray, Tyler, Lansing, & Bertschy, 1990). Clinicians also can access a wealth of therapy materials useful in this type of analytic approach from Analytika (Plant, 1994).

COMMUNICATION TRAINING AND THERAPY. This common form of audiologic rehabilitation emphasizes the role of communication strategies and pragmatics to facilitate successful communication. The adult with hearing impairment is coached regarding those factors in conversational situations that the listener can control or exercise that can maximize the opportunity to perceive what is spoken. Many of these factors are classified as being either anticipatory or repair strategies for the listener to use. Anticipatory strategies refer to things the listener can do to better prepare for communication or ensure that it will be successful. Some examples of anticipatory strategies that can be helpful are listed in Table 4.12.

Repair strategies involve techniques used to overcome a breakdown in communication that has already occurred. The person with hearing loss (and the speaker as well) can use one or more of these strategies to help with perceiving a given message. Examples of common repair strategies are also given in Table 4.12.

Table 4.13 demonstrates further how repair strategies can be used for specific communication problems. Persons with hearing impairment are encouraged to employ these communication strategies when necessary, which does require some degree of assertiveness on their part as they communicate with others. Successful use of communication strategies also requires that they be used in a diplomatic manner as well (see Conversational Styles box on page 145).

DeFilippo and Scott (1978) developed a technique called *speech tracking*, which can be used in therapy to provide practice in utilizing communication repair strategies in a conversation context. As it is used in therapy centered on improving auditory-speech perception, speech tracking involves having a listener repeat a phrase or sentence presented by a clinician in an auditory-only condition. To assist

TABLE 4.12

Examples of Anticipatory and Repair Strategies the Person with Hearing Loss Can Use to Enhance the Extent to Which Hearing Contributes to Speech Perception

Anticipatory Strategies
- Minimizing the distance from the speaker
- Optimizing the hearing aid volume setting
- Reducing the level of competing signals (stereo, TV) SNR
- Using situational cues to anticipate topics and words

Repair Strategies
- Asking the speaker to repeat all or part of a message
- Asking the speaker to rephrase or simplify the message
- Asking a follow-up question to either confirm the content of a previous message or to elaborate on it

TABLE 4.13

Some Communication Problems Commonly Experienced by Hearing Impaired People, and Associated (Specific) Requests for Clarification

WHAT WAS THE COMMUNICATION PROBLEM?	HOW YOU CAN ASK FOR HELP
You understood only part of the message.	Repeat the part you understood; ask for the part you didn't understand (e.g., "You flew to *Paris*?").
You couldn't see the speaker's mouth.	"Please put your hand down."
The person was speaking too fast.	"Please speak a little slower."
The person's speech was too soft.	"Please speak a little louder."
The sentence was too long.	"Shorter, please."
The person's speech was not clear.	"Speak a little more clearly, please."
The sentence was too complicated.	"Please say that in a different way."
You don't know what the problem was.	"Please say that again."

Source: Erber (1993).

in perceiving 100 percent of the message, the listener can use various repair strategies, such as requesting that the entire sentence, or portions, be repeated or rephrased, until the complete utterance is comprehended. Visual cues may be added for bisensory training as well. Performance in the speech tracking procedure is monitored by calculating the number of words or sentences correctly repeated by the listener per minute over a set period of time. An example of the tracking method as applied in a therapy session is provided below. (The topic of the sentence is fishing.)

> *Clinician:* Dry flies float on the surface.
> *Listener:* Dry . . . on the . . . ? Please repeat it.
> *Clinician:* Dry flies float on the surface.

See the text website to measure your own tracking score.

Listener: Dry flies . . . on the . . . ? Please repeat the word after "flies."
Clinician: Float.
Listener: Float?
Clinician: Yes.
Listener: Dry flies float on the water.
Clinician: No. On the surface of the water.
Listener: Oh. Dry flies float on the surface.
Clinician: Yes.

In recent years, audiologists have frequently included condensed variations of communication training and counseling as an important aspect of audiologic rehabilitation for adults at the time they are fitted with new hearing aids (Beyer & Northern, 2000). Many think that sharing information with the patient about the role of hearing and vision and the use of communication strategies in communicating is a timely and appropriate adjunct to the hearing aid orientation process, and audiologists have begun to do this on a more frequent basis (Schow, Balsara, Smedley, & Whitcomb, 1993). Montgomery (1994) discussed the rationale for providing a brief exposure to auditory rehabilitation at the time the patient who is hard of hearing is fitted with a hearing aid. Montgomery uses the acronym WATCH for his abbreviated program, which includes the following key elements of AR: W: Watch the talker's mouth (lipreading); A: Ask specific questions (conversation-repair strategies); T: Talk about your hearing loss (admission of hearing loss); C: Change the situation (situation control); and H: Health care knowledge (consumer education and awareness). The program, which takes about one hour to share with the new hearing-aid user, is designed to provide important tips for successful communication, as well as to "encourage or empower the hearing-impaired patient to take charge of his or her communication behavior and take responsibility for its success."

Conversational Styles

It's important to note that persons with hearing loss can react to their hearing problems either in a positive or negative fashion. This can result in the routine use of one of three general conversational styles for the listener with hearing impairment, as summarized below.

Passive: The listener has a tendency to withdraw from conversations and social situations. When unable to hear what is said, this person is prone to bluff or pretend to hear by simply smiling or nodding his or her head. Persons using this approach do very little to facilitate communication.

Aggressive: The listener routinely blames others for communication difficulties (e.g., "Everyone mumbles" or "He does not speak loudly enough"). It is common for listeners using this style to convey a hostile, negative feeling toward their communication partners.

Assertive: The listener takes responsibility for facilitating communication (e.g., turning down the television or stereo during conversation, sitting closer, acknowledging to communication partners that he or she has a hearing loss) and does so in a positive, diplomatic manner.

Three handouts called HIO BASICS, CLEAR, and SPEECH, developed by Schow (2001) and Brockett and Schow (2001), constitute another approach to providing short-term audiologic rehabilitation. Used *primarily* in conjunction with the fitting/ orientation process, these tools involve presenting key aspects of the rehabilitation process. HIO BASICS focuses on presenting information related primarily to the care and effective use of hearing aids. CLEAR provides suggestions for the person with a hearing impairment regarding the communication process, while SPEECH gives helpful suggestions for the significant other that are designed to facilitate communication. The latter two handouts are closely tied to Schum's (1989) Clear Speech. More detailed descriptions of all three of these handouts are found in Chapter 10.

Sweetow and Henderson-Sabes (2004) recently have introduced LACE, or Listening and Communication Enhancement, which is an interactive computer program designed to improve listening skills (www.neurotone.com). LACE is intended for use in the patient's home in a self-directed manner. Therapy sessions run thirty minutes a day, five days a week, for four weeks, and focus on perception of degraded speech, developing/refining certain cognitive skills important for listening, and the effective use of communication strategies. Immediate feedback is provided to the patient during the exercises, and progress is monitored electronically. The developers have shown that LACE improved patients' abilities to comprehend speech in noisy environments and increased their confidence in dealing with difficult listening situations.

Audiologists are encouraged to consider providing a form of brief AR *routinely* as they work with adults who are hard of hearing.

SUMMARY POINTS

- Basic oral (verbal) communication involves five key components: the speaker, a message (often with auditory and visual forms), a listener, feedback to the speaker, and the environment in which the communication takes place.
- Both the segmental and suprasegmental components found in speech contribute to speech perception.
- Hearing impairment results in the loss of varying degrees of segmental and suprasegmental information, which leads to problems with speech perception.
- Speech has quite a bit of built-in redundancy, making it possible to figure out what was said even though the listener did not perceive all the acoustical information produced by the speaker.
- Auditory training is intended to facilitate auditory perception in the listener with impaired hearing.
- Long-term auditory training therapy is not done routinely with a majority of cases with hearing loss. However, it can be a key component of audiologic rehabilitation for cochlear implant recipients, those with prelingual onset of hearing loss, and those with severe to profound impairments.
- Assessment of auditory skills can provide valuable information regarding candidacy for therapy, can help in identifying areas in need of work in therapy, and can be useful in outcomes assessment.

- Analytic, synthetic, and pragmatic approaches to auditory training currently are employed in a variety of forms for children and adults.
- Passive and aggressive conversational styles are negative, often counterproductive reactions to hearing loss, while the assertive conversational style is a more positive approach that places responsibility on those with hearing loss to assist in facilitating communication.
- Numerous forms of communication strategies are available to assist in making communication more successful.
- A number of models have been developed for providing AR on a short-term basis, and these usually are incorporated into the hearing aid fitting process.

RECOMMENDED READING

Blamey, P., & Alcantara, J. (1994). Research in auditory training. In J.-P. Gagne & N. Tye-Murray (Eds.), Research in audiological rehabilitation [Monograph]. *Journal of the Academy of Rehabilitative Audiology, 27,* 161–192.

Erber, N. (1982). *Auditory training.* Washington, DC: Alexander Graham Bell Association for the Deaf.

Erber, N. (1996). *Communication therapy for hearing-impaired adults.* Abbotsford, Victoria, Australia: Clavis Publishing.

Gagne, J.-P., & Jennings, M. (2000). Audiological rehabilitation intervention services for adults with acquired hearing impairment. In M. Valente, H. Hosford-Dunn, and R. Roeser (Eds.), *Audiology treatment.* New York: Thieme.

Kricos, P. (Ed.) (2000). Contemporary models of aural rehabilitation. *Seminars in Hearing, 21*(3).

Tye-Murray, N. (2004). *Foundations of aural rehabilitation* (2nd ed.). Clifton Park, NY: Delmar Learning.

REFERENCES

Alpiner, J., & McCarthy, P. (Eds.). (2000). *Rehabilitative audiology: Children and adults* (3rd ed.). Baltimore: Williams & Wilkins.

Beyer, C., & Northern, J. (2000). Audiologic rehabilitation support programs: A network model. *Seminars in Hearing, 21*(3), 257–266.

Bilger, R., Rzcezkowski, C., Nuetzel, J., & Rabinowitz, W. (1979, November). Evaluation of a test of speech perception in noise (SPIN). Paper presented at the convention of the American Speech–Language–Hearing Association, Atlanta, GA.

Blamey, P., & Alcantara, J. (1994). Research in auditory training. In J.-P. Gagne & N. Tye-Murray (Eds.), Research in audiological rehabilitation [Monograph]. *Journal of the Academy of Rehabilitative Audiology, 27,* 161–192.

Brockett, J., & Schow, R. (2001). Web site profiles common hearing loss patterns and outcome measures. *Hearing Journal, 54*(8), 20.

Carhart, R. (1960). Auditory training. In H. Davis & R. Silverman (Eds.), *Hearing and deafness* (2nd ed.). New York: Holt, Rinehart & Winston.

Clark, T., & Watkins, S. (1985). *Programming for hearing impaired infants through amplification and home visits* (4th ed.). Logan: Utah State University.

Davis, H., & Silverman, R. (1960). *Hearing and deafness* (2nd ed.). New York: Holt, Rinehart & Winston.

Davis, H., & Silverman, R. (1978). *Hearing and deafness* (4th ed.) New York: Holt, Rinehart & Winston.

Davis, J., & Hardick, E. (1981). *Rehabilitative audiology for children and adults.* New York: Wiley and Sons.

DeFilippo, C., & Scott, B. (1978). A method for training and evaluating the reception of ongoing speech. *Journal of the Acoustical Society of America, 63,* 1186–1192.

Denes, P., & Pinson, E. (1993). *The speech chain* (2nd ed.). New York: Freeman.

Durrant, J., & Lovrinic, J. (1995). *Bases of hearing science* (3rd ed.). Baltimore: Williams & Wilkins.

Erber, N. (1979). Speech perception by profoundly hearing-impaired children. *Journal of Speech and Hearing Disorders, 122,* 255–270.

Erber, N. (1982). *Auditory training.* Washington, DC: Alexander Graham Bell Association for the Deaf.

Erber, N. (1993). *Communication and adult hearing loss.* Abbotsford, Victoria, Australia: Clavis Press.

Erber, N. (1996). Communication therapy for hearing-impaired adults. Melbourne, Australia: Clavis Publishing.

Fletcher, H. (1953). *Speech and hearing in communication.* Princeton, NJ: D. VanNostrand.

Gagne, J.-P. (1994). Visual and audiovisual speech perception training: Basic and applied research needs. In J.-P. Gagne & N. Tye-Murray (Eds.), Research in audiological rehabilitation [Monograph]. *Journal of the Academy of Rehabilitative Audiology, 27,* 133–160.

Gagne, J.-P., & Jennings, M. (2000). Audiological rehabilitation intervention services for adults with acquired hearing impairment. In M. Valente, H. Hosford-Dunn, & R. Roeser (Eds.), *Audiology treatment.* New York: Thieme.

Goldstein, M. (1939). *The acoustic method of the training of the deaf and hard of hearing child.* St. Louis: Laryngoscope Press.

Hegde, M. (1995). *Introduction to communicative disorders* (2nd ed.). Austin, TX: Pro-Ed.

Hirsh, I., Davis, H., Silverman, S. R., Reynolds, E., Eldert, E., Bensen, R. (1952). Development of materials for speech audiometry. *Journal of Speech and Hearing Disorders, 17,* 321–337.

Kalikow, D., Stevens, K., & Elliott, L. (1977). Development of a test of speech intelligibility in noise using sentence materials with controlled word predictability. *Journal of the Acoustical Society of America, 61,* 1337–1351.

Katz, D., & Elliott, L. (1978, November). *Development of a new children's speech discrimination test.* Paper presented at the convention of the American Speech–Language–Hearing Association, Chicago.

Kricos, P., & Holmes, A. (1996). Efficacy of audiologic rehabilitation for older adults. *Journal of American Academy of Audiology, 7*(4), 219–229.

Lansing, C., & Bienvenue, L. (1994). Intelligent computer-based systems to document the effectiveness of consonant recognition training. *Volta Review, 96,* 41–49.

Lehiste, I. (1970). *Suprasegmentals.* Cambridge, MA: The MIT Press.

Lehiste, I. (1976). Suprasegmental features of speech. In N. J. Lass (Ed.), *Contemporary issues in experimental phonetics* (pp. 225–242). New York: Academic Press.

Ling, D. (1976). *Speech and the hearing-impaired child: Theory and practice.* Washington, DC: Alexander Graham Bell Association for the Deaf.

Ling, D. (1989). *Foundations of spoken language for hearing-impaired children.* Washington, DC: Alexander Graham Bell Association for the Deaf.

Ling, D., & Ling, A. (1978). *Aural rehabilitation.* Washington, DC: Alexander Graham Bell Association for the Deaf.

MacKay, I. (1987). *Phonetics: The science of speech production* (2nd ed.). Austin, TX: Pro-Ed.

Miller, G. (1951). *Language and communication.* New York: McGraw-Hill.

Miller, G., & Nicely, P. (1955). Analysis of perceptual confusions among some English consonants. *Journal of the Acoustical Society of America, 27,* 338–352.

Minifie, F. (1973). Speech acoustics. In F. Minifie, T. Hixon, & F. Williams (Eds.), *Normal aspects of speech, hearing and language.* Englewood Cliffs, NJ: Prentice-Hall.

Montgomery, A. (1994). WATCH: A practical approach to brief auditory rehabilitation. *The Hearing Journal, 47*(10), 53–55.

Montgomery, A., Walden, B., Schwartz, D., & Prosek, R. (1984). Training auditory–visual speech recognition in adults with moderate sensorineural hearing loss. *Ear and Hearing, 5,* 30–36.

Moog, J., Biedenstein, J., & Davidson, L. (1995). *The SPICE.* St. Louis: Central Institute for the Deaf.

Myatt, B., & Landes, B. (1963). Assessing discrimination loss in children. *Archives of Otolaryngology, 77,* 359–362.

Nilsson, M., Sali, S., & Sullivan, J. (1994). Development of the Hearing in Noise Test for the measurement of speech reception thresholds in quiet and noise. *Journal of the Acoustical Society of America, 87,* 1085–1099.

Northern, J., & Downs, M. (2002). *Hearing in children* (5th ed.). Baltimore: Williams & Wilkins.

Owens, E. (1978). Consonant errors and remediation in sensorineural hearing loss. *Journal of Speech and Hearing Disorders, 43,* 331–347.

Owens, E., Benedict, M., & Shubert, E. (1971). Further investigation of vowel items in multiple-choice discrimination testing. *Journal of Speech and Hearing Research, 14,* 814–847.

Owens, E., Benedict, M., & Shubert, E. (1972). Consonant phoneme errors associated with pure tone configurations and certain types of hearing impairment. *Journal of Speech and Hearing Research, 15,* 308–322.

Owens, E., Kessler, D., Telleen, C., & Shubert, E. (1985). The Minimal Auditory Capabilities (MAC) battery. *Hearing Journal, 34*(9), 32–34.

Owens, E., & Schubert, E. (1977). Development of the California Consonant Test. *Journal of Speech and Hearing Research, 20,* 463–474.

Oyer, H. (1966). *Auditory communication for the hard of hearing.* Englewood Cliffs, NJ: Prentice-Hall.

Peterson, G. E., & Barney, H. L. (1952). Control methods used in the study of the vowels. *Journal of the Acoustical Society of America, 32,* 693–703.

Plant, G. (1994). *Analytika.* Somerville, MA: Audiological Engineering Corp.

Ross, M., & Lerman, L. (1970). A picture identification test for hearing impaired children. *Journal of Speech and Hearing Research, 13,* 44–53.

Rubenstein, A., & Boothroyd, A. (1987). Effect of two approaches to auditory training on speech recognition by hearing-impaired adults. *Journal of Speech and Hearing Research, 30,* 153–160.

Sanders, D. (1971). *Aural rehabilitation.* Englewood Cliffs, NJ: Prentice-Hall.

Sanders, D. (1993). *Management of hearing handicap* (3rd ed.). Englewood Cliffs, NJ: Prentice-Hall.

Schow, R. L. (2001). A standardized AR battery for dispensers. *Hearing Journal, 54*(2), 10–20.

Schow, R., Balsara, N., Smedley, T., & Whitcomb, C. (1993). Aural rehabilitation by ASHA audiologists: 1980–1990. *American Journal of Audiology, 2,* 28–37.

Schum, D. (1989). *Clear and conversational speech by untrained talkers: Intelligibility.* Paper presented at the American Speech-Language-Hearing Association, Seattle, WA.

Schwartz, D., & Surr, R. (1979). Three experiments on the California Consonant Test. *Journal of Speech and Hearing Disorders, 44,* 61–72.

Sher, A., & Owens, E. (1974). Consonant confusions associated with hearing loss above 2,000 Hz. *Journal of Speech and Hearing Research, 17,* 669–681.

Stevens, S., & Davis, H. (1938). *Hearing: Its psychology and physiology.* New York: Wiley & Sons.

Stout, G., & Windle, J. (1994). *Developmental Approach to Successful Listening II.* Englewood, CO: Resource Point.

Sweetow, R., & Henderson-Sabes, J. (2004). The case for LACE: Listening and auditory communication enhancement training. *Hearing Journal, 57*(3), 32–38.

Tillman, T., & Carhart, R. (1966). *An expanded test for speech discrimination utilizing CNC monosyllabic words.* Northwestern University Auditory Test No. 6 (Technical Report No. SAM-TR55). Brooks Air Force Base, TX: USAF School of Aerospace Medicine.

Trammel, J. (1981). *Test of auditory comprehension (TAC).* North Hollywood, CA: Foreworks.

Tye-Murray, N. (2004). *Foundations of aural rehabilitation* (2nd ed.). San Diego, CA: Singular Publishing Group.

Tye-Murray, N., Tyler, R., Lansing, C., & Bertschy, M. (1990). Evaluating the effectiveness of auditory training stimuli using a computerized program. *Volta Review, 92,* 25–30.

Tyler, R., Preece, J., & Lowder, M. (1983). *The Iowa cochlear implant tests.* Iowa City: University of Iowa Press.

Walden, B., Erdman, I., Montgomery, A., Schwartz, D., & Prosek, R. (1981). Some effects of training on speech recognition by hearing-impaired adults. *Journal of Speech and Hearing Research, 24,* 207–216.

Walden, B., & Grant, K. (1993). Research needs in rehabilitative audiology. In J. Alpiner & P. McCarthy (Eds.), *Rehabilitative audiology: Children and adults.* Baltimore: Williams & Wilkins.

Watkins, S. (Ed.). (2004). *SKI-HI curriculum: Family-centered programming for infants and young children with hearing loss.* Logan, UT: Hope, Inc.

Watkins, S., & Clark, T. (1993). *SKI-HI resource manual: Family-centered home-based program for infants, toddlers and school-aged children with hearing impairment.* Logan, UT: Hope, Inc.

CHAPTER 5

Visual Stimuli in Communication

Nicholas M. Hipskind

CONTENTS

INTRODUCTION

When engaged in conversation, we tend to rely primarily on our hearing to receive and subsequently comprehend the message being conveyed. In addition, given the opportunity, we often look at the speaker in order to obtain further information related to the topic of conversation. The speaker's mouth movements, facial expressions, and hand gestures, as well as various aspects of the physical environment in which the communication takes place, are all potential sources of useful information. Humans learn to use their vision for communication to some extent, even though most of us enjoy the benefits of normal hearing and find it unnecessary in most situations to depend on vision to communicate effectively.

The hearing impaired person, on the other hand, is much more dependent on visual cues for communication. The degree to which the hearing impaired need visual information when conversing with someone is proportional to the amount of information that is lost due to hearing impairment. In other words, a person with a severe hearing loss is likely to be more dependent on visual information to communicate than an individual with a mild auditory impairment.

Visual information may be transmitted by means of a manual or an oral communication system. In oral communication, the listener uses visual cues by observing the speaker's mouth, facial expressions, and hand movements to help perceive what is being said. This process is referred to by such terms as lipreading, visual hearing, visual communication, visual listening, or speechreading. Among laypersons the most popular of these terms is *lipreading*. The term implies that only the lips of the talker provide visual cues. However, because the use of vision for communication involves more than merely watching the speaker's mouth, most professionals prefer the term *speechreading*. Thus, speechreading is used in the remainder of this chapter to refer to visual perception of oral communication.

Manual communication, or *signing*, also relies on a visual system. Manual communication is transmitted via special signs and symbols made with the hands and is received and interpreted visually. This complex form of communication allows for transfer of information via the visual channel when both the sender and the receiver are familiar with the same set of symbols.

The intent of this chapter is to discuss the advantages and limitations of vision as part of the audiologic rehabilitation process. Emphasis will be given to the factors that affect speechreading, as well as to a discussion of manual communication methods. The reader is reminded that the hearing impaired comprise two populations: the hard of hearing and the deaf. Although frequently classified under the generic term *hearing impaired*, these groups have different communication needs and limitations. Therefore, it is unrealistic to expect that a single rehabilitation method can satisfy all their communication needs. Ultimately, it is the clinician's responsibility to select appropriate strategies that will enable the hard of hearing and the deaf to use vision to effectively enhance their communicative skills, to achieve educational and vocational success, and to mature emotionally and socially.

> Speechreading involves attempting to perceive speech by using visual cues to supplement whatever auditory information is available.

■ FACTORS RELATED TO SPEECHREADING

The variables that affect the speechreading process usually fall in four general areas: the speaker, the signal code, the environment, and the speechreader. While research has contributed to a better understanding of how speech is processed visually, some of the findings are equivocal and have been found to be difficult to duplicate in the clinical setting. This is not to imply that professionals should ignore available laboratory findings; rather, they must realize the significance of these findings in order to provide individualized patient programming. The following section presents selected experimental evidence regarding factors that have been reported to influence the efficacy of speechreading. Figure 5.1 provides a summary of these factors.

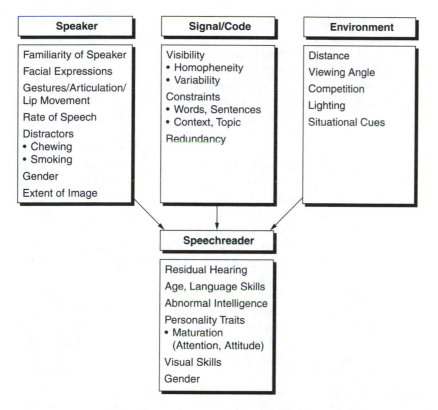

FIGURE 5.1

Summary of various factors related to speechreading performance. Arrows have been drawn from the Speaker, Signal/Code, and Environmental lists to Speech-reader to signify that all these factors influence the speechreader's performance, in addition to those variables that are directly related to the speechreader.

Speaker

Differences among speakers have a greater effect on speechreading than on listening. Over fifty years ago a positive correlation was shown to exist between speaker–listener familiarity and the information received from speechreading. That is, speechreading performance improves when the speaker is familiar to the receiver (speechreader). Speakers who use appropriate facial expressions and common gestures and who position themselves face to face or within a 45-degree angle of the listener also facilitate communication for the speechreader (Berger, 1972a).

The rate of normal speech results in the production of as many as 15 phonemes per second. Evidence suggests that the eye may be capable of recording only 8 to 10 discrete movements per second. Thus, at times a speaker's speaking rate may exceed the listener's visual reception capabilities. Although normal rate of speech may be too fast for optimal visual processing, extremely slowed and exaggerated speech production does not assure improved comprehension. It has been reported that

A slightly slower to normal speech rate with precise, not exaggerated, articulation is best for speech-reading.

speakers who use a slightly slower to normal speech rate accompanied by precise, not exaggerated, articulation are the easiest for the speechreader to understand. Recently, Montgomery and Houston (2000) noted that the rapidity of speech may not be as limiting a factor in determining speechreading success as was once thought, because each phoneme does not have a discrete visual image as speech is produced. Thus, the speechreader actually may not have to process as many visual stimuli per second as once thought. In addition, the speaker also should avoid simultaneous oral activities, such as chewing, smoking, and yawning, when conversing with a person with hearing impairment. Other potentially counterproductive postures include holding a hand near the mouth while talking and wearing sunglasses. While the masking effects of these coincidental activities have not been documented, they seem likely to complicate an already trying task. With respect to the gender of speakers, Daly, Bench, and Chappell (1996) were the most recent to demonstrate that female speakers are easier to speechread than are male speakers. Related to this finding, little evidence exists concerning the potential influence that gender-related variables associated with the speaker, such as a moustache or the use of lipstick, may have on speechreading success.

The speaker may enhance conversational efficiency by complementing speechreading with appropriate facial expressions and gestures (Sanders, 1993). From infancy, we learn that the spoken word "no" is accompanied by a stern facial expression and shaking of the head and/or index finger from side to side. Salutations are made in conjunction with a smile and the extension or wave of the hand, opening of the arms, and/or puckering of the lips. Similarly, shrugging of the shoulders has become a universal gesture that augments the verbal phrases "I don't know" or "I don't care." Consequently, appropriate nonverbal communication is closely associated with the verbal message and is used simultaneously with speech to provide emphasis and redundancy. This means that situations where the speechreader can observe both the head and body of the speaker generally will be more productive for the speechreader. Nitchie (1912) was one of the first teachers of speechreading to stress that the hearing impaired must learn to be cognizant of nonverbal cues, such as gestures, when attempting to understand speech.

Signal and Code

Distinctive features are unique characteristics of a given phoneme that distinguish one phoneme from another.

Speech consists of acoustic information that is efficiently received and effectively interpreted by the normal auditory mechanism. It possesses physical characteristics that are compatible with the receptive capabilities of the normal ear. The basic units of speech are consonants and vowels, classified as phonemes. A phoneme has distinctive acoustic features that enable the listener to distinguish it from all other speech sounds.

Vowels embody the major concentration of acoustic energy found in speech and are termed resonated phonemes. Vowel production is accomplished by directing vocalizations through the oral cavity, which is altered in shape and size by different tongue and lip positions. These subtle alterations are responsible for providing each vowel with specific acoustic features.

Consonants, which are primarily responsible for the intelligibility of speech, are termed articulated phonemes, because their production involves the manipulation of the various articulators: lips, tongue, and teeth. As pointed out in Chapter 4, these phonemes possess *distinctive features* that permit a listener to recognize them. Miller and Nicely (1955) classified these features as voicing, nasality, affrication, duration, and place of articulation. Except for place of articulation, the identifying characteristics of consonants are perceived well on the basis of acoustic information. Although difficult to distinguish acoustically, the place of articulation may be processed to some extent visually due to the visibility of the articulators.

Because many of the 40 or more phonemes used in English demonstrate ambiguous or very limited visible features, an individual who relies solely on vision to understand speech faces much uncertainty. Knowledge of the visual components of speech depends, for the most part, on research using small speech units, that is, consonant–vowel combinations or monosyllabic words (e.g., Jackson, 1988; Owens & Blazek, 1985).

VISEMES. The number of distinctive visual features of vowels and consonants is reduced to the shape of the mouth for vowels and the place of articulation for consonants. Because the perception of phonemes is primarily an auditory function based on acoustic features, Fisher (1968) coined the term *viseme* to indicate the distinguishable visual characteristics of speech sounds. A viseme, therefore, is a speech sound (phoneme) that has been classified by its place of articulation or by the shape of the mouth. This creates a major limitation for the observer of speech compared to that of the listener. Whereas combinations of auditory distinctive features are unique to each phoneme, several phonemes yield the same viseme, thus limiting the speechreader to the conclusion that one of a group of sounds was uttered.

> A viseme is a group of phonemes in which each looks alike when spoken.

Because groups of consonants are produced at the same points of articulation, the phonemes within these groups cannot be differentiated visually without grammatical, phonetic, or lexical information. These visually confusable units of speech are labeled *homophenes*, different speech sounds that look the same. Similarly, words that look alike are referred to as homophenous words. Look in the mirror and say aloud or have a friend utter the syllables /p/, /b/, and /m/. As you watch and listen simultaneously, the syllables sound so different that you may not notice their visual similarities. However, when these same syllables are formed without voice, you will note that their visual characteristics are indistinguishable. This same type of confusion often occurs among word groups (e.g., *pet, bed,* and *men; tip, limb,* and *dip;* and *cough* and *golf*). However, it has been demonstrated that talkers significantly influence the number of visemes produced (Kricos & Lesner, 1982). That is, some talkers are easier to speechread than are other talkers because they produce more distinctively different viseme groups. It has been estimated that, regardless of the number of viseme categories reported by various authors, in conversational speech nearly 50 percent of the words are indistinguishable visually; that is, they look like other words (Berger, 1972b).

> Homophenes are words that look alike when spoken, even though they sound different. Homophones are words that sound and look the same but are spelled differently.

CONSONANT VISEMES. A number of studies have been conducted to determine the number of visemes in spoken English. Woodward and Barber (1960), Fisher (1968), Erber (1974), Binnie et al. (1976), Jeffers and Barley (1971), Walden et al. (1977), Lesner et al. (1987), and Owens and Blazek (1985) have determined that there are a limited number of visually distinct patterns that can be made among spoken

English consonants. However, these authors do not agree on the number of visemes that can be recognized. Estimates vary from a low of four viseme groups to a high of nine viseme groups.

Table 5.1 lists the homophenous classifications proposed by several authors. Table 5.1 also illustrates the chance for error that a listener has when required to interpret phonemes visually. Except for the *independent visemes* of /l/, /h/, /r/, and /w/ reported by Erber (1974), Binnie et al. (1976), Walden et al. (1977), Owens and Blazek (1985), and Lesner et al. (1987) and the /j/ reported by Jeffers and Barley (1971), all viseme clusters contain at least two phonemes. Consequently, on the average, the speechreader has at best a 50 percent chance of correctly identifying a specific isolated phoneme within any group when relying solely on vision.

VOWEL VISEMES. Although vowels are not considered articulated phonemes, Jeffers and Barley (1971) suggested that vowels can be visually recognized by their movements, that is, by "a recognizable visual motor pattern, usually common to two or more speech sounds" (p. 42). These authors observed seven visually distinct movements when the vowels were produced at a slow rate accompanied with pronounced movement and normal rhythm. When the same phonemes were produced in conversational speech, the number of different movements was reduced to four.

Jeffers and Barley (1971) describe two viewing conditions based on speaker presentation that determine the visually distinct patterns among English phonemes produced in isolation. The first condition is referred to as *ideal*. Under this viewing condition the speaker provides the listener with essentially perfectly articulated

Ideal conditions include optimal distance, viewing angle, speech rate, and an unobstructed, well-lighted view of the speaker without auditory or visual distractions.

TABLE 5.1

Visemes for English Consonants Determined by Various Researchers

VISEME GROUPS			
Jeffers and Barley (1971)	Fisher (1968)		Binnie et al. (1976)
	Initial[a]	Final[b]	
1. /f, v/	1. /f, v/	1. /f, v/	1. /f, v/
2. /w, r/	2. /p, b, m, d/	2. /p, b/	2. /p, b, m/
3. /p, b, m/	3. /hw, w, r/	3. /ʃ, ʒ, dʒ, tʃ/	3. /w/
4. /θ, ð/	4. /ʃ, t, n, l, s, z, dʒ, j, h/	4. /t, d, n, θ, ð, s, z, r, l/	4. /l, n/
5. /ʃ, ʒ, tʃ, dʒ/	5. /k, g/	5. /k, g, ŋ, m/	5. /ʃ, ʒ/
6. /s, z/			6. /r/
7. /j/			7. /θ, ð/
8. /t, d, n, l/			8. /t, d, s, z/
9. /k, g, ŋ/			9. /k, g/

[a]Observed in the initial position.

[b]Observed in the final position.

Note: The order of the visemes is based on Binnie and coworkers' (1976) rank-ordering of the visual clustering of these phonemes.

speech that contains maximal visual cues. The second viewing condition is labeled *usual*. This condition occurs in what can be classified as everyday talking conditions. While the speaker does not intentionally distort his or her speech, he or she articulates in a typical manner that produces fewer visual cues. As can be seen in Table 5.2, these two conditions significantly influence which phonemes are included in which viseme cluster.

In general, it has been demonstrated that there are consistent visual confusions among vowels, frequently with vowels that have similar lip positions and movement (Jackson, Montgomery, & Binnie, 1976; Montgomery & Jackson, 1983). Furthermore, there are vowels that are seldom recognized visually and, as might be expected, the vowels that are perceived correctly in isolation are not necessarily comprehended visually in conversational speech.

In summary, most of the individual phonemes in our language are not unique visually, as they are when produced orally, resulting in considerable confusion and

Under ideal conditions, there are 14 total visemes, but under usual conditions there are 9, as compared to about 40 phonemes (see Table 5.2).

TABLE 5.2

Visemes for All Speech Sounds Combined in *Ideal* and *Usual* Viewing Conditions

COMBINED CONSONANT AND VOWEL SPEECHREADING MOVEMENTS
IDEAL VIEWING CONDITIONS

Visible	Obscure
1. Lower lip to upper teeth, /f, v/	10. Lips rounded, moderate opening to lips back, narrow opening, /ɔɪ/
2. Lips relaxed, moderate opening to lips puckered, narrow opening, /ɑu/	11. Tongue up or down, /t,d,n,l/
3. Lips puckered, narrow opening, /w,hw,r,u,ʊ,o,ou,ɝ/	12. Lips relaxed, moderate opening, /ɛ,æ,ɑ/
4. Lips together, /p,b,m/	13. Lips relaxed, moderate opening to lips back narrow opening, /ɑɪ/
5. Tongue between teeth, /θ,ð/	14. Tongue back and up, /k,g,ŋ/
6. Lips forward, /ʃ,ʒ,tʃ,dʒ/	
7. Lips back, narrow opening, /i,ɪ,eɪ,e,ʌ,j/	
8. Lips rounded, moderate opening, /ɔ/	
9. Teeth together, /s,z/	

COMBINED CONSONANT AND VOWEL SPEECHREADING MOVEMENTS
USUAL VIEWING CONDITIONS

Visible	Obscure
1. Lower lip to upper teeth, /f, v/	6. Lips forward, /ʃ,ʒ,tʃ,dʒ/
2. Lips puckered, narrow opening, /w,hw,r,u,ʊ,ou,ɝ/	7. Lips rounded, moderate opening, /ɔ,ɔɪ/
3. Lips together, /p,b,m/	8. Teeth approximated, /s,z; t,d,n,l; θ,ð; k,g,ŋ; j/
4. Lips relaxed, moderate opening to lips puckered, narrow opening, /ɑu/	9. Lips relaxed, narrow opening, /i,ɪ,eɪ,e,ʌ,ɛ,æ,ɑ,ɑɪ/
5. Tongue between teeth, /θ,ð/	

The movements are presented in an estimated order of relative visibility with 1 being most visible and 14 least visible.

Source: Adapted from Jeffers & Barley (1971).

Under ideal conditions, about 33% of speech is visible; with usual conditions, 10 to 25% is visible.

misperception on the part of the speechreader. Jeffers and Barley (1971) concluded that under optimal viewing conditions only about 40 percent of the information regarding consonant sounds provided by audition is available via vision. Furthermore, these authors demonstrated that the speechreader under ideal viewing conditions receives only about 33 percent of the information that is contained auditorily in conversational speech (vowels plus consonants). This visual information is reduced to approximately 17 percent (a range of 10 to 25 percent) when the speechreader is viewing conversations under everyday-type listening conditions.

VISIBILITY. In addition to the fact that a number of speech sounds and words look similar, another related problem for the speechreader is that many speech sounds are not very visible as they are produced. While phonemes like /p/ or /f/ can be seen quite well, other phonemes like /k/ or /t/ are produced in a far less visible manner. In addition, other features like *voicing* are not visible at all. It has been estimated that as many as 60 percent of the English phonemes are not readily visible (Woodward & Barber, 1960).

Visual Intelligibility of Connected Discourse. Researchers have determined the visemes that viewers can identify at the syllable and word levels, but they are less certain about what is visibly discernible when these speech elements are portions of lengthier utterances. The visual properties of isolated speech units change when placed in sentence form, as does the acoustic waveform itself. Unless there is a visible pause between words, a speechreader presumably perceives an uninterrupted series of articulatory movements of varying degrees of inherent visibility. This sequence is broken only when the speaker pauses, either deliberately or for a breath. As a result, the written message "There is a blue car in our driveway," is spoken /ðɛrIzəblukarInaʊɚdraɪvweI/. Connected speech contains numerous articulatory positions and movements that occur in a relatively short period of time. Consequently, the majority of phonemes in conversational speech occur in the medial position. The example just given contains an initial consonant /ð/, a final vowel /eI/, with numerous sounds (positions and movements) between these phonemes. Ironically, researchers have not determined the number of visemes that are identifiable when phonemes occur in the medial position.

Redundancy determines the predictability of a spoken message. The more redundancy present, the easier speechreading will be.

The nature of grammatical sentence structure imposes constraints on word sequences that are not present when the words are used in isolation. These word arrangement rules change the probabilities of word occurrence. Thus, the receiver's task is altered (theoretically made easier) because of the linguistic information and redundancy provided by connected discourse. Language is structured in a way that provides more information than is absolutely necessary to convey a given meaning or thought. Even if certain fragments of the spoken code are missed, cues or information inherent in the message may assist the receiver in making an accurate prediction of the missing parts. That is, oral language is an orderly process that is governed by the rules of pragmatic, topical, semantic, syntactic, lexical, and phonological constraints that are the sources for linguistic redundancy (Boothroyd, 1988). This redundancy creates the predictability of conversational speech. Table 4.4 summarizes several types of linguistic constraints that contribute to this.

Briefly, the pragmatic constraints of language allow for two or more individuals to share thoughts and information orally. Similarly, the topical constraints, which are also referred to as contextual and situational constraints, limit conversation to a specific topic, which, in turn, governs the vocabulary that is appropriate to describe the topic. We use this rule consistently, even though we frequently introduce it in a negative manner. For example, how many times have you said, "Not to change the subject," and then promptly deviated from the original topic of conversation? You are engaging the rule of contextual information and, regardless of how it is initiated, it provides your receiver with a preparatory set that allows her or him to expect a specific vocabulary concerned with a specific event. The situation or environment determines the manner in which the speaker will describe a certain event. Comedians are masters at using this rule; they alter the language of their "stories" based on the makeup of their audience. Contextual and situational constraints are closely allied and are used interchangeably by some authors. For example, during a televised sporting event, when a coach disputes a decision by a referee, have you noticed how well you perceive what the coach says, even though you only have limited auditory and visual cues available? Contextually, you perceive an argument while the situation causes the coach to express himself by using a rather limited and heated vocabulary that enables you to predict the words being used. As illustrated in this instance, the situation in which the conversation occurs provides information that otherwise you may not have been able to obtain by relying solely on the articulatory features of the message for perception.

Redundancy, the result of these constraints, contributes significantly to the information afforded by oral language. Thus, redundancy allows the receiver to predict missed information from the bits of information that have been perceived. To illustrate, "Dogs going" means the same as "The dogs are going away." The latter is grammatically correct and contains redundant information. Plurality is indicated twice (dogs, are), present tense twice (are, going), and the direction twice (going, away). Consequently, it would be possible to miss the words "are" and "away" while comprehending the message ("dogs are going"). If we miss part of a message, linguistic redundancy can enable us to synthesize correctly what we missed. However, as will be mentioned in the discussion of perceptual closure, a minimum amount of information must be perceived before accurate predictions can be made. In the preceding example, the words "dogs" and "away" would have to be processed visually in order for the speechreader to conceptualize the message "The dogs are going away."

Although the constraints of language do not enhance the physical visibility of oral sentences, they assist the receiver in visually understanding or speechreading what has been said. Albright, Hipskind, and Schuckers (1973) demonstrated that speechreaders actually obtain more total information from the redundancy and linguistic rules of spoken language than from phoneme and word visibility. Clouser (1976) concluded that the ratio between the number of consonants and vowels did not determine the visual intelligibility of sentences; rather, he found that short sentences were easier to speechread than longer sentences. In another study related to visual perception of speech, Berger (1972b) determined that familiar and frequently used words were identified visually more often than were words used infrequently. Additional information on redundancy is provided in Chapter 4 (see Tables 4.3 and 4.4).

Environment

Circumstances associated with the environments in which the speechreader must communicate can influence the speechreading process considerably. For example, investigators have demonstrated that such factors as distance and viewing angles between the speaker and receiver affect speechreading performance. Erber's (1971) study regarding the influence of distance on the visual perception of speech revealed that speechreading performance was optimal when the speaker was about 5 feet from the speechreader. Although performance decreased beyond 5 feet, it did not drop significantly until the distance exceeded 20 feet. Similarly, there is evidence that simultaneous auditory and visual competition can have an adverse effect on speechreading under certain conditions (O'Neill & Oyer, 1981). Although the amount of lighting is not an important factor in speechreading, provided a reasonable amount of light is present, Erber (1974) suggested that, for optimal visual reception of speech, illumination should provide a contrast between the background and the speaker's face.

Garstecki (1977) concluded that speechreading performance improved when the spoken message was accompanied by relevant pictorial and auditory cues. This finding was given further support by Garstecki and O'Neill (1980), whose subjects had better speechreading scores when the *CID Everyday Sentences* were presented with appropriate situational cues. In essence, environmental cues provide speechreaders with contextual and situational information, thereby increasing their ability to predict what is being conveyed verbally.

As noted earlier in the Speaker section, a 0 to 45 degree viewing angle is best; 90 degrees is not as good. Five to ten feet from the speaker is a good distance for speech reading.

Speechreader

Reduction of a person's ability to hear (auditory sensitivity) auditory stimuli is only one of several parameters that contribute to the disabling effects of hearing impairments. Other factors, such as auditory perception abilities (recognizing, identifying, and understanding), age of onset of the hearing loss, site(s) of lesions, and the educational and therapeutic management followed, all contribute toward making the hearing-impaired population extremely heterogeneous. This heterogeneity appears to extend to speechreading, because hearing-impaired individuals demonstrate considerable variability in their ability to use vision to speechread. Individual differences in speechreading abilities are large. This body of research is summarized by Dodd and Campbell (1987). Some persons possess amazing speechreading abilities, while others are able to perceive very little speech through the visual channel. Ever since speechreading has been included in audiologic rehabilitation, clinicians and researchers have attempted to determine what personal characteristics of the speechreader account for success or failure in speechreading, including variables such as age, gender, intelligence, personality traits, and visual acuity (O'Neill & Oyer, 1981). In general, it is impossible to totally clarify the characteristics associated with success in speechreading. The following is a sampling of the research that has been conducted in this area related to the speechreader.

AGE. There appear to be some interactions between a speechreader's age and other attributes that contribute to speechreading ability. Specifically, evidence suggests that speechreading proficiency tends to develop and improve throughout childhood and early adulthood and appears to be closely associated with the emergence of language skills. Even though their speechreading abilities are not fully developed, younger children, even infants, may use speechreading to some extent (Pollack, 1985).

Some older people demonstrate phonemic regression, that is, severe inability to understand speech via hearing, that is not consistent with their audiometric profiles (Gaeth, 1948). This same type of phenomenon may account, in part, for the finding that older individuals do less well in speechreading than their younger counterparts even when visual acuity is controlled. Hefler (1998) suggested that the elderly perform more poorly on experimental speechreading tasks because of the inability to process temporally changing visual information. Finally, it is important to note that decreased visual acuity may also contribute to reduced speechreading skill in the aged.

GENDER. This variable has been investigated thoroughly (Dancer et al., 1994). Overall, adult females consistently achieve higher speechreading scores than do males.

INTELLIGENCE. An abundance of research describes the relationship between speechreading and mental abilities. Generally, no demonstrable positive correlation has been found between understanding speech visually and intelligence, assuming intelligence levels in or above the "low normal" range (Lewis, 1972). However, a study conducted by Smith (1964) with a population of mentally impaired individuals revealed that much reduced intelligence levels did result in significantly poorer speechreading performance.

PERSONALITY TRAITS. As may be expected from the preceding discussion, investigators have not been able to ferret out specific personality traits that differentiate among levels of speechreading proficiency. While motivation is tenuous to assess, most clinicians intuitively concur that highly motivated (competitive) clients tend to speechread more effectively than do unmotivated clients. However, it is apparent that good and poor speechreaders generally cannot be stereotyped based on personality patterns (Giolas, Butterfield, & Weaver, 1974; O'Neill, 1951).

VISUAL SKILLS. Since speechreading is a visual activity, the acuity of vision is critical in the decoding process. As discussed in the Visual Assessment section of this chapter, vision has received meager attention from researchers in audiologic rehabilitation.

VISUAL ACUITY. In 1970, Hardick, Oyer, and Irion determined that they could rank successful and unsuccessful speechreaders based on their visual acuity. Furthermore, these authors observed a significant relationship between eye blink rate and speechreading ability, with poorer speechreaders demonstrating higher eye blink rates. Just prior to this research, Lovering (1969) demonstrated that even slight visual acuity problems (20/40 and poorer) had an appreciable, negative effect on speechreading scores. More recently, Johnson and Snell (1986) showed that distance and visual acuity have a significant effect on speechreading. These authors report that children with visual acuity of 20/80 or better should be able to speechread at 5 feet with an adequate degree of accuracy. When the speechreader is positioned

Speechreaders show better scores as they get older throughout childhood, if they are female, and if they have vision better than 20/40. IQ has little effect on speechreading as long as it is not below the normal range.

22 feet from the talker, then it is necessary that the speechreader have visual acuity no poorer than 20/30. If, however, the speechreader has one eye of 20/30 or better, then he or she should be able to speechread at a comparable level to those individuals with normal binocular vision under similar viewing conditions.

In support of the argument that good visual acuity is important for successful speechreading performance, Romano and Berlow (1974) concluded that visual acuity must be at least 20/80 before speech can be decoded visually. Recently, a line of research has compared visually evoked responses and speechreading ability. According to the results of this research, a viewer's ability to process speech visually is, in part, a function of the rapidity (latency) with which physical visual stimuli are transduced to neural energy for interpretation at the cortical level (Samar & Sims, 1983, 1984; Shepard, 1982; Shepard et al., 1977; Summerfield, 1992). While the clinical applicability of this research has not yet been fully realized, visually evoked responses can assist the clinician in understanding a client's ability to process visually oriented information. Potentially, visually evoked responses may provide audiologic rehabilitationists with information regarding a viewer's ability to speechread various types of oral stimuli.

VISUAL PERCEPTION. Based on Gibson's (1969) definition of perception, our eyes receive visual stimuli that are interpreted at a cortical level and provide us with visual information. This information, in turn, enables us to make a selective response to the original stimuli. Thus, when interpreting speech visually, the speechreader first "sees" the movement of the lips, which the cortex classifies as speech. The accuracy of the speechreader's response to these stimuli is partially a function of how well the peripheral-to-central visual process enables her or him to discriminate among the speaker's articulatory movements.

At present, explanations of the way in which the perceptual process develops are theoretical. However, two strategies appear relevant in connection with obtaining information from the environment. The first, figure–ground patterning, is achieved by identifying a target (meaningful) signal that is embedded in similar, but ambient, stimuli. Observe the following letters:

Figure–ground patterning involves an ability to focus on and perceive a target stimulus, or figure, from a background of other stimuli, or ground.

WABRIODRAZ

OPAIBLOHYE

LIPREADING

IRACRAXOLE

MUALYOCEPL

The letters within this rectangle are of the same case (capitals) and are placed in an order that meets the criterion of structural ordering. That is, all the letter combinations are possible and probable in written English. As noted, however, there is only one string of letters that creates a meaningful word, LIPREADING (see line 3). Thus, this sequence of printed symbols is the figure while all the other letters are merely spurious background stimuli. The development of figure–ground patterning permits the hearing impaired to separate meaningful visual and auditory events from ambient stimuli.

As early as 1912, Nitchie claimed that successful speechreaders are intuitive and able to synthesize limited visual input into meaningful wholes. Since then professionals have concurred that successful speechreaders possess the ability to visually piece together fragmented pictorial and spoken stimuli into meaningful messages. This ability, termed *closure,* is yet another strategy used to obtain information from environmental events. Before this strategy can be used effectively, a person must receive at least minimal stimulation and, more importantly, must have had prior experience (familiarity) with the whole. Both of the following sentences require that the reader use closure to obtain accurate information.

> Being able to combine or pull bits of information together in order to figure out what was said is termed *closure.*

1. Humpty _____ _____ _____ _____ wall.
2. When you _____ time, you murder _____.

In all probability you had little difficulty supplying the four words, *Dumpty sat on a,* to the first sentence. The second sentence may have been more difficult unless you are familiar with the adage, "When you kill time, you murder opportunity." The first sentence provides considerably fewer physical cues than does the second; but experience with and exposure to nursery rhymes permitted you to perceive the whole expression. Effective visual closure skills are essential for the hearing impaired, because, due to their disorder and the limited visual cues afforded by speech, they receive fragmented or distorted auditory and visual stimuli. In trying to understand the role of prediction or predictability, it is paramount to realize that we do not merely get some information by perception (processing the stimuli) and some from the context (prediction), and then add the two. If we did, the total information received would be equal to, or less than (because of redundancy or correlation), the sum of what we can get from either channel alone. The fact that the total is greater than the sum of both channels (as measured above) implies a facilitating or feedback effect from one to the other: The aural information facilitates visual processing, and the visual information enhances auditory processing.

HEARING. Unfortunately, the hearing impaired generally are not any better at speechreading than are those with normal hearing. Among the hearing impaired, however, there is a mild relationship between speechreading proficiency and the degree of hearing loss present. Those persons with significant amounts of residual hearing have the potential to speechread more successfully than those with very limited hearing. This occurs because speechreading is enhanced by the availability of simultaneous auditory cues contained in speech. This is especially apparent in persons beginning to use either a cochlear implant or tactile device, where speechreading performance often improves dramatically relative to what it was previously; because of the increased input provided by these devices, speechreading becomes easier.

> In general, those with hearing loss are not better speechreaders than those with normal hearing.

It is apparent that numerous factors have an impact on speechreading success. The successful clinician will be familiar with these and take each into account when assisting the hearing impaired in effectively using visual information for communication.

■ SPEECHREADING AND THE HEARING IMPAIRED

Assessing speechreading ability and providing effective speechreading instruction to the hearing impaired are two primary responsibilities of the aural rehabilitationist.

The next section outlines some of the ways in which a person's visual communication ability can be evaluated. It also describes several traditional and current approaches to speechreading instruction.

Assessment of Speechreading Ability

Because of the complexities associated with the process, accurate evaluation of speechreading performance is difficult. Professionals have attempted for several decades to develop a means of reliable and valid measurement, but to date no universally acceptable test or battery of tests has emerged for this purpose. Nevertheless, clinicians recognize the importance of assessing speechreading ability to determine if visual communication training is warranted for a particular individual, as well as to evaluate the effectiveness of speechreading training. Consequently, a number of formal and informal approaches for measuring speechreading ability are currently in use.

Vision-only refers to attempting to perceive speech via visual cues (without voice).

FORMAL SPEECHREADING TESTS. Since the mid-1940s, speechreading tests have been developed, published, and used. These tests, designed specifically to measure the speechreading abilities of adults or children, may consist of syllables, words, sentences, stories, or a combination of these stimuli. Speechreading tests are presented either in a vision-only condition without acoustic cues or in a combined visual–auditory test condition in which the stimuli are both seen and heard by the speechreader. These formal tests sometimes are presented via prerecorded videotape, but often are administered in a live, face-to-face situation, where the clinician presents the test stimuli. Although the test contents remain constant, the manner of presentation may vary considerably among clinicians when tests are administered live, which can make interpretation of the results less secure due to the variability created by using different speakers to present the test stimuli (Montgomery, Walden, Schwartz, & Prosek, 1984). Some of these tests are listed in Table 5.3 and in the appendixes of this chapter. It should be noted that several tests originally developed to assess auditory speech perception have also been used frequently to evaluate speechreading skills.

Speechreading and auditory assessment are both influenced by variables that raise or lower scores. These include vocabulary level, context, and response format (see Chapter 4).

INFORMAL SPEECHREADING TESTS. Informal tests are developed by the clinician, who selects stimulus materials of her or his choosing. Contents should vary as a function of the client's age and the information sought by the rehabilitationist. Clinicians use a variety of speech forms, including lists of words presented in isolation or in sentences. Sentence items may include statements like "What is your name?" or "Show me a toothbrush." Informal assessment allows the tester to select stimuli that are more pertinent for a particular client than items on formal speechreading tests. However, as a result of the loose format and the intent of these tests, the obtained results do not lend themselves well to comparative analysis.

Whether using formal or informal speechreading tests, it is important that the stimuli not be so difficult that they discourage the client nor so easy that test scores reflect a ceiling effect (100 percent correct for each viewer). Materials should be selected so that they approximate various types of stimuli encountered by the individual in everyday situations. For children and certain adults (such as those with

TABLE 5.3

Formal Speechreading Tests for Adults and Children

TITLE OF TESTS	AUTHOR(S)	CONTENT FORMAT
	Adults	
How Well Can You Read Lips?	Utley (1946)	Words Sentences Stories
Semi-Diagnostic Test	Hutton, Curry, & Armstrong (1959)	Words
Barley CID Sentences	Barley & Jeffers (1971)	Sentences
Lipreading Screening Test	Binnie, Jackson, & Montgomery (1976)	CV-Syllables
Denver Quick Test of Lipreading Ability[a]	Alpiner (1978)	Sentences
Assessment of Adult Speechreading Ability	New York League for the Hard of Hearing (1990b)	Sentences Paragraphs
Iowa Sentence Test	Tyler, Preece, & Tye-Murray (1986)	Sentences
	Children	
Craig Lipreading Inventory[a]	Craig (1964)	Words Sentences
Butt Children's Speechreading Test	Butt & Chreist (1968)	Questions Commands
Diagnostic Test of Speechreading	Myklebust & Neyhus (1970)	Words Phrases Sentences
The Children's Audiovisual Enhancement Test	Tye-Murray & Geers (2002)	Words

[a]See Appendixes 5B and 5C.

severe speech or writing problems), the response mode should involve pointing with a multiple-choice format; most adults are capable of responding to (writing or repeating) open-set tests. Because of the various shortcomings of existing speechreading tests, these instruments cannot be expected to provide completely valid measures of speechreading ability, but may yield data of some clinical usefulness.

The use of live, face-to-face presentation, although widespread, should be conducted carefully with optimal consideration for distance (5 to 10 feet), lighting (no shadows), and viewing angle (0 to 45 degrees). Even following these precautions, speaker variability will introduce uncertainty into the test situation. Not only will two speakers produce the same speech stimuli differently, but a single talker, producing the same stimuli twice, will not do so in precisely the same manner each time. Therefore, it is difficult to compare a person's skills from one testing to another (pre- and post-therapy) or to directly compare the performance of two individuals. Scores obtained through face-to-face test administration, although useful, need to be interpreted carefully.

Assessment of speechreading can involve the presentation of visual stimuli without any associated acoustic cues. Although this yields meaningful information regarding the basic skill of speechreading, additional testing of speechreading ability in a combined auditory–visual fashion is also advocated by many, because it more closely resembles ordinary person-to-person communication. Such testing provides a relevant measure of how well a person integrates visual and auditory information, which is how speech perception occurs in most real communication situations.

To estimate how a listener is using vision to supplement audition, present the listener with words and sentences in a vision-only mode, followed by another presentation in a vision-hearing combined (natural) mode. By subtracting the vision-only score from the vision-hearing score, a difference between these two presentation modalities will provide an estimate of the amount of information provided by speechreading for a given individual.

Speechreading abilities can also be assessed informally with speech tracking.

Schow (2005) noted that when college students with normal hearing are given his filmed version of Utley's (1946) *How Well Can You Read Lips?* test in a vision-only mode at a 0 degree azimuth, their performance is approximately as follows:

	SENTENCES	WORDS
Mean	35–45%	35–45%
Range	10–70%	25–70%

When given a similar filmed version of the *Semi-Diagnostic Test* (Hutton et al., 1959), these same students score as follows:

	WORDS	
	0 Degree Azimuth	90 Degree Azimuth
Mean	60–65%	50–60%
Range	25–90%	25–75%

The better *Semi-Diagnostic* scores are probably due to the closed response set, as opposed to the open response set in the Utley Test.

Visual Assessment and Speechreading Evaluation

It is important that assessment of speechreading skills be preceded by a measure of visual acuity. As discussed, there is clear evidence that even mild visual acuity problems can have adverse effects on speechreading performance. It is amazing, therefore, that audiologic rehabilitationists have given only limited attention to measuring basic visual abilities in connection with the assessment and instruction of speechreading with hearing-impaired persons. Concern for this is further reinforced by research on visual disorders among those with hearing loss. Evidence indicates that the incidence of ocular anomalies among hearing-impaired students is greater than for normally hearing children of the same age. Campbell and her associates (1981) surveyed the literature and found that 38 to 58 percent of the hearing impaired reportedly have accompanying visual deficiencies. Even more alarming are data from the National Technical Institute for the Deaf showing that, of the total number of students entering in the past, 65 percent demonstrated defective vision (Johnson et al., 1981). The elderly also present challenges, as their overall visual skills are declining at the same time as their hearing loss emerges. To maximize speech perception, both vision and auditory needs of the individual should be considered. Basic visual skills associated with the detection, recognition, resolution, and localization of visual stimuli are fundamental when assessing a person's visual acuity. Each of these measurements uses static stimuli; that is, the viewer describes specific characteristics of stationery targets that measure a certain aspect of the viewer's visual acuity. Although research on the relationship between visual acuity and speechreading has concentrated on visual *recognition* (commonly referred to as far visual acuity), at least for some clients it may be prudent to determine their ability to *detect, resolve,* and *localize* visual test stimuli prior to initiating speechreading therapy.

Hearing Impairment and Dependence on Vision

The degree to which the hearing impaired depend on vision for information is related to the extent of their hearing loss. To paraphrase Ross (1982), there is a world of difference between the deaf, who must communicate mainly through a visual mode (speechreading or manual communication), and the hard of hearing, who communicate primarily through an auditory mode (albeit imperfectly).

DEAF. The deaf, who receive quite limited meaningful auditory cues, must rely more on their vision to keep in contact with their environment. The deaf, by the nature of their disorder, use their vision projectively and are visually oriented. However, as stated throughout this chapter, vision generally is less effective than audition when used to decode spoken language. Furthermore, for the congenitally deaf, English usually is *not* their native language. Therefore, these individuals must learn to decode a foreign language without the benefit of auditory cues. English competency, which is most effectively and efficiently developed via the auditory channel, is essential to communication in our society. By definition, "speechreading is an inherently linguistic activity" (Boothroyd, 1988). The deaf therefore are further handicapped in that, before they can gain meaning from speechreading English, they must have developed the linguistic rules of English, which, in turn, are most naturally acquired through aural stimulation. In summary, to benefit from speechreading, the listener–viewers must have a fairly extensive language background. Without this they are not able to fill in the gaps providing them with information that cannot be obtained through speechreading or hearing (Bevan, 1988). Thus, the deaf face the monumental challenge of having to speechread words that they may never have conceptualized.

HARD OF HEARING. Hard of hearing individuals, by definition, possess functional residual hearing, which permits them to receive and ultimately perceive more auditory stimuli within their environment than those who are deaf. This enhanced ability would suggest that they are less dependent on their vision than are the deaf when perceiving speech. Even so, the hard of hearing, who employ their vision to supplement distorted and reduced acoustic stimuli, receive considerably more information from the spoken code than is provided solely by their auditory channel.

Various investigators have assessed the advantages that audition, vision, and a combination of these sensory modalities afford the receiver when decoding spoken stimuli (CHABA, 1991; Massaro, 1987). Few would disagree that using these two senses simultaneously produces better speech reception than using either alone. Likewise, it is clear that vision can provide information to the receiver when decoding speech in the absence of auditory cues. More importantly, however, even limited auditory input allows the listener to establish a referent from which additional information can be gained visually. Thus, the contributions made by these sensory mechanisms as receptors of speech fall into a hierarchy. That is, when both residual hearing and speechreading are available, the impaired listener tends to do better on a communicative task (see Figure 5.2). For example, if a person achieves a speech recognition score of 50 percent with hearing alone and a speechreading score of 20 percent using similar test material, this individual might achieve a combined auditory–visual score that could approach 80 to 90 percent. In other words, there is more than a simple additive effect from the combination of auditory and visual information. Therefore, the utility of vision in decoding speech should be exploited in audiological communication training.

FIGURE 5.2

Mean discrimination scores for normal hearing adults using audiovisual and audio-only speech stimuli (NU-6s).
Source: Binnie (1973).

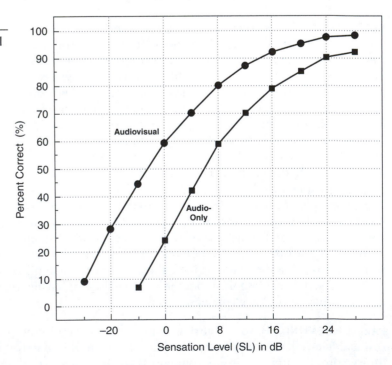

Traditional Speechreading Methods

During the early 1900s, four methods of teaching speechreading were popularized in the United States (O'Neill & Oyer, 1981). Three of these methods were nurtured by individuals who had normal hearing until adulthood, at which time they acquired significant hearing losses. Initially, they sought assistance to overcome the limitations placed on them by their sensory deprivation. Subsequently, they became interested in assisting other hearing-impaired persons in developing speechreading skills, eventually establishing methods that bear their names: the Bruhn method (1929), the Kinzie method (Kinzie & Kinzie, 1931), and the Nitchie method (1912). Later, Bunger (1944) wrote a book describing a speechreading method developed by Brauckman in Jena, Germany, the Jena method. Although these original four speechreading methods are seldom used now as they were originally conceived, it is recommended that the interested reader refer to French-St. George and Stoker (1988) for a historical chronicle of speechreading.

ANALYTIC AND SYNTHETIC APPROACHES. Each of the above original methods for teaching speechreading, as well as the recent approaches used currently, primarily makes use of one of two general approaches (analytic or synthetic) for speechreading instruction. However, for the most part, these incorporate the same general strategies as the analytical and synthetic approaches described in Chapter 4 for auditory training. The analytic approach to speechreading is based on the concept that, before an entire word, sentence, or phrase (the whole) can be identified, it is necessary to perceive visually each of its basic parts. That is, because a word is constructed by placing phonemes in a given sequential order and sentences (thoughts) are constructed by correctly ordering words, it is essential that the viewer initially identify phonemes visually in isolation before attempting to perceive words. Likewise, we must be able to identify individual words before attempting to recognize strings of words (sentences or phrases). Said differently, this approach to speechreading considers the phoneme and syllable to be the key units for visual perception; therefore, these units must be recognized in isolation before comprehension of the whole is probable.

Analytic speechreading centers around visually perceiving the details *found in speech.*

Conversely, the synthetic approach to speechreading emphasizes that the perception of the whole is paramount regardless of which of its parts is perceived visually. Consequently, the speechreader is encouraged to comprehend the general meaning of oral utterances, rather than concentrating on accurately identifying each component within the oral message. As noted earlier, a considerable number of English phonemes are not visible or distinguishable on the speaker's lips; thus, the receiver must predict and synthesize information from fragmented visual input and also use available contextual cues. The synthetic approach therefore considers speechreading key words and the sentence and phrase to be the basic units and backbone of visual speech perception.

Synthetic speechreading involves grasping the general thought of the speaker through intuitive thinking.

A procedure known as Continuous Discourse Tracking (CDT) developed by De-Filippo and Scott (1978) is being used in speechreading assessment and therapy. Tracking requires the hard of hearing listener to speechread verbatim passages presented by the clinician either in a vision-only or in a combined auditory–visual manner. A performance score is derived by counting the number of words per minute (wpm) the listener–viewer correctly identifies. Schow (2005) reported that his normally hearing college students, when presented combined auditory–visual stimuli, had CDT scores ranging from 76 to 102 wpm with a mean of 88 wpm. Patients who, after considerable exposure to CDT, still have very low scores (<20–25 wpm) may be candidates for cochlear implantation or training in ASL. Readers may assess their own CDT performance on the companion website (www.isu.edu/spchpath/rehab/). An example of how tracking is applied in a therapy session is presented in Chapter 4.

Table 5.4 contains examples of general speechreading therapy activities focused on emphasizing analytic and synthetic speechreading skills.

Recent Trends in Speechreading Instruction

The improvements in hearing aids, assistive listening devices (ALDs), vibrotactile devices, and cochlear implants that have occurred during the past two decades have made it possible for the hearing impaired, especially those with moderate-to-severe losses, to more effectively use their hearing than in the past in an integrated manner with speechreading. In a sense, this increased potential to greatly improve the communication abilities of those with hearing loss through hearing aids has, in part, led to much less emphasis on long-term speechreading therapy in rehabilitation programs for many individuals than in the past, particularly those with mild to moderate hearing impairments. Instead, what is done routinely with these individuals is to remind them of the importance of attending visually while communicating and encourage them to utilize this potentially helpful information as much as possible as another way, in addition to using hearing aids, to maximize overall speech perception. However, speechreading is still viewed as a useful component

---

TABLE 5.4

Examples of Analytical and Synthetic Speechreading Therapy Activities

ANALYTIC ACTIVITIES

1. Present syllable pairs with initial consonants that are the same or different (e.g., /ba/ and /ba/, or /la/ and /ba/) and ask the speechreader to discriminate if the initial consonant in the syllable pair is the same or different.
2. Present three or four words (e.g., *talk, tool, mop*) and have the speechreader determine which word has /m/ in the initial position.
3. Present single words and ask the speechreader to identify each word from a short list of printed words that the speechreader has in front of him.

SYNTHETIC ACTIVITIES

1. Show the speechreader a picture and ask her to provide four to six words that logically could be used by someone talking about the picture.
2. Name a topic (e.g., popular television shows) and have the speechreader identify the name of each show that you present.
3. Present a short paragraph and then ask the speechreader to answer three to four questions based on the content of the paragraph.

of audiological rehabilitation, and long-term therapy designed to facilitate speech-reading skills still is recommended on a selective basis for some persons with hearing impairment. The next two sections briefly discuss some of the more recent ways in which speechreading has been incorporated into rehabilitation strategies for both children and adults.

CHILDREN. There has been a dearth of information available concerning speech-reading strategies for this population (Yoshinaga-Itano, 1988). One probable explanation for this is that some therapeutic approaches used with hearing-impaired children have focused almost exclusively on maximizing the use of the auditory channel (Pollack, 1964, 1985; Wedenberg, 1951), with little if any attempt made to teach speechreading skills. This auditory-only unisensory philosophy of management for the hearing impaired is sometimes referred to as the auditory–verbal approach. Despite the unisensory orientation of these approaches, children trained in this manner often emerge with effective speechreading skills. Although this approach clearly focuses on processing and using auditory input, speechreading appears to develop synergistically with the acquisition of auditory and language skills (Pollack, 1964).

Other professionals believe that speechreading therapy has some relevance to a comprehensive plan for audiologic rehabilitation for children. Yoshinaga-Itano (1988) suggests using what she terms a *holistic approach* when teaching hard of

In the aural approach, auditory abilities are developed to the fullest extent possible. Consequently, formal speechreading training is not incorporated into a child's overall program, and speech-reading actually is prevented in some therapy activities.

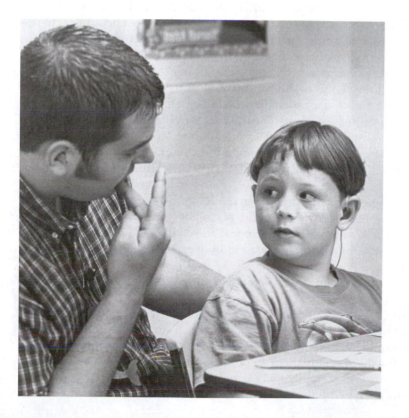

Analytic drill emphasizing visual cues associated with a consonant.

hearing children to speechread. This method differs from the traditional approaches to speechreading in that, rather than using a single technique for all young clients, it focuses on each individual child's motivation, tolerance, and sense of responsibility for communicating. Goals include building the child's knowledge base concerning the speechreading process and having the child develop an appreciation of the benefits that speechreading can provide in perceiving speech. Consequently, the stimuli used are client oriented, and therapy is based on each client's capabilities and needs in real-life situations, rather than just in canned exercises. Therefore, clinical activities must address the individual needs of each child. In addition, the speechreading activities must be interesting and give the child the opportunity to experience frequent success by correctly perceiving what is being presented. Figure 5.3 is an example of an activity that may be appropriate for *some* hard of hearing children. The child is given a worksheet with a picture on it and asked to speechread the key words presented by the clinician or by other children if it is being used in a group session. Beyond providing contextual and situational information, the picture has the potential to stimulate client motivation and interest. As a reward, the clinician may ask the child to color the picture. The clinician is reminded that this is only an example and the idea and format should be adapted to meet the needs and interests of her or his clients.

Children born with severe-to-profound hearing losses or who acquire the hearing loss prelingually become potential recipients of speechreading therapy if an oral–aural or total communication approach to management is followed. These children are fit as early as possible with hearing aids binaurally or cochlear implants. As part of an overall management approach, they also are encouraged to use vision and receive speechreading therapy, along with auditory training. Both analytic and synthetic training activities are used to develop visual as well as auditory skills. Although a portion of speechreading and auditory skill development is done in vision-only or auditory-only conditions, many professionals currently advocate using both vision and audition together. Expressions with visual and auditory stimuli presented simultaneously are more natural and provide an opportunity to integrate the auditory and visual cues that are available. More information on the application of speechreading with hearing-impaired children can be obtained in the publications by McCaffrey (1995), Tye-Murray (1993a, 1993b), or Haspiel (1987).

Auditory-only refers to attempting to perceive speech via hearing (without visual clues).

ADULTS. In the past, speechreading training was often provided to hearing-impaired adults in an intensive manner over a lengthy period of time, which sometimes extended for weeks and even months. This approach is still used selectively in some instances, such as with adults with severe, progressive hearing losses or some cochlear implant recipients. For these individuals, speech perception is challenging at best, and attempting to maximize the use of visual cues through extensive speechreading therapy is sometimes warranted, even if the benefits derived are limited.

Long-term speechreading therapy typically includes both analytic and synthetic training activities. In addition, clinicians are encouraged to use both visual-only and visual–auditory sensory modalities throughout the therapy program. The level of difficulty for the speechreader can be varied by degrading either the visual or auditory stimulus. For example, increasing the distance between the speechreader and the clinician will increase the level of difficulty for the speechreading

Space Patrol

FIGURE 5.3

Example of an exercise used
in speechreading therapy
with children.

space suit   space helmet

sky   sun

stop   stars

    Here is a space ship. Lets take a ride in it. Put on
your _____ and your _____ .
Step in and sit down. We will see the _____
and the _____ in the _____ . We will
not _____ for a long time.

task. Focused speechreading therapy of this nature can be done in either an individualized or group setting. However, group sessions afford an opportunity for the
participants to interact and learn from one another. In some instances, clinicians
elect to conduct programs that combine both individual and group sessions for the
participants to gain the benefits of each format. Guidance in this application of
speechreading, including useful information regarding therapy activities, can be
obtained from Wayner and Abrahamson (1996), Feehan, Samuelson, and Seymour
(1982), and Tye-Murray (1997). It should be noted that research by Walden and his
colleagues (1977, 1981) strongly suggests that demonstrable improvement in

speechreading skills occurs within the first 5 or 6 hours of training, but very little additional improvement (learning) is observed thereafter. Furthermore, it is suggested in the literature that sentence recognition by the hard of hearing is optimized immediately after training is started, regardless if this training is primarily auditory or visual (Walden et al., 1981). Therefore, the implication is that short-term involvement in speechreading therapy is usually the best approach, and long-term involvement should be conducted/pursued only rarely.

Even though long-term speechreading therapy generally is used only in isolated situations, there has been a growing interest in including limited speechreading instruction as part of a general orientation to effective communication skills. This approach is comparatively short term and typically emphasizes a number of key components of effective communication, including the importance of speechreading in communicating, as well as providing basic information about how to enhance speechreading performance in a variety of communicative situations. The intent here is not to engage the person with a hearing loss in therapy and drill-like activities in an attempt to improve visual perception of speech. Rather, it is to highlight to the individual the importance and benefits of using the visual skills that he or she already has in order to maximize speech perception abilities. This strategy has generally taken two different forms. In one of the approaches, clinicians organize small (6 to 12 members) groups of adults with hearing impairments. These groups typically meet once a week for 4 to 6 weeks, with each session devoted to a general topic related to enhancing overall communication skills. Among the more common topics included are the following:

Group AR sessions often focus on these four main topics.

1. Understanding hearing loss
2. Using assistive listening devices
3. Using communication strategies and speechreading
4. Effective use of hearing aids

The session devoted to speechreading often includes general information about the speechreading process, as well as tips for effective speechreading (Table 5.5).

Another approach used is to provide a streamlined and condensed version of the same type of communication-related information and helpful hints. This can be

TABLE 5.5

Tips for Speechreading

Be relatively close to the person(s) with whom you are communicating.

Watch the speaker's mouth, facial expressions, and hand gestures as much as possible.

Be aware of the topic of conversation and contextual cues.

Maximize your hearing (hearing aids and assistive listening devices at optimum volume and minimize background noise).

Let the talker know that you have a hearing loss and request that she or he face you as much as possible.

done in one session, often when the individual is fit with hearing aids. One example of this is the CLEAR program (Schow, 2001) described in Chapter 10. The "L" in CLEAR emphasizes the necessity to "look at" and "lipread" the talker. WATCH (Montgomery, 1994) is another method designed to help reinforce the importance of observing the talker. The "W" in this program is for "Watch the talker's mouth." Both CLEAR and WATCH are designed to illustrate the importance of seeing as well as listening during conversation.

Since hearing loss is an invisible disorder and since hard of hearing individuals comprehend much of what is said and yet misinterpret a significant amount of conversation, the general populace, and frequently significant others, are unaware of the deleterious effects of hearing loss, especially on oral communication. SPEECH (see Chapter 10) is a related program designed to help normally hearing people communicate effectively with individuals who have a hearing loss.

INNOVATIVE OPTIONS. Speechreading training can occur in formats other than the traditional face-to-face approach. For example, individuals can use videotapes as self-instructional programs to improve speechreading skills. Examples include *I See What You're Saying,* a two-volume series produced by the New York League for the Hard of Hearing (1990a) and the National Technical Institute for the Deaf (NTID) Speechreading Videotapes (1987).

Another innovative approach to speechreading training is referred to as computer-assisted interactive video (CAIV) instruction. The use of computers with computer-driven video and laser disc players has received considerable attention and application in hearing rehabilitation during the past decade. Mahshie (1987) defines interactive video as a "video program that can be controlled by the person using it."

Case 5.1

The importance of using a *preparatory set* with the hard of hearing during oral communication needs to be emphasized, because it is frequently underutilized. Tye-Murray (2004) refers to this as providing *topical cues* for the listener. In fact, normally hearing listeners use this strategy with regularity during conversation. They will say, "not to change the topic but. .." and proceed to change the topic. However, they have provided the listener with a "preparation" for the new topic, and generally the listener will be able to follow the ensuing conversation. As an example, in a recent audiologic rehabilitation adult support group a retired professor expressed that he was having great difficulty in most communication situations. He stated that he was not able to gain much information either from audition, via his digital hearing aids, or from his vision. However, when the audiologist said, "Let's talk about what you did yesterday," the patient had little difficulty conversing. When the audiologist injected, "Now let's talk about your favorite hobby—golf," the patient became even more accurate in his exchange of information. His ability to receive and express appropriately and accurately continued when the audiologist alerted him that they were now going to discuss current events. What became evident during this therapy session was that this hard of hearing person was able to use his audition and vision far more effectively to decode conversational speech if he knew the topic(s) to be discussed.

However, for this methodology to be useful, it must be capable of controlling complex protocols tailored to the rehabilitative needs of individual students or clients. Therefore, CAIV must incorporate a variety of teaching strategies and client response formats. The advantage of laser videodisc is the rapidity and accuracy with which specific stimuli can be accessed from the videodisc. Fifteen years ago the first interactive video for speechreading was developed at the NTID by Cronin (1979). This system was known as DAVID (Dynamic Audio Video Interactive Device). Since the initiation of this technology, researchers and clinicians have used interactive video systems to determine the benefits of cochlear implants and vibrotactile devices on speechreading. In 1986, laser videodisc technology was introduced as a speechreading training protocol (Kopra, Kopra, Abrahamson, & Dunlop, 1986). It is not within the scope of this chapter to discuss in detail the various CAIV programs now available. However, the following are examples of the more current interactive video speechreading programs: Auditory-Visual Laser Videodisc Interactive System (ALVIS), developed by Kopra et al. (1987); Computer-Assisted Speech Perception Evaluation and Training (CASPER), and CASPERSENT (sentences), designed by Boothroyd (Boothroyd, 1987; 2005) (with CASPERSENT, 60 sets of 12 sentences are available on DVD for adults to use in audio, visual, and audiovisual applications); Computer-Aided Speechreading Training Program (CAST), designed by Pichora-Fuller and Benguerel (1991); and Conversation Made Easy, developed at the University of Iowa Hospitals by Tye-Murray and her associates (2002a). Most of these CAIV programs include both analytic and synthetic-based activities for speechreading instruction, including a tracking component. There is little doubt that more computer-generated speechreading programs will be developed for use by the hearing impaired in the future. Tye-Murray (2004) lists several reasons to use computerized speechreading instruction to supplement the traditional forms of audiologic rehabilitation:

1. A variety of stimuli can be viewed by the patient in a short period of time.
2. The patient's responses are recorded within and between training sessions.
3. The patient may view a number of different talkers during a single session.
4. If the program is interactive, the patient's response determines the ensuing stimulus.
5. The patient determines the pace of the instruction.
6. The instruction occurs at the patient's convenience.

However, it also is clear that the traditional face-to-face format, involving both patient and clinician, will continue to be an important and viable format for audiologic rehabilitation as well.

■ MANUAL COMMUNICATION

Vision can be used by the hearing impaired for communication in another manner besides speechreading. Physical gestures and facial expressions have always been used by humans to express emotions and to share information. The transmission of thoughts in this manner undoubtedly preceded the verbal form of communication. As stated earlier in this chapter, manual communication is comprised of specific gestural codes. That is, a visual message is transmitted by the fingers, hands, arms, and bodily postures using specific signs or fingerspelling. In general, manual communication is used by a high percentage of the deaf to communicate with other individuals also having manual communication skills. The various forms of manual communication are used in isolation or in combination with speech.

Types of Manual Communication

Numerous forms of manual communication have evolved. The major types, along with spoken English, are briefly described and compared in Table 5.6 (Smith, personal communication, 1984). Smith pointed out that the only two pure languages represented in this group are English and American Sign Language.

AMERICAN SIGN LANGUAGE. American Sign Language, also referred to as ASL or Ameslan, was the first form of manual communication established, independent of existing oral languages, by the deaf. Consequently, the original sign language was indeed a unique "natural" language. Approximately one-half million deaf and hearing individuals use this language (Baker & Cokely, 1980). Interestingly, many individuals learn ASL via their deaf peers and associates rather than from their parents. Padden (1980) reports that it is probably the only language that is not learned from parents. Although most deaf adults are proud that they communicate via ASL and are annoyed by teachers and others who are averse to its use, the fact that they learned it from other children rather than from their parents influences their attitudes about sign language (Vernon & Andrews, 1990). The signs associated with ASL possess four identifying physical characteristics: hand configuration, movement, location, and orientation. In fact, Stokoe (1978) claims that there are 19 basic symbols for handshapes, 12 basic symbols for locations, and 24 basic symbols for movement. Although these parameters, referred to as *cheremes* by Stokoe, Casterline, and Croneberg (1965), are different from spoken lexical items, they may be viewed as analogous to the distinctive features of speech. These features are illustrated in Figure 5.4. The prosodic features of ASL are provided by facial expressions, head tilts, body movement, and eye gazes (Vernon & Andrews, 1990).

> Cheremes are the most basic and visually distinct units of sign language.

Because ASL is a language, it consists of words. However, there is not a corresponding sign to represent each English word, just as there is no unique relationship between the words used in English, French, Portuguese, Chinese, or Japanese. All languages were developed using a common code for the exchange of information. Also, the structure of each language is as unique as is its vocabulary (code). Thus, "Ni qui guo zhong-guo mei-you?" probably looks and sounds peculiar and unintelligible to those of us native to the United States, but the sentence is logical and meaningful to someone in Taiwan. Similarly, ASL is not a form of English, but rather a distinct language produced manually that requires just as unique a translation of English as does any foreign language.

> Iconic signs closely represent the respective actions or things. They are easily presented and understood, sometimes even by those not fluent in signing.

Some of the over 6,000 signs that are part of ASL can be decoded intuitively. These signs are classified as iconic, meaning that they are imageries of English words. The signs in Figure 5.5 will be familiar to most readers, even those who have never been exposed to manual communication, specifically ASL.

TABLE 5.6

Forms of Manual and Spoken Communication

AMERICAN SIGN LANGUAGE (ASL)	PIDGIN SIGNED ENGLISH (PSE)	SIGNED ENGLISH	LINGUISTICS OF VISUAL ENGLISH (LOVE)	SIGNING EXACT ENGLISH (SEE 2)	SEEING ESSENTIAL ENGLISH (SEE 1)	FINGER-SPELLING	CUED SPEECH	ENGLISH
Independent language; visual manual mode; own grammar; own syntax; signs are meaning based; has dialects, regionalisms, slang, puns; can be written; wide range of vocabulary covering minute differences in meaning; may borrow from other languages; is verbal, but also makes use of nonverbal elements.	A combination of elements from ASL and the sign systems, ranging from the more ASL-like (occasionally called Ameslish) to the more English-like (sometimes called CASE—Conceptually Accurate Signed English). Usually contains few if any sign markers (see Signed English), yet makes frequent use of fingerspelled English words. Used in conjunction with speech in interpreting and college teaching. Signs are meaning based.	Signed in accordance with English grammar, but signs are meaning based; specially invented sign markers for important affixes in English; invented by Bornstein; used widely in education.	Essentially the same as SEE 2, but has a method of writing each sign; used in education; invented by Wampler; usage is diminishing.	Signs are word based; special signs for all affixes in English; signed in strict accordance with English; invented by Zawolkow, Pfetzing, and Gustason; widely used in education; very influential.	Signs are based on word roots (morphemes) (trans/port/a/tion); an extreme form of word-based signs; invented by Anthony; not popular in United States, but still common in Iowa and Colorado schools for the deaf; signs for all affixes.	Manual representation of the written language; one hand shape for each letter of alphabet; used to borrow English words in ASL; when used with speech and speechreading, it is called the Rochester Method.	Employs 8 hand shapes in 4 positions on the face, and used in conjunction with lip movements to enable a deaf person to lipread more easily; based on sound with the syllable as the basic unit; devised by Orin Cornett at Gallaudet College.	Independent language; aural–oral mode; own grammar; own syntax; words are meaning based; contains dialects, regionalisms, slang, puns; can be written; wide range of vocabulary covering minute differences in meaning; may borrow from other languages; is verbal, but also makes use of nonverbal elements.

Artificial pedagogical systems, invented for educational purposes

Nonverbal communication: natural gestures, facial expression, body movements, body language, pantomime

Source: W. H. Smith, personal communication, 1984.

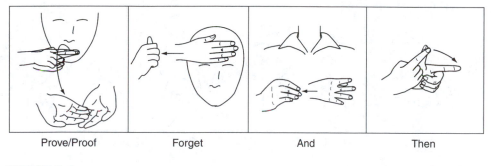

| Prove/Proof | Forget | And | Then |

FIGURE 5.4

Four signs used in ASL representing the features of handshape (DEZ), movement/signation (SIG), tabulation where sign is produced (TAB), and palmar direction of the hands.
Source: Riekehof, L. (1978). *The Joy of Signing.* Springfield, MO: Gospel Publishing House.

SIGNED ENGLISH SYSTEMS. There is evidence that only deaf adults are truly proficient at using ASL. When many hearing individuals attempt to communicate manually with the deaf using ASL, they often attempt to use the signs of ASL in a manner that more closely resembles English grammatically. This counterpart to ASL is commonly referred to as Pidgin Sign Language. In other words, Pidgin Sign Language involves combining ASL with English to some extent. If the signer makes considerable English-related modifications, then the result is Pidgin Signed English.

Other attempts have been made to seriously alter ASL so that it closely resembles English, and these are referred to as manually coded English or sign systems. Since sign systems more closely resemble English than ASL, they are often used in an educational setting to minimize the differences that exist between spoken and written English and ASL.

Signed English is a system in which the English words that appear in a message are signed in that same order. To indicate tense, person, plurality, and possession a sign marker is used as a suffix to the signed word. Seeing Essential English (SEE 1) was developed by David Anthony, a deaf individual, as a means of presenting English visually to the deaf as it is presented auditorily to normal hearing children. Anthony suggested that the word order of the message parallel the word order used in English. Signing Exact English (SEE II) is an outgrowth of SEE I. The purpose of this system is to maintain the syntactic structure of SEE I without making the system unintelligible for those using ASL. Linguistics of Visual English (LOVE) was established at approximately the same time as SEE II was initiated. Again, this was an attempt to refine another sign system aimed at approximating English. The vocabulary is more limited than that of SEE I and SEE II. It attempts to mirror spoken English by making signed movements that correspond to the number of syllables uttered in a spoken word. Yet LOVE is primarily a manual system identical to SEE II. The reader is urged to read the works of Scheetz (2001) and Vernon and Andrews (1990) for a historical and more detailed discussion of these systems.

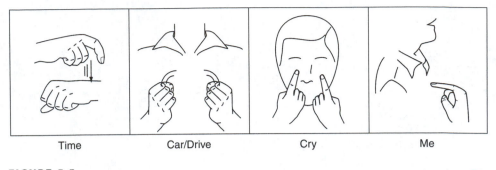

Time	Car/Drive	Cry	Me

FIGURE 5.5

Four iconic signs. The signs are visual images of the English words they represent.
Source: Riekehof, L. (1978). *The Joy of Signing.* Springfield, MO: Gospel Publishing House.

FINGERSPELLING. Another method of communicating manually is to have senders spell the words with their fingers. That is, instead of using pencil and paper, speakers spell their message in the air by using various handshapes to represent the letters in the English alphabet. This mode of communication, fingerspelling, represents the 26 letters of the English alphabet by 25 handshapes and 2 hand movements (see Figure 5.6). Collectively these are also referred to as the manual alphabet. The letters *i* and *j* are produced by the same handshape, with the *j* being produced by moving the hand in a hook or *j*-like motion. The letter *z* is made by moving a unique handshape in the form of a *z*. Although fingerspelling is an exact and effective means of communication, it is the least efficient form of manual communication; each letter of each word must be produced, which makes it a relatively laborious means of communicating. Because no additional characters are included in the alphabet nor digits in the numeric system, a person can learn to transmit a message via fingerspelling in a relatively short time. However, because of the rapidity with which one learns to "spell" a message and because of the similarity in the production of *e, o, m,* and *n* and between the letters *a* and *s*, the reception of fingerspelling requires considerable practice and concentration. As mentioned in the discussion of speechreading, the similarity among letters and sounds becomes more confounding during discourse than in isolation. But, as in every other form of communication, predictability mitigates this problem. Today, fingerspelling is used to supplement all forms of manual communication by expressing proper names, technical terms, and events that cannot be conveyed by signs. An application of fingerspelling is the Rochester Method, in which the teachers and students simultaneously "spell" what they are expressing orally.

Cued Speech also has applications for speech therapy.

CUED SPEECH. Some professionals have promoted the use of Cued Speech as an ancillary tool in speechreading instruction (Cornett, 1967, 1972). The intent of Cornett's (1967) Cued Speech system (some would prefer to classify it as a manual

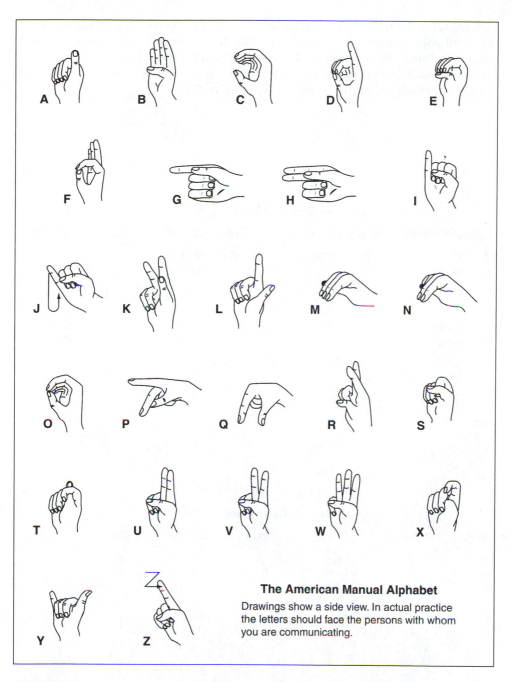

The American Manual Alphabet

Drawings show a side view. In actual practice the letters should face the persons with whom you are communicating.

FIGURE 5.6

American manual alphabet. The hand positions are shown as they appear to the person reading them.

Courtesy of Gallaudet College, Washington, DC.

system) is for the talker to use hand cues simultaneously while speaking to reduce the confusion produced by speechreading homophenous phonemes, making speechreading more accurate and effective. Cornett selected four hand positions and eight handshapes near the mouth to facilitate communication in the overall management of the hearing impaired (see Figure 5.7).

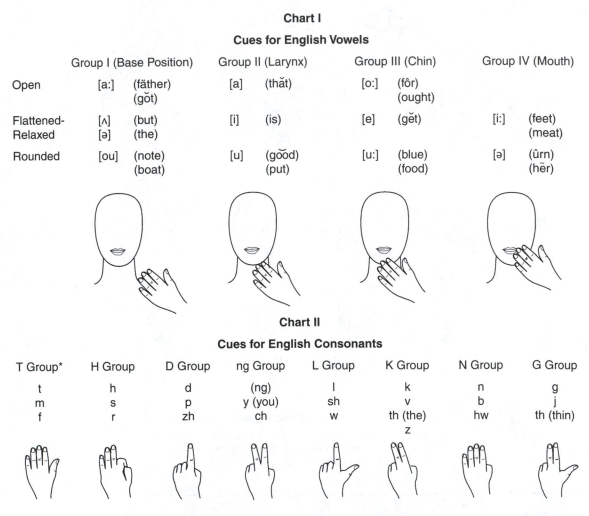

Chart I
Cues for English Vowels

	Group I (Base Position)		Group II (Larynx)		Group III (Chin)		Group IV (Mouth)	
Open	[a:]	(fäther) (gŏt)	[a]	(thăt)	[o:]	(fôr) (ought)		
Flattened-Relaxed	[ʌ] [ə]	(but) (the)	[i]	(is)	[e]	(gĕt)	[i:]	(feet) (meat)
Rounded	[ou]	(note) (boat)	[u]	(gŏod) (put)	[u:]	(blue) (food)	[ə]	(ûrn) (hẽr)

Chart II
Cues for English Consonants

T Group*	H Group	D Group	ng Group	L Group	K Group	N Group	G Group
t	h	d	(ng)	l	k	n	g
m	s	p	y (you)	sh	v	b	j
f	r	zh	ch	w	th (the)	hw	th (thin)
					z		

Note: The T group cue is also used with an isolated vowel—that is, an individual vowel not run with a final consonant from the preceding syllable.

FIGURE 5.7

Hand positions and handshapes used in cued speech.
Source: Cornett, R. (1967). Cued Speech. *American Annals of the Deaf, 112,* 3–13.

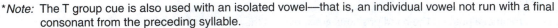

SUMMARY POINTS

- Speechreading and the use of manual communication are two important aspects of audiologic rehabilitation that involve the use of vision by those with hearing loss.
- Speechreading is a complex process that involves a large number of variables associated with the speechreader and other components of oral communication.
- Speechreading assessment can be done with a variety of formal and informal test protocols, using vision-only or combined vision–hearing conditions.
- Intensive training in speechreading is not frequently done. When carried out, both analytic and synthetic skill development activities are included.
- Shorter forms of audiologic rehabilitation are frequently used that encourage and assist those with hearing impairment to maximize the use of the speechreading skills that they already have.
- Manual communication consists of sign language, sign systems, and fingerspelling.
- American Sign Language, or ASL, is the language of the Deaf.
- Sign systems have been developed that modify ASL to make it more consistent with English. These systems are often used in educational programs.
- Fingerspelling, an adjunct to signing, uses the manual alphabet to spell out words in a message.

RECOMMENDED READING

Alpiner, J., & McCarthy, P. (Eds.). (2000). *Rehabilitative audiology: Children and adults* (3rd ed.). Philadelphia: Lippincott Williams & Wilkins.

Gagne, J. P., & Tye-Murray, N. (Eds.). (1994). Research in audiological rehabilitation: Current trends and future directions (Monograph). *Journal of the Academy of Rehabilitative Audiology, 27.*

Hipskind, N. (1978). Aural rehabilitation for adults. *Otolaryngologic Clinics of North America, 11,* 823–834.

Paul, P. (2001). *Language and deafness* (3rd ed.). San Diego, CA: Singular Publishing Group.

Scheetz, N. (2001). *Orientation to deafness* (2nd ed.). Boston: Allyn and Bacon.

Tye-Murray, N. (2004). *Foundations of aural rehabilitation* (2nd ed.). San Diego, CA: Singular Publishing Group.

Valente, M., Hosford-Dunn, H., & Roeser, R. (2000). *Audiology: Treatment.* New York: Thieme.

REFERENCES

Albright, P., Hipskind, N., & Schuckers, G. (1973). A comparison of visibility and speechreading performance on English and Slurvian. *Journal of Communication Disorders, 6,* 44–52.

Alpiner, J. G. (1978). *Handbook of adult rehabilitative audiology.* Baltimore: Williams & Wilkins.

Alpiner, J. (1982). Evaluation of communication function. In J. Alpiner (Ed.), *Handbook of adult rehabilitative audiology.* Baltimore: Williams & Wilkins.

Baker, C., & Cokely, D. (1980). *American sign language: A teachers resource test on grammar and culture.* Silver Spring, MD: T. J. Publishers.

Berger, K. (1972a). *Speechreading: Principles and methods*. Baltimore: National Educational Press.

Berger, K. (1972b). Visemes and homophenous words. *Teacher of the Deaf, 70,* 396–399.

Bevan, R. C. (1988). *Hearing-impaired children: A guide for parents and concerned professionals*. Springfield, IL: Charles C. Thomas.

Binnie, C. (1973). Bi-sensory articulation functions for normal hearing and sensorineural hearing loss patients. *Journal of the Academy of Rehabilitative Audiology, 6,* 43–53.

Binnie, C. A., Jackson, P., & Montgomery, A. (1976). Visual intelligibility of consonants: A lipreading screening test with implications for aural rehabilitation. *Journal of Speech and Hearing Disorders, 41,* 530–539.

Boothroyd, A. (1987). CASPER, computer-assisted speech perception evaluation and training. In *Proceedings of the 10th Annual Conference of the Rehabilitation Society of North America*. Washington, DC: Association for Advancement of Rehabilitation Technology.

Boothroyd, A. (1988). Linguistic factors in speechreading. In C. L. DeFilippo & D. G. Sims (Eds.), New reflections on speechreading (Monograph). *Volta Review, 90*(5), 77–87.

Boothroyd, A. (2005). *Computer-Assisted Speech Perception Testing and Training: Sentence Level*. Accessed 2005 from www.arthurboothroyd.com

Bruhn, M. E. (1929). *The Mueller–Walle method of lip reading for the deaf*. Lynn, MS: Nicholas Press.

Bunger, A. M. (1944). *Speech reading—Jena method*. Danville, IL: The Interstate Co.

Butt, D., & Chreist, F. (1968). A speechreading test for young children. *Volta Review, 70,* 225–239.

Campbell, C., Polomeno, R., Elder, J., Murray, I., & Altosaar, A. (1981). Importance of an eye examination in identifying the cause of congenital hearing impairments. *Journal of Speech and Hearing Disorders, 46,* 258–261.

CHABA, Working Group on Communication Aids for the Hearing-Impaired. (1991). Speech-perception aids for hearing impaired people: Current status and needed research. *Journal of the Acoustical Society of America, 90,* 637–685.

Clouser, R. A. (1976). The effects of vowel consonant ratio and sentence length on lipreading ability. *American Annals of the Deaf, 121,* 513–518.

Cornett, R. (1967). Cued speech. *American Annals of the Deaf, 112,* 3–13.

Cornett, R. O. (1972). *Cued speech parent training and follow-up program*. Washington, DC: Bureau of Education for the Handicapped, DHEW.

Craig, W. (1964). Effects of preschool training on the development of reading and lipreading skills of deaf children. *American Annals of the Deaf, 109,* 280–296.

Cronin, B. (1979). The DAVID system: The development of an interactive video system at the National Institute for the Deaf. *American Annals of the Deaf, 124,* 615–618.

Daly, N., Bench, J., & Chappell, H. (1996). Gender differences in speechreadability. *Journal of the Academy of Rehabilitative Audiology, 29,* 27–40.

Dancer, J., Krain, M., Thompson, C., Davis, P., & Glenn, J. (1994). A cross-sectional investigation of speechreading in adults: Effects of age, gender, practice and education. *Volta Review, 96,* 31–40.

DeFilippo, C., & Scott, B. (1978). A method for training and evaluating the reception of ongoing speech. *Journal of the Acoustical Society of America, 63*(4), 1186–1192.

Dodd, B., & Campbell, R. (1987). *Hearing by eye: The psychology of lip-reading*. London: Erlbaum.

Erber, N. P. (1971). Effects of distance on the visual reception of speech. *Journal of Speech and Hearing Research, 14,* 848–857.

Erber, N. P. (1974). Effects of angle, distance and illumination on visual reception of speech by profoundly deaf children. *Journal of Speech and Hearing Research, 17,* 99–112.

Feehan, P., Samuelson, R., & Seymour, D. (1982). *CLUES: Speechreading for adults*. Austin, TX: Pro-Ed.

Fisher, C. G. (1968). Confusions among visually perceived consonants. *Journal of Speech and Hearing Research, 12,* 796–804.

French-St. George, M., & Stoker, R. (1988). Speechreading: An historical perspective. In C. L. DeFilippo & D. G. Sims (Eds.), New reflections on speechreading (Monograph). *Volta Review, 90*(5), 17–31.

Gaeth, I. H. (1948). *A study of phonemic regression in relation to hearing loss.* Unpublished doctoral dissertation, Northwestern University.

Garstecki, D. (1977). Identification of communication competence in the geriatric population. *Journal of the Academy of Rehabilitative Audiology, 10,* 36–45.

Garstecki, D., & O'Neill, J. J. (1980). Situational cues and strategy influence on speechreading. *Scandinavian Audiology, 9,* 1–5.

Gibson, E. J. (1969). *Principles of perceptual learning and development.* New York: Appleton-Century-Crofts.

Giolas, T., Butterfield, E. C., Weaver, S. J. (1974). Some motivational correlates of lipreading. *Journal of Speech and Hearing Research, 17,* 18–24.

Hardick, E. J., Oyer, H. J., & Irion, P. E. (1970). Lipreading performance is related to measurements of vision. *Journal of Speech and Hearing Research, 13,* 92.

Haspiel, G. (1987). *Lipreading for children.* Washington, DC: Alexander Graham Bell Association for the Deaf.

Hefler, K. (1998). Auditory and auditory–visual recognition of clear and conversational speech by older adults. *Journal of the American Academy of Audiology, 9,* 234–242.

Hutton, C., Curry, E., & Armstrong, M. (1959). Semi-diagnostic test material for aural rehabilitation. *Journal of Speech and Hearing Disorders, 24,* 319–329.

Jackson, P. L. (1988). The theoretical minimal unit for visual speech perception: Visemes and coarticulation. *Volta Review, 90,* 99–115.

Jackson, P. L., Montgomery, A. A., & Binnie, C. A. (1976). Perceptual dimensions underlying vowel lipreading performance. *Journal of Speech and Hearing Research, 19,* 796–812.

Jeffers, J., & Barley, M. (1971). *Speechreading.* Springfield, IL: Charles C. Thomas.

Johnson, D., Caccamise, F., Rothblum, A., Hamilton, L., & Howard, M. (1981). Identification and follow-up of visual impairments in hearing-impaired populations. *American Annals of the Deaf, 126,* 321–360.

Johnson, D., & Snell, K. B. (1986). Effects of distance visual acuity problems on the speechreading performance of hearing-impaired adults. *Journal of the Academy of Rehabilitative Audiology, 19,* 42–55.

Kinzie, C. E., & Kinzie, R. (1931). *Lipreading for the deafened adult.* Chicago: John C. Winston.

Kopra, L., Kopra, M., Abrahamson, J., & Dunlop, R. (1986). Development of sentences graded in difficulty for lipreading practice. *Journal of the Academy of Rehabilitative Audiology, 19,* 71–86.

Kopra, L., Kopra, M., Abrahamson, J., & Dunlop, R. (1987). Lipreading drill and practice software for an auditory–visual videodisc interactive system (ALVIS). *Journal for Computer Users in Speech and Hearing, 3,* 58–68.

Kricos, P., & Lesner, S. (1982). Differences in visual intelligibility across talkers. *Volta Review, 84,* 219–225.

Lesner, S., Sandridge, S., & Kricos, P. (1987). Training influences on visual consonant and sentence recognition. *Ear and Hearing, 8,* 283–287.

Lewis, D. (1972). Lipreading skills of hearing impaired children in regular schools. *Volta Review, 74,* 303–311.

Lovering, L. (1969). *Lipreading performance as a function of visual acuity.* Unpublished doctoral dissertation, Michigan State University.

Mahshie, J. J. (1987). A primer on interactive video. *Journal for Computer Users in Speech and Hearing, 3,* 39–57.

Massaro, D. M. (1987). Speech perception by ear and eye: A paradigm for psychology inquiry. Hillsdale, NJ: Lawrence Erlbaum.

McCaffrey, H. (1995). Techniques and concepts in auditory training and speech-reading. Chapter 15 in R. Roeser & M. Downs (Eds.), *Auditory disorders in school children* (3rd ed.). New York: Thieme.

Miller, G. A., & Nicely, P. E. (1955). An analysis of the perceptual confusions among some English consonants. *Journal of the Acoustical Society of America, 27,* 338–352.

Montgomery, A. (1994). WATCH: A practical approach to brief auditory rehabilitation. *Hearing Journal, 10,* 10–55.

Montgomery, A., & Houston, T. (2000). The hearing-impaired adult: Management of communication deficits and tinnitus. In J. Alpiner, and P. McCarthy (Eds.), *Rehabilitative audiology: Children and adults* (3rd ed.). Philadelphia: Lippincott Williams & Wilkins.

Montgomery, A. A., & Jackson, P. L. (1983). Physical characteristics of the lips underlying vowel lipreading performance. *Journal of the Acoustical Society of America, 73,* 2134–2144.

Montgomery, A. A., Walden, B. E., Schwartz, D. M., & Prosek, R. A. (1984). Training auditory–visual speech reception in adults with moderate sensorineural hearing loss. *Ear and Hearing, 5,* 30–36.

Myklebust, H., & Neyhus, A. (1970). *Diagnostic Test of Speechreading.* New York: Grune & Stratton.

National Technical Institute for the Deaf. (1987). *NTID speechreading videotapes.* Washington, DC: Alexander Graham Bell Association for the Deaf.

New York League for the Hard of Hearing. (1990a). *I see what you're saying.* New York: Author.

New York League for the Hard of Hearing. (1990b). *Assessment of adult speechreading ability.* New York: Author.

Nitchie, E. B. (1912). *Lip reading: Principles and practice.* New York: Frederick A. Stokes.

Nitchie, E. B. (1950). *New lessons in lip reading.* Philadelphia: J. B. Lippincott.

O'Neill, J. J. (1951). An exploratory investigation of lipreading ability among normal-hearing students. *Speech Monographs, 18,* 309–311.

O'Neill, J. J., & Oyer, H. J. (1981). *Visual communication for the hard of hearing* (2nd ed.). Englewood Cliffs, NJ: Prentice-Hall.

Owens, E., & Blazek, B. (1985). Visemes observed by hearing-impaired and normal hearing adult viewers. *Journal of Speech and Hearing Research, 28,* 381–393.

Padden, C. (1980). The deaf community and the culture of deaf people. In C. Baker & R. Battison (Eds.), *Sign language and the deaf community: Essays in honor of William Stokoe.* Silver Spring, MD: National Association of the Deaf.

Pichora-Fuller, M. K., & Benguerel, A.-P. (1991). The design of CAST (computer-aided speechreading training). *Journal of Speech and Hearing Research, 34,* 202–212.

Pollack, D. (1964). Acoupedics. *Volta Review, 66,* 400.

Pollack, D. (1985). *Educational audiology for the limited hearing infant and preschooler* (2nd ed.). Springfield, IL: Charles C. Thomas.

Romano, P., & Berlow, W. (1974). Vision requirements for lipreading. *American Annals of the Deaf, 119,* 393–396.

Ross, M. (1982). *Hard of hearing children in regular schools.* Englewood Cliffs, NJ: Prentice-Hall.

Samar, V. J., & Sims, D. G. (1983). Visual evoked response correlates of speechreading performance in normal-hearing adults: A replication and factor analytic extension. *Journal of Speech and Hearing Research, 26,* 2–9.

Samar, V. J., & Sims, D. G. (1984). Visual evoked response components related to speechreading and spatial skills in hearing and hearing impaired adults. *Journal of Speech and Hearing Research, 27,* 23–26.

Sanders, D. A. (1993). *Aural rehabilitation* (3rd ed.). Englewood Cliffs, NJ: Prentice-Hall.

Scheetz, N. A. (2001). *Orientation to deafness* (2nd ed.). Boston: Lenstok Press.

Schow, R. (2001). A standardized AR battery for hearing aid dispensers. *Hearing Journal, 54*(8), 10–20.

Schow, R. (2005). Personal Communication.

Shepard, D. C. (1982). Visual–neural correlate of speechreading ability in normal-hearing adults: Reliability. *Journal of Speech and Hearing Research, 25,* 521–527.

Shepard, D. C., DeLavergne, R. W., Fruek, F. X., & Clobridge, C. (1977). Visual–neural correlate of speechreading ability in normal-hearing adults. *Journal of Speech and Hearing Research, 20,* 752–765.

Smith, R. (1964). *An investigation of the relationships between lipreading ability and the intelligence of the mentally retarded.* Unpublished master's thesis, Michigan State University.

Stokoe, W. C. (Ed.). (1978). *Sign and culture, a reader for students of American sign language.* Silver Spring, MD: Lenstok Press.

Stokoe, W., Casterline, D., & Croneberg, C. (1965). *A dictionary of American sign language on linguistic principles.* Washington, DC: Gallaudet College Press.

Summerfield, Q. (1992, January 29). Lipreading and audio-visual perception. *Philosophical Transactions of the Royal Society of London,* 71–78. Royal Society of London.

Tye-Murray, N. (1993a). *Cochlear implants: Audiological foundations.* San Diego, CA: Singular Publishing Group.

Tye-Murray, N. (1993b). *Communication training for hearing-impaired children and teenagers: Speechreading, listening and using repair strategies.* Austin, TX: Pro-Ed.

Tye-Murray, N. (1997). *Communication training for hard-of-hearing adults and older teenagers: Speechreading, listening, and using repair strategies.* Austin, TX: Pro-Ed.

Tye-Murray, N. (2002a). *Conversation Made Easy.* Available through Central Institute for the Deaf, St. Louis, MO.

Tye-Murray, N. (2004). *Foundations of aural rehabilitation* (2nd ed.). San Diego, CA: Singular Publishing Group.

Tye-Murray, N., & Geers, A. (1997). *The Children's Speechreading Enhancement Test (CHIVE).* St. Louis, MO: Central Institute for the Deaf.

Tye-Murray, N., & Geers, A. (2002). *The Children's Enhancement Test (CAVET).* St. Louis, MO: Central Institute for the Deaf.

Tyler, R., Preece, J., & Tye-Murray, N. (1986). *The Iowa phoneme and sentence tests.* Iowa City: University of Iowa Hospitals and Clinics.

Utley, J. (1946). A test of lipreading ability. *Journal of Speech and Hearing Disorders, 11,* 109–116.

Vernon, M., & Andrews, J. F. (1990). *The psychology of deafness: Understanding deaf and hard-of-hearing people.* New York: Longman.

Walden, B., Erdman, S., Montgomery, A., Schwartz, D., & Prosek, R. (1981). Some effects of training on speech perception by hearing-impaired adults. *Journal of Speech and Hearing Research, 24,* 207–216.

Walden, B., Prosek, R., Montgomery, A., Scharr, C., & Jones, C. (1977). Effects of training on the visual recognition of consonants. *Journal of Speech and Hearing Research, 20,* 130–145.

Wayner, D., & Abrahamson, J. (1996). *Learning to hear again.* Austin, TX: Hear Again.

Wedenberg, E. (1951). Auditory training of deaf and hard of hearing children. *Acta Otolaryngology* (Suppl. 94), *39,* 1–139.

Woodward, M. F., & Barber, C. G. (1960). Phoneme perception in lipreading. *Journal of Speech and Hearing Research, 3,* 212–222.

Yoshinaga-Itano, C. (1988). Speechreading instruction for children. In C. L. DeFilippo & D. G. Sims (Eds.), New reflections on speechreading (Monographs). *Volta Review, 90*(5), 241–254.

■ APPENDIXES

Appendix 5A: Utley—How Well Can You Read Lips?

This text, commonly referred to as the *Utley Test*, consists of three subtests: Sentences (Forms A and B), Words (Forms A and B), and Stories accompanied by questions that relate to each of the stories. Utley (1946) demonstrated that the Word and Story subtests are positively correlated with the Sentence portion of the test. Therefore, these are the stimuli most often used and associated with the *Utley Test*.

Utley evaluated her viewers' responses by giving one point for each word correctly identified in each sentence. A total of 125 words are contained in the 31 sentences on each form (Form A and B). Consequently, a respondent's score may range from 0 to 125 points. Utley suggested that homophenous words not be accepted when scoring the sentence subtest.

Utley administered the sentence subtest to 761 hearing-impaired children and adults, and the following descriptive statistics summarize her findings:

	FORM A	FORM B
Range	0–84	0–89
Mean	33.63	33.80
SD	16.36	17.53

PRACTICE SENTENCE

1. Good morning.
2. Thank you.
3. Hello.
4. How are you?
5. Goodbye.

UTLEY SENTENCE TEST—FORM A

1. All right.
2. Where have you been?
3. I have forgotten.
4. I have nothing.
5. That is right.
6. Look out.
7. How have you been?
8. I don't know if I can.
9. How tall are you?
10. It is awfully cold.
11. My folks are home.
12. How much was it?
13. Good night.
14. Where are you going?
15. Excuse me.
16. Did you have a good time?
17. What did you want?
18. How much do you weigh?
19. I cannot stand him.
20. She was home last week.
21. Keep your eye on the ball.
22. I cannot remember.
23. Of course.
24. I flew to Washington.
25. You look well.
26. The train runs every hour.
27. You had better go slow.
28. It says that in the book.
29. We got home at six o'clock.
30. We drove to the country.
31. How much rain fell?

Source: Utley, J. (1946). A test of lipreading ability. *Journal of Speech and Hearing Disorders, 11,* 109–116. Reprinted by permission.

Appendix 5B: The Denver Quick Test of Lipreading Ability

The *Denver Quick Test* is designed to measure adult ability to speechread 20 common everyday sentences. Sentences are presented "live" or taped by the tester and are scored on the basis of meaning recognition. No normative data are available to which individual scores may be compared; however, when the Quick Test was given without acoustic cues to 40 hearing-impaired adults, their scores were highly correlated (0.90) with their results on the *Utley Sentence Test* (Alpiner, 1982).

THE DENVER QUICK TEST OF LIPREADING ABILITY

1. Good morning
2. How old are you?
3. I live in (state of residence).
4. I only have one dollar.
5. There is somebody at the door.
6. Is that all?
7. Where are you going?
8. Let's have a coffee break.
9. Park your car in the lot.
10. What is your address?
11. May I help you?
12. I feel fine.
13. It is time for dinner.
14. Turn right at the corner.
15. Are you ready to order?
16. Is this charge or cash?
17. What time is it?
18. I have a headache.
19. How about going out tonight?
20. Please lend me 50 cents.

Source: Alpiner, J. (1982). Evaluation of communication function. In J. Alpiner (Ed.), *Handbook of Adult Rehabilitative Audiology* (pp. 18–79). Baltimore: Williams & Wilkins.

Appendix 5C: Craig Lipreading Inventory

The Craig Lipreading Inventory consists of two forms of 33 isolated words and 24 sentences. The vocabulary for these stimuli was selected from words used by children enrolled in kindergarten and first grade. A filmed version of the test is available. The test is usually presented "live," but may be videotaped by a clinician.

The viewer should be positioned 8 feet from the speaker. Each of the isolated words is preceded by a contextually meaningless carrier phrase, "show me." The respondent is provided with answer sheets that contain four choices for each stimulus. A single point is awarded for each of the words and sentences identified correctly. Consequently, maximum scores are 33 and 24 for the word test and sentence test, respectively.

Individual performances may be compared to the following mean scores obtained by Craig with deaf children:

	PRESCHOOL	NONPRESCHOOL
Words	62.5%–68%	68%–69%
Sentences	52.5%–62%	61.5%–63%

CRAIG LIPREADING INVENTORY

Word Recognition—Form A

1. white	12. woman	23. ear
2. corn	13. fly	24. ice
3. zoo	14. frog	25. goat
4. thumb	15. grapes	26. dog
5. chair	16. goose	27. cat
6. jello	17. sled	28. nut
7. doll	18. star	29. milk
8. pig	19. sing	30. cake
9. toy	20. three	31. eight
10. finger	21. duck	32. pencil
11. six	22. spoon	33. desk

SENTENCE RECOGNITION—FORM A

1. A coat is on a chair.
2. A sock and shoe are on the floor.
3. A boy is flying a kite.
4. A girl is jumping.
5. A boy stuck his thumb in the pie.
6. A cow and a pig are near the gate.
7. A man is throwing a ball to the dog.
8. A bird has white wings.
9. A light is over the door.
10. A horse is standing by a new car.
11. A boy is putting a nail in the sled.
12. A big fan is on a desk.
13. An owl is looking at the moon.
14. Three stars are in the sky.
15. A whistle and a spoon are on the table.
16. A frog is hopping away from a boat.
17. Bread, meat and grapes are in the dish.
18. The woman has long hair and a short dress.
19. The boys are swinging behind the school.
20. A cat is playing with a nut.
21. A man has his foot on a truck.
22. A woman is carrying a chair.
23. A woman is eating an apple.
24. A girl is cutting a feather.

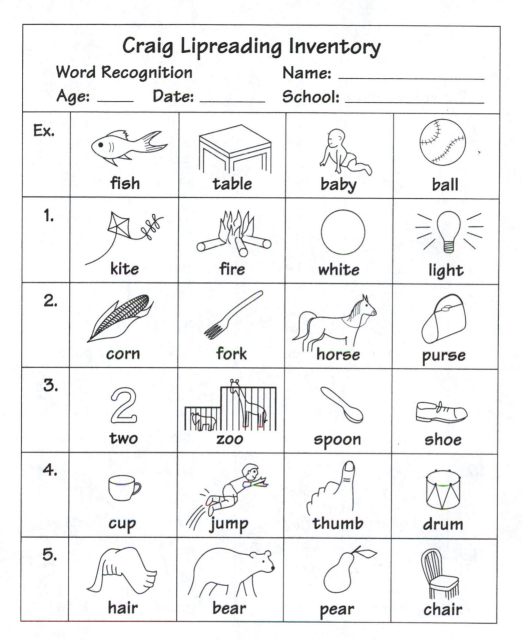

Craig Lipreading Inventory

Word Recognition

Name: _____

Age: ____ **Date:** _____ **School:** _____

Ex.	fish	table	baby	ball
1.	kite	fire	white	light
2.	corn	fork	horse	purse
3.	two	zoo	spoon	shoe
4.	cup	jump	thumb	drum
5.	hair	bear	pear	chair

Word Recognition   Page 2

6.	yoyo	hello	jello	window
7.	doll	ten	nail	suit
8.	pig	pie	book	pear
9.	two	toe	tie	toy
10.	flower	finger	fire	feather
11.	six	sing	sit	kiss

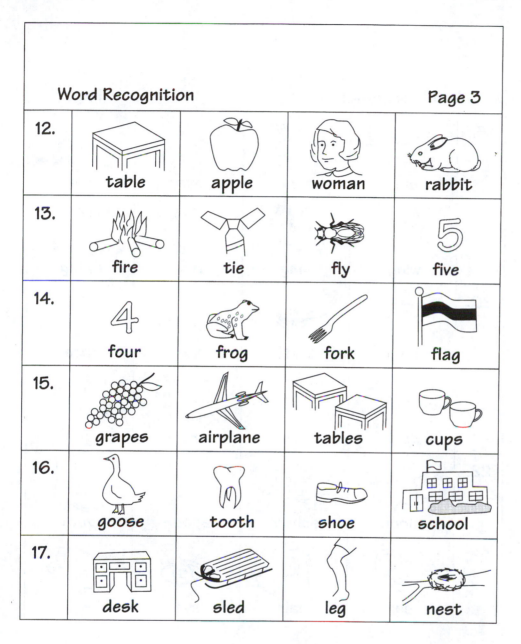

Word Recognition   Page 3

12.	table	apple	woman	rabbit
13.	fire	tie	fly	five
14.	four	frog	fork	flag
15.	grapes	airplane	tables	cups
16.	goose	tooth	shoe	school
17.	desk	sled	leg	nest

Word Recognition			Page 4
18. dog	sock	star	car
19. wing	sing	ring	swing
20. three	teeth	key	knee
21. duck	rug	truck	gun
22. moon	school	spoon	boot
23. ear	hair	eye	egg

Word Recognition   Page 5

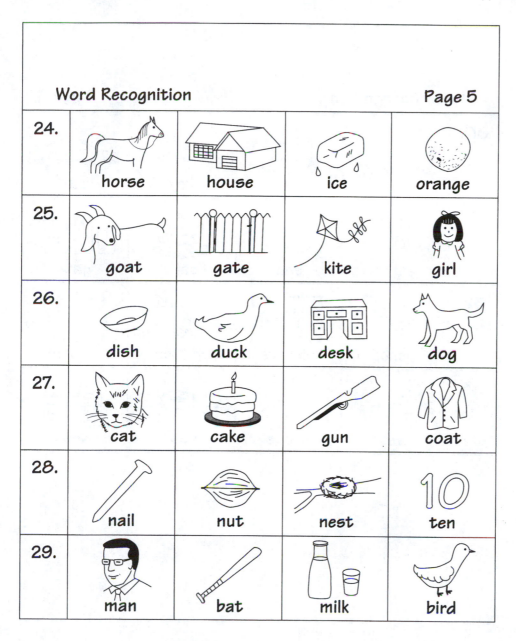

24.	horse	house	ice	orange
25.	goat	gate	kite	girl
26.	dish	duck	desk	dog
27.	cat	cake	gun	coat
28.	nail	nut	nest	ten
29.	man	bat	milk	bird

Word Recognition   Page 6

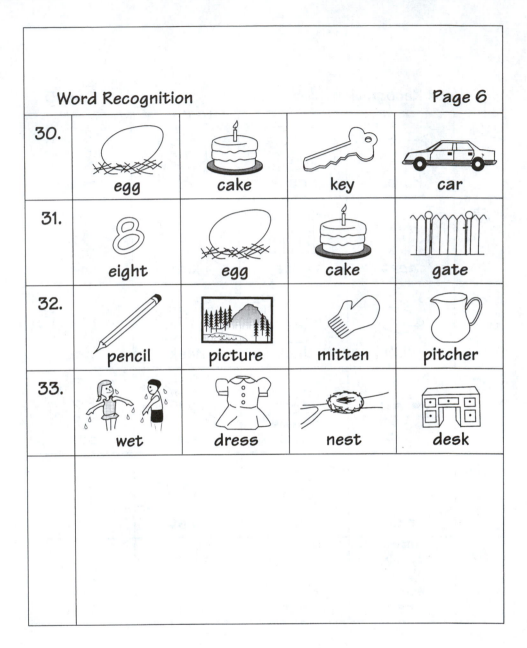

30.	egg	cake	key	car
31.	eight	egg	cake	gate
32.	pencil	picture	mitten	pitcher
33.	wet	dress	nest	desk

CHAPTER 6

Language and Speech of the Deaf and Hard of Hearing

Deborah S. Culbertson

CONTENTS

■ INTRODUCTION

All of us possess personal attitudes toward language and modes of communication. These feelings form a basis for the way we choose to view the language abilities of persons with hearing loss. For example, a father of a child with profound hearing loss and a cochlear implant states, "I won't respond to my daughter unless she uses

Language is a broad term to describe a system of symbols used as a social tool for the exchange of information.

spoken words." In contrast, a family with a young daughter with severe hearing impairment realizes that she is not responding well to amplified spoken language. Mom, Dad, and the two siblings go to the library, borrow all the sign language books, and start signing. An adolescent who is deaf begins a course of study at Gallaudet University and chooses not to use spoken language because it is not accepted by the Deaf community. All of these examples reflect "family" and personal attitudes toward language.

Professionals may respond to such family attitudes and choices toward language use in various ways. For many years, professionals established language programs based on their own principles and beliefs. Since the passage of PL 99-457, however, our profession has been moving in a new direction toward family-centered language programs (Roush & McWilliams, 1994). In family-centered programs, families are to be equal partners in language assessment, intervention, and decision making.

Morphology is the study of the minimal units of language that are meaningful, such as bug, -s for plural nouns or third-person verb tenses, -ing for present progressive, and -ed for past tense.

■ LANGUAGE AND COMMUNICATION

Factors Affecting Language Acquisition

It is essential for parents and professionals to consider how hearing loss affects the acquisition of spoken language. The deteriorated speech signal resulting from hearing loss robs the child with hearing impairment of information regarding the form (phonology, syntax, morphology), content (semantics), and use (pragmatics) of language. Not surprisingly, language delay is a consequence of this information loss.

Phonology is the study of sound systems used in languages.

It must be stressed that, despite their language learning difficulties, children with hearing loss are not a homogeneous group when it comes to language acquisition. The three most obvious factors that might account for differences in language acquisition among children with hearing impairment are the degree of loss, age of onset, and whether other disabilities are present.

Pragmatics refers to the functional use of language.

OTHER HANDICAPPING CONDITIONS. Almost 40 percent of children with hearing loss have other special needs: 10.0 percent with learning disability, 9.1 percent with mental retardation, 6.6 percent with attention deficit, 4.5 percent with visual impairment, 3.2 percent with cerebral palsy, 2.0 percent with emotional disturbance, and 13.3 percent with other conditions (Gallaudet Research Institute, 2005). The impact of other handicapping conditions is not fully known. However, cognitive impairment has been found to have a significant negative impact on language development in children with hearing loss (Yoshinaga-Itano, Sedey, Coulter, & Mehl, 1998), and learning disability has also been documented to have a negative impact on auditory perception and linguistic competence in children with cochlear implants (Isaacson et al., 1996).

Semantics is the study of word meanings and word relations.

Syntax is the aspect of language that governs the rules for how words are arranged in sentences.

Family status can also significantly impact language abilities of children with hearing loss. For example, reading scores are poorer for families with low socioeconomic status and can be related to factors such as unstable housing, family stress, and greater incidence of problems with health and transportation (Connor & Zwolan, 2004).

PREDICTORS. Mayne, Yoshinaga-Itaro, Sedey, and Carey (2000) reported that the significant predictors of early expressive language development in children who are deaf or hard of hearing included the child's age, the age of identification of the child's hearing loss (before or after 6 months), the child's cognitive status, and the presence or absence of one or more disabilities in addition to hearing loss.

In general, the greater the hearing loss, the greater the expected language delay. However, language abilities cannot be predicted solely on the basis of severity of hearing loss. Often, a range of language abilities can be observed in children with similar unaided audiograms. Surprisingly, some children with severe hearing impairment have age-appropriate language skills, while others have language difficulties that far exceed what would be expected for a given level of hearing loss. Even children who, at an early age, have mild fluctuating hearing losses secondary to otitis media may evidence significant delays in language development.

Since the 1990s, three key factors have greatly impacted the speech and language outcomes for children with hearing loss: (1) increased client diversity, (2) early intervention, and (3) availability of cochlear implants for use in children with severe-to-profound hearing loss. Each of these issues will be addressed in the following sections.

CULTURAL AND LINGUISTIC DIVERSITY. In the United States, English-speaking individuals from families of Western European origin have been considered the majority or mainstream culture. However, the number and impact of individuals from other linguistic and cultural backgrounds is increasing. It has been estimated that by 2050, the proportion of individuals from other linguistic and cultural backgrounds will increase to approximately 50 percent of the total U.S. population (Caeser & Williams, 2002). The 2000 U.S. Census requested that respondents classify themselves as either of Hispanic or Non-Hispanic ethnic origin and indicate their racial classification as (1) White, (2) Black, (3) American Indian or Alaska Native, or (4) Asian or Pacific Islanders. The largest groups, other than White, in order of occurrence were (1) Hispanic/Latino Americans, (2) African Americans, and (3) Asian Americans (U.S. Bureau of the Census, 2000). These top three groups were also reflected in the 2003–2004 Regional and National Summary report of data from the Annual Survey of Deaf and Hard of Hearing Children and Youth (Gallaudet Research Institute, 2005). The most common language spoken in the homes of children with hearing loss, besides English, is Spanish (Gallaudet Research Institute, 2005). When families from diverse cultural and language backgrounds are seen for speech and language services, all stages of service delivery from case history through follow-up counseling and management are impacted. Needs and issues related to serving these families are discussed by Wyatt (2002) and by Rhoades, Price, and Perigoe (2005).

Children and adults from other linguistic backgrounds have varying proficiencies in Standard American English ranging from none to limited to fluent to native proficiency. When families have limited or no proficiency in Standard American English, the need for an interpreter during assessment and management is a key consideration. Because of the increasing diversity of clinical populations, it is essential to seek out information on determining the need for and working with

Important language acquisition information on the impact of hearing loss has arisen from research concluded over the past sixty years.

interpreters to serve bilingual children and families (e.g., Langdon, 2003). If the clinician is not proficient in the family's native language, then best practice would dictate referral to a clinician who has proficiency in that language or the hiring of an interpreter. Use of a family member proficient in English and the native language is a less desirable alternative and should only be pursued if an interpreter cannot be secured. Unlike a hired interpreter, a family member is more likely to introduce his or her biases into the case history, assessment, and follow-up counseling. Use of an interpreter is supported by IDEA, which mandates that assessment be conducted in the child's native language. According to Langdon (2003), a first step in the use of an interpreter is to brief him or her as to the specific components of the case history interview, the formal and informal assessment measures, and the overall format of the session. The interpreter would serve as a cultural informant and assist with identifying materials and test items that might not be familiar to the child so that alternate materials and test responses can be identified in advance. The clinician may need to rely heavily on informal rather than formal standardized tests because few standardized tests are available in other languages. During the assessment session, the clinician would direct questions to the parents during the case history and then rely on the interpreter to administer the assessments to the child in his or her native language. Following the assessment, the interpreter and clinician would debrief by reviewing the session, including the overall quality of the session and the findings of the session. Then the interpreter would assist in translating the clinical report. Because children often have some level of proficiency in Standard American English, it often will be necessary to evaluate English language abilities in another diagnostic session.

If a form of manual communication is chosen for use with a child, some families find themselves challenged with the need for developing their child's proficiency in three different languages: the native language of the family, Standard American English, and sign language. The speech-language clinician would then be challenged to evaluate and assist with development in multiple languages.

EARLY INTERVENTION. Several researchers have offered evidence related to the benefits of early identification and management of hearing loss in children. Different researchers have examined different time frames for early versus later identification, for example, identification within the first 6 months compared to after 6 months (Yoshinaga-Itano et al., 1998a), and identification within the first 24 months compared to after 24 months (Calderon, 1998). As a group, early-identified children without other handicapping conditions have been reported to show age-appropriate language abilities and continue to maintain age-appropriate language abilities (Yoshinaga-Itano et al., 1998a). One cautionary note is that some studies have tended to use receptive and expressive vocabulary measures as an index of overall "language ability," and further study is needed to explore other areas of language. For example, early identification is not a strong predictor of speech intelligibility. Better speech intelligibility is predicted by more advanced language development, lesser degree of hearing loss, an oral mode of communication, and increased age (Yoshinaga-Itano et al., 1998a).

Duncan (1999) reported that kindergartners with early-identified hearing loss had conversational skills comparable to their normal hearing peers. She examined the conversational skills of eleven kindergarteners with normal hearing and of eleven with severe-to-profound hearing loss who had received early intervention. Communication samples were recorded and conversational skills were rated using a checklist procedure. The two groups were found to have highly similar conversational skills with respect to initiating, maintaining, shifting, and terminating conversations. The children with hearing loss, however, showed significantly greater physical initiations of conversations than those with normal hearing.

COCHLEAR IMPLANT USE. The 1990 FDA approval of multichannel cochlear implant use in children has offered greater access to acoustic speech information for children with severe and profound hearing loss. In many implanted children, cochlear implant use results in spoken language development that surpasses that typically seen with the use of power hearing aids. The age at which implantation occurs is a critical factor. In reviewing data from 181 children, Geers, Nicholas, and Sedey (2003) concluded that implantation at or before 5 years of age offers the potential for children to develop age-appropriate English language abilities. Svirsky et al. (2002) have also noted that children receiving cochlear implants before the age of 6 years with effective implant use and language stimulation perform at least as well as hearing aid users with pure tone averages in the 90 to 100 dB HL range in speech perception, speech production, and language development. It is important to remember that children with cochlear implants still receive an impoverished acoustic signal that puts them at risk for listening, language, and academic difficulties. Early identification, family-based language stimulation programs, effective cochlear implant use, and school support services are needed to allow these children to fully develop their abilities.

For children with cochlear implants, some aspects of language development may occur at normal or above normal rates of development after implantation,

---

Case 6.1. BR

BR had meningitis at age 7 months, and a severe-to-profound hearing loss was subsequently identified. BR was immediately fit with hearing aids, and home intervention based on auditory verbal (AV) principles was initiated. At the age of 14 months, BR received a cochlear implant. At the age of 3, BR began receiving AV services through the public schools. BR is now 7 years of age, and he has been placed in a regular classroom in the public schools for kindergarten and first grade. While in school, he has received AV services from a teacher of the hearing impaired and from the outpatient clinic. He has also had a classroom language facilitator, but there are plans to phase out this support provider in the upcoming school year. BR's mother is highly involved in his AV therapy and in fostering his educational success. She has integrated language stimulation and communication strategies into his everyday life. Her influence is judged to be an enormous factor in his overall success as an oral communicator. While he is delayed in receptive and expressive language, his speech is 100 percent intelligible. Current therapy goals include use of possessive and plural /s/ marker, use of *the* and *a,* and understanding telephone conversation from a disclosed topic.

> ## Case 6.2. FM
>
> FM, a male child, and his twin brother were born at 26 weeks gestation. While his brother was found to have normal hearing, FM was found to have severe-to-profound hearing loss and cerebral palsy. FM was aided at 5 months of age, and at 22 months of age FM received a cochlear implant. FM is now 28 months of age. He is showing signs of developing auditory awareness and is showing increased vocalizations. Evaluation at this point indicates that he is exhibiting a severe delay in both expressive and receptive language abilities. He receives services based on auditory-verbal therapy principles once a week at home through a state early invention program and twice a week from a speech language pathologist.

while other aspects of language may be delayed. Ertmer, Strong, and Sadagopan (2003) illustrated this through a case study of a child implanted at 20 months whose language was evaluated periodically out to 42 months. This child showed normal or above normal rates of development with respect to decreased use of nonwords, increased receptive vocabulary, type–token ratio, increased use of word combinations, and in the comprehension of phrases. The child showed below normal rates of development in speech intelligibility, number of word types and tokens, and mean length of utterance. Results may be better for children implanted at earlier ages. Miyamoto et al. (2003) reported language results for a child implanted at 6 months that suggested nearly age-equivalent receptive language and beyond the expected age equivalent score for expressive language measured at 2 years of age.

Spencer, Barker, and Tomblin (2003) examined the expressive and receptive language, reading comprehension, and writing of 16 school-age children with cochlear implants and 16 children with normal hearing. All children with implants were implanted between the ages of 30 and 76 months. The children with cochlear implants performed within one standard deviation of their age-matched normal hearing peers in language comprehension, reading comprehension, and writing accuracy. The children with implants scored significantly poorer on sentence formulation and number of words used in the written narrative.

Geers, Nicholas, and Sedey (2003) examined 181 children between the ages of 8 and 9 years who had been implanted by 5½ years of age. They found that the strongest predictors for language ability were greater nonverbal intelligence, smaller family size, higher socioeconomic status, and female gender. More than half of the children with implants had language skills similar to those of normal hearing peers in verbal reasoning, narrative ability, utterance length, and lexical diversity. Children from oral communication programs had significantly better narratives, breadth of vocabulary, use of bound morphemes, length of utterance, and complexity of syntax in spontaneous language. In the area of speech production, the average intelligibility for the children was 63.5 percent, with children showing better consonant than vowel production and those from oral communication programs demonstrating better speech intelligibility. Chin (2003) found that school-age children with implants produce non-English sounds in their speech (e.g., uvular stops), but that non-English sounds are more prevalent in children from total communication programs.

> ## Case 6.3. JZ
>
> JZ, a male child, had meningitis when he was 9 months of age. Testing initially revealed a moderate-to-severe sensorineural hearing loss. Seven days after recovery from the meningitis, JZ was aided, and speech-language therapy was initiated. At age 2 years, hearing re-evaluation indicated that the hearing loss in the right ear had progressed to a profound hearing loss. At age 2½ years, JZ received a cochlear implant. JZ is now 6 years of age and is fully mainstreamed into a regular first-grade classroom. He exhibits a severe language disorder with deficits in vocabulary, concepts, and conversational abilities. He is receiving services from a speech–language pathologist and a teacher of the deaf and hard of hearing. He uses spoken language only to communicate, and his speech is judged to be 70 percent intelligible to others. His current speech goals include production of /s/, /z/, and s-blends.

When comparing implanted children from oral and total communication programs, there is evidence for better speech production for those in oral communication (OC) programs, and an early advantage in receptive communication for children in total communication (TC) programs (Connor et al., 2000). Tye-Murray (2003) found that when participating in an oral conversation, children from OC programs spend less time in communication breakdown than children from TC programs. Because children are not randomly assigned to OC and TC programs, other factors can contribute to language outcomes in this population, and recent research studies have attempted to statistically control for some of these other factors (Connor et al., 2000). Another complication is the variability with respect to emphasis placed on spoken language use in TC programs. This can range from TC programs with a sign emphasis, to TC programs with equal emphasis on sign and speech, to TC programs with a speech emphasis. It might be expected that children who use spoken language would have better spoken language skills.

The following sections will discuss language characteristics for children with hearing impairment in two general age ranges: preschool (birth to age 5) and school age (age 5 through adolescence). Issues related to language assessment and management for all children are presented next. While speech is the oral means for expressing language, its separate presentation in latter sections is intended to simplify the discussion.

Language Characteristics of Preschool Children with Hearing Impairment

Carney and Moeller (1998) provide a thorough discussion of the impact of early onset hearing loss on language and literacy skills. The presence of hearing loss during the critical early periods of a child's development may deprive the child of unambiguous auditory and linguistic cues from the language models in his or her daily environment. The lack of opportunities to hear auditory language on a consistent basis may severely compromise the child's ability to develop the semantic, syntactic, morphologic, pragmatic, and phonologic aspects of language, which in turn greatly increases the likelihood of subsequent reading and academic difficulties. Although many children with hearing impairment, even of a severe degree, may have language skills commensurate with their age peers, many evidence delays in the various facets of language comprehension and production. Some common language characteristics of children who are hearing impaired are shown in Table 6.1.

Importance of Parent–Child Interactions

Several authors have compared parent–child interactions of hearing parents with children who are normal hearing with those of hearing parents with children who are hearing impaired. These researchers have suggested that a child's hearing handicap can have a detrimental effect on parental communication styles. Goss (1970) was one of the first researchers to express concern regarding the verbal behavior of mothers with children who are hearing impaired. He observed that mothers of deaf children were less likely to use verbal praise, to ask for opinions and suggestions, and to use questions. He also noted that mothers of children who are hearing impaired were more likely to show disagreement, tension, and antagonism and to give more suggestions than were mothers of hearing children.

TABLE 6.1

Some Common Characteristics of Language Usage by Children Who Are Hearing Impaired

Syntax

Shorter sentences (reduced mean length of utterances)
Simpler sentences (e.g., reduced use of complex syntactical constructions such as passive tense and relative clauses)
Overuse of certain sentence patterns (particularly subject–verb–object patterns)
Infrequent use of adverbs, auxiliaries, and conjunctions
Inappropriately constructed sentences (e.g., "The girl she want few some bread."
Non-English word order
Incorrect usage of irregular verb tense

Semantics

Reduced expressive and receptive vocabulary
Limited understanding of metaphors, idioms, and other figurative language
Difficulty with multiple meanings of words (e.g., *row, run*)

Pragmatics

Restricted range of communicative intents (e.g., conversational devices, performatives, requests) in preschool children with hearing impairment
Lack of knowledge regarding conversational conventions, such as changing the topic or closing conversations
Limited knowledge and use of communication repair strategies

Despite the concerns expressed by Goss (1970) and others, the professional must not assume that parental interactions will be aberrant. Lederberg and Everhart (1998) found that mothers of deaf and hearing children communicated with their children to the same extent, and that the mothers of the children with hearing impairment exhibited a number of functional adaptations to their children's hearing loss, such as using visual communication and tactile attention-getting strategies.

KNOWLEDGE OF SCHEMA IN PRESCHOOL CHILDREN. It has been suggested that early child language development is established through the use of daily routines in the child's life (Schirmer, 1994). The child, for example, experiences typical sequences of events and communication at dinner time, bath time, and bed time. Over time, the child stores and remembers a body of knowledge (called "schema") about these events and forms (Yoshinaga-Itano & Downey, 1986). Children with impaired hearing often have limited schemata for two main reasons. First, they have limited access to the language used by parents and siblings during daily routines. Second, children with hearing loss miss out on incidental learning opportunities. The child with normal hearing can overhear mom and dad talking about cleaning up the dinner dishes. The child with hearing loss may hear little of conversations unless they are directed toward him or her. In addition, parents using simultaneous communication may not sign communications if they are not directed toward their child.

Family-centered intervention involves shared responsibility with the parents for the child's intervention, with the family retaining the ultimate decision making regarding intervention goals and services. A major goal of family-centered intervention is to strengthen family functioning, thus empowering the family to capitalize on its unique strengths when addressing the needs of the child with hearing impairment.

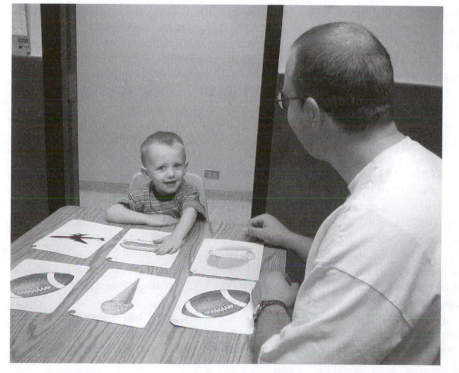

A young child works on communication skills in a therapy setting.

Thus, children with hearing impairment have reduced language input, and the language they miss leads them to miss out on knowledge about their world.

SEMANTIC AND PRAGMATIC FUNCTIONS IN PRESCHOOL CHILDREN. Several investigators have reported that preschool children with hearing impairment exhibit a full range of pragmatic functions but limited semantic functions using nonverbal and verbal communication behaviors (Skarakis & Prutting, 1977).

Yoshinaga-Itano and Stredler-Brown (1992) provided data concerning the frequency of use of different nonverbal and verbal communicative intentions (e.g., comment on object–action, request object–action–information, answer, acknowledgment, and protest) for children with hearing impairment during parent-child play sessions. Data were provided for the following age ranges in months: 6–12, 13–18, 19–24, 25–30, and 31–36. All 82 children in this cross-sectional sample were hard of hearing (better ear pure-tone averages better than 70 dB HL, 44 percent) or deaf (better ear pure-tone averages greater than 70 dB HL, 56 percent) and were enrolled in the Colorado Department of Health Home Intervention Program. Results showed that the overall number of nonverbal communicative intentions across categories increased with age. Children who were hard of hearing or deaf used a similar number of nonverbal communications. Verbal communication behaviors began to appear at 19 months of age, stabilized through 30 months, and then showed significant growth between 30 and 36 months. The children who were hard of hearing, however, showed significantly more verbal communications than the children who were deaf.

Nicholas and Geers (2003) examined communication samples from child–caregiver play interactions for a range of pragmatic functions (requesting, answering, calling attention to an event or action, directing, acknowledging, attempting to get information) in children with severe-to-profound hearing loss ranging in age from 1 to 4 years. The average age of identification of hearing loss was approximately 10 to 12 months. When compared to normal hearing peers, deaf children evidenced far fewer communicative acts, reduced utterance length, significantly reduced vocabulary use (words or signs), and significantly fewer informative functions (response, statement, question). The pattern of communication functions for deaf children was similar to that of younger normal hearing children.

EARLY VOCABULARY IN PRESCHOOL CHILDREN. Few studies have investigated the early vocabulary of children with hearing loss. Normative data for the expressive vocabulary development of children who are deaf or hard of hearing were provided by Mayne et al. (2000). These investigators found that, on average, children whose cognitive quotients were 80 or greater and whose hearing losses had been identified by 6 months of age had a rate of vocabulary growth similar to children with normal hearing. Children whose hearing loss was identified after 6 months and/or whose cognitive status was compromised evidenced significant delays in their language acquisition rates.

The dramatic impact that early identification of hearing loss has on language acquisition was highlighted in what is sure to be considered a classic study by Yoshinaga-Itano and her co-authors (1998). The results of these authors' investigation of

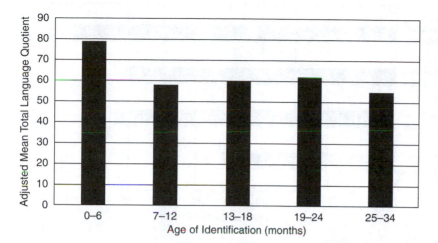

FIGURE 6.1

Adjusted mean total language quotients for groups based on age at identification of hearing loss.

Source: Reprinted with permission from Yoshingo-Itano, C., Sedey, A. L., Coulter, D. K., & Mehl, A. L. (1998). Language of early- and later-identified children with hearing loss. *Pediatrics, 102,* 1161–1171.

the language competence of early- and late-identified children with hearing loss clearly showed the advantages in language learning that are evident for children whose hearing loss is identified by 6 months of age. Figure 6.1 shows significantly better language competence in young children (1 to 3 years of age at the time of this study) whose losses were identified early. Figure 6.2 shows language acquisition as a function of both age of identification and cognitive status. What is particularly stunning in this figure is the fact that early-identified children with lower cognitive levels achieved essentially the same language levels as late-identified children with higher cognitive skills. These results should provide a strong impetus for the implementation of universal newborn hearing screening across the United States.

As of 2005, 38 states have passed legislation requiring hearing screening for all babies born in the state.

Language Characteristics of School-Age Children with Hearing Impairment

The literature pertaining to the acquisition and use of language by school-age children who have hearing impairment is extensive and establishes a number of important concerns. One important caveat in reviewing the literature discussed in this section is that the impact of early intervention has generally been limited to young children in early identification programs and to children receiving cochlear implants. Consequently, most of the information presented hereafter represents that from children whose hearing losses were identified beyond 2 years of age. Based on preliminary data related to early intervention, we may expect significantly better language outcomes for early-identified school-age children with lesser degrees of hearing loss. Three major aspects of language have been evaluated in this population: (1) lexical–semantic skills, (2) syntactic–morphologic skills, and (3) pragmatic, or functional communication, skills. Each of these will be briefly discussed.

LEXICAL–SEMANTIC SKILLS OF SCHOOL-AGE CHILDREN. The acquisition of the semantic component of language by children with hearing impairment may be mildly

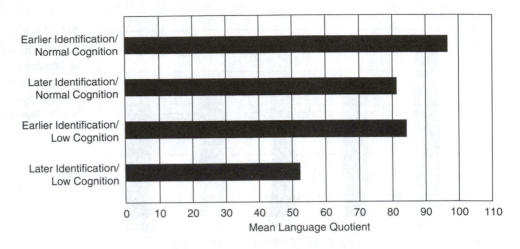

FIGURE 6.2

Mean total language quotient scores at 31 to 36 months by age at identification of hearing loss and cognition.

Source: Reprinted with permission from Yoshingo-Itano, C., Sedey, A. L., Coulter, D. K., & Mehl, A. L. (1998). Language of early- and later-identified children with hearing loss. *Pediatrics, 102,* 1161–1171.

to profoundly delayed. Reduced vocabulary is common among individuals with hearing loss. Moeller, Osberger, and Eccarius (1986) and Osberger et al. (1986) administered a large battery of expressive- and receptive-language tests to children and young adults ranging in age from 4.5 to 20 years. Severe delays in the acquisition of lexical–semantic skills were observed across all age groups. On the average, the children's performance on the various measures of word knowledge was similar to that of a 6- to 8-year-old child with normal hearing. Marked difficulties with the semantic–lexical aspects of language have been documented by other investigators (Brenza, Kricos, & Lasky, 1981; Yoshinago-Itano, Snyder, & Mayberry, 1996).

SYNTACTIC–MORPHOLOGIC SKILLS OF SCHOOL-AGE CHILDREN. The difficulties in acquisition of English syntactic–morphologic skills by children who have hearing impairment have been extensively documented and are even more pronounced than this population's difficulties with the semantic–lexical aspects of language. Descriptive studies of the syntactic abilities in this population have shown evidence of the following:

1. Restricted knowledge of word classes as evidenced by overuse of nouns and verbs and omission of function words.
2. Restricted knowledge of syntax as evidenced by overuse of the subject-verb-object sentence structure.
3. Syntactic delay with subsequent plateau in regard to syntactic abilities.
4. Deviant syntax in children with profound hearing impairment, e.g., misuse of morphological markers, omission of major sentence constituents, and asequential word order.

In their study of 145 children and young adults, ages 4.5 to 20 years, Moeller et al. (1986) found that few students evidenced language ages greater than 5 to 7 years in receptive syntax. Children who are hearing impaired have substantial difficulties with the more complex, subtle aspects of syntax (Yoshinago-Itano et al., 1996). Given the seeming inconsistencies in English syntax, it is not surprising that such difficulties are experienced by individuals with severe hearing impairment. Consider, for example, the following sentences: "I am going home."—"I am going to school."—"I am going to the store." It is no wonder that individuals with impaired hearing have difficulty sorting through the irregularities of the English language, ultimately generating sentences such as "I am going school" or "I am going to home."

PRAGMATIC SKILLS OF SCHOOL-AGE CHILDREN. The abilities of school-age children with impaired hearing to control the pragmatic aspects of language have, until fairly recently, received less attention from researchers. The limited research that has been conducted with older children, however, has delineated a number of concerns with the pragmatic aspects of language. Duchan (1988) reviews these studies, which show that many school-age children with hearing loss have difficulties with conversational turntaking and topic initiations and maintenance. Studies of the pragmatic abilities of children who have been educated in a *total communication* program were reviewed by Johnson (1988). Although difficulties in turn-taking, topic identification, and communication repair were noted in these studies, there is at least some evidence that there is a steady progression of conversational skills in children with hearing impairment as they become older. Prinz and Prinz (1985) found that children's communication competence increased from ages 3 to 11 years (the ages of their subjects) as a result of their improved American Sign Language discourse strategies.

> *Total communication* is a philosophy of communicating with children who are deaf using one or several modes of communication, including oral language, signed communication, written language, fingerspelling, gestures, facial expression, and Cued Speech, depending on the child's needs.

PLATEAU IN LANGUAGE ACQUISITION FOR SCHOOL-AGE CHILDREN. More disturbing than the delays in the development of language skills in children with hearing impairment is the apparent plateau in development of these skills, which has been documented in numerous studies (Boothe, Lasky, & Kricos, 1982). For example, Moeller, et al. (1986) found little growth in semantic and syntactic skills of children with severe hearing losses after 12 to 13 years.

Yoshinaga-Itano and Downey (1996) caution, however, that it would be erroneous to assume that *no* language growth occurs after age 12 years. Although a decrease in skills for both metacognitive processing strategies and semantic language may occur for many children who are hearing impaired around 12 years of age, these authors point out that significant developmental increases will most likely occur in both semantic and syntactic skills after age 12.

> *Metacognition* refers to the child's knowledge and awareness of the thinking process and is tied closely to the child's use of higher symbolic language for reasoning and problem solving.

PRELITERACY AND LITERACY ISSUES. Another issue in language development for the child with impaired hearing is the development of literacy (reading and writing) skills. Low reading and writing proficiency skills for children with hearing impairment have been related to limited oral language skills that serve as a base for literacy. Children with hearing loss also may not be exposed to the range and amount of prereading and reading activities as children with normal hearing (Limbrick,

McNaughton, & Clay, 1992). Unfortunately, little attention has been directed toward establishing the precursors to reading and writing in this population.

Onsets and *rimes* are the terms frequently used by reading specialists to denote the parts of words that children must learn to segment as they develop their phonological awareness skills. In words such as *bat, cat, that, flat, rat,* and *mat,* the onset of the word is the initial consonant or consonant blends, and the rimes are the rhyming word endings (*-at*).

An important precursor to reading ability is the development of phonological awareness. Phonological awareness is the ability to recognize that words consist of individual syllables, onsets and rimes, and phonemes and is related to the success with which children learn to read and spell. According to Miller (1997), prelingual deafness may inhibit phonemic awareness, although it does not preclude its formation. The ability to speechread does not provide enough phonological information to eliminate the need to access the acoustic parameters of speech. Although speechreading ability appears to be a good predictor of later phonological development, it is not adequate for complete development of phonological awareness (Dodd, McIntosh, & Woodhouse, 1998; Laybaert, 1998).

Children with normal hearing learn about printed materials when they are very young. Infants and toddlers see and are shown letters and words on pictures, toys, and television, and in books. Parents read storybooks, traffic signs, and television ads. In contrast, children with hearing impairment may not have the same amount of exposure to these literacy experiences. This may be due to an unintentional overemphasis on spoken-language development in the early years with the expectation that reading and writing will be taught later in the elementary school setting. Literacy development and literacy facilitation activities are discussed in van Kleeck and Schuele (1987) and Schuele and van Kleeck (1987). Ewoldt (1985) has described a school-based literacy program for children with hearing impairment that included storytelling, story creation, and free time for drawing and writing. Such activities may be crucial because reading is a critical skill for the child with hearing impairment. It provides for vocabulary expansion throughout life. Reading skills also allow the child who is deaf access to captioned television and the teletype device for the deaf (TDD).

Language Assessment

Measures used for assessing the language of children with hearing impairment can be categorized as follows: (1) communication checklists, (2) formal language tests, and (3) communication/language sample analyses. Many of the assessments most commonly used with young children with hearing impairment are those developed and standardized for use with children with normal hearing. Use of these assessments allows one to consider the language skills of children with hearing loss with reference to their normal-hearing peers. One could determine, for example, that Johnny, age 7, who has hearing impairment, has a vocabulary score typical of a 4.5-year-old child with normal hearing. Standard assessments typically indicate that spoken-language proficiency is usually delayed in children with impaired hearing. Assessments standardized on children with hearing impairment do exist. These assessments are likely to be most available to clinicians working in settings with a steady caseload of children with hearing impairment.

Because relatively few measures of language are specifically designed for children with hearing impairment, the clinician often needs to consider use of language-evaluation measures that were devised for and standardized with children with normal hearing. Language measures such as the *Peabody Picture Vocabulary*

Test (*PPVT;* Dunn & Dunn, 1997), the *Expressive One-Word Picture Vocabulary Test-Revised* (*EOWPVT-R;* Gardner, 1990), and the *Test of Language Development* (*TOLD;* Newcomer & Hammill, 1977) can be administered to children with impaired hearing. However, caution in the administration, scoring, and interpretation of test results is warranted when these tests are administered to children who have impaired hearing. For example, one should not compute or use mental ages or IQ scores for the child with impaired hearing, because low scores usually reflect only the child's language delay. A few language assessment tests have been developed for and normed on children with hearing impairment (Table 6.2).

LIMITATIONS AND CAUTIONS IN USING FORMAL LANGUAGE MEASURES. Receptive language tests typically involve oral presentation of a word or sentence and require a picture-pointing response by the child. If a child with impaired hearing responds incorrectly, it is difficult to determine whether a language or a perceptual problem is responsible. Using printed stimulus items puts too much reliance on the child's reading abilities, making it difficult to ascertain whether a language or a reading problem is responsible for the child's errors. Even signing of the stimulus items is not without difficulties. The iconic nature of some signs may help the child to match the sign with the pictured response; thus, a true measure of the child's linguistic skills is not accomplished.

Formal measures may not provide a true measure of a child's linguistic skills in everyday conversations, in which the child has access to situational and linguistic cues to help decipher what is being said. The need to combine formal and informal strategies for language assessment of children with hearing impairment is delineated in an excellent article by Moeller (1988).

Assessment of conversational and narrative skills is also important in reflecting the language abilities of children with hearing loss. Conversational abilities typically are evaluated through videorecording play interactions or natural conversations. Narrative abilities can be evaluated by asking children to review wordless picture stories and then either tell the story (oral narration) or write the story (written narration). Analysis of conversational and narrative samples often includes consideration of syntactic and morphologic forms used, communicative functions, vocabulary, and length of utterances or sentences. Tur-Kaspa and Dromi (1998) found distinct differences between the spoken and written narratives of children with normal hearing and early-identified children with severe-to-profound hearing loss. The children with hearing loss used less complex syntactic forms than the normal hearing children.

ESSENTIAL CONDITIONS FOR EVALUATING LANGUAGE ABILITIES. Several factors must be kept in mind when evaluating the language of a child with hearing impairment. First, sensory devices such as hearing aids or cochlear implants should be checked for proper function. Second, the test environment should be optimized by reducing noise and other environmental distractions. Third, when spoken language is used during testing, the clinician should make a conscious effort to allow the child full access to speechreading cues. This might necessitate allowing the child time to look down at a picture and then look back at the tester's face prior to presentation of the test item.

An extremely important factor in language evaluation is that persons administering language tests be proficient users of the child's primary communication

Cued Speech involves the use of hand positions and shapes to resolve some of the ambiguities associated with trying to speechread words that look alike on the lips. Unlike fingerspelling, which is based on letters, the hand supplements associated with Cued Speech are based on sounds.

TABLE 6.2

Language Assessment Tests Designed for Children with Hearing Impairment

TEST	NORMED	SCREENING VERSION AVAILABLE	NUMBER OF SUBTESTS	NUMBER OF VERSIONS	FORMAT	MODE OF COMMUNICATION
Test of Syntactic Ability (TSA) (Quigley, Steinkamp, Power, & Jones, 1976)	Normal hearing and hearing impaired	Yes (2 different versions)	20	1	Paper and pencil	Written
Grammatical Analysis of Elicited Language (GAEL) (Moog & Geers, 1979; Moog, 1983)	Hearing impaired	No	0	3 (presentence, simple sentence, and complex sentence)	Props, modeled scripts, imitation	Oral, total communication
Teacher Assessment of Grammatical Structures (TAGS) (Moog & Kozak, 1983)	Normal hearing	No	0	3 (presentence, simple sentence, complex sentence)	Teacher rates child using sentences in daily classroom activities	Oral, signed English
Spontaneous Language Analysis Procedure (SLAP) (Kretschmer & Kretschmer, 1978)	Hearing impaired	No	6	1	Child in conversation	Any
Carolina Picture Vocabulary Test (Layton & Holmes, 1985)	Hearing impaired	No	0	1	Picture pointing	Total Communication
Rhode Island Test of Language Structure (Engen & Engen, 1983)	Normal hearing and hearing impaired	No	0	1	Picture pointing	Any
Scales of Early Communication Skills (Moog & Geers, 1975)	Hearing impaired	No	3	1	Demonstration and observation	Any
SKI-HI Language Development Scale (Tonelson & Watkins, 1979)	Hearing impaired	No	2	1	Parent observation	Any

mode and language, whether that be spoken language only, spoken language + Cued Speech, spoken language + Signed English, or American Sign Language. Otherwise, test results will be invalid, reflecting misunderstanding of test instructions and desired responses rather than language ability.

American Sign Language is frequently referred to as ASL. It is a form of manual communication used by culturally Deaf individuals in the United States and has a unique grammar that is not based on English.

Communication and Language Management for Preschool and School-Age Children with Hearing Impairment

Carney and Moeller (1998) describe a number of treatment goals for language development of deaf children, including the following:

1. Enhanced parent–child communication in the chosen communication modality or language
2. Understanding of increasingly complex concepts and discourse
3. Acquisition of lexical and world knowledge
4. Development of verbal reasoning skills as a foundation for literacy attainment
5. Enhanced self-expression and acquisition of pragmatic, syntactic, and semantic language rules
6. Development of spoken, written, and/or signed narrative skills

Discourse refers to an extended verbal act, such as a conversation.

Two traditional intervention formats have predominated in language intervention with children with hearing impairment: One emphasizes syntactic mastery and stresses the need for drill and practice, and the other emphasizes the need for a more natural or experiential approach to language learning. While language drills may be employed in the elementary and upper school years, they are of little meaning or interest to the young child with hearing impairment. In addition, heavy use of highly structured drills does not allow children time for social interaction and conversation.

Children with normal hearing have a wide range of conversational skills that children with hearing impairment may not have. Drilling on vocabulary labels or simple sentence forms does not allow a child with hearing loss to discover how to hold and maintain a conversation. Consequently, exposure to communication functions, forms, and structures in everyday contexts should be the primary goal of early communication development programs. As noted previously, children with hearing impairment may miss out on a great deal of incidental learning (e.g., others' conversations). Thus, an important part of language facilitation with the young child with impaired hearing is creating experiences that allow the child to discover and learn about a wide range of everyday events and reasons to communicate about them. Language facilitation strategies are applicable to all children with hearing impairment regardless of whether they are developing spoken and/or signed language.

It is important for parents, teachers, and clinicians to facilitate rather than directly teach language targets and forms. Rather than drill or dictate what the child says, adults can learn to facilitate the child's use of conversational skills. True conversation is characterized by contingent and relevant responses, shared topics, and a mutual frame of reference. For example, instead of requiring the child to label all the fruit in the fruit bowl, Mom can show the child the bowl of fruit and follow the child's conversational lead.

Contingent responding means that what caregivers say to (or do for) their young language-learning children depends on the children's preceding utterances. For example, caregiver imitation of or response to the child's utterances can be reinforcing to the child, resulting in the child's repetition of the utterance or continued engagement in dialogue with the caregiver.

Adults may need to learn to be responsive and contingent. Parents who talk, talk, talk may believe that they are teaching lots of language. In the meantime, where is the child's opportunity to talk or communicate? The parents can miss out on the child's special interest and focus, or on the child's attempt to enter the conversation. If the child does use words and/or gestures, then the adult needs to acknowledge the communication. For example, if the child reaches for the apple in the fruit bowl, the parent could respond, "Oh, you want the red apple," rather than ignoring the child and continuing to instruct, "Now, this is a red apple, and this a green pear, and this is a yellow banana."

Even with knowledgeable language modelers and an abundance of contextually rich communication exchanges, some structure and practice will be necessary for language to develop in children who are hearing impaired, especially those with more severe losses. However, syntactic and semantic principles must be presented under appropriate pragmatic conditions. Wilbur, Goodheart, and Fuller (1989) attribute many of the difficulties children with impaired hearing have with linguistic structures to the practice of teaching them language using sets of unrelated sentences, with each sentence presented in isolation, devoid of any pragmatic or semantic context. A focus on isolated sentences may ultimately teach the child syntactic word order for certain syntactical devices, such as determiners, indefinite pronouns, and modals, but fails to teach the child under what pragmatic situation it would be appropriate and useful to employ the device.

The signing abilities of parents, instructors, and clinicians is critical to language development for children using a total communication approach. Moeller and Luetke-Stahlman (1990) studied parental use of simultaneous communication with their preschoolers who were deaf. All parents had sign language mean length utterances (MLUs) that were lower than their own child's MLU. Parents rarely signed or spoke syntactically or semantically complex utterances. And, unlike parents who were deaf, these parents with normal hearing rarely used fingerspelling to introduce new words. This writer remembers the comment of one father of a deaf child who said, "I don't need to know much sign language because my son only knows five signs." Clinicians and educators need to find ways to help parents gain,

---

Case 6.4. MW

MW is a child who was diagnosed at 2 years of age with a hearing loss that was believed to possibly have been progressive since birth. He has a moderate sensorineural hearing loss in the right ear and a moderate to severe sensorineural hearing loss in the left ear. Immediately following this diagnosis, amplification and auditory verbal therapy were initiated. From the onset, his parents were highly involved in maintaining effective amplification use and in offering home-based language stimulation. At age 6, MW was discharged from therapy because he had age-appropriate speech, language, and auditory skills. During kindergarten and first grade he was fully mainstreamed in regular classrooms and received no support services. At the end of first grade, he was performing above grade level in reading and math. His speech is judged to be 90 to 100 percent intelligible. If his hearing loss continues to progress, he may become a candidate for a cochlear implant.

and understand the importance of, sign language proficiency. For example, video-tape sign series are now available to help families learn sign language (e.g., *Sign with Me: A Family Sign Language Curriculum;* Moeller & Schick, 1993). Challenging as it may be, the instructor(s), parents, and siblings must be proficient in sign language in order for the child to develop language at a normal rate. If those communicating with the child are proficient in signing, every conversation can serve to aid language proficiency in the child with hearing impairment.

STRATEGIES FOR DEVELOPING CONVERSATIONAL SKILLS. Schirmer (1994) discusses several conversational approaches that facilitate language development. These approaches encourage the child's practice as a conversation partner learning how and when to initiate, take turns, and end conversations. The strategies employ real and role-played conversations. As such, they help the child become more communicatively proficient with all language aspects, not just syntax or morphology.

One technique discussed by Schirmer was *recasting.* Adults communicating with the child target syntactic–semantic structures for development. If and when the child uses incomplete or inappropriate forms during conversation, the adult recasts the utterance maintaining the child's meaning but providing the appropriate form. For example, if the child says, "Daddy eated cookie" the parent responds, "Yes, daddy ate the cookie." The parent does not require the child to correct his or her original utterance. This technique has been found to facilitate language development in children with hearing impairment.

Children with hearing impairment often have underdeveloped schema or limited knowledge concerning everyday events like what happens during a trip to the doctor's office (Yoshinaga-Itano & Downey, 1986). Schema can be developed by purposefully planning experiential learning events. For example, Dad could read a book about a trip to the doctor for a checkup, Dad and child could talk about visiting the doctor for a checkup, prepare for the trip to the doctor (e.g., take a bath and leave at the appointed time), visit the doctor and talk about the office and checkup, and later remember and tell Mom about the visit to the doctor's office.

When real-life schema-building experiences cannot be arranged, adults can set up conversational scenarios or imaginary play scenes. The child and adult can pretend a "going-to-the-doctor scene" including what happens prior to and during the visit. The role-played scene still allows the child to learn about language and conversation in that setting.

Practical suggestions for teaching language use, content, and form are also provided by Luetke-Stahlman and Luckner (1991). They point out that much of the success in teaching the pragmatic aspects of language will depend on the teacher's and caretaker's ability to create an abundance of meaningful language opportunities for the child to communicate in routine situations. Several saboteur strategies are suggested to provide the child with opportunities to use language that has been mastered. One type of activity, for example, is to violate a routine event. At the dinner table, set the table by placing the plates and silverware on the chairs, or forget to put the child's favorite, mashed potatoes, on the table. These sabotaging activities provide opportunities for the child to protest, request, comment, and tease, and ensure that the child has ample opportunity to use language in a meaningful context.

Sabotage activities provide motivation and opportunity for children to use and practice their emerging language skills. For example, a child may be presented with a desirable object that has been placed in a clear jar with a lid that is childproof. This increases the likelihood that the child will engage in communicative interaction with the caregiver, and the caregiver is provided with an opportunity to stimulate the child with the language needed to make a request for assistance, such as "open please."

The same requirement to create real needs in the context of natural settings is stressed by Luetke-Stahlman and Luckner (1991) for the semantic and syntactic aspects of language. Suggestions for helping children expand their English vocabularies are provided. One technique is the use of semantic mapping, in which a new word, such as *satisfactory,* is explained in graphic form using words the child already knows, such as *excellent* and *terrible.* Communication games, such as barrier games, can provide opportunities for children to use their emerging syntactic skills in a fun, meaningful way.

PRELITERACY AND LITERACY ACTIVITIES. In addition to facilitating conversational skills, parents and clinicians will also want to provide early preliteracy and literacy activities for the young child with hearing impairment. Words on labels and traffic signs can be pointed out to the child, and story reading and retelling can be used to develop early awareness of reading and print. Children should also be allowed the opportunity to draw pictures, trace letters, and watch their stories be written down by their parents. Literacy activities for children with hearing impairment have been presented by Truax (1985) and Staton (1985).

BILINGUAL EDUCATION FOR CHILDREN WHO ARE DEAF. In recent years, some educators have embraced a bilingual–bicultural approach to communication with education of deaf children. Interest in the bilingual approach was sparked by Johnson, Liddell, and Erting (1990), who suggested that the academic curriculum would be more accessible to children who are deaf if it was presented in American Sign Language (ASL), which they felt should be the child's primary language. Under the model proposed by Johnson et al. (1990), ASL would be used for academic instruction and interpersonal communication in the classroom. English skills would be taught through written language, with explanations given using ASL. Johnson et al. (1990) argue that acceptance of ASL as the primary language of children who are deaf will yield better academic success *and* ultimately greater English language competency than presenting instruction solely in English. An excellent discussion of rehabilitative issues in the bilingual education of children who are deaf is presented by Lieberth (1990). She poses a number of unanswered questions regarding

Bilingual–Bicultural

There is considerable controversy in deaf education regarding the bilingual–bicultural approach to education of children with severe and profound hearing losses. This method is based on the premise that American Sign Language (ASL) is the native language of children with hearing losses and therefore should be the primary teaching language in school programs for children with hearing loss. Under this model, English is taught as a second language in written form, and the culture of Deaf individuals is emphasized in the curriculum. At this time, there is some evidence to support the efficacy of this approach, with several studies currently underway. Implementation of this model is another matter, however. For example, the majority of deaf children have hearing parents with no prior signing experience, and thus there should be concern about a lack of early exposure in ASL for these children.

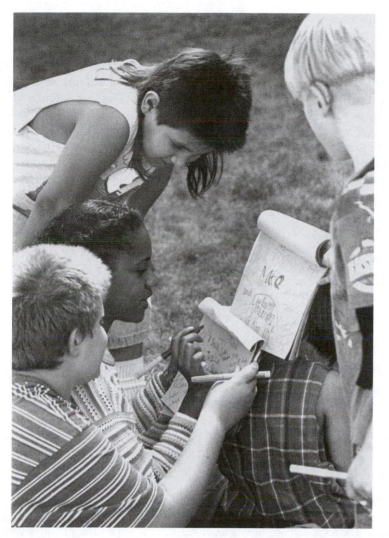

Real-life activities are helpful in building language skills.

Should the clinician assume that *all* children with hearing loss will show language learning difficulties and delays? Not at all! The children who are least likely to evidence significant language delays are those whose hearing loss is in the mild-to-moderate range who have above-average cognitive and linguistic processing skills and supportive learning environments (Gilbertson & Kamhi, 1995). And at the other end of the spectrum are children with hearing impairment who have additional learning disabilities that exacerbate their language-learning difficulties. It is imperative that each child be evaluated without prior expectations of how children with hearing loss should or will perform in the language arena. Because language delay is prevalent in this population, full-time use of appropriate sensory devices (hearing aids, FM systems, and/or cochlear implants) and aggressive speech–language therapy is often a necessity.

the bilingual education model, including whether competency in English can be developed through writing, how parents with normal hearing will acquire competency in sign language, and how the relationship between children who are deaf and their parents with normal hearing will be affected by the child's bilingualism. Stewart (1993) emphasizes that bilingual–bicultural programs should not have exclusive use of ASL as the ultimate goal, but rather should provide for consistent and complete linguistic input in the target language as well. Thus, ASL and English-based signing could serve as complementary communication tools. Like Lieberth (1990), Stewart (1993) raises a number of questions regarding the current move in deaf education toward a bilingual education model. It is only through the gathering of data from controlled investigations that we will be able to answer these questions and to document the efficacy of a bilingual model of education for children who are deaf.

SPEECH CHARACTERISTICS, ASSESSMENT, ■ AND MANAGEMENT

General Considerations

Early identification: Identification of hearing loss prior to 6 months of age.

Early management: Speech–language–hearing intervention provided prior to 6 months of age.

Many parents, teachers, and clinicians advocate the development of oral communication skills to the greatest extent possible. The focus of this section reflects that attitude. However, this perspective is not meant to deny that other means of communication, such as sign language, are beneficial and essential. Indeed, not all children with hearing loss will be predominately oral communicators. The following discussion will address hearing as a foundation for speech sound development, early vocalizations of the child with hearing loss, speech intelligibility, speech characteristics of those with hearing loss, and considerations for speech assessment and management.

HEARING AS THE FOUNDATION FOR SPEECH SOUND DEVELOPMENT. Infants do not produce intelligible words until about 1 year of age. However, their early ability to recognize and differentiate speech sounds is a critical precursor to the production of those words (Sininger, Doyle, & Moore, 1999). In fact, a fetus hears speech at approximately 28 weeks gestation (Moore, Perazzo, & Braun, 1995), and by 6 months of age the child has learned to discriminate the sounds of his or her native language (Downs & Yoshinaga-Itano, 1999). Normal hearing allows for the development of speech perception. What are the effects of early auditory deprivation such as that produced by hearing loss? Studies of early auditory deprivation in animals show changes in the morphology and function of the central auditory system through which speech acoustic information is carried and processed.

Evidence suggests that babies are learning to listen to and differentiate the speech sounds of their own language during the first six months of life. Is this first six months a critical period for the development of spoken language? Downs and Yoshinaga-Itano (1999) reviewed the speech and language abilities of children with hearing loss identified prior to age 6 months and those identified later. Amazingly, children who were identified early and had no other complicating conditions typically had speech

> Early and appropriate intervention is the most effective strategy for developing normal speech and language in children with hearing loss (Downs & Yoshinaga-Itano, 1999).

and language abilities *within the normal range* for their age. Downs and Yoshinaga-Itano proposed that identification and management of hearing loss by 6 months of age are the most effective strategy for developing normal speech and language. They found that many children whose hearing loss had been identified and managed prior to 6 months developed normal speech by age 5 years.

EARLY VOCALIZATIONS OF THE CHILD. In order to consider early vocalizations of the child with hearing loss, review of normal infant vocalizations is necessary. Normal-hearing babies develop vocalizations in an ordered sequence from birth to their first words (Stoel-Gammon & Otomo, 1986). They move through the following sequence of sound productions: crying and vegetative sounds (burps, coughs, sneezes), cooing and laughing, reduplicated babbling (same consonant–vowel syllable produced in a repetitive string, babababa), and variegated babbling (change in consonant–vowel syllable in a string, *badabada*) with sentence-like intonation (Oller, 1980). Between 11 and 14 months, children produce some speech sound combinations called *vocables* to consistently represent meaning (Owens, 1990). For example, the child may call her blanket "bee" on a consistent basis. Some time around the first birthday the child will begin producing her first words.

Infants with hearing loss vocalize also. Like normal-hearing babies they coo, squeal, growl, babble (Stoel-Gammon & Otomo, 1986); produce similar vowel positions and a greater proportion of velar–back consonants at 12 to 15 months (Smith, 1982); and show similar development of place of articulation of consonants and in the frequency of babbling. In contrast to infants with normal hearing, they produce fewer consonantlike sounds from 6 to 10 months of age (Oller & Eilers, 1988; Stoel-Gammon & Otomo, 1986). Oller and Eilers, for example, reported that whereas babies with normal hearing started canonical babbling (reduplicated babbling) between 6 and 10 months of age, babies with hearing loss showed onsets between 11 and 25 months and showed fewer instances of canonical babbling. Until the 1990s and the increased use of universal newborn hearing screening, relatively few children with hearing loss were identified within the first year of life, much less studied with respect to vocal behaviors. Research in this area should expand, given the widespread use of universal newborn hearing screening.

SPEECH INTELLIGIBILITY. Speech intelligibility refers to the proportion of speech that can be understood by a listener. Typically, speech intelligibility is evaluated by requiring a speaker to produce sentences that are recorded. The recording is then played to listeners who are asked to identify the words in the sentences, with percent of correct word identification indicating overall intelligibility. Two main factors affect intelligibility: the experience of the listener with deaf speech and the difficulty level of the vocabulary and sentence structure for the speaker. Listeners experienced with deaf speech yield higher intelligibility scores, and simpler vocabulary and sentences yield higher intelligibility scores (Monsen, 1975). Monsen, for

Infant vocalizations: Sounds such as crying, coughing, cooing, laughing, babbling, and vocables (word approximations) that precede spoken words.

Speech intelligibility: Proportion of speech understood by a listener.

example, reported that, although many studies indicated an average of 20 percent intelligibility for those with severe-to-profound hearing loss, his use of simpler sentence materials resulted in an average of 76.7 percent intelligibility. Also, the typical measure of speech intelligibility involves listener identification of words in unrelated sentences from a tape recording. This task does not allow face-to-face clues and context that can add substantially to real-world speech intelligibility.

Not only does intelligibility affect daily conversation, but it also affects perceptions of a speaker's cognitive competence and personality. Speakers who have good or moderately good speech intelligibility are perceived much more positively than speakers with poor intelligibility (Most, Weisel, & Matezky, 1998). This is true for listeners who both have and have not had experience in listening to deaf speech. This may explain why some deaf speakers choose not to use speech, even though they may be capable of producing some intelligible words. Plant (1999), for example, reported on a deaf speaker who exhibited 80 to 90 percent intelligibility with contextual and face-to-face cues to listeners and yet who still chose not to use his speech in daily life.

Levitt (1987) studied the speech and language of 120 children 10 to 14 years of age and found that speech intelligibility was directly related to the degree of hearing loss. However, there is considerably greater variability in speech intelligibility for children whose hearing losses are at or exceed 90 dB HL.

Svirsky et al. (2002) evaluated the speech intelligibility of 151 prelingually deafened children ranging in age from 1 to 15 years of age, all of whom were using hearing aids. Speech intelligibility was found to be related to degree of profound loss with the children who had more residual hearing tending to be more intelligible. However, deaf children whose pure-tone averages exceeded 110 dB HL seldom had intelligibility scores higher than 20 percent (i.e., fewer than 1 in 5 words that might be understood in an utterance).

Although unaided hearing thresholds might allow for some prediction of speech intelligibility, aided audiometric thresholds and tests of speech perception abilities (Smith, 1975) should provide a better indicator of a given child's speech intelligibility. Plotting of the aided audiogram on a Familiar Sounds Audiogram (see Figure 6.3), for example, can allow one to predict what speech sounds might be available through audition to serve as a basis for speech development.

One highly controversial issue related to speech intelligibility is the effect of communication mode. Some argue that the early use of sign language diverts attention from spoken language, resulting in poor speech intelligibility. Others argue that competence in sign language might have little impact on speech intelligibility, whereas competency in a language might benefit reading and writing performance

Does early sign language use inherently limit the development of intelligible speech? Or are children in total communication environments simply limited in their exposure to and use of speech?

FAMILIAR SOUNDS AUDIOGRAM

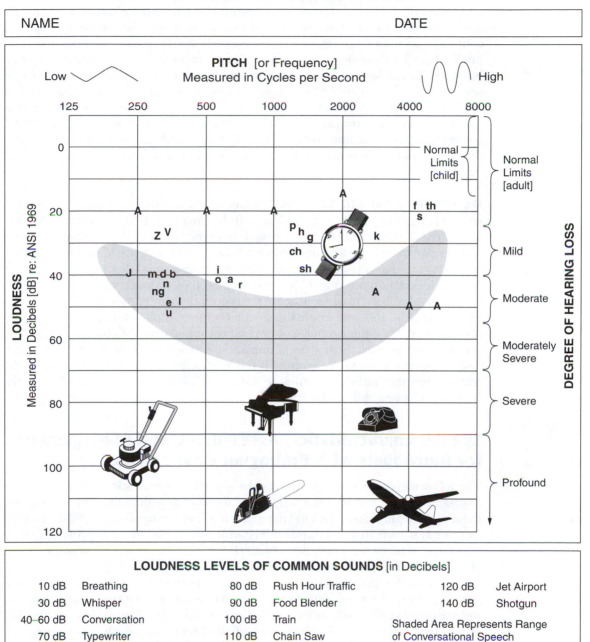

FIGURE 6.3

Aided thresholds (A) plotted on the Familiar Sounds Audiogram.

(Stuckless & Birch, 1997). Osberger and Robbins (1994) compared the speech intelligibility of children with cochlear implants using total communication and children with cochlear implants using oral communication. The children using oral communication had significantly better intelligibility. Potential causes of improved intelligibility for those using oral communication included (1) more intensive speech training, (2) teachers in total communication programs not having expertise in speech training, (3) higher expectations for oral communication set by parents and teachers, and (4) peer use of speech. There is no evidence that the use of sign language itself detracts from speech intelligibility. However, it appears that some total communication programs give little attention to speech use and development and that this could easily explain why children in these programs have poorer speech intelligibility.

SPEECH PERCEPTUAL ABILITIES. One key factor that is not always established is the speech perceptual abilities of children with hearing loss. Blamey, Sarant, Paatsch, and Barry (2001) and others have strongly asserted that speech perceptual abilities (e.g., as evidenced by scores on word identification and sentence identification tests) are related to the language levels and speech production abilities of children with hearing loss. Miyamoto et al. (2003) have reported on a visual habituation test procedure that has been used to evaluate the speech discrimination abilities of infants with normal hearing and infants receiving cochlear implants. Early data suggests that within the first three months of implant use infants are not able to discriminate sounds, but that after six months of implant use they begin to show signs of speech discrimination. It would be exciting if this type of procedure could be used to determine whether individual children with cochlear implants are developing the speech perception abilities necessary for the development of spoken language.

Speech Characteristics, Assessment, and Management for Individuals with Prelingual Hearing Loss

The following discussion will address the speech characteristics, assessment, and management concerns for two categories of individuals with prelingual hearing loss: those with hearing loss in the mild to moderately severe range (i.e., unaided pure tone thresholds ≤70 dB HL) and those with hearing loss in the severe-to-profound range (i.e., unaided pure tone thresholds >70 dB HL). A final section will address the speech of persons with acquired hearing loss (i.e., onset after 5 years of age).

Prior to this discussion, it is important to present two key tenets related to speech concerns for those with hearing loss. These tenets have been summarized by Robbins (1994). First, advancements in hearing aid technology and the availability of multichannel cochlear implants have allowed those with profound hearing loss greater access to speech acoustic cues than ever before. Despite these technological advances, the development of intelligible speech in children with prelingual profound hearing loss is still a challenge. Second, speech training must be fit into the realm of establishing overall communicative competence. Robbins suggested six guidelines for achieving this: (1) integrate auditory and speech goals, (2) follow a "dialogue" rather than "tutorial" format, (3) use bridging activities to promote real-world carryover, (4) practice communication sabotage, (5) use contrasts in perception and production, and (6) select speech goals that enhance communicative competence. One enjoyable and meaningful way to develop and practice speech sound listening discrimination and production with young children is to establish associations between familiar toys or actions and their sounds. Srinivasan (1996) provides a chart for clinicians and parents (see Table 6.3). The child can listen to family members "moo" when playing with the toy cow and be encouraged to "moo" also. (See Robbins, 1994, and Estabrooks, 1994, for sample speech activities.)

INDIVIDUALS WITH MILD-TO-MODERATELY SEVERE PRELINGUAL HEARING LOSS

SPEECH CHARACTERISTICS OF INDIVIDUALS WITH PRELINGUAL MILD-TO-MODERATELY SEVERE HEARING LOSS. Although published data are sparse, children with mild-to-moderately severe hearing loss generally have intelligible speech (Elfenbein, Hardin-Jones, & Davis, 1994; Jensema, Karchner, & Trybus, 1978). The predominant speech errors of this population are related to the misarticulation of single consonants (Elfenbein et al., 1994) and consonant blends (Cozad, 1974).

Knowledge of speech acoustics and the typical sloping audiometric configuration would suggest that errors might be most common for speech sounds of low intensity, high frequency, and/or short duration. Complexity of formation, visibility, and developmental order of acquisition are also considerations in the speech errors of this population. Sounds most commonly in error are the affricates, fricatives, and blends (Elfenbein et al., 1994). Elfenbein, Hardin-Jones, and Davis found that the most common error types were substitutions (57 percent), followed by distortions (29 percent), and omissions (14 percent). The types of speech errors made by children with mild-to-moderately severe hearing loss resemble the errors made by younger children with normal hearing.

Phonologic assessments have been made of children with hearing loss to indicate rule-governed speech behaviors. Two sets of researchers have reported phonologic analyses of children with hearing loss in the mild-to-moderately severe range (Oller & Kelly, 1974; West & Weber, 1974). They found that these children were producing accurate vowels and were showing phonological processes used by younger children with normal hearing (e.g., voicing avoidance, fronting of consonants). Oller and Kelly proposed that children who are hard of hearing develop and use speech sounds in the same order as children with normal hearing.

SPEECH ASSESSMENT OF INDIVIDUALS WITH MILD-TO-MODERATELY SEVERE LOSS. The child with hearing loss in the mild-to-moderately severe range typically has speech errors comparable to normal-hearing children with articulation or phonological delays. Therefore, the practice of using standard articulation tests and phonologic analyses appears justified. One caution for the tester is to consider the vocabulary level of the stimulus words or items used and the need for replacing words or items not within the child's vocabulary. Formal assessments of vowel production, voice quality, and suprasegmental features may not be called for, given that these speech characteristics are less likely to be problematic for children with mild to moderately severe hearing losses. However, possible evaluation procedures are discussed in the assessment section for children with severe to profound hearing loss.

TABLE 6.3			
Listening Sounds List			
SOUND	**ASSOCIATED OBJECT**	**ASSOCIATED ACTION**	**ASSOCIATED PHRASE**
ah	airplane (high pitch) truck (low pitch)		
oo	train (*woo woo*), owl (*hoot hoot*), ghost (*boo!*), cow (*moo*), dog (*woof woof*)		"Oops!"
ee	mouse (*ee ee ee*), bird (*cheep cheep*),	sweep down the slide ("Whee!")	
ai			"Hi!" "Bye bye!"
au	cat (*meow*),	down, around	"Ouch!"
o	rabbit (*hop hop*),	hop	hot, pop, "All gone!" knock (on the door)
oe		open, roll over	"Row, row the boat" "Roll (the ball)"
ay	horse (*neigh*)		"Hooray!"
a	duck (*quack*) sheep (*baaa*)		
u	up	run	"Uh oh!"
oi	pig (*oink*)		
m	ice cream (*Mmm!*)		"Mama," more, "Yumm! Yumm!"
n		knock	"No!"
w		walk, wind, wash, wipe	
b	bubbles, bus (*buh buh buh*)		"Bye! Bye!"
p	pop boat (*putt putt*)	pour, pat, pull/push	
t	clock (*tick tock*)	turn, tiptoe	
d	hammer (*duh duh duh*)		
k		cut	
g		go, drinking (*guh guh guh*)	
sh		Sleeping (*shh!*)	
s	snake (*sss*)		
f		off (take ___ *off*)	
l		lalling to a tune (*lah lah lah . . .*)	
z	bee (*zzzz*)		
h	witch (*hee hee hee*)	laughing ("Ha! Ha! Ha!")	"It's hot!"
y	yo yo		"Yuk", yes

Source: Srinivasan (1996).

> ### Case 6.5. JF
>
> JF is a child with mild autism whose mild sensorineural hearing loss was first identified at age 7. Use of an FM system was initiated at school, and use of personal hearing aids was implemented at home. JF's language abilities are age-appropriate with the exception of pragmatics. He has difficulty in communicating effectively with children his age, but this has been related to his mild autism. JF's speech is fully intelligible and no articulation or phonological problems were noted. However, JF tends to use breathy, whispered speech, and voice therapy was initiated to resolve that problem. There is evidence of prior vocal nodules, and a recurrence of nodules or some other vocal cord pathology is now suspected.

SPEECH MANAGEMENT OF INDIVIDUALS WITH MILD-TO-MODERATELY SEVERE LOSS. With early and appropriate amplification, many children with hearing loss in the mild-to-moderately severe range can be expected to have highly intelligible speech. However, children whose losses remain undetected and/or not amplified may be expected to manifest more extensive speech errors. Gordon-Brannan, Hodson, and Wynne (1992), for example, presented a case of a child in phonological treatment who showed significant gains only after his trough-shaped hearing loss was identified and he was fitted with hearing aids. In many cases, the clinician's major efforts will be directed toward articulation and/or phonological treatment. Standard articulation and/or phonological treatment techniques are generally appropriate with some special considerations and modifications to programming.

Several considerations should be kept in mind while undertaking such treatment. First, children with normal hearing who have articulation or phonologic disorders are capable of using auditory feedback cues. Children with hearing loss may need visual, tactile, and/or kinesthetic cues to compensate for their inability to hear certain speech sound distinctions.

Second, the clinician must be familiar with the child's aided hearing thresholds in order to identify which speech sounds are not likely to be within the child's residual hearing range. This information can be gained by plotting the child's aided hearing thresholds on the Familiar Sounds Audiogram (see Figure 6.3). For sounds not within the child's aided hearing range, nearly total reliance on other cues for speech sound production is likely.

Third, the clinician should be familiar with the impact of co-articulation, since speech sounds change when paired with different speech sounds. Consequently, training on isolated speech sound productions should be limited and instead should move quickly to the production of sounds in meaningful words and phrases. For children with hearing loss in the birth to 3-year age range, Cole (1992) advocates use of the following guidelines:

1. Selecting and sequencing the child's speech targets based on normal developmental information
2. Maximizing and ensuring optimal residual hearing
3. Having parents and clinicians target spoken language goals during normal everyday activities (p. 74)

> ## Case 6.6. EF
>
> EF is the 3 ½-year-old sister of JF. Her mild-to-moderate sensorineural hearing loss was iden-tified at age 3 when her hearing was tested after the identification of her brother's hearing loss. She was immediately fit with powder-pink hearing aids. EF is highly communicative, and her language abilities are within the normal range. Her primary deficit is in the area of articulation, and she is receiving speech therapy to address that.

INDIVIDUALS WITH PRELINGUAL HEARING LOSS IN THE SEVERE TO PROFOUND RANGE. Historically, children with severe-to-profound hearing loss have demonstrated significant deficits in speech production. With the availability of cochlear implants, improved speech production is generally expected. The discussion below pertains mainly to children wearing hearing aids.

SPEECH CHARACTERISTICS OF INDIVIDUALS WITH PRELINGUAL HEARING LOSS IN THE SEVERE TO PROFOUND RANGE. Studies have indicated that the average intelligibility of children with severe to profound hearing loss is approximately 20 percent, although individual ratings vary from 0 to 100 percent (Carney, 1986). These children may exhibit difficulties with consonant production, vowel and diphthong production, and voice quality (Hudgins & Numbers, 1942). For purposes of discussion, speech characteristics in this population will be discussed under the categories of respiration, resonance, phonation, and articulation and phonology. Because this categorization simplifies the discussion, we must remain aware that respiratory, resonatory, phonatory, and articulatory and phonologic behaviors are interactive and co-occur during ongoing speech. Smith (1982) cautions that the speech of children who are deaf actually represents "stacks of errors which are complex and interrelated" (p. 27). Children with severe-to-profound hearing loss also exhibit faulty suprasegmental features. The discussion of suprasegmental errors will be followed by assessment and management considerations.

RESPIRATION. Clinicians and investigators have observed that individuals with severe-to-profound hearing loss may speak only a few syllables on a single exhalation of air (Forner & Hixon, 1977). Hutchinson and Smith (1976), for example, noted high airflow rates (i.e., air wastage) during production of some consonant segments. Forner and Hixon (1977) studied abdomen and ribcage movement in ten young adult males with severe-to-profound hearing losses. Unlike speakers with normal hearing, these subjects, who had poor speech intelligibility, initiated speech at low lung volumes, uttered only a few syllables at a time with air wastage during the pauses between segments, and continued to speak with lung volumes well below functional residual capacity. Cavallo, Baken, Metz, and Whitehead (1991) studied chest wall movements before vowel production in seven adult males. Ribcage and abdominal movements were recorded, and lung volume was estimated based on measures from a mercury strain gauge. Before vowel production, the speakers with hearing loss demonstrated expansion of the ribcage and contraction of the diaphragm comparable to that seen in speakers with normal hearing. However, speakers with hearing loss lost significantly more air during the short adjustment period immediately prior to vowel production. These investigators proposed that speakers with hearing loss delay the adduction of vocal folds prior to phonation that would normally limit loss of air. They further suggested that this might explain why some speakers with hearing loss initiate speech at or below functional residual capacity for the lungs.

RESONANCE. Both hyponasality and hypernasality have been observed in the speech of those with severe to profound hearing loss (Smith, 1975). The presence of resonance problems is interesting, given that acoustic information on nasality is found in the lower frequencies, where speakers with hearing loss may have more residual hearing (Borden, Harris, & Raphael, 1994). In these cases, individuals might be trained to make use of auditory cues to nasality, resulting in improved resonance.

> Resonance: Vibration of air in the throat, oral cavity, and/or nasal cavity; resonance problems include hypernasality and hyponasality.

PHONATION. Studies of respiration led investigators to link air wastage prior to and during the production of speech with insufficient vocal fold adduction, rather than to respiratory difficulties. Inadequate vocal fold adduction has been directly observed in speakers with hearing loss when producing vowels (Metz, Whitehead, & Whitehead, 1984). This incomplete closure can result in the overall perception of breathy voice quality and in the perception of voiceless sounds being substituted for voiced sounds (McGarr & Whitehead, 1992).

Control of fundamental frequency of the voice is also primarily a function of laryngeal events. When compared to normal-hearing peers, persons who are deaf may use higher average fundamental frequency, as observed by Angelocci, Kopp, and Holbrook (1964). However, some do retain normal average fundamental frequency, as observed by Monsen (1979). Another observation is that the range of fundamental frequencies produced across utterances is reduced in the speech of the deaf.

Speech intensity, another aspect of phonation, is also primarily a function of laryngeal activity. Unfortunately, data on voice intensity for speakers with hearing loss are limited. Reduced intensity, excessive intensity, and reduced intensity variations across utterances have all been observed in this population. Reduced intensity and lack of intensity variation have been related to pervasive breathiness and low lung volume during speech. Excessive intensity has been related to excessive glottal resistance.

> Phonation: Vocalizations produced with vocal fold vibration; problems with phonation include breathy voice quality with inadequate vocal fold adduction, abnormally high fundamental voice frequency, and excessive voice intensity with excessive vocal fold resistance.

ARTICULATION AND PHONOLOGY. Variability seems to be one of the hallmarks of speech production among those with severe-to-profound hearing loss. Despite the variability, some typical errors have been identified. First, patterns of consonant and vowel errors can be identified. Second, consonant misarticulation is much more common than vowel or diphthong misarticulation.

The following categorizations of vowel error patterns, offered originally by Hudgins and Numbers (1942), have been substantiated in more recent research:

1. Vowel neutralization (i.e., the tendency for all vowels to resemble the neutral schwa)
2. Diphthong and vowel confusions (e.g., /aI/ for /a/ or /a/ for /ai/)
3. Nasalization of vowels

The perception of vowel neutralization has been verified by acoustic and physiologic studies, including studies indicating centralized or static tongue position across vowels (Tye-Murray, 1991).

Children with hearing loss produce consonants less accurately than vowels on both spontaneous and imitative tasks (Geffner & Freeman, 1980). Hudgins and Numbers (1942) categorized the most common consonant errors of children who are deaf in the following way:

1. Voicing errors (e.g., substitution of /b/ for /p/)
2. Omission and distortion of consonants (e.g., omission of velars and final consonants)
3. Omission of consonants in blends (e.g., /tap/ for /stap/)
4. Nasalization of consonants

Voicing errors may include voiced or voiceless confusions, devoicing of final consonants, and omission of final voiced consonants (Hutchinson et al., 1978).

Studies of tongue placement during consonant production have been conducted using a technique called *palatometry*. Palatometry involves the placement of a thin custom-fit pseudopalate over the child's hard palate and maxillary teeth. The pseudopalate has a set of 96 electrodes, which, when contacted by the tongue, show as contact points on a display screen. Figures 6.4 and 6.5 (Dagenais, 1992), respectively, show the pseudopalate and the computer's visual display targets for a selected

Palatometry: A pseudopalate with 96 contact electrodes is fit like a dental retainer against the speaker's hard palate, and the speaker then views a computer display that shows the appropriate tongue to palate contacts while adjusting her tongue to match the target.

FIGURE 6.4

Palatometry pseudopalate showing the 96 contact electrodes.

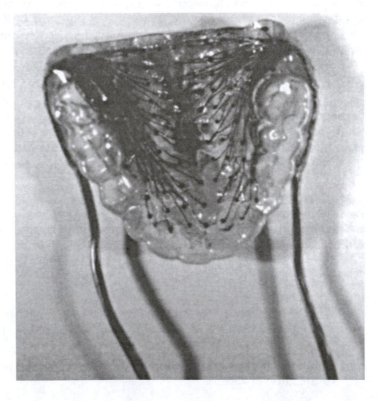

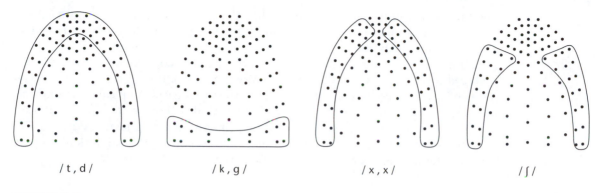

/ t , d /   / k , g /   / x , x /   / ʃ /

FIGURE 6.5

Contact patterns used for training consonants with palatometry.

set of consonants. Results of palatometry studies have indicated that children with profound hearing loss have idiosyncratic tongue-to-palate contacts as compared to speakers with normal hearing (Dagenais & Critz-Crosby, 1991).

In addition to individual phoneme errors, speech of persons who are deaf is sometimes characterized by reduced co-articulatory movements. The production of a speech sound in an utterance can be influenced by both preceding sounds and subsequent sounds. Reduced co-articulation in deaf speakers has been related to slower and less precise movement of the tongue (Okalidou & Harris, 1999).

Data suggest that cochlear implants allow for the greatest speech acoustic information for the development of speech sound production in children with profound hearing loss. Toby, Geers, and Brenner (1994) compared matched groups of hearing aid users, cochlear implant users, and tactile device users across a three-year period and found significantly better speech sound production in children with cochlear implants. Children with cochlear implants showed significantly greater overall improvement in their production of intelligible vowels and consonants and were more accurate in producing some of the less visible place features (e.g., velars) and manner features (e.g., glides).

SUPRASEGMENTAL ASPECTS. Suprasegmental features include changes in duration, intensity, and fundamental frequency across syllables in an utterance. Suprasegmentals are important because they communicate an individual's emotional intent, the urgency of a message, and linguistic stress. Suprasegmental problems in deaf speakers can contribute substantially to poor intelligibility (Gold, 1980).

Individuals who are deaf speak at an overall rate 1.5 to 2 times slower than that of speakers with normal hearing (Tye-Murray, 1992). Slow speaking rate has been related to prolongation of individual phonemes and the presence of lengthy pauses within utterance. It is interesting to note that some investigators have reported improved intelligibility for slower speaking rates (Osberger & Levitt, 1979). Thus, overall slow speaking rate may, in part, serve as an appropriate compensatory adjustment.

Speakers with hearing loss have been found to use more and longer pauses in addition to within-phrase pauses during utterances. Speakers with normal hearing

Suprasegmental features: Variations in intensity, fundamental frequency, and duration of syllables and pauses across an utterance; problems with suprasegmentals include overall slow speaking rate, within-phrase pauses, excessive fundamental frequency variation, and less than normal fundamental frequency variation.

tend to avoid within-phrase pauses. Although speakers who are deaf often exhibit abnormal pause behaviors, Osberger and Levitt (1979) found little associated effect on speech intelligibility.

Differences in intonation of deaf speakers have been consistently associated with reduced speech intelligibility (Formby & Monsen, 1982). Both excessive pitch variation and less than normal pitch variation have been observed. Atypical intonation has been associated with lower overall speech intelligibility (Formby & Monsen, 1982).

In summary, speakers who are deaf may have difficulty adjusting duration, intensity, and intonation within an utterance. These suprasegmental difficulties may result in faulty linguistic stress and reduce overall speech intelligibility.

Speech Assessment of Individuals with Severe or Profound Hearing Loss

Comprehensive speech evaluation of those with severe or profound hearing loss should include perceptual measures of intelligibility, articulation and phonology, suprasegmental features, and voice characteristics. The additional use of acoustic and/or physiologic measures is typically restricted to those who have access to the instrumentation. In this section, four general areas of evaluation will be considered.

MEASURES OF SPEECH INTELLIGIBILITY. Assessment and improvement of speech intelligibility would appear to be important goals for speakers with severe or profound hearing loss. Percent of intelligible word scores and intelligibility ratings are the most widely used measures, and difficulties arise with each.

As indicated previously, often speakers are required to produce sentences and listeners later identify the words that they hear, with percent of correct words

Adult deaf individuals may undertake speech therapy to improve intelligibility.

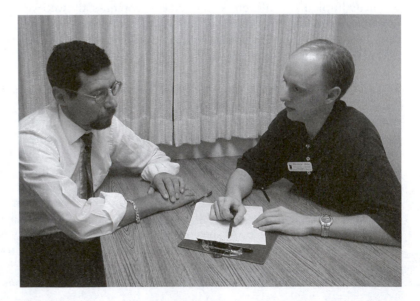

reflecting percent of speech intelligibility. However, the speech intelligibility score can vary widely depending on the following:

1. Complexity of vocabulary and sentences spoken
2. Presence or absence of contextual cues
3. Presence or absence of visual and lipreading cues
4. Listener experience with deaf speech

Thus, one score will typically represent the intelligibility only for that speaking–listening situation (Monsen, 1979).

Another type of assessment tool, the rating scale, has been presented by the National Technical Institute for the Deaf (NTID; Subtelny, 1977). This procedure requires a set of listeners who first are trained in the use of a 5-point rating scale. The scale ranges from 1 (speech cannot be understood) to 5 (speech is completely intelligible). Obviously, most clinicians would probably have only one listener—herself—to make these rating judgments.

Requiring deaf children to read sentences may underestimate intelligibility due to a child's difficulty in reading fluently. Assessment of intelligibility for picture description tasks or conversational samples, instead, can indicate how the child's knowledge of spoken language affects speech intelligibility. We can use these samples to calculate the number of totally intelligible utterances, number of totally unintelligible utterances, and number of intelligible and unintelligible words.

MEASURES OF ARTICULATION AND PHONOLOGY. Standard articulation tests have been used in the assessment of children with hearing loss (Abraham, Stoker, & Allen, 1988). Although these tests are not normed for children with hearing loss, they do indicate phonemes produced accurately, phonemes produced inaccurately, and the types of speech sound errors (substitution, distortion, omission).

Clinicians who have larger numbers of children with hearing loss may choose to obtain assessment tools specific to this population. Some evaluations, that is, phonetic evaluations, address whether the child is capable of producing a speech sound through imitation or in conversational speech. Ling (1976) developed the Phonetic Level Evaluation specifically for children with severe-to-profound hearing loss. On the Phonetic Level Evaluation, the child imitates nonsense syllables. Imitative target syllables include consonants and consonant blends in the initial and final positions of syllables and vowels and diphthongs. Toby, Geers, and Brenner (1994) reported on the use of the CID Phonetic Inventory, an evaluation tool that includes imitation of suprasegmentals, vowels and diphthongs, initial consonants, initial consonants with alternating vowels, final consonants, and final alternating consonants. Miccio, Ingrisano, and Balkany (1990) cautioned that deaf children may be able to imitate or spontaneously produce a large range of speech sounds and yet not use these sounds contrastively to produce words in ongoing speech.

A second type of evaluation, phonologic evaluation, indicates whether speech sounds are produced accurately and contrastively in conversation. Phonologic evaluation typically uses a speaking sample other than that produced through imitation of the clinician or through reading sentences. Ling (1976) suggested that in order to obtain a valid picture of phonologic skills a tape recording should be made of the

Phonetic repertoire: A set of speech sounds that a child can produce regardless of whether they are used appropriately in everyday speech.

Phonologic system: Speech sounds that are used in a rule-based way in everyday speech.

child in all five of the different types of discourse: conversation, description, narration, question, and explanation. The clinician would then analyze the tape-recorded sample to determine which speech sounds are and are not used accurately and consistently.

PERCEPTUAL ASSESSMENT OF SUPRASEGMENTALS AND VOICE CHARACTERISTICS. Speech and voice characteristics are most often assessed by clinicians who listen to and rate the characteristics of a spoken passage or spontaneous speech sample. Some clinicians, for example, may use Wilson's voice rating system (1977) in which judgments are made related to laryngeal valving, pitch, nasality, intensity variability, and pitch variability. In addition, Wilson urges clinicians to check for the presence of voice deviations such as diplophonia, audible inhalation, pitch breaks, and phrasing irregularities.

ACOUSTIC AND PHYSIOLOGIC DISPLAYS. Instrumentation providing displays of acoustic characteristics of speech are generally more likely to be available to clinicians than physiologic instrumentation. Commonly used equipment that displays acoustic features includes the Visi-Pitch (Kay Elemetrics, Inc.), which can indicate fundamental frequency and intensity, and the IBM SpeechViewer, which can indicate the mean frequency and standard deviation of frequency across an utterance, mean intensity and standard deviation of intensity across an utterance, and percentage of utterance voiced. Physiologic instrumentation can be used to assess respiratory function, nasality, and tongue-to-palate contacts. A spirometer can be used to assess speech initiatory lung volumes and other patterns of respiratory adjustment. A nasometer can be used to determine the presence of hyponasality or hypernasality, and a palatometer can be used to indicate whether an individual is making appropriate tongue-to-palate contacts.

Speech Management for Individuals with Severe or Profound Hearing Loss

Nearly all investigators who have studied speech production in persons who are deaf are struck by the extreme variability in error patterns among individuals. Such differences highlight the importance of individualizing speech management procedures. With the advent of universal newborn screening comes the opportunity to potentially prevent speech and language delay in children born with hearing loss. Yoshinaga-Itano and Apuzzo (1998a, 1998b) again remind us that children identified and provided appropriate amplification and family-centered intervention no later than 6 months of age typically develop speech and language in the normal range.

A critical concern with speech training is that it be as meaningful as possible. Speech is used to express meaning. Speech sounds that cannot be heard and developed through the use of optimal amplification or cochlear implant use may require the use of additional visual and/or tactile cues. However, training should not focus on lengthy motor drills of sounds in meaningless syllables. Speech sound training should move quickly to the use of meaningful words. In accordance with a whole-language philosophy, speech targets should appear in words that a child would learn about in natural contexts. A child, for example, would not simply learn the label "duck" when working on production of the /d/ and produce it each time the clinician showed a toy duck. The child would read about ducks, play with ducks, go see ducks at the duck pond, and talk about birds that are ducks and birds that are not ducks. In addition, the development of sounds in different phonetic contexts is also important to ensure the development of coarticulation.

Four major approaches may enhance speech training in persons with hearing loss: (1) early and consistent use of devices to provide optimal use of residual hearing, (2) anatomic and pictorial monitoring, (3) visual cues, and (4) use of complex feedback aids.

Most individuals with hearing loss possess some residual hearing, and its use should be maximized. This is the primary and best means for providing feedback for the development of speech. An important question to ask is whether the client's hearing aid, FM system, cochlear implant, or vibrotactile system provides her or him with as many speech sounds as possible. It would be ideal if clinicians could assume that clients are receiving the most speech sounds possible with the assistance of their sensory devices. But the fitting of devices, particularly in children, can be a tricky bit of educated guesswork. If the clinician questions the audibility of speech for a given client, consultation and possibly referral to the child's audiologist would be appropriate. Another related question is whether the client has the best device for allowing speech development. Tobey, Geers, and Brenner (1994) reported on three matched groups of children with profound hearing loss that received intensive speech training, but who were fit with either hearing aids, cochlear implants, or vibrotactile devices. All three groups showed improvement in imitative speech production and percent of intelligible words, but the children with cochlear implants showed the greatest gains. And yet it should be noted that children with cochlear implants still have difficulty in developing intelligible speech (Robbins, 1994).

Anatomic and pictorial monitoring has also been used to help establish speech sound production. Anatomic charts, sagittal sections of the head with a mobile tongue, and pictures of tongue shape may be useful in some cases. Some of these models are available commercially, but they can also be made without undue expense. The problem with these aids is that they provide a static picture, whereas the production of a speech sound is not static. It may be wise to use these types of models only in the initial stages of sound production and only as a last resort.

Another approach to improving speech production is visual stimulation by the clinician and/or visual monitoring with the use of a mirror. Some information concerning speech production is available visually. However, excessive attention to visual feedback may be hazardous. The visual characteristics of sounds dramatically change as a function of context. For example, /ʃ/ looks considerably different in the words *shoe* and *she.*

Complex feedback aids or devices have also been used to assist in training speech production. Most devices provide for visual monitoring of acoustic features of speech, such as the VisiPitch and IBM SpeechViewer. The VisiPitch allows for display of fundamental frequency of the voice and intensity variation across an utterance. The IBM SpeechViewer allows for child-friendly displays, with loudness

Providing feedback is an important element of speech therapy with the hearing impaired.

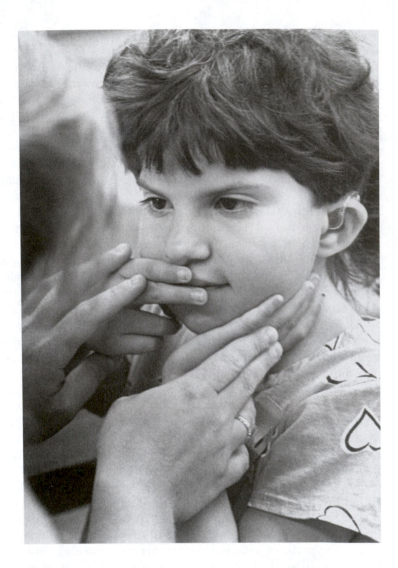

indicated by the changing size of a balloon, pitch indicated as changes on a thermometer, and vowel accuracy indicated by a monkey dropping a coconut from a tree. Vowel production and fundamental frequency treatment benefits have been documented with the use of the IBM SpeechViewer (Pratt, Heintzelmann, & Deming, 1993; Ryalls, LeDorze, Boulanger, & Larouche, 1995). However, there is no proof that the system is more effective than traditional therapy approaches or that it produces carryover to everyday speech. In addition, children appear to lose interest in the displays across multiple sessions. Consequently, these types of devices may be of greatest benefit as a supplementary treatment tool and in providing objective measures of treatment efficacy.

One type of feedback display shows tongue placement. The palatometer, described earlier, gives feedback on contact points of the tongue. Reports of palatometry training with children who are deaf have been promising, but the system is not widely available for use (Dagenais, 1992). Dagenais suggested that speech training might begin with the use of these systems to establish correct articulatory placement for sounds in nonsense syllables and single-syllable words and then move to more traditional approaches that emphasize words and phrases.

TECHNOLOGY. Massaro and Light (2004) reported on the use of Baldi, a computer-animated talking head with transparent skin that allows for visualization of the tongue, teeth, and palate and visual cues for neck vibration and airflow for frication. Seven students with hearing loss and related speech production errors were selected to participate in this study to determine the impact of speech perception and production training based on watching and hearing Baldi (animatedspeech.com/Research/research_effectiveness.html) producing sounds and words. Students sat at a desk with a laptop computer, external speakers, and an external microphone. During this training, Baldi would produce the sounds and words while the children watched the movements of his tongue, hard palate, and teeth. Perceptual training consisted of watching and hearing Baldi's productions and then identifying the sounds or words heard. Speech production training involved students' producing sounds and words while attempting to match their speech movements to those of Baldi. Students were trained on syllables and words that exhibited voiced versus voiceless distinctions, consonant cluster distinctions, and fricative versus affricate distinctions. These researchers reported significant improvements in the perception and production of trained speech sounds.

Speech Characteristics of Individuals with Postlingual Profound Hearing Loss

Descriptions of speech abilities in individuals with acquired hearing loss have been limited. Acquired deafness in those with well-developed speech appears to produce a gradual rather than immediate deterioration of speech. Hearing plays a role in the long-term monitoring and maintenance of speech coordination (Zimmerman & Rettaliata, 1981). A wide variation in speech production abilities has been observed in this population. Cowie and Douglas-Cowie (1983), for example, reported intelligibility scores ranging from 10 to above 90 percent in a sample of thirteen adults. These investigators also reported that reduced intelligibility and voice quality or slurring resulted in negative reactions by the listeners judging the speech samples. The wide variation in speech production has been related primarily to age at onset of hearing loss, although degree of hearing loss and hearing aid history also have been considered secondary factors (Cowie, Douglas-Cowie, & Kerr, 1982). The following specific speech errors were observed in this population according to Kishon-Rabin, Taitelbaum, Tobin, and Hildesheimer (1999): (1) decreased vowel space due to centralization of the first two formants, (2) inaccurate production of /s/ and /sh/, (3) similar voice onset time values for voiced and voiceless plosives, (4) substitution of /r/ with /w/, and (5) tendency to omit consonants in the final position of words. Kishon-Rabin et al. also reported that after receiving cochlear implants their postlingually deafened adults showed significant improvements in speech and voice quality over a two-year period.

SUMMARY

Who should be responsible for speech and language intervention for individuals with hearing loss? The audiologist, speech–language pathologist, teacher of the hearing impaired, and family members will all have a role in the management of the child with hearing loss. All have complementary and sometimes overlapping contributions toward language facilitation. The audiologist will have the greatest expertise in monitoring the child's hearing loss, establishing and ensuring that sensory devices are providing the maximum amount of speech acoustic cues, and communicating to others about the aspects of speech that may be inaudible to the child. The speech–language pathologist will have the strongest background and training in current language intervention techniques, including ways to establish more family-centered intervention. The teacher of the hearing impaired will offer means of tutorial and educational support and may be the most proficient of the professionals with respect to knowledge and use of sign language. The family is the constant in the child's life (Crais, 1991); as such, the family's needs and choices are critical to the success and carryover of language and speech intervention. The true challenge of family-centered intervention is working out the collaboration and consultation between the family and professionals involved in the management of the child with hearing loss.

SUMMARY POINTS

- The presence of hearing loss in children does not preclude language development, although it can have a serious impact on the child's overall language competence.
- The inability to hear spoken language on a consistent, unambiguous basis may severely compromise the child's ability to develop the semantic, syntactic, pragmatic, and phonologic aspects of language.
- Although there are several language measures specifically designed for children with hearing impairment, the clinician will probably need to supplement these measures with assessment tools that were designed and standardized with children who have normal hearing.
- For most children with severe hearing loss, a combination of language drill and experiential language stimulation will be necessary to enhance language development.
- Early identification and intervention are essential to optimize the child's chance of developing age-appropriate language skills.
- Because hearing is the foundation for speech development, hearing aid and/or cochlear implant use must be implemented as soon as possible to provide children with hearing loss access to speech acoustic information.
- The development of speech in children with congenital hearing loss can best be promoted when hearing loss identification, home intervention, and amplification are provided within the first six months of life.
- Infants with hearing loss do vocalize. However, studies suggest differences in their babbling behaviors when compared to normal-hearing babies.

- Children with mild to moderately severe hearing losses (up to 70 dB HL) typically have highly intelligible speech with predominately articulation and phonological errors.
- Children with severe and profound hearing losses (>70 dB HL) are much more variable with respect to speech intelligibility and speech errors. Intelligibility in this population ranges from 0 to 100 percent, with possible errors in vowel and diphthong production, consonant production, respiration for speech, resonance, phonation, and suprasegmental speech characteristics.

RECOMMENDED READING

Caesar, L. G., & Williams, D. R. (2002). Socioculture and the delivery of health care: Who gets what and why? *The ASHA Leader, 7*(6), 6.

Estabrooks, W. (1994). *Auditory–verbal therapy for parents and professionals.* Washington, DC: Alexander Graham Bell Association for the Deaf.

Ewolt, C. K. (1985). A descriptive study of the developing literacy of young hearing-impaired. In R. Kretchmer (Ed.), Learning to write and writing to learn. *Volta Review* [Special issue], *87.* Washington, DC: Alexander Graham Bell Association for the Deaf, pp. 109–126.

Isaacson, J. E., Hasenstab, M. S., Wohl, D. L., & Williams, G. H. (1996). Learning disability in children with postmeningitic cochlear implants. *Archives of Otolaryngology Head and Neck Surgery, 122*(9), 929–936.

Levitt, H. (1987). Interrelationships among the speech and language measures. In H. Levitt, N. McGarr, & D. Geffner (Eds.), Development of language and communication skills of hearing-impaired children. *ASHA Monographs, 26,* 123–139.

Ling, D. (1989). *Foundations of spoken language for hearing-impaired children.* Washington, DC: Alexander Graham Bell Association for the Deaf.

Mayne, A. M., Yoshinaga-Itano, C., Sedey, A. L., & Carey, A. (2000). Expressive vocabulary development of infants and toddlers who are deaf or hard of hearing. *Volta Review, 100*(5) (monograph), 1–28.

Osberger, M. J., & Robbins, A. M. (1994). Speech intelligibility of children with cochlear implants. *Volta Review, 96*(5), 169–181.

Rhoades, E. A., Price, F., & Perigoe, C. B. (2005). The changing American family and ethnically diverse children with hearing loss and multiple needs. *The Volta Review, 104*(4) (monograph), 285–305.

Robbins, A. M. (1994). Guidelines for developing oral communication skills in children with cochlear implants. *Volta Review, 96*(5), 75–82.

Srinivasan, P. (1996). *Practical aural habilitation for speech–language pathologists and educators of hearing-impaired children.* Springfield, IL: Charles C. Thomas.

Svirsky, M. A., Robbins, A. M., Kirk, K. I., Pisoni, D. B., & Miyamoto, R. T. (2000). Language development in profoundly deaf children with cochlear implants. *Psychological Science, 11,* 153–158.

Tomblin, J. B., Spencer, L., Flock, S., Tyler, R., & Gantz, B. (1999). A comparison of language achievement in children with cochlear implants and children using hearing aids. *Journal of Speech Language and Hearing Research, 42,* 497–511.

Yoshinaga-Itano, C. (2003). From screening to early identification and intervention: Discovering predictors to successful outcomes for children with significant hearing loss. *Journal of Deaf Studies and Deaf Education, 8*(1), 11–30.

Yoshinaga-Itano, C., & Downey, D. M. (1996). Development of school-aged deaf, hard-of-hearing, and normally hearing students' written language. *Volta Review, 98,* 3–7.

Alexander Graham Bell Association for the Deaf and Hard of Hearing:
www.agbell.org

Resources for families of children with hearing loss:
www.gohear.org
www.helpkidshear.org
www.raisingdeafkids.org

Free videos and library on oral deaf education:
www.oraldeafed.org

Early Intervention for Deaf and Hard of Hearing Children:
www.center.uncg.edu/index.asp
www.ibwebs.com/hearing/htm

REFERENCES

Abraham, S., Stoker, R., & Allen (1988). Language assessment of hearing-impaired children and youth: Patterns of test use. *Language, Speech, and Hearing Services in the Schools, 19,* 160–173.

Angelocci, A. A., Kopp, G. A., & Holbrook, A. (1964). The vowel formants of deaf and normal-hearing eleven-to-fourteen-year-old boys. *Journal of Speech and Hearing Disorders, 29,* 156–170.

Bankson, N. (1977). *Bankson Language Screening Test.* Baltimore: University Park Press.

Blamey, P. J., Sarant, J. Z., Paatsch, L. E., & Barry, J. G. (2001). Relationships among speech perception, production, language, hearing loss, and age in children with impaired hearing. *Journal of Speech, Language, and Hearing Research, 44*(2), 264–286.

Boothe, L., Lasky, E., & Kricos, P. (1982). Comparison of the language abilities of deaf children and young deaf adults. *Journal of Rehabilitation of the Deaf, 15,* 10–15.

Borden, G. J., Harris, K. S., & Raphael, L. J. (1994). *Speech science primer: Physiology, acoustics, and perception of speech* (3rd ed.). Baltimore: Williams & Wilkins.

Brenza, B. A., Kricos, P. B., & Lasky, E. Z. (1981). Comprehension and production of basic semantic concepts by older hearing-impaired children. *Journal of Speech and Hearing Research, 24,* 414–419.

Calderon, R. (1998). Further support for the benefits of early identification. *Volta Review, 100*(5), 53–85.

Carney, A. E. (1986). Understanding speech intelligibility in the hearing impaired. *Topics in Language Development, 6*(3), 47–59.

Carney, A. E., & Moeller, M. P. (1998). Treatment efficacy: Hearing loss in children. *Journal of Speech, Language, and Hearing Research, 41,* S61–S84.

Cavallo, S. A., Baken, R. J., Metz, D. E., & Whitehead, R. L. (1991). Chest wall preparation for phonation in congenitally profoundly hearing-impaired persons. *Volta Review, 12,* 287–299.

Chin, S. B. (2003). Children's consonant inventories after extended cochlear implant use. *Journal of Speech, Language, and Hearing Research, 46*(4), 849–864.

Cole, E. B. (1992). Promoting emerging speech in birth to three-year-old hearing-impaired children. *Volta Review, 94,* 63–77.

Connor, C. Mc., Hieber, S., Arts, H. A., & Zwolan, T. A. (2000). Speech, vocabulary, and the education of children using cochlear implants: Oral or total communication? *Journal of Speech, Language, and Hearing Research, 43*(5), 1185–1204.

Connor, C. Mc., & Zwolan, T. A. (2004). Examining multiple sources of influence on the reading comprehension skills of children who use cochlear implants. *Journal of Speech, Language, and Hearing Research, 47*(3), 509–527.

Cowie, R. I. D., & Douglas-Cowie, E. (1983). Speech production in profound post-lingual deafness. In M. E. Lutman & M. P. Haggard (Eds.), *Hearing science and hearing disorders.* New York: Academic Press.

Cowie, R. I. D., Douglas-Cowie, E., & Kerr, A. G. (1982). A study of speech deterioration in post-lingually deafened adults. *Journal of Laryngology and Otology, 96,* 101–112.

Cozad, R. L. (1974). *The speech clinician and the hearing-impaired child.* Springfield, IL: Charles C. Thomas.

Crais, E. R. (1991). Moving from "parent involvement" to family-centered services. *American Journal of Speech-Language Pathology, 9,* 5–8.

Dagenais, P. A. (1992). Speech training with glossometry and palatometry for profoundly hearing-impaired children. *Volta Review, 94,* 261–282.

Dagenais, P. A., & Critz-Crosby, P. (1991). Consonant lingual–palatal contacts produced by normal-hearing and hearing-impaired children. *Journal of Speech and Hearing Research, 34,* 1423–1435.

Dodd, B., McIntosh, B., & Woodhouse, L. (1998). Early lipreading ability and speech and language development of hearing-impaired pre-schoolers. In R. Campbell, B. Dodd, & D. Burnham (Eds.), *Hearing by ear and eye II: Advances in the psychology of speechreading and auditory–visual speech* (pp. 283–301). United Kingdom: Psychology Press.

Downs, M. P., & Yoshinaga-Itano, C. (1999). The efficacy of early identification and intervention for children with hearing impairment. *Pediatric Clinics of North America, 46*(1), 79–87.

Duchan, J. F. (1988). Assessing communication of hearing-impaired children: Influences from pragmatics. In R. R. Kretschmer & L. W Kretschmer (Eds.), Communication assessment of hearing-impaired children: From conversation to classroom [Monograph]. *Journal of the Academy of Rehabilitative Audiology, 21*(Suppl.), 19–41.

Duncan, J. (1999). Conversational skills of children with hearing loss and children with normal hearing in an integrated setting. *Volta Review, 101*(4), 193–203.

Dunn, L., & Dunn, L. (1997). *Peabody Picture Vocabulary Test–Revised (PPVT-3).* Circle Pines, MN: American Guidance Service.

Elfenbein, J. L., Hardin-Jones, M. A., & Davis, J. M. (1994). Oral communication skills of children who are hard of hearing. *Journal of Speech and Hearing Research, 37,* 216–226.

Engen, E., & Engen, T. (1983). *Rhode Island Test of Language Structure.* Austin, TX: Pro-Ed.

Ertmer, D. J., Strong, L. M., & Sadagopan, N. (2003). Beginning to communicate after cochlear implantation: Oral language development in a young child. *Journal of Speech, Language, and Hearing Research, 46*(2), 328–342.

Formby, C., & Monsen, R. B. (1982). Long-term average speech spectra for normal and hearing-impaired adolescents. *Journal of the Acoustical Society of America, 71,* 196–202.

Forner, L. L., & Hixon, T. J. (1977). Respiratory kinematics in profoundly hearing-impaired speakers. *Journal of Speech and Hearing Research, 20,* 373–407.

Gallaudet Research Institute. (2005). *Regional and national summary report of data from the 2003–2004 Annual Survey of Deaf and Hard of Hearing Children and Youth.* Washington, DC: GRI, Gallaudet University.

Gardner, M. E. (1990). *Expressive One-Word Picture Vocabulary Test–Revised.* Novato, CA: Academic Therapy Publications.

Geers, A., Brenner, C., & Davidson, L. (2003). Factors associated with development of speech perception skills in children implanted by age five. *Ear and Hearing, 24*(1), 24S–35S.

Geers, A. E., Nicholas, J. G., & Sedey, A. L. (2003). Language skills of children with early cochlear implantation. *Ear and Hearing, 24*(1), 46S–58S.

Geffner, D. S., & Freeman, L. R. (1980). Assessment of language comprehension of six-year-old deaf children. *Journal of Communication Disorders, 13,* 455–470.

Gilbertson, M., & Kamhi, A. G. (1995). Novel word learning in children with hearing impairment. *Journal of Speech, Language, and Hearing Research, 38,* 630–642.

Gold, T. (1980). Speech production in hearing-impaired children. *Journal of Communication Disorders, 13,* 397–418.

Gordon-Brannan, M., Hodson, B., & Wynne, M. K. (1992). Remediating unintelligible utterances of a child with a mild hearing loss. *American Journal of Speech Language Pathology,* 28–37.

Goss, R. (1970). Language used by mothers of deaf children and mothers of hearing children. *American Annals of the Deaf, 115,* 93–96.

Hudgins, C. V., & Numbers, E. C. (1942). An investigation of the intelligibility of speech of the deaf. *Genetic Psychology Monographs, 25,* 289–392.

Hutchinson, J. M., & Smith, L. L. (1976). Aerodynamic functioning during consonant production by hearing-impaired adults. *Audiology and Hearing Education, 2,* 16–24.

Hutchinson, J. M., Smith, L. L., Kornhauser, R. L., Beasley, D. S., & Beasley, D. C. (1978). Aerodynamic functioning in consonant production in hearing-impaired children. *Audiology and Hearing Education, 4,* 23–31.

Jensema, C. J., Karchmer, M. A., & Trybus, R. J. (1978). *The rated speech intelligibility of hearing-impaired children: Basic relationships.* Washington, DC: Gallaudet College Office of Demographic Studies.

Johnson, H. A. (1988). A sociolinguistic assessment scheme for the total communication student. In R. R. Kretschmer & L. W. Kretschmer (Eds.), Communication assessment of hearing-impaired children: From conversation to classroom [Monograph]. *Journal of the Academy of Rehabilitative Audiology, 21*(Suppl.), 101–129.

Johnson, R. E., Liddell, S. K., & Erting, C. J. (1990). *Unlocking the curriculum: Principles for achieving access in deaf education.* Gallaudet Research Institute Working Paper 89-3. Washington, DC: Gallaudet University.

Kishon-Rabin, L., Taitelbaum, R., Tobin, Y., & Hildesheimer, M. (1999). The effect of partially restored hearing on speech production of postlingually deafened adults with multichannel cochlear implants. *Journal of the Acoustical Society of America, 106*(5), 2843–2857.

Kretschmer, R. R., & Kretschmer, L. W. (1978). *Language development and intervention with the hearing impaired.* Baltimore: University Park Press.

Langdon, H. (2003). *Working with interpreters to serve bilingual children and families.* Rockville, MD: ASHA.

Laybaert, J. (1998). Phonological representation in deaf children: The importance of early linguistic experience. *Scandinavian Journal of Psychology, 39,* 169–173.

Layton, T. L., & Holmes, D. W. (1985). *Carolina Picture Vocabulary Test.* Austin, TX: Pro-Ed.

Lederberg, A. R., & Everhart, V. S. (1998). Communication between deaf children and their hearing mothers: The role of language, gesture, and vocalizations. *Journal of Speech, Language, and Hearing Research, 41,* 887–899.

Lieberth, A. K. (1990). Rehabilitative issues in the bilingual education of deaf children. *Journal of the Academy of Rehabilitative Audiology, 23,* 53–61.

Limbrick, E. A., McNaughton, S., & Clay, M. M. (1992). Time engaged in reading: A critical factor in reading achievement. *American Annals of the Deaf, 137*(4), 309–314.

Ling, D. (1976). *Speech and the hearing-impaired child: Theory and practice.* Washington, DC: Alexander Graham Bell Association for the Deaf.

Luetke-Stahlman, B., & Luckner, J. (1991). *Effectively educating students with hearing impairments.* New York: Longman.

Massaro, D. W., & Light, J. (2004). Using visible speech to train perception and production of speech for individuals with hearing loss. *Journal of Speech, Language, and Hearing Research, 47*(2), 304–321.

Mayne, A. M., Yoshinaga-Itano, C., Sedey, A. L., & Carey, A. (2000). Expressive vocabulary development of infants and toddlers who are deaf or hard of hearing. *Volta Review, 100*(5) (Monograph), 1–28.

McGarr, N. S., & Whitehead, R. (1992). Contemporary issues in phoneme production by hearing-impaired persons: Physiologic and acoustic aspects. *Volta Review, 94,* 33–45.

Metz, D., Whitehead, R., & Whitehead, B. (1984). Mechanics of vocal fold vibration and laryngeal articulatory gestures produced by hearing-impaired speakers. *Journal of Speech and Hearing Research, 27,* 62–69.

Miccio, A., Ingrisano, D., & Balkany, T. (1990). *Emergence of phonological contrasts following cochlear implantation.* Paper presented at the annual meeting of the American Speech–Language–Hearing Association.

Miller, P. (1997). The effect of communication mode on the development of phonemic awareness in prelingually deaf students. *Journal of Speech, Language, and Hearing Research, 40,* 1151–1163.

Miyamoto, R. T., Houston, D. M., Kirk, K. I., Perdew, A. E., & Svirsky, M. A. (2003). Language development in deaf infants following cochlear implantation. *Acta Otolaryngologica, 123,* 241–244.

Moeller, M. P. (1988). Combining formal and informal strategies for language assessment of hearing-impaired children. Communication assessment of hearing-impaired children: From conversation to classroom. In R. R. Kretschmer & L. W. Kretschmer (Eds.), Communication assessment of hearing-impaired children: From conversation to classroom [Monograph]. Supplement, *Journal of the Academy of Rehabilitative Audiology, 21,* 73–101.

Moeller, M. P., & Luetke-Stahlman, B. (1990). Parents' use of signing exact English: A descriptive analysis. *Journal of Speech and Hearing Disorders, 55,* 327–338.

Moeller, M. P., Osberger, M. J., & Eccarius, M. (1986). Receptive language skills [Monograph 231]. *Language and learning skills of hearing-impaired students, Asha Monographs,* 41–54.

Moeller, M. P., & Schick, B. (1993). *Sign with me parent workbook.* Omaha, NE: Center for Hearing Loss in Children.

Monsen, R. B. (1979). Acoustic qualities of phonation in young hearing-impaired children. *Journal of Speech and Hearing Research, 22,* 270–288.

Moog, J. S., & Geers, A. E. (1975). *Scales of early communication skills for hearing impaired children.* St. Louis: Central Institute for the Deaf.

Moog, J. S., & Geers, A. E. (1979). *Grammatical analysis of elicited language—simple sentence level.* St. Louis, MO: Central Institute for the Deaf.

Moog, J. S., & Geers, A. E. (1983). *Grammatical analysis of elicited language–presentence level.* St. Louis, MO: Central Institute for the Deaf.

Moog, J. S., & Kozak, V. J. (1983). *Teacher assessment of grammatical structures.* St. Louis, MO: Central Institute for the Deaf.

Moore, J. K., Perazzo, L. M., & Braun, A. (1995). Time course of axonal myelination in the human brainstem auditory pathway. *Hearing Research, 87,* 21.

Most, T., Weisel, A., & Matezky, A. (1996). Speech intelligibility and the evaluation of personal qualities by experienced and inexperienced listeners. *Volta Review, 98*(4), 181–190.

Newcomer, P., & Hammill, D. (1977). *Test of Language Development.* Los Angeles: Western Psychological Services.

Nicholas, J. G., & Geers, A. E. (2003). Hearing status, language modality, and young children's communicative and linguistic behavior. *Journal of Deaf Studies and Deaf Education, 8*(4), 422–437.

Okalidou, A., & Harris, K. S. (1999). A comparison of intergestural patterns in deaf and hearing adult speakers: Implications from an acoustic analysis of disyllables. *Journal of the Acoustical Society of America, 106*(1), 394–409.

Oller, D. K. (1980). The emergence of speech sounds in infancy. In G. Yeni-Komishan, J. Kavanaugh, & C. A. Ferguson (Eds.), *Child phonology: Vol 1. Production* (pp. 93–112). New York: Grune and Stratton.

Oller, D., & Eilers, R. E. (1988). The role of audition in infant babbling. *Child Development, 59,* 441–449.

Oller, D., & Kelly, C. A. (1974). Phonological substitution processes of a hard-of-hearing child. *Journal of Speech and Hearing Disorders, 39,* 65–74.

Osberger, M. J., & Levitt, H. (1979). The effect of timing errors on the intelligibility of deaf children's speech. *Journal of the Acoustical Society of America, 66,* 1316–1324.

Osberger, M. J., Moeller, M. P., Eccarius, M., Robbins, A. M., & Johnson, D. (1986). Expressive language skills [Monograph 23]. In M. J. Osberger (Ed.), *Language and learning skills of hearing-impaired students* (pp. 54–65). Asha Monographs. Washington, DC: Asha.

Owens, R. E. (1990). Development of communication, language, and speech. In G. H. Shames & E. H. Wiig (Eds.), *Human communication disorders* (pp. 30–73). Columbus, OH: Merrill Publishing.

Plant, G. (1999). Speech training for young adults who are congenitally deaf: A case study. *Volta Review, 100*(1), 5–17.

Pratt, S. R., Heintzelmann, A. T., & Deming, S. E. (1993). The efficacy of using the IBM SpeechViewer Vowel Accuracy Module to treat young children with hearing impairment. *Journal of Speech and Hearing Research, 36,* 1063–1074.

Prinz, P. M., & Prinz, E. A. (1985). If only you could hear what I see: Discourse development in sign language. *Discourse Processes, 8,* 1–19.

Quigley, S. P., Steinkamp, M., Power, D., & Jones, B. (1978). The test of syntactic abilities. Beaverton, OR: Dormac.

Robinshaw, H. M. (1995). Early intervention for hearing impairment: Differences in the timing of communicative and linguistic development. *British Journal of Audiology, 29,* 315–334.

Roush, J., & McWilliams, R. A. (1994). Family-centered early intervention: Historical, philosophical, and legislative issues. In J. Roush & N. D. Matkin, (Eds.), *Infants and toddlers with hearing loss: Family-centered assessment and intervention* (pp. 3–23). Baltimore, MD: York.

Ryalls, J. LeDorze, G., Boulanger, H., & Laroche, B. (1995). Speech therapy for lowering vocal fundamental frequency in two adolescents with hearing impairments: A comparison with and without the IBM SpeechViewer. *Volta Review, 97,* 243–250.

Schirmer, B. R. (1994). *Language and literacy development in children who are deaf.* New York: Maxwell Macmillan International.

Schuele, M. A., & van Kleeck, A. (1987). Precursors to literacy: Assessment and intervention. *Topics in Language Disorders, 7*(2), 32–44.

Skarakis, E. A., & Prutting, C. A. (1977). Early communication: Semantic functions and communication intentions in the communication of the preschool child with impaired hearing. *American Annals of the Deaf, 122,* 392–394.

Smith, B. L. (1982). Some observations concerning pre-meaningful vocalization of hearing-impaired infants. *Journal of Speech and Hearing Disorders, 47,* 439–441.

Smith, C. R. (1975). Residual hearing and speech production in deaf children. *Journal of Speech and Hearing Research, 18,* 795–811.

Spencer, L. J., Barker, B. A., & Tomblin, J. B. (2003). Exploring the language and literacy outcomes of pediatric cochlear implant users. *Ear and Hearing, 24*(3), 236–247.

Srinivasan, P. (1996). on disc. Practical aural rehabilitation for speech–language pathologists and educators of hearing-impaired children. Springfield, IL: Charles C. Thomas.

Staton, J. (1985). Using dialogue journals for developing thinking, reading, and writing with hearing-impaired students. *Volta Review, 87*(5), 127–153.

Stewart, D. A. (1993) Bi bi to MCE? *American Annals of the Deaf, 138,* 331–337.

Stoel-Gammon, C., & Otomo, K. (1986). Babbling development of hearing-impaired and normally hearing subjects. *Journal of Speech and Hearing Disorders, 51,* 33–41.

Stuckless, E. R., & Birch, J. W. (1997). The influence of early manual communication on the linguistic development of deaf children. *American Annals of the Deaf, 142*(3), 71–78.

Subtelny, J. D. (1977). Assessment of speech with implications for training. In F. Bess (Ed.), *Childhood deafness: Causation, assessment, and management* (pp. 183–194). New York: Grune & Stratton.

Svirsky, M. A., Chin, S. F., Miyamoto, R. T., Sloan, R. B., & Caldwell, M. D. (2002). Speech intelligibility of profoundly deaf pediatric hearing aid users, *Volta Review, 102*(4), 175–198.

Tobey, E. A., Geers, A., Brenner, C., Altuna, D., & Gabbert, G. (2003). Factors associated with development of speech production skills in children implanted by age five. *Ear and Hearing, 24*(1), 36S–45S.

Tonelson, S., & Watkins, S. (1979). *SKI*HI language development scale.* Logan, UT: Hope, Inc.

Truax, R. (1985). Linking research to teaching to facilitate reading–writing–communication connections. *Volta Review, 87*(5), 155–169.

Tur-Kaspa, H., & Dromi, E. (1998). Spoken and written language assessment of orally trained children with hearing loss: Syntactic structures and deviations. *Volta Review, 100*(3), 186–203.

Tye-Murray N. (1991). The establishment of open articulatory postures by deaf and hearing talkers. *Journal of Speech and Hearing Research, 34,* 453–459.

Tye-Murray, N. (1992). Articulatory organizational strategies and the roles of auditory information. *Volta Review, 94,* 243–260.

Tye-Murray, N. (2003). Conversational fluency of children who use cochlear implants. *Ear and Hearing, 24*(1), 82S–89S.

U.S. Bureau of the Census. (2000). *Statistical abstract of the United States, 2000 (120th ed.).* Washington, DC: Author.

van Kleeck, A., & Schuele, C. M. (1987). Precursors to literacy: Normal development. *Topics in Language Disorders, 7*(2), 13–31.

West, J. J., & Weber, J. L. (1974). A phonological analysis of the spontaneous language of a four-year-old hard-of-hearing child. *Journal of Speech and Heating Disorders, 38,* 25–35.

Wilbur, R., Goodhart, W., & Fuller, D. (1989). Comprehension of English modals by hearing-impaired students. *Volta Review, 91,* 5–18.

Wilson, F. B. (1977). *Voice disorders.* Austin, TX: Learning Concepts.

Wyatt, T. A. (2002). Assessing the communicative abilities of clients from diverse cultural and language backgrounds. In D. E. Battle (Ed.), *Communication disorders in multicultural populations* (3rd ed.; pp. 415–460). Boston: Butterworth-Heinemann.

Yoshinaga-Itano, C. (2003). From screening to early identification and intervention: discovering predictors to successful outcomes for children with significant hearing loss. *Journal of Deaf Studies and Deaf Education, 8*(1), 11–30.

Yoshinaga-Itano, C., & Apuzzo, M. L. (1998a). Identification of hearing loss after age 18 months is not early enough. *American Annals of the Deaf, 143*(5), 380–387.

Yoshinaga-Itano, C., & Apuzzo, M. L. (1998b). The development of deaf and hard of hearing children identified early through the high-risk registry. *American Annals of the Deaf, 143*(5), 416–424.

Yoshinaga-Itano, C., & Downey, D. M. (1986). A hearing-impaired child's acquisition of schemata: Something's missing. *Topics in Language Disorders, 7*(1), 45–57.

Yoshinaga-Itano, C., & Downey, D. M. (1996). Development of school-aged deaf, hard-of-hearing, and normally hearing students' written language. *Volta Review, 98,* 3–7.

Yoshinaga-Itano, C., Sedey, A. L., Coulter, D. K., & Mehl, A. L. (1998). Language of early- and later-identified children with hearing loss. *Pediatrics, 102,* 1161–1171.

Yoshinaga-Itano, C., Snyder, L. S., & Mayberry, R. (1996). How deaf and normally hearing students convey meaning within and between written sentences. *Volta Review, 98,* 9–38.

Yoshinaga-Itano, C., & Stredler-Brown, A. (1992). Learning to communicate: Babies with hearing impairments make their needs known. *Volta Review, 94,* 107–129.

Zimmerman, G., & Rettaliata, P. (1981). Articulatory patterns of an adventitiously deaf speaker: Implications for the role of auditory information in speech production. *Journal of Speech and Hearing Research, 24,* 169–178.

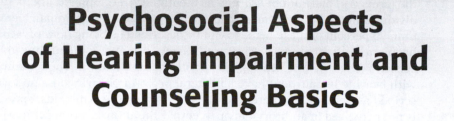

CHAPTER 7

Psychosocial Aspects of Hearing Impairment and Counseling Basics

Kris English

CONTENTS

INTRODUCTION

Adjusting to hearing impairment and accepting recommendations regarding audiologic rehabilitation can be a difficult process for many individuals, as well as for their families. This chapter will describe a range of psychological, social, and emotional difficulties frequently experienced by persons with hearing impairment across the lifespan. In addition, a description of basic counseling concepts will be provided to demonstrate how professionals can help individuals with hearing loss to contend with the problems of living with hearing loss and identify and assume ownership of their individual solutions.

PSYCHOSOCIAL ASPECTS
■ OF HEARING IMPAIRMENT

No hearing loss is exactly like another, but there are some ways to organize our understanding of this impairment. First to be recognized is the distinction between the terms *deaf* and *hard of hearing*. As mentioned in Chapter 1, about 30 million individuals in the United States have some degree of hearing impairment, and more than 90 percent of these persons can be described as being *hard of hearing:* that is, having a mild, moderate, or severe hearing loss and some ability to understand speech with the use of hearing aids or other amplification. The remaining persons with hearing impairment have a bilateral profound hearing loss and would be described as being *deaf,* whereby, even with powerful hearing aids, speech generally is not perceived in auditory-only perceptual situations. Another important distinction is needed between the concepts of *being deaf* (having a bilateral profound hearing loss) and *being Deaf.* The latter phrase, with the capital D, refers to a cultural identification with the Deaf community; this distinction and the unique concerns of cultural Deafness will be reviewed in a later section.

deaf: Profound degree of hearing loss, whereas *Deaf* connotes a pride in associating with a group who share the same culture (i.e., the Deaf community).

Initially, however, we will consider some general psychosocial and emotional implications of living with hearing loss, first among children and adolescents (that is, growing up with hearing impairment) and then among adults (acquiring hearing impairment). This first section expands upon the CORE model described in Chapter 1. Specifically, we will consider how hearing loss affects, and is affected by, **O**verall Participation Variables (psychoemotional and social) and **R**elated Personal Factors.

Growing Up with Hearing Loss

The most significant consequence of growing up with a hearing loss is the difficulty in perceiving others' words, because this limitation has a direct effect on the ability to develop one's own words and subsequent language skills. Even a mild degree of hearing loss can adversely affect vocabulary development and the subtle intricacies of language use. When language development is delayed, there is a cascading effect on many aspects of a child's psychosocial development, including self-concept, emotional development, family concerns, and social competence.

Self-concept or self-image: How one sees oneself.

SELF-CONCEPT. Individuals are not born with their self-concepts intact; rather, *self-concept is learned* by absorbing the input, feedback, and reactions from those around us. Children typically internalize such reactions without question, and allow others' attitudes to define themselves to themselves. Children are likely to think these thoughts: "I see myself the way you tell me you see me. If you see me as loved or unlovable, capable or not capable, a delight or a trial—this is how I see myself."

It appears that children with hearing loss are at risk for developing a relatively poor self-concept, most likely from negative reactions regarding their communication difficulties and also from being perceived differently as hearing aid users. For example, Cappelli and colleagues (1995) collected information from 23 hard of hearing children, ages 6 to 12, as well as from 23 children with no hearing loss, matched by sex and classroom. From a "Self-Perception Profile for Children," it was found that children with hearing impairment perceived themselves as less socially accepted than their non-hearing-impaired peers. Another recent study (Bess, Dodd-Murphy, & Parker, 1998) asked more than 1,200 children with mild hearing loss to answer questions such as this: "During the past month, how often have you felt badly about yourself?" Overall, children with mild hearing loss exhibited significantly higher dysfunction in self-esteem than children without hearing loss (self-esteem or self-regard being an evaluative component of self-concept). The researchers concluded that "even mild losses can be associated with increased social and emotional dysfunction among school aged children" (p. 350).

Children who grow up with hearing loss not only receive negative feedback and reactions because of their communication difficulties, but also because of the cosmetic issue of looking different. Our society has yet to accept hearing aids as a neutral technical device; instead, there tends to be a negative association with hearing aid use, with biased assumptions of reduced abilities, attractiveness, and intelligence. Many studies have examined this phenomenon, often called the *hearing aid effect* (Blood, Blood, & Danhauser, 1977), by showing subjects a set of pictures of individuals, some wearing visible hearing aids and some not. All characteristics were identical except for the presence of hearing aids; yet when the instruments were visible, individuals were given lower scores in almost every category of intelligence, personality, attractiveness, and capability. It appears that the very presence of a hearing aid can cause overall negative reactions.

> **Hearing aid effect:** A psychological reaction to the presence of a hearing aid; the viewer has negative assumptions about the hearing aid user.

It is encouraging to note that preschool children seem less likely to hold these negative and preconceived notions (Riensche, Peterson, & Linden, 1990) and that teens may be becoming more accustomed to and accepting of hearing aids among their peers (Stein, Gill, & Gans, 2000). But, in general, if the appearance of a device on or in the ears creates a negative reaction among people who see it, their reaction is likely to be perceived by the hearing aid user, which can adversely affect the user's self-concept. We would do a disservice to children growing up with hearing loss to dismiss society's reactions to hearing aids as a non-issue or to downplay it as "only the other person's problem." Edwards (1991) reminds us that "it is the wearing of the device which 'amplifies' the difference between the child with hearing loss and his or her peers" (p. 7), and children deserve our honesty in acknowledging that this difference does exist. (To experience the hearing aid effect firsthand, college students [with normal hearing] are frequently assigned to wear a very visible pair of hearing aids for a full day around their community and record their subjective impressions of those around them as well as their own reactions.)

Since "the acquisition of language is essential for the development of self" (Garrison & Tesch, 1978, p. 463), it follows that a delay in language acquisition would adversely affect the development of self. This correlation, in fact, has been demonstrated in several studies, described in the next section.

EMOTIONAL DEVELOPMENT. An individual uses language to describe, interpret, and ultimately understand the abstract nature of his or her emotions. Because of concomitant language deficits, children growing up with hearing loss may have limited experience in self-expression and a subsequent delay in awareness and understanding of their own emotions, as well as the emotions of others. By virtue of having a

FIGURE 7.1

Missing out on adult conversations about emotions.

> Aunt Betty reminded me that this is the anniversary of her father's death. She is a little shaky, but she does feel better remembering all the good times while growing up. Still, that explains why she was so subdued the other day, I was pretty worried about that . . . .

Affective vocabulary: Words and phrases that describe feelings or emotional reactions (e.g., discouraged, elated, bored, upset).

hearing loss, they frequently miss overhearing adults and older children talk about and verbally manage their feelings about situations (see Figure 7.1).

Researchers have shown that children with hearing loss are often less accurate in identifying others' emotional states than children without hearing loss and have a poorer understanding of affective words. Understanding affective vocabulary has been positively related to personal adjustment (Greenberg & Kusche, 1993), so these findings reinforce our understanding of the contributions of communication to self-understanding. (For further information about the importance of general emotional development, readers are referred to Goleman, 1995.) Figure 7.2 shows how these issues adversely affect a child's emotional and social development.

FAMILY CONCERNS. More than 90 percent of children with hearing loss are born into families with normal-hearing parents. The vast majority of these parents have little or no experience with hearing loss, so the diagnosis of hearing loss is devas-

FIGURE 7.2

Hearing loss in children can have a "domino effect."

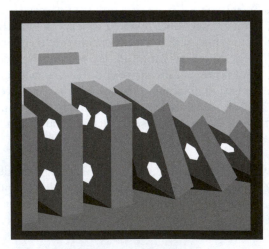

When children can't express their feelings, they are unable to understand those feelings; an inability to understand one's feelings impairs the ability to understand how others feel (empathy); understanding how others feel is a prerequisite for friendship development.

tating news, a moment frozen in time that they never forget. Even if parents have suspected hearing loss for some time before the diagnosis, they still report experiencing sadness, as well as relief, for having their suspicions confirmed. From their reports, it appears that most parents experience emotional reactions consistent with the stages or phases of the "grief cycle" (Kübler-Ross, 1969). The grief cycle includes a progressive set of emotional reactions, starting with *shock,* because the information generally was not expected, and *denial,* because the information does not reconcile with one's dreams for the future. When the reality of the situation begins to sink in, parents in grief may find themselves feeling *depressed* or helpless for a time while they attempt to cope with the implications of the diagnosis. The final stage of this cycle is *acceptance,* but more than one parent has been heard to say that they feel the term *resignation* is more accurate. Other reactions include depression, sorrow, confusion, and vulnerability, and they have been known to resurface at unexpected times in the family's development. Luterman (2001) reminds us that it is inappropriate for a professional to expect families to be "over their grief by now"; families have the right to feel the way they feel, and professionals must refrain from passing judgment. It is important to keep in mind that we do not predictably "march through" stages of grief and ultimately recover to be the same person as before. Parents report moving back and forth within these emotional reactions during different stages of their child's development, and often they find themselves almost as grieved by a new event as when they first received the diagnosis of hearing loss.

> Grief cycle: A pattern of reaction and adjustment to loss.

Case 7.1. Ms. Carlow

Ms. Carlow had been surprised but not worried when she had been told that her new daughter did not pass a hearing screening—after all, no one in the family had any hearing problems. So, when the audiologist told her that the more advanced tests indicated hearing loss in both ears, she was stunned. She held her baby close while the audiologist talked, but she couldn't pay attention. Her mind immediately jumped to her husband: He will say the test results must be wrong, that they must get a second opinion. That is always a good idea anyway, right? She picked up isolated words as the audiologist talked, something about more appointments and—what else? Impressions—of what? And why was she talking about fruit? A year later, Ms. Carlow realized, at a moment when all she wanted to do was hold her baby and think, the audiologist had been explaining the "speech banana."

Over time, parents work their way past their own anticipated self-concept of being parents of a "perfect" child to the new reality of being parents of a child who has a hearing loss, and this process can be harder for some parents than for others. Kricos (2000) writes about professionals' perceptions of parents who are struggling with acceptance:

> Parents in the denial stage may appear to clinicians to be blocking efforts to initiate the intervention program. However, it should be remembered that this initial reaction to the diagnosis may provide a time for parents to search for inner strength and accumulate information. The goal for clinicians during this stage of grieving is to find

ways of not merely tolerating parental denial but accepting it, while still offering, to the best of their abilities, the services the child needs. Unfortunately, parents who appear to be denying their child's hearing impairment are often perceived by clinicians as foolish and stubborn, when they should be perceived as loving parents who, for the time being, cannot accept the professional's diagnosis of such a severe disability in their child. (pp. 279–280)

Even as parents work through their emotional reactions, difficulties may persist, again because of communication. Several studies have described a tendency in mother–child interactions to be more rigid and more negative when the child has a hearing loss. Verbal exchanges are briefer and more directive and include less praise compared to mothers whose children have normal hearing (Pipp-Siegel & Biringen, 2000). Without intervention, these communication styles can have an impact on the quality of parent–child attachment.

Professionals may inadvertently contribute to parental confusion or stress by emphasizing issues that are not at the forefront of parents' concerns. For instance, upon first fitting hearing aids on a child, professionals are likely to intone these instructions: "Mrs. Tomas, you will want to make sure that Isabella wears these hearing aids every waking hour. That way, she will have the best conditions to develop speech and language." Although an accurate statement, this clinical approach may miss the mark for many parents; it might be more helpful to "speak their lan-

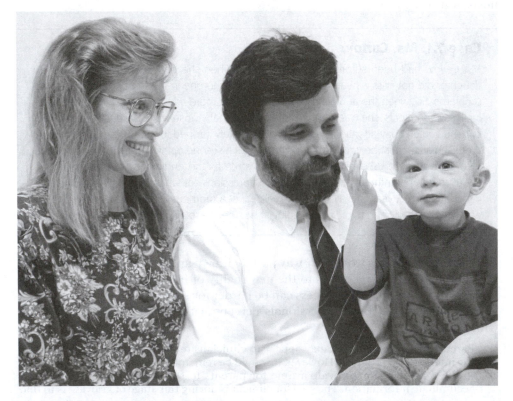

Family counseling can assist in establishing successful parent–child attachment.

guage" by "saying the same thing differently." For example,

> Mrs. Tomas, the more Isabella wears her hearing aids, the more she will learn from your voice how much you love her and cherish her; the more she will learn when you are teasing and when you are serious about obeying you; the more she will be part of family jokes and family lessons and family history . . .

At the time that all this is happening, Isabella will also have optimal conditions to develop speech and language, but it has been presented in a context that families can understand and use. In addition, the undue pressure of "pleasing the professional" has been removed; instead, the parent has been acknowledged as a competent adult who has a lot to manage and who will do her best for her child as her energy level allows.

SOCIAL COMPETENCE. As children grow up, their social world expands to include same-age peers. Here, too, difficulties have been observed among children with hearing loss: Because of their delay in developing communication skills, children with hearing loss have fewer opportunities for peer interactions, making it difficult to learn "the social rules governing communication" (Antia & Kreimeyer, 1992, p. 135). Poor and limited communication results in poor social competence, which includes these skills (Greenberg & Kusche, 1993):

Social competence: Skills for successful and satisfying personal relationships.

- Capacity to think independently
- Capacity for self-direction and self-control
- Understanding the feelings, motivations, and needs of self and others
- Flexibility
- Ability to tolerate frustration
- Ability to rely on and be relied on by others
- Maintaining healthy relationships with others

It would appear that children with hearing loss are at risk in developing these social competencies. For instance, a group of parents of 40 children with hearing impairment completed a questionnaire that indicated overall that their children had more than typical problems interacting with others and establishing friendships (Davis, Elfenbein, Schum, & Bentler, 1986). The children themselves were interviewed, and 50 percent ($N = 20$) expressed their own concerns about peers and social relationships. Most children stated that they would not mention wearing hearing aids because of "a fear of being teased and embarrassed, and many others reported spending most of their time alone" (p. 60). The researchers wondered if these social problems were typical among most preadolescents, so they conducted the same interview among fifty-eight children without hearing loss. After factoring out the responses from two children who had just moved to a new school, only 12 percent ($N = 7$) of these children reported having difficulty with making friends or getting teased.

SPECIAL ISSUES IN ADOLESCENCE. Most of the information reviewed so far has focused on elementary school children. The teen years present new challenges and heighten the intensity of existing ones. Adolescence is a stage of life with important developmental tasks, including peer group affiliation, identity formation, occupational preparation, and adjustment to physiologic changes (Altman, 1996). During these turbulent times, self-consciousness increases, as well as uncertainty and

Peer groups provide safe environments for adolescents to practice important life skills, including communication, cooperation, and compromise.

mood swings. All teens, with or without hearing loss, may feel besieged with emotions that they find hard to articulate, and the presence of hearing loss can exacerbate teens' struggles for self-awareness and self-expression.

Peer relationships take paramount importance for teens, yet these relationships may be strained when hearing loss is involved. Mothers have reported that their teenage children seemed less emotionally bonded to their friends when hearing loss was a variable and also rated these friendships as higher in aggression (Henggeler, Watson, & Thelan, 1990). Being with other teens with hearing loss may be more important than expected, when we consider how peer relationships help teens to define themselves. Most of the 220 mainstreamed students in one study indicated that they preferred to spend most of their time with other students with hearing impairment, finding these relationships deeper and more satisfying (Stinson, Whitmore, & Kluwin, 1996).

The desire to conform to group expectations seems to peak in ninth grade (Kimmel & Weiner, 1995). For teens with hearing loss, this desire will probably include the desire to reject amplification for the sake of conformity. This desire may also represent a struggle to accept oneself as a person with a disability. The hearing aid effect is probably still in play, although there is some evidence that the magnitude of negative effect has lessened in the last ten years (Stein et al., 2000). Overall, however, it is agreed that "during adolescence, being different is generally not valued" (Coyner, 1993, p. 19).

During these years, students need to develop appropriate social or interpersonal skills to advocate for their needs as they transition to college or work settings. This developmental task frequently is not supported, resulting in high school graduates who move on to higher education or work placements without learning how to describe and request the services that they need to succeed (English, 1997; Flexer, Wray, & Leavitt, 1990). Professionals who serve adolescents face the challenge of helping with the here and now issues of self-identity, as well as concerns of the imminent future, and the former may seem so paramount that the latter is overlooked.

SUMMARY. This section described a range of possible psychosocial and emotional difficulties that might occur as a result of growing up with a hearing loss. Self-concept can be affected because of communication limitations, as well as parental attachment, emotional development, and social competency. Interventions are available to help to reduce these effects, and they should be used when concerns arise (English, 2002). The following section will consider how similar psychosocial issues can affect persons who acquire hearing loss in their adult years.

Acquiring Hearing Loss

Although relatively few children are born with hearing loss, most individuals, if they live long enough, acquire some degree of hearing loss as part of the aging process. Occasionally, adults also acquire hearing loss as a side effect of some medications or as a result of head injury or noise exposure. Adults are not immune to the psychological, emotional, and the previous social effects described with respect to children. Parallel categories will be considered here as they apply to adults: self-concept, psychoemotional reactions, and family and social concerns.

SELF-CONCEPT. It has long been noted that adults can be reluctant to admit to having a hearing loss and to take steps toward remediation. When people seek help from an audiologist, they have usually waited an average of seven years from the time that they first noticed hearing problems. During these years, they may attempt to dismiss the problem as the fault of others (e.g., accusing people of mumbling) or using other avoidance techniques. Another indicator that adults have a difficult time adjusting to their self-concept of a person with hearing loss is the fact that only about 20 percent of the population who would benefit from the use of hearing aids actually obtain and use them. When asked, people in the remaining 80 percent indicate cosmetic concerns as second only to the cost of hearing aids (Kochkin, 1996).

To underscore the effect of hearing aids on self-concept, consider the following study: A group of older women with hearing loss was divided in half, but only the women in one group were fit with hearing aids (Doggett, Stein, & Gans, 1998). All subjects then interacted with unfamiliar same-age peers who later rated them on attractiveness, friendliness, confidence, and intelligence. The subjects who wore the hearing aids were rated as less confident, less friendly, and less intelligent than the subjects not wearing hearing aids. The remarkable point about this study is that the raters did not even notice the hearing aids and so were not responding to their appearance! The authors surmised that the subjects wearing hearing aids displayed less confidence, friendliness, and intelligence because they projected a negative self-image. Again, as with children, ignoring the hearing aid effect with adults is akin to ignoring the proverbial elephant standing in the middle of the living room. It would be naïve to assume that, because they are self-confident adults in most other aspects of their lives, they are invulnerable to this undeniable cosmetic concern.

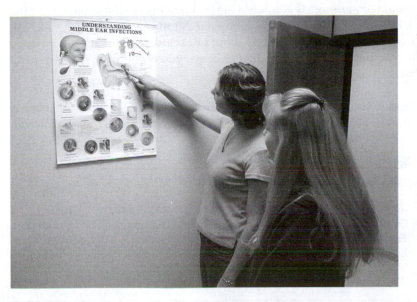

Helping the person to understand the underlying basis for a hearing disability facilitates adjustment to it.

PSYCHOEMOTIONAL REACTIONS. In addition to avoidance and worry about cosmetics, adults have reported a full range of other emotions and psychological reactions to hearing loss, including anger ("Why is this happening?"), anxiety and insecurity ("What will this mean about my future?"), stress (especially before the effects of the hearing loss are well understood, for instance, in understanding speech in restaurants), resentment, depression, and grief. See Table 7.1 for a list of typical emotional reactions to hearing loss. The grief cycle was mentioned earlier with respect to parents and the diagnosis of hearing loss in children, but adults also experience a type of grief when their suspicions about deteriorating hearing have been confirmed. Its expression can be very subtle, as depicted in the following scenario.

Case 7.2

A 92-year-old man sought a hearing evaluation to address recent listening difficulties. Test results confirmed that he had a mild-to-moderate hearing loss, and hearing aids were recommended to help him to meet his listening goals. Upon hearing this, he lowered his head, sighed deeply, and said, "I've always thought of hearing aids as only for old people." His audiologist waited with him quietly, and in less than one minute he raised his head, shook himself slightly, and asked, "Well, what do we do first?" That moment was a very brief but real expression of grief: "I am vulnerable, mortal, getting farther and farther away from my youth."

When we are excluded from a conversation, it is human nature (because we are naturally egocentric) to suspect that the conversation is about us. Adults with hearing loss struggle regularly with *conversational exclusion,* which can lead to behaviors that would suggest paranoia. However, it is vital that we do not confuse these reactions with the paranoia associated with schizophrenia and other mental health problems; this kind of paranoia is actually a natural reaction to the situation. At the same time, such reactions should not be dismissed as unimportant: If persons with hearing loss feel actively ignored or talked about or excluded, they may not have associated these reactions with the existence of hearing loss and may experience an undefined sense of disquiet or confusion.

FAMILY CONCERNS. Family members take the brunt of the stress while a member is coming to accept the fact that his or her hearing is changing. They are blamed for not

---

TABLE 7.1
Common Psychoemotional Reactions to Hearing Loss

Alienated	Angry	Annoyed	Anxious	Bewildered	Bitter
Cheated	Confused	In denial	Depressed	Disturbed	Drained
Enraged	Fearful	Frustrated	Guilty	Hopeless	Impatient
Insecure	Lonely	Lost	Nervous	Overwhelmed	Panicked
Sad	Skeptical	Suspicious	Tense	Upset	Vulnerable
Weary	Withdrawn	Worried			

speaking clearly or for purposefully leaving the person with hearing loss out of the conversation. Because communication is difficult, families do tend to talk around the patient or, if asked to repeat something, to minimize the effort by responding, "Never mind, it wasn't really important." Significant others (particularly spouses) often assume the responsibility of "hearing" for the family member, by explaining what was missed, covering up for miscommunications, taking responsibility for all telephone contacts, or worrying about possible social embarrassment when a response is unrelated to the comment made. In half-jest, adults with hearing loss have been known to introduce their spouses this way: "Have you met my hearing aid?"

The person with hearing loss usually does not realize the burden that this spouse carries. When the patient and spouse take identical surveys to describe the effects of the hearing loss on their lives, the spouse usually reports greater problems before a hearing aid fitting and greater benefit after the hearing aid fitting than the patient does. These reports tell us a great deal about the stress of the hearing loss on the nonimpaired spouse or significant other.

Other family members may experience frustration and disappointment when communication by phone or in person is ineffective, and the person with the hearing loss may internalize these problems as a rejection of themselves rather than of the communication problems. A downward spiral can occur: "It's too hard to talk to Dad so I'll keep the details to a minimum." Dad resents the limitation and contributes even less to the communication efforts.

SOCIAL CONCERNS. When communication becomes gradually more difficult, our social world can constrict accordingly. The adult with hearing loss may opt out of favorite activities because the listening challenges are too stressful. When efforts are made to interact as if no hearing loss exists, misunderstandings typically occur (believing a comment was a joke when it was meant to be serious or completely misunderstanding a comment); this may result in embarrassment, possible blame directed to the communication partner, and eventually the use of avoidance techniques. Regular attendance at religious, family, and leisure activities becomes curtailed, often with excuses about losing interest, rather than recognizing the root of the problem. This social withdrawal has been shown to lead to depression. It is not uncommon to find adults not making the connection between the change in their lifestyles and their gradual hearing loss.

Avoidance techniques: Strategies used to postpone acknowledgment of a difficult situation.

SUMMARY. Acquiring hearing loss in adulthood is usually a gradual, insidious process and is usually recognized by family and friends before being recognized by the person whose hearing is becoming impaired. Before, during, and after confirmation of hearing loss, adults may experience many of the same psychosocial difficulties that children do.

About Being Deaf

So far we have considered the psychosocial and emotional effects of hearing loss in general. Several studies have noted that the more severe the hearing loss, the more severe the psychosocial and emotional problems can be (Warren & Hasenstab,

1986). These kinds of severe difficulties have been described by Meadow (1976, 1980), who reported how deaf children and adults have been characterized as compulsive, egocentric, and rigid. Deficits in empathy have been described (Bachara, Raphael, & Phelan, 1980), as well as higher than expected levels of anxiety (Harris, Van Zandt, & Rees, 1997) and a condition called "primitive personality" among deaf individuals (Vernon, 1996):

> This disorder involves a combination of extreme educational deprivation (usually functional illiteracy), miniscule social input and knowledge, including awareness of appropriate social behavior, immaturity, and a generally psychologically barren life. While not psychotic, individuals with primitive personalities are not able to cope with life in our complex modern society. When the communication handicap of deafness is not dealt with, educationally and psychologically, primitive personality is a frequent result. (p. 237)

Although few deaf people experience a genuinely "extreme deprivation," most do contend with limited language input that can result in a reduced repertoire of coping skills. Frustrations and worries that cannot be verbally expressed can escalate into impulse disorder behaviors or depression. It must be understood that psychological difficulties are not caused by the hearing loss per se, but rather by the communication problems that result from hearing loss. If these kinds of concerns present themselves, a referral to a qualified psychologist or other counselor is in order.

Impulse disorder:
Having difficulty controlling one's initial reactions or impulses; acting without considering consequences.

BEING DEAFENED. The previous paragraphs focused on issues of individuals who were born deaf. Persons who become deafened in their adult years (late-onset deafness) have a uniquely stressful situation, because they have no preestablished ties to the Deaf community, yet also face challenges in maintaining their ties to the hearing world. Communication may be limited to writing notes or speechreading, neither procedure being very conducive to spontaneous or lengthy conversation. A sense of isolation is likely to occur, as well as anger, frustration, denial, or depression (Zarrella, 1995).

Depression may result not only from the difficulties in communication, however. Speech communication occurs at a "symbolic" level of hearing, as defined by Ramsdell (1960). But there are other levels of hearing as well, including the *warning* or environmental level and the *primitive* level, which means hearing sounds so basic to our lives that we are not even aware of their occurrence. Virtually every action we make, every activity in our environment, produces a sound to which we react, often unconsciously. Persons who suddenly lose their hearing frequently report that the world has become "dead" to them. For example, to see a door shut forcefully and not hear the anticipated slam tend to make deafened people feel they are no longer interacting with the world around them. Even more distressing may be the absence of sound produced by the self, such as our own footsteps or voices. Ramsdell stressed that the depression of a deafened person occurs because he "is not aware of the loss he has suffered at the primitive level. . . . He is unaware that there is such a thing as this primitive level in the first place" (p. 464).

Fortunately, hearing aids and cochlear implants often provide much psychological relief to many deafened adults. Recovering some degree of sound perception, even if only at the primitive level, can result in reduced anxiety and depression.

"Deafness with a Capital D"

About 1 million people in the United States not only have a profound hearing loss and derive no benefit from hearing aids (i.e., being audiologically deaf), but they also identify themselves as members of the Deaf community (being culturally deaf). This cultural affiliation is described by Vernon and Andrews (1990):

> Membership in the deaf community involves identification with deaf people, shared experiences in school and work, and active participation in group activities with other deaf people. . . . Most notably, deaf community members share frustrating experiences trying to communicate in the hearing world. . . . [S]ome hearing individuals, such as educators, counselors, and spouses, can be "courtesy" members. However, only deaf persons can really know what deafness means. Neither social class nor sex nor religion are important attributes for membership; the most distinguishing criteria are communication skill and preference. (pp. 7–8)

Communication within the Deaf community is based on the use of American Sign Language (ASL), a manual language with its own syntax and rules of use (with roots in French and English) (see Chapter 5). Deaf theater and Deaf poetry thrive across the country, notably at Gallaudet University in Washington, DC, the only liberal arts university for the Deaf in the world. In addition to having its own language, like other cultures the Deaf community has its own traditions, mores, and values. The passing on of these values and traditions and even ASL is not accomplished through the more common vertical enculturation process from parent to child, because only about 10 percent of deaf children are born to deaf parents (a phrase usually shortened as "deaf of deaf"). Instead, the transference of culture has occurred horizontally, among peers in residential schools or in postsecondary settings like colleges or communities.

Deaf persons tend to marry other Deaf persons and usually (but not always) would prefer to have children who also have profound hearing loss, like themselves (see the following Case Study). Connections to the Deaf community are usually lifelong, and elderly deaf individuals typically maintain friendships established in their childhood (Becker, 1980).

Deaf community: A group of individuals who share cultural similarities in language (ASL), mores, traditions, and values.

Enculturation process: Shaping or raising children according to values defined by a culture.

Case 7.3. Tony

The topic for the day in Audiology 101 was the early identification of hearing loss. A young man named Tony sat in the front of the class to follow the sign language interpreter. He raised his hand and explained with both speech and sign language, "This topic is particularly important to me because my wife and I just had a baby last Saturday." The class applauded, and he continued, "Yes, because both she and I are deaf, they tested our baby's hearing. Unfortunately, he didn't pass the test." The class responded with silent nods of the head to show they were sorry. But he wasn't done—with a twinkle in his eye, he added, "Yes, he can hear." The collective jaw of the entire class dropped, and a few students laughed uncomfortably. Even though it was said teasingly, he wanted the class to understand that their preference would have been for a child who was deaf as they were, and the fact that the baby had normal hearing was a type of "failed test" to them.

The psychological, emotional, and social development of Deaf individuals will be influenced by all the same variables as those who are not culturally Deaf. Are they raised in families that accept them for who they are? Is communication easy to establish and sustain? Is the ability to express oneself and be understood and accepted part of one's experience? The topic of "being Deaf" is far too complex to cover in depth here; for more information about the psychology of deafness, the reader is referred to the Recommended Reading at the end of this chapter. Readings on the phenomenon of Deaf culture are also provided.

"KNOWING IS NOT ENOUGH": ■ COUNSELING BASICS

Having an understanding of the psychological, social, and emotional effects of living with hearing loss ("knowing" about its effects) satisfies one level of professional development. However, persons with hearing loss expect more from the professionals who serve them: They expect active support as they adjust to their situation and have consistently expressed disappointment that, in general, they do not receive it (Glass & Elliot, 1992). Clearly, then, "knowing" about these concerns is not enough. The next step in professional development is to advance from "knowing" to "know-how," as in knowing how to provide the personal adjustment support that our patients and their families need and expect. Extensive materials are available on developing this know-how, but this section will provide only highlights on counseling basics. Readers are strongly encouraged to seek formal coursework in counseling as it relates to their disciplines, both in their training program and in informal training throughout their professional careers.

Important Distinctions

Audiologic counseling: Helping patients "own their hearing loss" and advance to problem solving.

Before proceeding, we must be clear about the following terms. When we refer to counseling, we are not referring to psychotherapy or psychoanalysis, whereby mental health professionals (i.e., psychiatrists and psychologists) use their professional training to help clients to find ways to solve pervasive life problems. *Psychotherapy* helps patients to explore unconscious behavior patterns in order to alter ways of relating and functioning by examining and challenging personal history and by analyzing the meanings of one's responses (Cormier & Hackney, 1999; Crowe, 1997). Psychotherapy generally views the patient as being ill and searches for the cause of a person's problems, which might be rooted in family relationships or childhood trauma.

Counseling, in comparison, is designed to help people to develop "here-and-now strategies for coping with life, decision making, and current problems" (Shames, 2000, p. 6). Social workers, school counselors, ministers, and other spiritual leaders are professional counselors. Whereas psychotherapy attempts to effect major personality changes, counseling focuses on supporting personal adjustments to situations by helping a person to understand his or her feelings and engage in problem solving (see Figure 7.3).

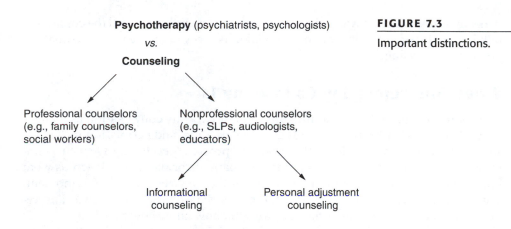

FIGURE 7.3

Important distinctions.

Nonprofessional counseling may not be as familiar a concept, but it occurs routinely: A financial planner will counsel on tax problems, a teacher will counsel on test-taking strategies, an audiologist will counsel on hearing conservation, and so on (Kennedy & Charles, 2001). These examples involve content or *informational counseling,* which is one facet of nonprofessional counseling; but all professionals on occasion will work with clients or students facing emotional crises as well (e.g., the stress associated with financial risk or the despair and discouragement from failing an important exam). When the emotional crisis is related to the professional's specialty, *nonprofessional personal adjustment support* becomes a second facet of nonprofessional counseling.

Professional boundaries must be respected, of course. Nonprofessional counselors must define relationships by boundaries that clarify the roles and functions of individuals in the relationship (Stone & Olswang, 1989). When a professional begins to feel uncomfortable with either the content or the intensity of the interaction, he or she can assume that a boundary is being approached, and it is probably an appropriate time to refer the patient or parent to a professional counselor.

Professional boundaries: Notable distinctions between professions as they approach common areas of concern.

What We May Think Counseling Is

Counseling is often narrowly perceived as *explaining:* A professional talks while a patient or parent listens to information about the audiogram, the anatomy of the ear, the benefits and limitations of hearing aids and cochlear implants, and the range of communication options. Undoubtedly, explaining is an essential aspect of service delivery, because patients, parents, and family members want and need information. Providing this information is called *content counseling* or *informational counseling* and is vital to audiologic rehabilitation.

The primary characteristic of content counseling is its tendency to become a one-way direction of communication (i.e., the professional talks and the patient or parent listens). If a patient or parent wants to talk about any of the psychosocial or emotional concerns discussed previously, how is he or she to interact with this one-way stream of information? It isn't possible; so when personal adjustment issues present themselves, another direction in communication needs to be made available, a two-way conversation in which the parent or client can talk more and the counselors talk less. This two-way direction of interaction is a key component of personal adjustment counseling.

What Counselors Say Counseling Is

The counseling profession describes this kind of two-way conversation as a facilitative process, whereby the patient is given room, time, and permission to "tell his story." Stone, Patton, and Heen (1999) call this process "developing a learning conversation." In our context, we encourage the patients or parents to teach us what life with hearing loss is like for them and what their concerns are at that moment. This approach respects patients and parents as the experts of their lives and requires us to drop our assumptions that we somehow know how they feel.

The Counseling Process

The facilitative or counseling process (Figure 7.4) involves the following steps (adapted from Egan, 2002):

1. Help patients tell their story
2. Help patients clarify their problems
3. Help patients take responsibility for their listening problems (challenge themselves)
4. Help patients establish their goals
5. Develop an action plan
6. Implement the plan
7. Conduct ongoing evaluation

Readers will notice that the CARE model described in Chapter 1 includes these steps under **C** for Counseling. Without care and reflection, audiological rehabilitation may rush through steps 1 and 2, bypass step 3, and pick up again at step 4; in other words, the professional may assume he or she already knows the patient's story and begin setting goals immediately (taking over the rehabilitation or adjustment process, rather than developing a partnership with the patient).

Long-term success in adjusting to hearing loss may ultimately depend on the effective management of the first three steps, because they usually involve an understanding of the psychosocial and emotional impact of living with a hearing loss.

FIGURE 7.4

Counseling process as it might be applied to some audiologic rehabilitation situations.

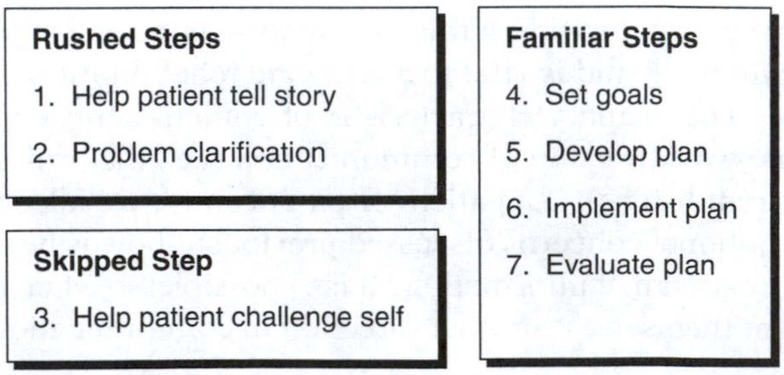

Rushed Steps

1. Help patient tell story
2. Problem clarification

Skipped Step

3. Help patient challenge self

Familiar Steps

4. Set goals
5. Develop plan
6. Implement plan
7. Evaluate plan

This chapter will conclude with a discussion of how to incorporate these steps in audiological rehabilitation.

HELP PATIENTS (OR PARENTS) TELL THEIR STORY. Every patient and every parent has a unique perspective on living with a hearing loss. There is an inherent danger for professionals to assume that "we've heard it all before," and therefore we truly understand their struggles and frustrations and fears. This tendency is called *habituation.* While we surely have a general impression of these problems, we can never know what it is really like, exactly, for Ms. Juarez or Mr. Percy or 10-year-old Isaac. It is essential first that professionals conscientiously ask each patient, "What is it like for you?" And then listen carefully to each individualized response.

If a patient says, "No one understands how hard this is for me," it is not helpful to say that we do understand, because in fact we do not know how it is for this patient. A response such as "Most people with hearing loss experience these difficulties" does not help the patient feel personally understood, but only clumped into an impersonal category of "others." A response that focuses only on the patient, such as "You are having a tough time right now," gives the patient the message that she was heard and understood.

Using a self-assessment instrument can be very helpful in providing the opportunity for a patient to tell his or her story. While a patient takes the time to consider and describe his or her communication problems (part of step 2), that person is also provided the opportunity to expand on the items that are of particular concern. Describing one's communication difficulties is an act of personal self-disclosure that may make a patient feel uncomfortable; however, the exercise of reading and talking about a standardized, neutral set of questions can take the pressure off, because both patient and professional are looking at the instrument, rather than at each other.

> **Self-assessments:** Paper and pencil questionnaires or surveys to help persons to describe their listening problems to themselves and others.

HELP PATIENTS CLARIFY THEIR PROBLEMS. Because the development of hearing loss in adults can occur slowly over several years, or because parents of children with hearing loss have a complicated life to juggle, or because children with hearing loss have limited experience in expressing their feelings and concerns, considerable time is needed to help individuals to describe and clarify their actual communication problems, as well as their emotional reactions to them and the psychosocial ramifications. Earlier, self-assessment instruments were mentioned as a strategy to help patients to tell their stories—and, as they tell their stories, not only are they being heard but they are getting clear in their minds what these problems are. Many instruments are available, and the reader is referred to Geier (1997) for a compilation of more than thirty of them. For example, the *Abbreviated Profile of Hearing Aid Benefit (APHAB)* (Cox & Alexander, 1995) poses twenty-four statements in the areas of ease of communication and communicating in adverse conditions (background noise, reverberation, etc.). An example of such a statement is "I have trouble hearing a conversation when I am with family at home." The patient describes his or her perception from "Always" to "Never" and receives the opportunity to recognize that such difficulties are a common aspect of living with a hearing loss. Many instruments open the door to a discussion about psychosocial reactions to hearing loss; for instance, the *Self-Assessment of Communication (SAC)* (Schow & Nerbonne,

1982) asks this question: "Does any problem or difficulty with your hearing upset you?" Responses range from "Almost always" to "Almost never," and it is up to the patient to decide whether he or she is comfortable with this kind of self-disclosure.

Self-assessments are not the only way to help patients to clarify their problems; conversation and carefully selected questions can also provide this opportunity. The point here is that patients need to understand their problems before they can develop solutions for them.

HELP PATIENTS TAKE RESPONSIBILITY FOR THEIR LISTENING PROBLEMS. Once patients clarify their communication and/or interpersonal problems, it might be assumed that they are ready to solve them. However, we have already learned that the psychosocial and emotional aspects of hearing loss can interfere with logical problem solving (using hearing aids to their best advantage, etc.). There is a real risk at this stage for the professional to take over and tell the patient or parent what to do: Obtain and use hearing aids, learn sign language, or enroll in speechreading classes, for example. But like any other personal problem, the patient has to accept responsibility for the problem in order to commit herself to the solution. Far too often, patients agree to purchase hearing aids, but with no personal commitment or sincere intention to use them. It is probable that there are more hearing aids in drawers than on ears.

Another behavior that indicates that patients are not yet assuming the responsibilities of living with hearing loss is the common complaint that communication breakdowns occur because other people speak too softly, or they mumble, or children speak too quickly and with high voices. As long as the patient insists that everyone else should just speak more clearly, he or she is shirking his or her own role in

Good communication between marriage partners is vital in understanding the impact of hearing loss.

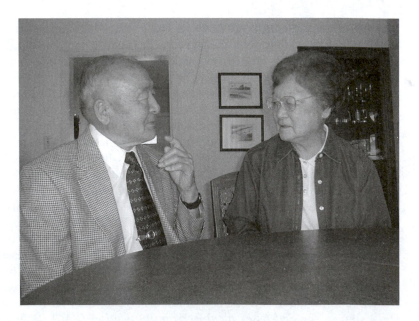

successful communication. To help patients move past this stage of inaction, audiological rehabilitation must take its cue from other helping professions and place responsibility for successful rehabilitation squarely on the patient. Once the problems have been clarified, we must ask, "And now, what are *your* listening goals? As you identify them, I will support you in attaining these goals."

This may be the point where the adult patient says, "I want to hear my grandchildren when they visit—but I won't wear hearing aids." He has identified two goals and (for the purpose of our discussion), unfortunately, they are incompatible. The ultimate decision is still his: He won't be able to hear his grandchildren without amplification, so what does he want to do about that? No amount of persuading will make a genuine difference; the patient has to find the internal resources to commit to his decision.

Not all adults struggle with the cosmetics of hearing aids, but, if they do, they can be encouraged to conduct a type of cost–benefit analysis: that is, compare the social costs of hearing aid use to the listening benefits that they seek. Which provides the outcome more valuable to them? If the listening benefits are perceived as greater, they might be more willing to tolerate the social costs of hearing aid appearances. Figure 7.5 gives an example of this activity.

Another way to describe this thought process is called "substituting *and* for *but*"; that is, trade the word *but* for the word *and*. Initially, an adult may believe, "I want to hear my grandchildren better *but* I dislike how these hearing aids look." This way of thinking pits one condition against the other, and they mutually exclude each other. The adult could be asked to try thinking in these terms: "I want to hear my grandchildren better *and* I dislike how these hearing aids look." Including the possibility of both conditions coexisting at the same time gives the adult another way to look at the situation, one that could move her past a mental block to one that could help her to meet her goals (Kelly, 1992).

The CORE model of assessment considers patient attitudes, including readiness for change. Professionals must appreciate that some patients struggle with

Patients must assume responsibility for their hearing problem before they will genuinely engage in the effort to improve their situation.

Some amplification goals can be accomplished with assistive devices when hearing aids are not accepted.

Using Hearing Aids		Not Using Hearing Aids	
+	–	+	–

FIGURE 7.5

Articulating the "pluses and minuses" of a decision.

change and would rather avoid it if possible. An empathetic, nonjudgmental attitude on our part can help patients face their fears and consider "taking the plunge."

When to Refer

It is not uncommon for patients and parents to present with difficulties that cannot be accounted for by the hearing loss alone. Marital problems, family dissension, parenting dilemmas, financial or legal stress, fragile emotional and mental health, all these situations can be exacerbated by the presence of hearing loss; but treating the hearing loss will not resolve the fundamental problems. There is no easy answer to the question "When should I refer to a professional counselor?"; however, the answer is apparent when the professional sees a situation outside his or her expertise and scope of practice. It is strongly recommended that a referral system be established in advance so that, when the need to refer arises, a phone contact is immediately provided to the patient. This preparation will suggest to the patient that an outside referral is not rare and that the professional is aware of and is adhering to his or her professional boundaries.

SUMMARY

The second half of this chapter takes the reader beyond an awareness of patients' psychosocial difficulties with hearing loss to an awareness of how the professional's interactions with patients can support (or hinder) their adjustment process. The basic concepts were these: Listen carefully as the patient tells her story, help her to identify her listening problems, and help her to assume ownership for her problems so that she can commit to the solutions. If a professional finds herself wondering, "If this patient didn't want these hearing aids, why did she come for an evaluation in the first place?" the professional did not spend time in the beginning to hear the patient's story (i.e., her perception of her problems) and whether she was ready to take on the challenge of adjusting to hearing aid use. Following the counseling process through each step will lead to a deeper and more accurate understanding between patient and professional and facilitate the development of a therapeutic relationship with mutual goals.

SUMMARY POINTS

- Many persons with hearing loss experience a range of psychological, social, or emotional difficulties, although it is impossible to know exactly how a hearing loss affects a particular individual unless he or she specifically tells us.
- Because of resultant language delays, children with hearing loss may experience difficulties with self-expression and self-awareness, which can affect their ability to empathize with others and to achieve age-appropriate social skills.
- Adults who acquire hearing loss may also experience problems as they adjust to the consequences of the disability, including the acceptance of hearing aids.

- The Deaf culture does not see hearing loss as a disability, but rather a difference in abilities. Like other communities, its members share core values and traditions and also share the use of a common language (ASL).
- Counseling techniques are often used to help patients to accept and develop solutions for their listening problems.
- Self-assessments give patients an opportunity to tell their story and clarify their problems.
- Patients are more likely to accept recommendations if they feel they have been listened to and respected.

RECOMMENDED READING

AUDIOLOGIC COUNSELING

Clark, J., & English, K. (2004). *Audiologic counseling: Helping patients and families adjust to hearing loss.* Boston: Allyn and Bacon.

English, K. (2002). *Counseling children with hearing impairment and their families.* Boston: Allyn and Bacon.

Flasher, L., & Fogel, P. (2004). *Counseling skills for speech-language pathologists and audiologists.* New York: Thomson/Delmar Learning.

Luterman, D. M. (2001). *Counseling persons with communication disorders and their children* (4th ed.). Austin, TX: Pro-Ed.

Shames, G. H. (2000). *Counseling the communicatively disabled and their families: A manual for clinicians.* Boston: Allyn and Bacon.

PSYCHOLOGY OF DEAFNESS

Harvey, M. (2003). *Psychotherapy with deaf and hard of hearing persons: A systemic model* (2nd ed.). Mahwah, NJ: Lawrence Erlbaum.

Marschark, M. (1993). *Psychological development of deaf children.* New York: Oxford University Press.

Shirmer, B. (2001). *Psychological, social, and educational dimensions of deafness.* Boston: Allyn and Bacon.

DEAF CULTURE

Greenberg, J. (1970). *In this sign.* New York: Holt, Rinehart and Winston.

Holcomb, R. (1996). *Deaf culture our way.* San Diego, CA: Dawn Sign Press.

Padden, C., & Humphries, T. (2005). *Inside deaf culture.* Cambridge, MA: Harvard University Press.

Preston, P. (1995). *Mother father deaf: Living between sound and silence.* Cambridge, MA: Harvard University Press.

RECOMMENDED WEBSITES

Association of Late Deafened Adults:
www.alda.org

Hearing Loss Association of America (formerly SHHH):
www.shhh.org

"Beyond Hearing" listserv, Duke University:
www.saywhatclub.com/r-bh.htm

National Association of the Deaf:
www.nad.org

Gallaudet University:
www.gallaudet.edu

National Technical Institute for the Deaf:
www.ntid.edu

REFERENCES

Altman, E. (1996). Meeting the needs of adolescents with impaired hearing. In F. Martin & J. G. Clark (Eds.), *Hearing care for children* (pp. 197–210). Boston: Allyn and Bacon.

Antia, S., & Kreimeyer, K. (1992). Social competence intervention for young children with hearing impairments. In S. Odom, S. McConnell, & M. McEvoy (Eds.), *Social competence of young children with disabilities: Issues and strategies for intervention* (pp. 135–164). Baltimore: Paul H. Brookes.

Bachara, G., Raphael, J., & Phelan, W. (1980). Empathy development in deaf preadolescents. *American Annals of the Deaf, 125,* 38–41.

Becker, G. (1980). *Growing old in silence.* Berkeley: University of California Press.

Bess, F. H., Dodd-Murphy, J., & Parker, R. (1998). Children with minimal sensorineural hearing loss: Prevalence, educational performance, and functional status. *Ear and Hearing, 19*(5), 339–355.

Blood, G. W., Blood, M., & Danhauser, J. L. (1977). The hearing aid "effect." *Hearing Instruments, 20,* 12.

Cappelli, M., Daniels, T., Durleux-Smith, A., McGrath, P. J., & Neuss, D. (1995). Social development of children with hearing impairments who are integrated into general education classrooms. *Volta Review, 97,* 197–208.

Cormier, S., & Hackney, H. (1999). *Counseling strategies and interventions* (5th ed.). Boston: Allyn and Bacon.

Cox, R., & Alexander, O. (1995). The abbreviated profile of hearing aid benefit. *Ear and Hearing, 16,* 176–186.

Coyner, L. (1993). Academic success, self-concept, social acceptance, and perceived social acceptance for hearing, hard of hearing, and deaf students in a mainstream setting. *Journal of the American Deafness and Rehabilitation Association, 27*(2), 13–20.

Crowe, T. (1997). Approaches to counseling. In T. Crowe (Ed.), *Applications in counseling in speech–language pathology and audiology* (pp. 80–117). Baltimore: Williams & Wilkins.

Davis, J., Elfenbein, J., Schum, R., & Bentler, R. (1986). Effects of mild and moderate hearing impairments on language, educational, and psychosocial behavior of children. *Journal of Speech and Hearing Disorders, 51,* 53–62.

Doggett, S., Stein, R., & Gans, D. (1998). Hearing aid effect in older females. *Journal of American Academy of Audiology, 9*(5), 361–366.

Edwards, C. (1991). The transition from auditory training to holistic auditory management. *Educational Audiology Monograph, 2,* 1–17.

Egan, G. (2002). *The skilled helper* (7th ed.). Pacific Grove, CA: Brooks/Cole.

English, K. (1997). *Self-advocacy for students who are deaf and hard of hearing.* Austin, TX: Pro-Ed.

English, K. (2002). *Counseling children with hearing impairment and their families.* Boston: Allyn and Bacon.

Flexer, C., Wray, D., & Leavitt, R. (1990). *How the student with hearing loss can succeed in college: A handbook for students, families, and professionals.* Washington, DC: Alexander Graham Bell Association for the Deaf.

Garrison, W. M., & Tesch, S. (1978). Self-concept and deafness: A review of research literature. *Volta Review, 80,* 457–466.

Geier, K. (1997). *Handbook of self-assessment and verification measures of communication performance.* Columbia, SC: Academy of Dispensing Audiologists.

Glass, L., & Elliot, H. (1992). The professional told me what it was but that was not enough. *Shhh, 13*(6), 26–28.

Goleman, D. (1995). *Emotional intelligence: Why it can matter more than IQ.* New York: Bantam Books.

Greenberg, M. T., & Kusche, C. A. (1993). *Promoting social and emotional development in deaf children: The PATHS project.* Seattle: University of Washington Press.

Harris, L. K., Van Zandt, C. E., & Rees, T. H. (1997). Counseling needs of students who are deaf and hard of hearing. *School Counselor, 44,* 271–279.

Henggeler, S. W., Watson, S. M., & Thelan, J. P. (1990). Peer relations of hearing-impaired adolescents. *Journal of Pediatric Psychology, 15*(6), 721–731.

Kelly, L. J. (1992). Rational–emotive therapy and aural rehabilitation. *Journal of the Academy of Rehabilitative Audiology, 25,* 43–50.

Kennedy, E., & Charles, S. (2001). *On becoming a counselor: A basic guide for non-professional counselors* (3rd ed.). New York: Crossroads Publishing.

Kimmel, D. C., & Weiner, I. B. (1995). *Adolescence: A developmental transition.* New York: Wiley & Sons.

Kochkin, S. (1996). Customer satisfaction and subjective benefit with high performance hearing aids. *Hearing Review, 3*(12), 16–26.

Kricos, P. B. (2000). Family counseling for children with hearing loss. In J. Alpiner & P. A. McCarthy (Eds.), *Rehabilitative audiology: Children and adults* (3rd ed.; pp. 275–302). Philadelphia: Lippincot Williams & Wilkins.

Kübler-Ross, E. (1969). *On death and dying.* New York: Macmillan Publishing.

Luterman, D. L. (2001). *Counseling persons with communication disorders and their families* (4th ed.). Austin, TX: Pro-Ed.

Meadow, K. (1976). Personality and social development of deaf persons. *Journal of Rehabilitation of the Deaf, 9,* 3–16.

Meadow, K. (1980). *Deafness and child development.* Berkeley: University of California Press.

Pipp-Siegel, S., & Biringen, Z. (2000). Assessing the quality of relationships between parents and children: The Emotional Availability Scales. *Volta Review, 100*(5) (monograph), 237–249.

Ramsdell, P. (1960). The psychology of the hard of hearing and the deafened adult. In H. Davis & S. Silverman (Eds.), *Hearing and deafness* (pp. 459–473). New York: Holt, Rinehart and Winston.

Riensche, L., Peterson, K., & Linden, S. (1990). Young children's attitudes toward peer hearing aid wearers. *Hearing Journal, 43*(10), 19–20.

Schow, R., & Nerbonne, M. (1982). Communication screening profile: Use with elderly clients. *Ear and Hearing, 3,* 135–147.

Shames, G. H. (2000). *Counseling the communicatively disabled and their families: A manual for clinicians.* Boston: Allyn and Bacon.

Stein, R., Gill, K., & Gans, D. (2000). Adolescents' attitudes toward their peers with hearing impairment. *Journal of Educational Audiology, 8,* 1–6.

Stinson, M. S., Whitmore, K., & Kluwin, T. N. (1996). Self perceptions of social relationships in hearing-impaired adolescents. *Journal of Educational Psychology, 88*(1), 132–143.

Stone, D., Patton, B., & Heen, S. (1999). *Difficult conversations: How to discuss what matters most.* New York: Viking Press.

Stone, J. R., & Olswang, L. B. (1989). The hidden challenge in counseling. *Asha, 31,* 27–31.

Vernon, M. (1996). Psychosocial aspects of hearing impairment. In R. Schow & M. Nerbonne (Eds.), *Introduction to audiologic rehabilitation* (3rd ed.; pp. 229–263). Boston: Allyn and Bacon.

Vernon, M., & Andrews, J. (1990). *The psychology of deafness: Understanding deaf and hard of hearing people.* New York: Longman.

Warren, C., & Hasenstab, S. (1986). Self-concept of severely to profoundly hearing impaired children. *Volta Review, 88,* 289–296.

Zarrella, S. (1995, November 20). Providing services for adults with late-onset hearing loss. *Advance for Speech–Language Pathologists and Audiologists, 11.*

8

Audiologic Rehabilitation Services in the School Setting

Kris English

CONTENTS

INTRODUCTION

Recent data have indicated that when a hearing loss is identified early and when amplification and early intervention are in place by 6 months of age, a child is much more likely to acquire age-level language and learning milestones (Downs & Yoshinaga-Itano, 1999). This kind of aggressive management is just the start of many years of audiologic rehabilitative services as a child progresses through the educational system. Readers are encouraged to relate this chapter's content to the two rehabilitation models discussed in Chapter 1. For example, education is one of the variables included in the O in CORE, for **O**verall Participation Variables, and in both the CORE and CARE models, the E (**E**nvironment) is addressed when considering a classroom's acoustics.

This chapter will examine school-based audiologic rehabilitative (AR) services by addressing three questions:

- *Why* are AR services required in school settings?
- *What* AR services are provided in schools?
- *Who* is responsible for AR services in the school environment?

WHY AR SERVICES ARE REQUIRED IN SCHOOL SETTINGS: THE EDUCATIONAL CONSEQUENCES ■ OF HEARING IMPAIRMENT

Hearing impairment is considered to be an educationally significant disability. Unless immersed at home and at school in a signing environment, children learn language through the auditory system. If the auditory input is distorted or inconsistent, the child can experience a variety of difficulties in language development, such as reduced vocabulary development, delayed syntax development, and inappropriate use of morphological markers and figurative speech (Kuntze, 1998; Lederberg & Prezbindowski, 2000; Musselman & Kircaali-Iftar, 1996; Paul, 1998). Table 8.1 provides a set of typical language milestones and how they can be delayed by a profound hearing loss. Chapter 6 provides more detailed information as well.

Because most academic success depends on a competent use of language, these deficits in a child's language development can have a direct effect on cognitive development (learning). Children with profound hearing impairment (HI) have often been found to have depressed math scores and reading levels that plateau at the fourth- or fifth-grade reading level (Davis, Shepard, Stelmachowitz, & Gorga, 1982; Holt, 1995; Kelly, 1993; Paul, 1998). In the twenty-first century, our futures depend on the ability to acquire and use a broad information base; thus, children with hearing impairment start out with a marked disadvantage. Audiologic rehabilitative services are needed now more than ever to help children to stay competitive in school and in the marketplace.

Degree of Loss: Terminology

deaf: Having a bilateral profound hearing loss; Deaf: Having a cultural identification with the Deaf community.

This chapter conforms to terminology found in federal law when describing hearing loss. The term *hearing impairment* is nonspecific in that it only indicates that some kind of hearing loss is present, but it does not describe the degree or nature of the loss (conductive, sensorineural, mixed) or whether it is unilateral or bilateral. The term *hard of hearing* describes a child who has mild-to-severe loss in one or both ears.

TABLE 8.1

Impact of Profound Hearing Loss on Language Development

AGE	CHILD WITH NORMAL HEARING	CHILD WITH PROFOUND HEARING LOSS
18 months	Vocabulary of 25 words	No words
2–3 years	Understands directions, uses short sentences, asks questions	Few words, yells and points to express desires
3–4 years	Makes long sentences	Some single words
4–5 years	Uses "why" and "how," past and future tense; 2,000-word vocabulary	Has more single words
5–6 years	Grammar and syntax used correctly	Asks the names of things
6–7 years	Approximately 16,000 words	Asks questions
7–8 years	22,000 words	Uses mostly nouns, some verbs, pronouns, articles
9–10 years	Sentence length of approximately 12 words	Reading vocabulary at approximately 15 percent of normal
17 years	>80,000 words	Vocabulary <third grade

The term *deaf* is synonymous with severe to profound bilateral hearing loss (meaning that the child obtains very little benefit from amplification in understanding speech). (When the term *Deaf* appears with a capital D, it is meant to denote a cultural identification with the Deaf community, described more fully in Chapter 7.)

There is a strong relationship between the degree of hearing loss and the degree of educational impact: the more severe the loss, the more difficult learning can be. However, it would be a mistake to assume that a mild hearing loss would have little or no impact on learning; even a mild loss can put a child at risk for academic failure. A study of 1,218 children with minimal hearing loss showed that 37 percent had failed a grade (Bess, Dodd-Murphy, & Parker, 1998). In addition, a statistically high number had poorer communication skills than children with no hearing loss, and, as a group, they exhibited more problems in stress, social support, and self-esteem. These authors cited another study (Davis, Elfenbein, Schum, & Bentler, 1986) that found that children with minimal hearing loss "could have as much or more difficulty on verbal, educational, and psychosocial tasks as a child with a mild or moderate loss" (p. 340). We are learning that any type of hearing loss presents the risk of academic failure and psychosocial difficulties, and no loss can be discounted as insignificant.

We cannot even assume that children with hearing impairment in only one ear, with normal hearing in the other ear (unilateral hearing loss), are not experiencing academic difficulties. It was once thought that one normal ear was sufficient; however, it has been found that children with unilateral hearing loss are ten times more likely to fail a grade by age 10 compared to normal-hearing children (Bess,

Minimal hearing loss: Lacking the ability to hear most pure tones softer than 20 dB.

Klee, & Culbertson, 1986; English & Church, 1999). *The degree of hearing loss, by itself, cannot be used as a predictor of academic achievement or as a determiner of the level of support provided in a school.*

The exact prevalence rate depends on how hearing loss is defined; for instance, some states include in their census children with unilateral hearing loss or mild conductive hearing loss while others do not. Some states consider hearing loss to be present when a child does not respond to a pure tone at 15, 20, or 25 dB HL. Depending on the screening methods and definitions of hearing loss, studies have described incidence rates ranging from 3 to 15 percent (Johnson, 2000). If a conservative estimated prevalence rate of 3 to 4 percent is used, this would mean that among the 50 million schoolchildren in the United States, approximately 1 to 2 million children, have some degree of hearing impairment.

Mandated by Law

Because hearing loss is an educationally significant disability, by federal law these children are entitled to a free appropriate public education (FAPE), which means access to "special education and related services which are provided at public supervision and direction, and without charge" (34 CFR § 300.4[a]). In other words, the services needed to support the education of a child with hearing loss are paid for by public funds, rather than by parents. The term *appropriate* is intentionally left undefined, with the understanding that each child's educational program will be based on individual requirements. Some of the related services include a range of audiologic rehabilitative services, to be discussed in a subsequent section.

IDEA: Individuals with Disabilities Education Act: Guarantees educational rights to children with disabilities.

The law under discussion is called the *Individuals with Disabilities Education Act* (IDEA). It was first enacted in 1975 as the Education for All Handicapped Children Act (PL 94-142). Before PL 94-142 was passed, parents who had children with disabilities were frequently denied the right to enroll their children in the public school system. The passage of PL 94-142 was a milestone in ongoing efforts to protect the rights of all persons with disabilities. The actual law can be located in Volume 34 of the *Code of Federal Regulations* (CFR), found in all law school libraries and many general university and public libraries. The volume is divided into sections, designated with this § symbol. Readers are encouraged to refer to this original source as they develop a background in special education issues.

The mandate of a free appropriate public education was described earlier as a key component of this law. A second mandate, directly related to our discussion of audiologic rehabilitative services, can be found in 34 CFR § 300.303: "Each public agency shall insure that the hearing aids worn in school by children with hearing impairment, including deafness, are functioning properly." This requirement has often been the door-opener to audiologic rehabilitative services in school settings. If a parent asks, "How is your school meeting this requirement?" the school (the "public agency") must demonstrate that it has a program in place to monitor and check hearing aid and classroom amplification systems.

The U.S. Congress is required to reauthorize this law every few years, which allows for the opportunity to refine, update, and possibly expand on the original version. The first reauthorization occurred in 1986, when the Education of the Handicapped Amendments (PL 99-457) were passed. All educational services, including audiologic rehabilitation, were expanded to include children from birth to 5 years of age. This development formally brought audiologic rehabilitation into the area of early intervention services for infants and toddlers and their families.

The next reauthorization occurred in 1990. At this time, the law (PL 101-476) was renamed the Individuals with Disabilities Education Act (IDEA). This law used the term "disability" rather than handicap, and substituted the term "children with disabilities" for "handicapped children," codifying the use of *people-first* language. Persons with disabilities asked for this change, preferring to be considered persons first, who also happen to have a disability. Terms such "mentally retarded children" or "the hearing impaired" are now revised to say "children with mental retardation" or "individuals with hearing impairment."

> **People-first language:** An identification of an individual before the mention of a disability.

Amendments to IDEA were passed in 1997, and the changes included requirements to make educational goals as functional as possible (i.e., related to classroom performance and classroom expectations). It also required programs to provide progress reports at least as often as parents are informed of the progress of children without disabilities and to include the general education teacher in meetings to ensure integration of special education goals into the general education curriculum. The 2004 amendments align IDEA with the 2001 No Child Left Behind (NCLB) Act. By law, the IDEA will continue to be reexamined every four or five years to ensure that children with hearing loss and other disabilities receive an appropriate education. A timeline of these legislative events can be found in Table 8.2.

Key Components of Individuals with Disabilities Education Act (IDEA)

Throughout these reauthorizations, three critical components have remained constant. The first was the guarantee of a free appropriate public education (FAPE), which was discussed previously. The other two components are these:

- That FAPE is to be provided in the least restrictive environment (LRE)
- That a child's educational program will be documented with the use of the Individual Education Program (IEP)

TABLE 8.2

Time Line of Special Education Legislative Acts

YEAR	LAW
1975	PL 94-142: Education of All Handicapped Children Act
1986	PL 99-457: Education of Handicapped Act Amendments (including services to children from birth to age 5)
1990	PL 101-476: Individuals with Disabilities Education Act (IDEA)
1997	PL 105-71: IDEA 1997 Amendments (IEPs must have functional goals, etc.)
2004	PL 108-446: IDEA Improvements Act (aligns IDEA with NCLB)

Least Restrictive Environment (LRE)

LRE: Least restrictive environment: Where the child has most access to academic, social, and emotional support.

The concept of LRE is often considered to be synonymous with mainstreaming, or educating children with disabilities in a local public school among children without disabilities. However, it is important to note that IDEA does not mandate mainstreaming per se, but simply the consideration of the least restrictive environment for the most appropriate education. Therefore, LRE is essentially open to interpretation and consequently remains imprecise.

EDUCATIONAL OPTIONS. To help schools make educational placement decisions, the Code of Federal Regulations states the following: "Each public agency shall insure that a continuum of alternative placements is available to meet the needs of children with disabilities for special education and related services" (34 CFR § 300.551[a]). Placement options include variations of the following settings:

- Full-time regular education classroom in the child's neighborhood school.
- Regular education with in-class support, such as instruction from a speech–language pathologist or teacher of children who are deaf or hard of hearing.
- Regular education, with pull-out sessions held in another classroom.
- Part-time regular education classroom; part-time special education in a resource room.
- Full-time special education in a separate or self-contained classroom held by a teacher of children with hearing loss, with a small number of other children with hearing loss, often in the child's general neighborhood.
- Full-time special education in a separate facility (often called a *center-based program*), not necessarily in the child's neighborhood.
- Residential school, with a large number of children with hearing loss and many teachers of children with hearing loss. Some children live on campus during the week; some attend as day students.

LRE continuum: A range of educational options, from regular education in one's neighborhood to a residential school.

The LRE continuum is represented in Figure 8.1.

Case 8.1. Laurie

Laurie is 5 years old and has a severe bilateral hearing loss, identified before her first birthday. She has received a range of services from that time, wears two hearing aids all day, and is currently enrolled in a kindergarten program in her neighborhood and is also receiving therapy consistent with an auditory–verbal approach (i.e., a strong emphasis on developing listening skills) in a private clinic. Her language development is delayed but measurably improving, and her social skills are age appropriate. Her mother has been told by school officials that the first-grade placement should be at a specialized program, which would involve a bus ride of over an hour both ways. This placement would use sign language in its instruction, but Laurie's parents have been committed to an auditory–verbal approach for four years. They are therefore opposed to this placement recommendation because of the distance and because of the communication methods used. They will have to meet with the school administrators to make their case, and because they have learned their rights, they expect their understanding of the term "least restrictive environment" to carry the day.

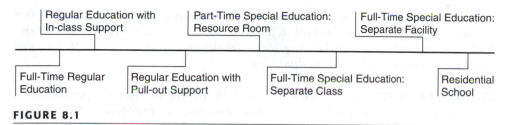

FIGURE 8.1

Continuum of educational placements.

In the first fifteen years of special education, placement decisions considered the concept of mainstreaming as a move from special education to regular education. That is, children with hearing loss would most likely be placed in a special education environment, and as the child demonstrated grade-level competencies in math or in reading, he or she would gradually spend more time in a regular education class-room. In the last decade, there has been a reconsideration of this concept, and now the philosophy of *inclusion* is being applied, resulting in an initial placement of the child in a regular education program and the provision of supports or special services to help the child succeed in this placement. Only when it is clear that individualized or small-group instruction is necessary is the child taken from the class and provided help in resource room instruction or other educational placement.

Figure 8.2 gives the current distributions of students with hearing impairment across a variety of educational placements (U.S. Department of Education, 2002a). It shows a growing trend toward placing children with hearing loss in regular education classrooms. Research supports the effectiveness of inclusive

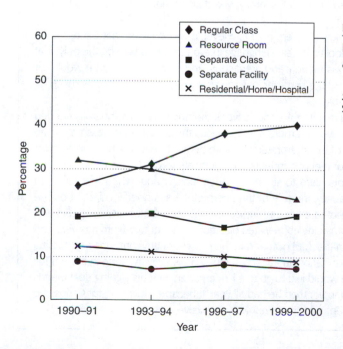

FIGURE 8.2

Percentage of students with hearing impairment ages 6 to 21 by type of educational environment: 1990–1991 to 1999–2000.

Source: U.S. Department of Education, Office of Special Education Programs.

classroom placements, but the concept is not without its dissenters. Interpreters of this regulation repeatedly caution that it is not appropriate to generalize about LRE among children with hearing loss. *The determination of the LRE for each child must be made on an individual basis.*

LRE FOR A CHILD WITH HI. For a child with a hearing impairment, the preceding interpretation of least restrictive environment may not be appropriate. A child with a mild to moderately severe hearing loss may succeed in a regular education classroom if full support is provided to address the variety of language and listening needs that can impede learning. Because so much learning (social as well as academic) is language based, it is impossible to generalize about the appropriate environment for individuals who are hard of hearing.

The appropriate environment becomes a more complicated issue for the child who is deaf. The Commission on Education of the Deaf (1988) held that placement of a deaf child in a regular classroom, even with an interpreter, may be more restrictive than placement in a fully signing environment with deaf peers. Because of communication difficulties, a deaf child may experience unique academic, social, and emotional complications in the regular classroom. If such is the case, the regular

---

Case 8.2. Carlos

Carlos was identified as having a bilateral profound hearing loss at age 6 months. His family decided on total communication as his primary mode of communication and began to attend sign classes offered by the Early Intervention program. He attended a preschool that included many other deaf children and had developed several friendships there. By the time he was ready for kindergarten, most of his family were fairly fluent in sign, and Carlos was developing early reading skills.

Because his preacademic skills were near age level, it was decided that Carlos would attend his neighborhood school with a sign language interpreter. He was to be the only deaf child in the school, but he was friendly and gregarious, and it was assumed he would "fit right in." His new teacher spent the summer learning sign language to achieve as much direct communication as possible.

Everyone was surprised that it took Carlos several months to acquire the skills needed to use an interpreter effectively. Even more surprising was the difficulty his classmates had in adjusting to the presence of the interpreter. Although he tried to be inconspicuous, most of Carlos's classmates did not feel comfortable communicating with Carlos through the interpreter. Their initial attempts were to speak to Carlos directly and, when that failed, to mime their intentions. Eventually, the role of the interpreter was understood, but both he and the classroom teacher noted that communication between Carlos and his peers was restricted to the essentials: providing abbreviated directions, one- or two-word answers, and so on. The natural interaction that had occurred in the preschool environment was missing here. Because of the communication limitations, Carlos was effectively alone in a room full of people. When asked if he would like to go to a kindergarten with his signing deaf friends from preschool, he looked happier than he had all year. It became clear that, for Carlos, the regular education environment was more, not less, restrictive.

classroom is not the LRE for a deaf child: "Placing a deaf child in the regular classroom without the language needed to function as a participant seriously impedes, if not precludes, the child from receiving any worthwhile education in the class" (p. 33).

In response to these concerns, the U.S. Department of Education (DOE) issued "policy guidance" to states and school districts regarding the LRE for children with severe-to-profound hearing loss (*Federal Register,* October 30, 1992, *57*[211], pp. 49274–49276). Noting that "the communicative nature of the disability is inherently isolating" (p. 49274), the DOE advised that the LRE provisions of the IDEA may be incorrectly interpreted for children who are deaf. The following factors are of paramount importance when determining the LRE for a child who is deaf:

- Communication needs and the child's and family's preferred mode of communication
- Linguistic needs
- Severity of hearing impairment and potential for using residual hearing
- Academic level
- Social, emotional, and cultural needs of the child, including opportunities for peer interactions and communications

The DOE reminded educators that "The provision of FAPE is paramount, and the individual placement determination about LRE is to be considered within the context of FAPE" (p. 49275). In other words, no interpretation of LRE is meant to override the provision of an appropriate education. See Ramsey (1997) for more information on this issue.

The Individualized Education Program (IEP)

The services to be provided to a child with a hearing loss are described in a document called an Individualized Education Program (IEP). It has been said that the IEP is not only a collection of forms, but also a *process:* That is, a group of interested persons (parents, teachers, school administrators, and related service providers such as audiologists, speech–language pathologists, school nurses, etc.), referred to as the Individualized Education Program Committee (IEPC), spend considerable time reviewing a child's current level of skills, and decide on reasonable goals for the upcoming year. The process involves a great deal of sharing, learning, and ultimately agreeing on how to implement the child's educational program. Parents can request a revisit of this process at any time to consider changes in the child or other variables.

IEP: Individualized Educational Program: A written report describing a child's current level of performance, annual goals, and procedures used to meet these goals.

As mentioned earlier, services are available to families as soon as a disability has been identified. From birth to age 3, services are tailored to the needs of the child within the context of the family (rather than the need of the child alone), so the document used to describe these services is called the Individualized Family Service Plan (IFSP).

The Communication Debate

Perhaps the most important consideration regarding educational placement is the communication method used. Unfortunately, this is a very complex matter, involving one of the oldest debates in education regarding the best way to teach a child with hearing impairment. This *communication debate* focuses on how to provide language instruction to children who are deaf. Students of audiologic rehabilitation will want to have a working knowledge of the issues; however, the choice of approach ultimately lies with parents, and professionals do not serve parents well by persuading them to adapt an approach that does not fit with their family. See Recommended Reading at the end of this chapter for more information on these topics.

The communication options include an oral–aural approach (i.e., using speech and hearing), a combination of signing with speech and hearing (total communication), a system called Cued Speech, and the use of sign only. Each approach is briefly described here.

ORAL–AURAL APPROACH. This method emphasizes speech communication (oral), optimal use of amplified residual hearing (aural), and the development of speechreading (also known as lipreading), while discouraging the use of sign language. This approach was espoused by Alexander Graham Bell (1847–1922), who, in addition to his other accomplishments, was a skilled speech teacher. Supporters of the oral–aural approach feel that "with spoken language, opportunities for higher education are less restricted, a more extensive range of careers is open, and there is greater employment security. Those who can talk also face fewer limitations in the personal and social aspects of their lives" (Ling, 1990, p. 9).

A relatively recent refinement of the oral–aural approach is the *auditory–verbal approach.* The primary difference between these approaches is that the auditory–verbal approach makes a concerted effort during aural rehabilitation therapy to remove visual cues, encouraging the child to develop the auditory system with directed listening practice. Speechreading is used as a secondary rather than primary teaching strategy. To stimulate auditory development, the therapist reduces or eliminates visual information by covering most of his or her face while presenting the speech stimuli (Estabrooks, 2004).

Approximately 30 percent of the schoolchildren with hearing loss in the United States are instructed in the oral–aural or auditory–verbal approaches.

TOTAL COMMUNICATION. To capitalize on the visual information provided by sign language, *total communication* (TC) was introduced in the 1960s. TC incorporates the use of many modalities at once: signing, speech, listening, and speechreading, as well as the contributions of nonverbal communication (body language and facial expressions). The nature of the signing depends on the background of the educator, who may use American Sign Language (ASL), or a sign system such as Signed Exact English (SEE), or a combination of ASL and SEE called Pigeon Sign, described in detail in Chapter 5. Briefly, ASL is recognized as a legitimate language with a rich lexicon and a fully developed linguistic structure. Its roots are in French Sign Language, and it has been in existence for over 200 years. Unlike most languages, ASL has the unique characteristic of being learned from deaf peers rather than from hearing family members (Hoffmeister, 1990). Because fewer than 10 percent of deaf children are born of deaf parents, ASL is typically learned from deaf friends and other adults, rather than from parents. In spite of this limited access to ASL, supporters feel that it should be the language of instruction for all children who are deaf.

Whereas ASL has evolved as a natural *sign language*, SEE is a *sign system* (i.e., a way to sign English words) created in the 1960s to address concerns regarding low reading and writing skills. SEE uses manual markers for linguistic concepts (e.g., plurality and tense) to correspond directly to the structures of the English language and follows the exact word order of English. SEE is just one of several artificial systems; readers of historical records will come across references to many versions. The use of these systems has diminished since the 1980s, for the most part being replaced with Pidgin Sign.

Like other pidgin languages, Pidgin Sign combines elements of different languages, in this case a manual language (ASL) and a spoken language (English). Pidgin Sign is a "contact language . . . a result of something that occurs when two groups of people need or desire to communicate" (Luetke-Stahlman & Luckner, 1991, p. 10). In an exchange, a hearing person communicating with Pidgin Sign is likely to omit articles such as "the" or "a/an" or the "ing" endings of gerund verbs as in ASL. The word order, however, is usually identical to English, while in ASL the word order could be quite different (e.g., adjectives following rather than preceding nouns, as in "shoes brown").

Although the type of sign will vary from one classroom to another, total communication (TC) is the general practice found around the country; it is used in about 66 percent of classroom instruction for children with hearing loss.

> **Sign system:** Not a language, but a method of depicting an oral language like English with manual symbols.

CUED SPEECH. Another approach developed in the 1960s is called *Cued Speech*. Cued Speech is not a language but a visual support system to facilitate speechreading. Hand shapes made close to the face represent phonemes, which helps the speechreader discriminate between similar phonemes. For example, the phonemes /k/ and /g/ require distinct handshapes (/k/ as if pointing to the throat with the index and middle fingers, while the /g/ points with all five fingers), thus providing the speechreader with a visual cue to the voiced or unvoiced component of the phonemes. Cued Speech can be found in concentrated areas across the United States, but only in about 1 percent of classroom instruction (Gallaudet Research Institute, 2005).

> **Cued Speech:** A set of handshapes to help with speechreading sounds that look virtually identical (compare "Friday" to "fried egg").

USING SIGN ONLY (BI–BI). In 1988, the Commission on the Education of the Deaf recommended yet another approach, called a *bilingual–bicultural* ("bi–bi") approach. This approach advocates teaching ASL as a deaf child's first language and that written English be taught as a second language. Speech production and listening skills are not emphasized. Its implementation requires teachers to be native or fluent users of ASL, and, as one might expect, not many teachers are so well qualified. Approximately 1 percent of students are immersed in the bi–bi approach (Coryell & Holcomb, 1997).

■ AR SERVICES PROVIDED IN SCHOOLS

This section will describe a range of school-based audiologic rehabilitative services (American Speech–Language–Hearing Association, 2002):

- Screening and assessment of hearing impairment
- Management of amplification

- Direct instruction and indirect consultation
- Hearing conservation
- Evaluation and modification of classroom acoustics
- Transition planning to postsecondary placements

Ideally, these services are provided by an audiologist. As noted in Chapter 1, when audiologists provide these services, there are five times as many children with hearing impairments served, and two-and-a-half times more hearing aids and other forms of amplification in use as compared to when others provide the services (Downs, Whitaker, & Schow, 2003).

Screening and Assessment

EARLY IDENTIFICATION OF HEARING LOSS. Most children are now screened for hearing loss at birth. When newborns do not pass the screening, their parents are referred to a hospital or clinic for a comprehensive assessment. If a hearing loss is confirmed, parents are referred to their local early intervention program. That program will provide auditory training, speech and language therapy, and also other supports (for example, physical therapy) if needed.

SCREENING IN KINDERGARTEN THROUGH GRADE 12. Schools are usually required by law to screen all school-age children at select grades to determine the existence of unidentified hearing loss (e.g., in kindergarten and grades 1–3, and 12). Because more and more children are demonstrating mild hearing loss in the high frequencies (most likely due to high levels of noise exposure), these screening programs have become more valuable than ever in identifying hearing problems that may not be evident to parents, teachers, or the child.

Play audiometry provides useful information concerning hearing loss with preschoolers.

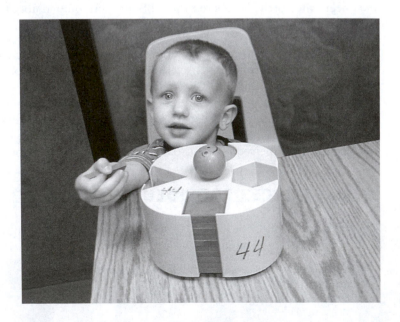

In addition to screening, children with *known* hearing loss must have an annual hearing assessment to determine the stability of the loss and to reconsider the appropriateness of the child's hearing aids and other amplification systems. Assessment information should include conventional hearing test information, speech recognition and speechreading abilities in quiet and in noise, and functional performance with amplification.

Management of Amplification

Managing amplification is a critical audiologic rehabilitative service. Amplification includes personal hearing aids, personal FM systems, cochlear implants, sound field amplification, and assistive devices. Without a systematic monitoring program, hearing aids and personal FM systems can be expected to have a 50 percent failure rate of operation (Lipscomb, Von Almen, & Blair, 1992; Robinson & Sterling, 1980). Educational audiologists have agreed that, given the high and unacceptable likelihood of malfunction, a monitoring program should be established, consisting of a daily visual inspection and listening check and at least one electroacoustic analysis every semester of each hearing aid and FM device (English, 1991). When such a program is rigorously applied, the malfunction rate can be as low as 1 percent (Langan & Blair, 2000). Given the importance of amplification to a child's academic success, a zero tolerance for malfunction rates should be established in each school.

The day-to-day management of amplification depends primarily on teachers, classroom aides, and speech–language pathologists. The audiologist must appreciate that these professionals' days are already crowded with countless responsibilities. The request to include yet another task might be received with skepticism, doubt, or worry. The technical aspects of the request also can be intimidating: Typically, classroom professionals have little or no background in amplification, and they might worry that they will break something. Therefore, the audiologist must consider strategies that will not only train but also motivate school professionals to provide consistent amplification management. If developing an inservice, the audiologist should remember that active learning is more likely to effect changes than traditional lecture (Naeve-Velguth, Hariprasad, & Lehman, 2003). Whether training is formal or informal, procedures should be reviewed on a regular basis to confirm that details are not forgotten or misapplied. Every time the student changes teachers, of course, the process needs to be repeated.

The audiologist should combine classroom records with his or her own (e.g., in chart or spreadsheet format) to document that the program is doing everything possible to help the student hear well, and then share these data with parents and administrators while giving full credit to the classroom professionals. This public acknowledgment will help classroom professionals perceive the value of their role in this long-term team effort.

Direct Instruction and Indirect Consultation

When children have hearing loss, they usually need direct instruction in developing their listening skills, speech production, and use of language. These supports may be provided within the classroom, one on one, or in small groups, or children may leave the classroom to join a teacher, SLP, or audiologist in another (resource) room.

When a child is deaf, this type of direct instruction may not have as much relevance given the level of hearing loss and limits of amplification. Audiologists and SLPs may then pay particular attention to a child's communication strategies in a broader view. An educational audiologist at the Governor Baxter School for the Deaf in Maine described its Communication Strategies curriculum with these four categories (Snow, 2000):

PRAGMATICS

Kindergarten: Identify strangers versus friends versus family; express wants, needs, and preferences.

Grades 5 and 6: Support and justify actions and answers; understand and use hints; recognize sarcastic comments by wording and facial expressions.

LITERACY

Kindergarten: Recognize and practice writing phone numbers; use name signs for all classmates; recognize written names of classmates.

Grades 5 and 6: Read English and change to ASL; give basic directions in ASL.

LIFE SKILLS

Kindergarten: Order food successfully, using picture-pointing menu; speech-read one's name.

Grades 5 and 6: Carry on a conversation with a hearing peer via print.

DEAF CULTURE

Kindergarten: Identify self and familiar people as Deaf or hearing; introduce self using name sign.

Grades 5 and 6: Understand the purpose of interpreters; learn significance of Deaf theatre and poetry.

If a child's needs are not very involved or if personnel are not available for direct support, indirect consultation may take place among teachers and related service providers. As mentioned earlier, an audiologist may train the teacher how to do a daily hearing aid check, because it is not possible for the audiologist to do it him- or herself every day, or an SLP may provide an informal inservice on how to develop language skills within the curriculum, rather than work with the child directly.

Hearing Conservation

Because society is becoming increasingly noisy and because children are being exposed to ever-higher noise levels, the incidence of high-frequency noise-induced hearing loss in children is on the rise. Noise exposure comes from toys, snowmobiles, and other engines, but most often from music through headphones. The output from personal radio systems through headphones can exceed 115 dB. The hearing loss caused by this noise trauma is permanent and entirely preventable; therefore, school programs are required to develop educational training programs to teach all children about hearing health and hearing loss prevention. Health textbooks typically do not cover this topic, so it is usually left to the communication disorders specialist (audiologist, speech–language pathologist, teacher of children with hearing impairment) to develop age-appropriate lessons. Programs typically include a description of the auditory system, the effects of noise on this system, and a review of preventive measures. These programs have proved to be very effective (Bennett & English, 1999; Chermak, Curtis, & Seikel, 1996), but they are also time intensive and are often considered a luxury item on the menu of services delivered.

Hearing conservation: Teaching children how to protect their hearing from high noise levels.

Evaluation and Modification of Classroom Acoustics

Classroom acoustics is the up-and-coming topic in audiologic rehabilitative services in schools. The reason why will be provided later, but first we need to consider the three variables that can affect the acoustic environment of a classroom: noise levels, reverberation, and distance between teacher and student. The *noise level* of the typical classroom can be very high, often louder than the teacher's voice. Children talk while working in small groups, feet shuffle on linoleum floors, heat and air conditioning systems turn on and off, computers hum, and so on. The higher the noise level, the harder it is for children with hearing impairment to hear oral instruction. In fact, when the noise level is just slightly higher than the teacher's voice, a child with hearing loss will understand very little of what he or she says. Unfortunately, most classrooms currently have background noise levels that exceed acceptable levels.

Even if a room is quiet, it can still have problems with *reverberation*. Reverberation is another word for *echo* and refers to the prolongation of sound as sound waves reflect off the hard surfaces in a room. Excessive reverberation occurs when floors have linoleum or tile instead of carpet or the walls and ceilings are covered with plaster instead of acoustic tile. Reverberation interferes with speech perception by overlapping with the energy of the direct signal of the teacher's voice. A child with hearing impairment cannot interpret this distorted speech quickly enough, so reverberation is as much a problem as high noise levels. *Reverberation time* (RT) is a value used to indicate the amount of time it takes for a sound to decay 60 dB from its initial onset. For optimal perception of speech, it has been recommended that the RT in a classroom not exceed 0.3 second; however, the RT for most classrooms typically ranges from 0.4 to 1.2 seconds (Crandell, Smaldino, & Flexer, 2005).

The third variable to consider with respect to classroom acoustics is the *distance* between teacher and student. Teachers move around the room most of the day, so the distance between teacher and student will vary from one minute to the next. The distance will affect the perceived sound level of the teacher's voice: The sound level for most conversational speech is approximately 60 dB SPL measured from 6 feet away, but this level drops as the distance between speaker and listener increases. When teachers stand a distance away, their voices may become too soft for most HI children to hear and understand, even with good hearing aids.

Hearing aids are limited not only by distance, but also by their nonselective amplification of all sounds in the classroom. Background noise sources such as overhead fans, buzzing fluorescent lights, and shuffling feet all contribute to the auditory input, and it can be very difficult to discriminate speech from this noise. An ideal solution to these listening challenges is the use of wireless FM (frequency modulated) amplification systems. There are two kinds of FM systems: *personal* systems used by individual students, and *sound field* systems designed to amplify the teacher's voice throughout the entire classroom (i.e., the sound field).

FM: A radio signal that carries the speaker's voice directly to a receiver.

PERSONAL FMS. Personal FMs have two components. The first is the teacher's microphone and transmitter unit, which picks up and transmits the teacher's voice. The microphone may be attached to a lapel or worn on a neck loop or headset.

The second component of the system is the student's unit, a device that picks up the FM signal carrying the teacher's voice, amplifies it, and delivers it to the student's ears. This receiver can be an attachment to a personal hearing aid or a small unit resembling a personal radio or cassette player (see Chapter 2).

With an FM system, the teacher's voice is transmitted by a frequency-modulated (FM) signal to the student's receiver, which works very much like a personal radio station. The teacher's mouth is approximately 6 to 8 inches away from the microphone and, because the teacher's voice is transmitted by FM signal rather than airwaves, the student perceives this voice as if the teacher were always speaking 6 to 8 inches away from his or her hearing aid microphone (overcoming the limitation of distance). Reception stays consistent up to a distance of 200 feet. With an FM system, the problem of direction of the speaker is also eliminated. The clarity of the teacher's voice is not affected as she turns away from the listener (changing directions).

In addition to overcoming the problems of distance and direction, FM systems also address the problem of hearing in noise. FM systems are designed to amplify and transmit the teacher's voice at intensity levels well above the environmental noise, creating a favorable signal-to-noise listening condition. Controls are available to receive input from the FM microphone only (e.g., to listen to a lecture when the teacher is the only one talking), hearing aid plus FM input together (to hear both teacher and classroom conversation), or hearing aid microphone only (to hear class discussion only when the teacher is working with other students).

The FM advantage: Amplifying a speaker's voice above background noise, while not being affected by distance or direction.

These factors combine in what is called *the FM advantage* (Flexer, Wray, & Ireland, 1989, p. 14). The FM advantage consists of overriding the negative effects of noise by increasing the teacher's voice, as well as eliminating the adverse effects of distance and direction.

Sound field amplification: Amplifying an entire area (the sound field), such as a classroom or auditorium.

SOUND FIELD FM SYSTEMS. Another way of improving classroom acoustics is to amplify the teacher's voice for the entire classroom with the use of sound field amplification, usually recognized as a type of PA system. By amplifying the teacher's voice via loud speakers placed around the classroom, the problems with background noise and distance can be reduced. With a sound field system, the teacher wears a wireless microphone (an FM transmitter), and her or his voice is transmitted to an FM receiver and amplifier and one or more speakers placed around the room. The teacher is free to move as before, but, regardless of her or his position, the teacher's voice will be amplified to all corners of the room. Sound field amplification has been found to enhance academic performance not only for children with hearing loss, but also for children whose first language is not English, who have language disorders, or who have mild mental retardation (Rosenberg et al., 1999).

A new variation of the concept of amplifying the whole classroom is to amplify the small area around the student. Desktop speakers are being used with students who change rooms across the day; they take both the microphone and book-sized speaker with them as they move from math to science class, for example.

It is important to note that amplifying the sound field (the classroom area) does not completely overcome reverberation problems, so a classroom would still need to be evaluated to determine how to reduce the amount of hard surfaces. The usual first modifications are to carpet the floor and to install acoustic tile on the ceiling.

Why the current interest in classroom acoustics? Because the overall record of poor acoustic environments has attracted the interest of the federal government as an issue of access for persons with disabilities. Just as restaurants are required to provide menus in Braille and government offices must have restroom facilities that can accommodate wheelchairs, so, it is reasoned, the acoustics of a school should allow full *acoustic access* to oral instruction. Acoustic standards have been developed and can be found on the website for the Federal Architecture and Transportation "Access" Board (www.access-board.gov/acoustics/index.htm). The evaluation of classroom acoustics will be an increasing responsibility for persons providing audiologic rehabilitative services in the school setting and an exciting opportunity to positively affect the education of children with hearing loss. And as mentioned at the beginning of this chapter, attention paid to a student's classroom environment addresses both of the Es described in the CORE and CARE models.

Transition Planning to Postsecondary Placements

Ultimately, audiologic rehabilitative services are expected to support a child through to a successful high school graduation, but even here planning for the future is required. Once students graduate, the special education safety net is no longer in place for students with hearing loss. To prepare for the transition to placements after high school (college, vocational training, and work settings), students are required to meet with teachers and parents to develop an Individualized Transition Plan (ITP). If the student plans on attending a particular college, a representative of the college should attend this meeting; likewise, representatives from vocational training programs or work settings should provide input, as deemed necessary. The purpose of this transition planning is to ensure that the student has time to prepare for the requirements needed to enter college or vocational training or for job placement. The law reads "The IEP for each student, beginning no later than age 16 (and at an earlier age, if deemed appropriate), must include a statement of each public agency's and each participating agency's responsibilities, or linkages, or both, before the student leaves the school setting" (34 CFR § 300.45).

ITP: Individualized Transition Plan: A long-term plan to arrange for further education or job training after high school.

This transition planning is especially important when we consider college placements. Although students with hearing loss enter college programs at the same rate as students without hearing loss, their dropout rate is much higher (71 percent compared to 47 percent) (Bullis & Egelston-Dodd, 1990; Welsh, 1993). It would appear that college career success depends as much on the ability to develop a social support system and to obtain and use support systems (interpreters, note takers, FM systems) as on the ability to earn good grades. Materials are available to help students to prepare for college, particularly in the area of being one's own advocate for supports and services (DuBow, Geer, & Strauss, 2000; English, 1997).

Deaf students may be particularly interested in attending colleges with an emphasis in Deaf culture, such as Gallaudet University (the only liberal arts college for the Deaf in the world) in Washington, DC, or the National Technical Institute for the Deaf (NTID) in Rochester, New York. On the west coast of the United States, the California State University at Northridge (CSUN) also has a large Deaf student enrollment. Transition to these environments requires planning as well, and students need a great deal of support during this process (English, 1993).

How Services Are Provided

Although these AR responsibilities are carefully described, they are not implemented as widely as one would expect. Earlier it was mentioned that 1 to 2 million schoolchildren are estimated to have some degree of hearing loss; however, according to annual data collected by the U.S. Department of Education, fewer than 10 percent of children with hearing loss receive the audiologic services to which they are entitled (U.S. Department of Education, 2002b) (see Table 8.3). The reasons why children with hearing loss are underserved vary from one region to the next, but a common reason seems to be that parents are not fully aware of their rights to these services.

■ AR SERVICE PROVIDERS IN SCHOOL SETTINGS

School-based AR services are provided in a team approach, with the following professionals working as team members.

Teachers

Not too long ago, most children with hearing impairment were taught in small, self-contained classes run by teachers specially trained to teach them. This model still exists, but now, because of the movement toward inclusion (discussed earlier), many of these teachers may be assigned to several schools to provide support to children as they attend their neighborhood schools. Support may consist of direct instruction, individually or in small groups, or indirect consultation with the general classroom teacher. This collaboration is essential since most regular education teachers receive little training about hearing loss. Information on adapting curriculum, verifying hearing aid function, and the like is shared, as well as reports on student progress.

TABLE 8.3

Number of Children Ages 6 to 21 Served under IDEA, Part B, by Disability during the 2000–2001 School Year

STATE	MULTIPLE DISABILITIES	HEARING IMPAIRMENTS	ORTHOPEDIC IMPAIRMENTS	OTHER HEALTH IMPAIRMENTS	VISUAL IMPAIRMENTS
Alabama	1,356	975	603	3,994	427
Alaska	484	222	69	932	45
Arizona	2,513	1,456	721	1,788	564
Arkansas	1,087	592	190	5,636	191
California	5,366	9,336	11,455	18,426	3,687
Colorado	2,989	1,221	5,569	0	309
Connecticut	2,197	751	218	7,830	326
Delaware	0	219	1,118	0	51
District of Columbia	408	83	83	162	18
Florida	0	3,134	4,276	8,246	1,100
Georgia	0	1,466	947	13,720	602
Hawaii	271	370	133	1,338	77
Idaho	500	299	117	1,203	114
Illinois	0	3,343	2,766	7,618	1,020
Indiana	1,208	1,711	1,358	3,641	780
Iowa	282	554	680	129	136
Kansas	1,992	576	452	5,258	211
Kentucky	2,409	649	443	6,781	424
Louisiana	951	1,324	1,389	7,769	424
Maine	2,728	247	76	2,554	87
Maryland	6,098	1,211	477	7,469	515
Massachusetts	2,687	1,399	884	1,192	616
Michigan	2,838	3,006	12,970	0	873
Minnesota	0	1,896	1,480	7,767	382
Mississippi	480	589	1,705	0	236
Missouri	880	1,182	663	7,846	418
Montana	573	195	76	1,145	63
Nebraska	379	592	451	2,388	206
Nevada	660	424	284	1,427	136
New Hampshire	381	260	141	3,600	137
New Jersey	19,518	1,524	609	6,684	335

(continued)

TABLE 8.3

Continued

STATE	MULTIPLE DISABILITIES	HEARING IMPAIRMENTS	ORTHOPEDIC IMPAIRMENTS	OTHER HEALTH IMPAIRMENTS	VISUAL IMPAIRMENTS
New Mexico	1,116	515	267	2,093	181
New York	21,768	5,647	2,783	25,215	1,902
North Carolina	1,751	2,011	1,046	13,211	621
North Dakota	0	127	126	619	55
Ohio	13,320	2,495	2,267	6,554	1,085
Oklahoma	1,611	775	482	3,449	353
Oregon	0	981	747	4,835	321
Pennsylvania	1,986	2,648	1,263	2,203	1,152
Puerto Rico	1,146	847	508	1,525	506
Rhode Island	300	238	121	2,541	68
South Carolina	261	1,070	785	3,546	312
South Dakota	566	136	95	574	47
Tennessee	1,743	1,303	1,095	8,876	776
Texas	8,629	5,519	5,486	36,539	2,289
Utah	1,256	575	171	1,154	232
Vermont	113	212	111	1,197	50
Virginia	2,392	1,315	756	13,930	474
Washington	2,724	1,486	845	17,763	314
West Virginia	0	393	192	2,315	213
Wisconsin	0	1,394	1,325	6,269	409
Wyoming	37	169	137	883	57
American Samoa	20	2	1	3	4
Guam	60	33	13	58	10
Northern Marianas	40	10	9	10	5
Palau	5	4	6	4	1
Virgin Islands	22	18	1	33	7
Bureau of Indian Affairs	458	38	16	268	21
U.S. and Outlying Areas	122,559	70,767	73,057	291,850	25,975
50 States, D.C., P.R.	121,954	70,662	73,011	291,474	25,927

Source: U.S. Department of Education, 2002b.

Audiologists

School-based audiologists have developed a specialty called educational audiology, often considered to be audiology *plus,* that is, clinical audiology skills *plus* an understanding of the school culture, legal mandates, and the roles and responsibilities unique to the school setting (Berg, Blair, Viehweg, & Wilson-Vlotman, 1996; English, 1995). A primary limitation to the provision of these services has been the relatively small number of audiologists hired to serve children in schools. The American Speech–Language–Hearing Association (ASHA) (2002) has conservatively estimated the need to be one audiologist for every 12,000 schoolchildren. This 1:10K ratio would necessitate hiring at least 5,000 audiologists, but for over a decade only about 1,000 educational audiologists have been employed by schools. Because of this hiring shortage, provision of services may be shared by any of the following professional colleagues. As noted earlier, audiologists are much more effective in providing these services.

Speech–Language Pathologists

Speech–language pathologists (SLPs) are the professionals most likely to provide speech and language therapy and auditory training. They may be the persons responsible for ensuring that a child's hearing aids are functioning, troubleshooting basic problems, and reporting any problems to the audiologist. SLPs usually provide support to the classroom teacher by describing how to provide visual cues,

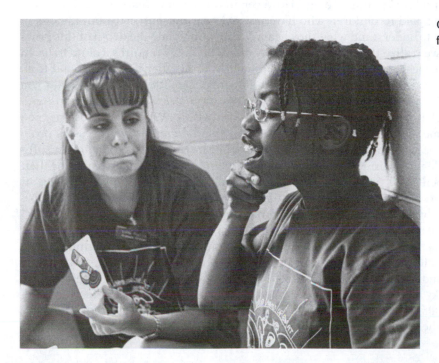

One-on-one speech therapy focused on articulation.

promote speechreading opportunities, control for acoustic problems, and so on. SLPs also often conduct hearing screening programs.

Related Support Personnel

Approximately 30 to 40 percent of children with hearing loss have additional disabilities, such as vision loss, autism, and learning disabilities (Gallaudet Research Institute, 2005). Therefore, associated AR services are also provided by the following, as well as others:

- School nurses, for medications and other health concerns, as well as hearing screening
- School psychologists, for assessment of verbal and nonverbal intellectual abilities
- Adaptive physical education teachers, for large motor and balance development
- Mobility and orientation specialists, for children with visual impairments

It is not at all unusual for these professionals to have a limited background in the area of hearing loss, which makes it all the more important to take a team approach in providing services.

■ SERVICES FOR CHILDREN WITH AUDITORY PROCESSING PROBLEMS

Up to this point, we have considered the audiologic rehabilitative services only for children with hearing impairment. However, in the last few years, increased attention is being paid to children who have normal hearing sensitivity, but deficits in their ability to understand what they hear. We can appreciate the depth of this problem when we realize that the vast majority of a school day requires a child to listen to his or her teacher's instruction, understand it, remember it, and respond to it. Imagine a classroom teacher giving the following instructions: "Class, I want you to take out your yellow math book and turn to page 197. Do only the even-numbered problems and then leave your paper on my desk. When you are done, you may do some silent reading until 10:40." A child with an auditory processing problem might be easily confused with this long set of instructions, or she might sufficiently understand until other children start making noise as they reach for their books, pencils, and paper. Such a child may look distracted or "off task" as he or she looks around trying to figure out what to do, and to a teacher the child's behaviors might appear hyperactive or immature.

Because auditory processing (listening) is an invisible behavior, it may be difficult for teachers to realize that it involves instantaneous complex cognitive activity, specifically, receiving, symbolizing, comprehending, interpreting, storing, and recalling auditory information or, put more simply, "what we do with what we hear" (Lasky & Katz, 1983, p. 5). The American Speech–Language–Hearing Association (2005) described APD to include problems in several listening domains, including these three:

- *Temporal aspects of hearing or pattern recognition:* The ability to rapidly and accurately sequence auditory information.
- *Monaural discrimination:* The ability to perceive degraded words or words in competion when signal and competition are present in one ear.
- *Understanding binaural acoustic information* such as a signal in one ear by ignoring competition in the other, or different *(dichotic) information* when both parts are useful and heard in two ears at once.

When a child has problems with one or more of these listening challenges, he or she may have an *auditory processing disorder* (APD). Until recently, the term *central auditory processing disorder* (CAPD) has been used, but since "central" and "processing" are redundant words, some professionals now prefer that the term APD be used (Jerger & Musiek, 2000).

APD: Auditory processing disorder: A range of difficulties with auditory information, in spite of normal hearing acuity.

The overall impression of a child with APD is one who seems generally inattentive, "out of it," restless, forgetful, or impatient or acts socially inappropriately. Listening difficulties often surface in third grade, when classroom instruction becomes less directed, and this has been recommended as a good time for screening these children. Such difficulties may even be apparent from the first days of formal schooling, because listening is the mode by which a prereader acquires information. As of now, there is no general consensus on how to diagnose this condition, but screening instruments such as the S.I.F.T.E.R. (Anderson, 1989) found in Figure 8.3, MAPA, and SAB (Schow & Seikel, in press) found in Chapter 9 may be used by audiologists to determine that a child's listening behaviors are outside normal limits.

As mentioned, secondary behaviors that arise as a consequence of listening problems provide us with clues to the possible presence of APD. Adults are first alerted to listening difficulties when they observe the following in a child:

1. Responding inconsistently to auditory stimuli. For example, sometimes a child successfully follows a set of directions, yet other times becomes confused with the same task.
2. Demonstrating a relatively short attention span or becoming easily fatigued when confronted with long or complex listening activities.
3. Appearing overly distracted by both auditory and visual stimuli. Some children with APD feel compelled to respond immediately and fully to everything they hear, see, and touch and are unable to filter out relevant from irrelevant stimuli. Among auditory stimuli, the hum of a computer and the bubbling of a fish-tank in class may command as much attention as the teacher's voice, and the child is unable to ignore the background noises as irrelevant. These behaviors are also consistent with attention deficit hyperactivity disorder (ADHD), and a differential diagnosis can be difficult to achieve.
4. Frequently requesting that information be repeated: Saying "huh?" more often than other children.
5. Having problems with short- and long-term memory skills, such as counting; reciting the alphabet or the days, weeks, and months of the year; or recalling a home address or phone number.

S.I.F.T.E.R.

by Karen L. Anderson, Ed.S., CCC-A

STUDENT _____ TEACHER _____ GRADE _____

DATE COMPLETED _____ SCHOOL _____ DISTRICT _____

The above child is suspect for hearing problems that may or may not be affecting his/her school performance. This rating scale has been designed to sift out students who are educationally at risk possibly as a result of hearing problems. Based on your knowledge from observations of this student, circle the number best representing his/her behavior. After answering the questions, please record any comments about the student in the space provided on the reverse side.

1. What is your estimate of the student's class standing in comparison of that of his/her classmates?	UPPER 5	4	MIDDLE 3	2	LOWER 1
2. How does the student's achievement compare to your estimation of his/her potential?	EQUAL 5	4	LOWER 3	2	MUCH LOWER 1
3. What is the student's reading level, reading ability group or reading readiness group in the classroom (e.g., a student with average reading ability performs in the middle group)?	UPPER 5	4	MIDDLE 3	2	LOWER 1

ACADEMICS ☐

4. How distractible is the student in comparison to his/her classmates?	NOT VERY 5	4	AVERAGE 3	2	VERY 1
5. What is the student's attention span in comparison to that of his/her classmates?	LONGER 5	4	AVERAGE 3	2	SHORTER 1
6. How often does the student hesitate or become confused when responding to oral directions (e.g., "Turn to page . . . ")?	NEVER 5	4	OCCASIONALLY 3	2	FREQUENTLY 1

ATTENTION ☐

7. How does the student's comprehension compare to the average understanding ability of his/her classmates?	ABOVE 5	4	AVERAGE 3	2	BELOW 1
8. How does the student's vocabulary and word usage skills compare with those of other students in his/her age group?	ABOVE 5	4	AVERAGE 3	2	BELOW 1
9. How proficient is the student at telling a story or relating happenings from home when compared to classmates?	ABOVE 5	4	AVERAGE 3	2	BELOW 1

COMMUNICATION ☐

FIGURE 8.3

Screening Instrument for Targeting Educational Risk

10. How often does the student volunteer information to class discussions or in answer to teacher questions?	FREQUENTLY 5	OCCASIONALLY 4	3	2	NEVER 1	
11. With what frequency does the student complete his/her class and homework assignments within the time allocated?	ALWAYS 5	4	USUALLY 3	2	SELDOM 1	
12. After instruction, does the student have difficulty starting to work (looks at other students working or asks for help)?	NEVER 5	4	OCCASIONALLY 3	2	FREQUENTLY 1	

CLASS PARTICIPATION □

13. Does the student demonstrate any behaviors that seem unusual or inappropriate when compared to other students?	NEVER 5	4	OCCASIONALLY 3	2	FREQUENTLY 1	
14. Does the student become frustrated easily, sometimes to the point of losing emotional control?	NEVER 5	4	OCCASIONALLY 3	2	FREQUENTLY 1	
15. In general, how would you rank the student's relationship with peers (ability to get along with others)?	GOOD 5	4	AVERAGE 3	2	POOR 1	

SCHOOL BEHAVIOR □

Teacher Comments

Has this child repeated a grade, had frequent absences, or experienced health problems (including ear infections and colds)? Has the student received, or is he/she now receiving, special services? Does the child have any other health problems that may be pertinent to his/her educational functioning?

The S.I.F.T.E.R. Is a Screening Tool Only

Any student failing this screening in a content area as determined on the scoring grid below should be considered for further assessment, depending on his/her individual needs as per school district criteria. For example, failing in the Academics area suggests an educational assessment, in the Communication area a speech–language assessment, and in the School Behavior area an assessment by a psychologist or a social worker. Failing in the Attention and/or Class Participation area in combination with other areas may suggest an evaluation by an educational audiologist. Children placed in the marginal area are at risk for failing and should be monitored or considered for assessment depending upon additional information.

(continued)

FIGURE 8.3

Continued

Scoring

Sum the responses to the three questions in each content area and record in the appropriate box on the reverse side and under Total Score below. Place an **X** on the number that corresponds most closely with the content area score (e.g., if a teacher circled 3, 4, and 2 for the questions in the Academics area, an X would be placed on the number 9 across from the Academics content area). Connect the **X**s to make a profile.

CONTENT AREA	TOTAL SCORE	PASS	MARGINAL	FAIL
ACADEMICS		15 14 13 12 11 10	9 8	7 6 5 4 3
ATTENTION		15 14 13 12 11 10 9	8 7	6 5 4 3
COMMUNICATION		15 14 13 12 11	10 9 8	7 6 5 4 3
CLASS PARTICIPATION		15 14 13 12 11 10 9	8 7	6 5 4 3
SOCIAL BEHAVIOR		15 14 13 12 11 10	9 8	7 6 5 4 3

FIGURE 8.3

Continued

It is also imperative to remember that the types of behaviors listed previously are seen in all children at some time, depending on general health and energy levels, personal worries or other distractions, a variety of other learning disabilities, or the presence of temporary hearing loss due to ear infections and allergies (Chermak & Musiek, 1997).

Because APD is difficult to diagnose and because there is no standard definition of the disorder, there is no specific count of the number of children who have auditory processing problems. Approximately 8 million to 12 million schoolchildren in the United States have learning disabilities, and many of them have APD. It appears that more boys have APD than girls, and many have allergies and a positive history of chronic ear infections (Keith, 1995). APD is typically considered a learning disorder and is often just one aspect of a more complex language–learning disorder. There are different kinds of processing problems, including the following:

■ Difficulties attending to speech with competing noise in the background (important when we consider the usual noise level in classrooms)
■ Difficulties hearing the differences in sounds and words (an essential skill for phonetic reading and spelling)

In addition to these kinds of problems, there is evidence that some children's auditory systems are not as efficient in the speed of transmission (slower neural activity) and that it may take longer than normal for signals to travel from the outer ear to the brain. If a delay like this is occurring, it could be said that a child cannot listen as fast as a teacher is talking (Bellis, 2002).

Providers of AR services in schools may be called on to make a diagnosis of APD and provide remediation as needed. Traditional auditory training techniques have been successfully applied to help children with normal hearing to develop listening skills: for example, learning to discriminate differences in long versus short tones or high versus low tones, as well as the sounds in words. Computer games (e.g., Earobics) have been designed to help a child to listen and discriminate between these kinds of sounds (see the end of the chapter for website information). If a child has difficulties ignoring background noise, many listening activities are presented while a tape of white noise or cafeteria noise is played as a method of desensitization. Activities are also provided to develop auditory memory, and to help a child "listen faster" by presenting stimuli with increasing speed. An innovative program called FastForward has been designed to help children to improve this last auditory skill: By logging onto the Internet, a child uses a computer to work through a series of games that are individualized to his or her processing speed. Speech sounds are electronically altered and are made increasingly more challenging to perceive. Scores are entered to the FastForward's mainframe, and subsequent games are modified to increase or decrease the level of difficulty as needed. Readers are referred to the end of the chapter for website information.

In addition to direct therapy, environmental modifications have been suggested, such as minimizing the negative effects of noise by eliminating unnecessary noise sources (replacing buzzing fluorescent lightbulbs or placing carpet on the floor to absorb chair and feet noise) and increasing the "signal" of a teacher's voice by installing classroom amplification. Coping and problem-solving strategies

---

Case 8.3. Kim

Kim is 7 years old and is in second grade. His classmates had been acquiring beginning reading skills for several months, but he did not understand the teacher's instruction about "letter sounds," and he was getting farther and farther behind. He was discouraged and struggling with his self-perception of "being stupid." He had been seeing a reading tutor for two months and was not making any progress. His motivation to learn was almost nonexistent.

He was diagnosed as having an auditory processing problem, specifically with not being able to hear the subtle differences in sounds. Using several modalities (visual cues, kinesthetic cues, etc.), he was taught first to recognize and describe the differences between long and short tones on a keyboard and between low and high frequencies. He was taught to perceive the differences between similar consonants and vowels and consonant–vowel combinations.

In the beginning, he was not eager to "work on listening." However, he enjoyed the one-on-one interaction and soon changed his attitude about learning. By the end of the twelve-week session, he had learned how to translate these listening games to reading skills and was dismissed from the program.

are usually taught, such as learning how to make lists and use calendars, pretutoring key vocabulary and concepts, and using a "study buddy" (Masters, Stecker, & Katz, 1998).

Children with APD can usually improve their listening skills and become actively engaged in communication and learning. However, after experiencing repeated failure and fatigue from effort, children with APD can present motivational problems, creating a downward spiral of discouragement even when they try hard. Remediation must include opportunities to promote and reward a student's efforts to persist when faced with a difficult task.

SUMMARY POINTS

- Hearing loss has educational significance, and children with hearing loss are entitled to AR services to support their educational programs.
- AR services include testing, amplification management, modified instruction, and consideration of classroom acoustics.
- Classroom acoustics can adversely affect learning, especially when there are high levels of noise and reverberation. Federal standards have been developed to help programs improve classroom acoustics.
- To reduce listening challenges, technologies such as personal and group FM systems are used to amplify the teacher's voice and deliver that signal directly to students' ears.
- AR services are documented in a child's IEP and are intended to provide a free appropriate public education in the least restrictive environment.
- Children with normal hearing and auditory processing problems benefit from many of the same AR services.
- AR services in school settings are provided to children by a team of professionals: primarily teachers, audiologists, and speech–language pathologists.

RECOMMENDED READING

Bellis, T. J. (2002). *When the brain can't hear: Unraveling the mysteries of auditory processing disorder.* New York: Pocket Book.

Cohen, L. (1995). *Train go sorry: Inside a Deaf world.* New York: Vintage Books.

Cohen provides a unique insider's perspective of Deaf culture. Although hearing, she grew up in a residential school for the deaf in New York as the daughter of a teacher there. She was generally accepted by the Deaf community, but at the same time was aware of a vast cultural divide.

Commission on Education of the Deaf. (1988). *Toward equality: Education of the deaf.* Washington, DC: U.S. Government Printing Office.

Crandell, C., Smaldino, J., & Flexer, C. (2005). *Sound field amplification: Applications to speech perception and classroom acoustics.* Clifton Park, NY: Thomson Delmar Learning.

English, K. (1995). *Educational audiology across the lifespan: Serving all learners with hearing loss.* Baltimore: Paul H. Brookes.

Johnson, C. (2000). Management of hearing in the educational setting. In J. Alpiner & P. McCarthy (Eds.), *Rehabilitative audiology: Children and adults* (3rd ed.). Baltimore: Lippincott Williams & Wilkins.

Oliva, G. (2004). *Alone in the mainstream: A deaf woman remembers public school.* Washington, DC: Gallaudet University Press.

Roeser, R., & Downs, M. (Eds.). (1995). *Auditory disorders in children* (3rd ed.). New York: Thieme.

Sheetz, N. (2001). *Orientation to deafness* (2nd ed.). Boston: Allyn and Bacon.

Winefield, R. (1987). *Never the twain shall meet: Bell, Gallaudet, and the communications debate.* Washington, DC: Gallaudet University Press.

> The author provides an objective review of the issues dividing the oral–aural and manual approaches by presenting a historical account of the beginning of the communications debate and its long-term ramifications with respect to Deaf culture and deaf identity.

RECOMMENDED RESOURCES

SOFTWARE

Earobics: A CD program designed to help children improve their listening skills. www.scicom.com

FastForward: An Internet-based auditory training program designed for children with auditory processing problems: www.scienticlearning.com

Johnson, C., Seaton, J., & Benson, P. (1997). *Educational audiology handbook.* San Diego, CA: Singular Group Publications.

> This text gives an in-depth review of the roles and responsibilities of the audiologist in school settings, it also has a CD with more than 500 pages of forms to help to document services and provide a standardized method of service delivery.

WEBSITES

Acoustics Standards Update:
www.edfacilities.org/lr/acoustics.cfm

Alexander Graham Bell Association:
www.agbell.org

Auditory Verbal International:
www.auditory-verbal.org

Educational Audiology Association:
www.eduaud.org

Hands and Voices:
www.handsandvoices.org

IDEA Amendments:
www.ed.gov/policy/speced/guid/idea/idea2004.html

National Association of the Deaf:
www.nad.org

National Cued Speech Association:
www.cuedspeech.org

REFERENCES

American Speech–Language–Hearing Association. (2002). *Guidelines for audiology service provision in and for the schools* (pp. 109–125). Rockville, MD: Author.

American Speech-Language-Hearing Association. (2005). *(Central) auditory processing disorders: The role of the audiologist [Position Statement].* Accessed 2005 from http://www.asha.org/members/deskref-journals/deskref/default

Anderson, K. (1989). Screening Instrument for Targeting Educational Risk (SIFTER). Accessed 2005 from http://www.hear2learn.com

Bellis, T. J. (2002). *When the brain can't hear: Unraveling the mysteries of auditory processing disorder.* New York: Pocket Book.

Bennett, J. A., & English, K. (1999). Teaching hearing conservation to school children: Comparing the outcomes and efficacy of two pedagogical approaches. *Journal of Educational Audiology, 7,* 29–33.

Berg, F., Blair, J., Viehweg, S., & Wilson-Vlotman, A. (1986). *Educational audiology for the hard of hearing child.* Orlando, FL: Grune & Stratton.

Bess, F. H., Dodd-Murphy, J., & Parker, R. A. (1998). Children with minimal sensorineural hearing loss: Prevalence, educational performance, and functional status. *Ear and Hearing, 19*(5), 339–354.

Bess, F., Klee, T., & Culbertson, J. L. (1986). Identification, assessment, and management of children with unilateral sensorineural hearing loss. *Seminars in Hearing,* 7(1), 43–50.

Bullis, M., & Egelston-Dodd, J. (1990). Priorities in the school-to-community transition of adolescents who are deaf. *Career Development for Exceptional Individuals, 13*(10), 71–82.

Chermak, G., Curtis, L., & Seikel, J. (1996). The effectiveness of an interactive hearing conservation program for elementary school children. *Language, Speech, and Hearing Services in Schools, 27*(1), 29.

Chermak, G., & Musiek, F. (1997). *Central auditory processing disorders: New perspectives.* San Diego, CA: Singular Group Publishing.

Commission on Education of the Deaf. (1988). *Toward equality: Education of the deaf.* Washington, DC: U.S. Government Printing Office.

Coryell, J., & Holcomb, T. K. (1997). The use of sign language and sign systems in facilitating the language acquisition and communication of deaf students. *Language, Speech, and Hearing Services in Schools, 28,* 384–394.

Crandell, C., Smaldino, J., & Flexer, C. (2005). *Sound field amplification: Applications to speech perception and classroom acoustics.* Clifton Park, NY: Thomson Delmar Learning.

Davis, J., Elfenbein, J., Schum, R., & Bentler, R. (1986). Effects of mild and moderate hearing impairments on language, educational, and psychosocial behavior of children. *Journal of Speech and Hearing Disorders, 51,* 53–62.

Davis, J., Shepard, N., Stelmachowicz, P., & Gorga, M. (1982). Characteristics of hearing impaired children in the public schools: Part I. Psychoeducational data. *Journal of Speech and Hearing Disorders, 46,* 130–137.

Downs, M., & Yoshinaga-Itano, C. (1999). The efficacy of early identification and intervention for children with hearing impairment. *Pediatric Clinics of North America, 46*(1), 79–87.

Downs, S. K., Whitaker, M. M., & Schow, R. L. (2003). Audiological services in schools that do and do not have an audiologist. Educational Audiology Association Summer Conference, St. Louis.

DuBow, S., Geer, S, & Strauss, K. (2000). *Legal rights: The guide for deaf and hard of hearing people* (5th ed.). Washington, DC: Gallaudet University Press.

English, K. (1991). Best practices in educational audiology. *Language, Speech, and Hearing Services in Schools, 22,* 283–286.

English, K. (1993). Students with hearing impairment in higher education: A follow-up study. *Educational Audiology Monograph, 3,* 27–31.

English, K. (1995). *Educational audiology across the lifespan: Serving all learners with hearing impairment.* Baltimore: Paul H. Brookes.

English, K. (1997). *Self-advocacy skills for students who are deaf and hard of hearing.* Austin, TX: Pro-Ed.

English, K., & Church, G. (1999). Unilateral hearing loss in children: An update for the 1990s. *Language, Speech, and Hearing Services in Schools, 30,* 26–31.

Estabrooks, W. (2004). *The ABCs of auditory-verbal therapy.* Washington, DC: Alexander Graham Bell Association for the Deaf.

Flexer, C., Wray, D., & Ireland, J. (1989). Preferential seating is NOT enough: Issues in classroom management of hearing impaired students. *Language, Speech, and Hearing in Schools, 20,* 11–21.

Gallaudet Research Institute. (2005). *Regional and national summary of data from the 2003–2004 annual survey of deaf and hard of hearing children and youth.* Washington, DC: Author.

Hoffmeister, R. (1990). ASL and its implications for education. In H. Bornstein (Ed.), *Manual communication: Implications for education* (pp. 108–127). Washington, DC: Gallaudet University Press.

Holt, J. (1995). Classroom attributes and achievement test scores for deaf and hard of hearing students. *American Annals of the Deaf, 139,* 430–437.

Individuals with Disabilities Education Act (IDEA), PL 101-476. (October 30, 1990). Title 20, U.S.C. 1400 et seq: *US Statutes at Large, 104,* 1103–1151.

Jerger, J., & Musiek, F. (2000). Report of the Consensus Conference on the diagnosis of auditory processing disorders in school-aged children. *Journal of the American Academy of Audiology, 11*(9), 467–474.

Johnson, C. D. (2000). Management of hearing in the educational setting. In J. Alpiner & P. McCarthy (Eds.), *Rehabilitative audiology: Children and adults* (3rd ed.). Baltimore: Lippincott Williams & Wilkins.

Keith, R. (1995). Tests of central auditory processing. In R. Roeser & M. Downs (Eds.), *Auditory disorders in children* (3rd ed.; pp. 101–116). New York: Thieme.

Kelly, L. (1993). Recall of English function words and inflections by skilled and average deaf readers. *American Annals of the Deaf, 138,* 282–296.

Kuntze, M. (1998). Literacy and deaf children: The language question. *Topics in Language Disorders, 184,* 1–15.

Langan, L., & Blair, J. C. (2000). "Can you hear me?" A longitudinal study of hearing aid monitoring in the classroom. *Journal of Educational Audiology, 8,* 24–26.

Lasky, E. Z., & Katz, J. (1983). *Central auditory processing disorders: Problems of speech, language, and learning.* Baltimore: University Park Press.

Lederberg, A., & Prezbindowski, A. (2000). Impact of child deafness on mother-toddler interaction: Strengths and weaknesses. In P. Spencer, C. Erting, & M. Marschark (Eds.), *The deaf child in the family and at school* (pp. 73–92). Mahwah, NJ: Lawrence Erlbaum Associates.

Ling, D. (1976). *Speech and the hearing impaired child.* Washington, DC: Alexander Graham Bell Association for the Deaf.

Ling, D. (1990). Advances underlying spoken language development: A century of building on Bell. *Volta Review, 92*(4), 8–20.

Lipscomb, M., Von Almen, P., & Blair, J. C. (1992). Students as active participants in hearing aid maintenance. *Language, Speech, and Hearing Services in Schools, 23*(3), 208–213.

Luetke-Stahlman, P., & Luckner, J. (1991). *Effectively educating students with hearing impairments.* New York: Longman.

Masters, M. G., Stecker, N. A., & Katz, J. (1998). *Central auditory processing disorders: Mostly management.* Boston: Allyn and Bacon.

Musselman, C., & Kircaali-Iftar, G. (1996). The development of spoken language in deaf children: Explaining the unexplained variance. *Journal of Deaf Studies and Deaf Education, 11,* 108–121.

Naeve-Velguth, S., Hariparsad, D., & Lehman, M. (2003). A comparison of lecture and problem-based instructional formats for FM inservices. *Journal of Educational Audiology, 11,* 5–14.

Paul, P. (1998). *Literacy and deafness: The development of reading, writing, and literate thought.* Boston: Allyn and Bacon.

Ramsey, C. (1997). *Deaf children in publics schools: Placement, context, and consequences.* Washington, DC: Gallaudet University Press.

Robinson, D. O., & Sterling, G. R. (1980). Hearing aids and children in school: A follow-up study. *Volta Review, 82,* 229–235.

Rosenberg, G., Blake-Rahter, T., Heavner, J., Allen, L., Redmond, B., Phillips, J., & Stigers, K. (1999). Improving classroom acoustics (ICA): A three-year FM sound field classroom amplification study. *Journal of Educational Audiology, 7,* 8–28.

Schow, R. L., & Seickel, J. A. (in press). Screening for (C)APD. In F. Musiek & G. Chermak (Eds.), *CAPD Handbook: Volume 1.* Baltimore: Williams & Wilkins.

Snow, L. (2000). Educational audiology at a bilingual school for the Deaf: An identity crisis? *Educational Audiology Review, 17*(1), 4–5.

U.S. Department of Education. (2002a). *Elementary and secondary educational statistics: School year 1999–2000.* Washington, DC: U.S. Department of Education National Center for Educational Statistics.

U.S. Department of Education. (2002b). *Twenty-fourth annual report to Congress on the implementation of the Individuals with Disabilities Education Act.* Washington, DC: U.S. Government Printing Office.

Welsh, W. (1993). Factors influencing career mobility of deaf individuals. *Volta Review, 95,* 329–339.

Comprehensive Approaches to Audiologic Rehabilitation

CHAPTER 9

Audiologic Rehabilitation for Children
Assessment and Management

Mary Pat Moeller
Ronald L. Schow
Mary M. Whitaker

CONTENTS

INTRODUCTION

This chapter will provide a comprehensive discussion of audiologic rehabilitation for children as provided at two major levels: (1) parent–infant/preschool and (2) the school years. Before specific components that constitute the rehabilitation process are addressed, however, the reader will get a brief overview of prevalence and service delivery statistics, applicable definitions and terms, a general profile of the client, typical rehabilitation settings at various age levels, and the identification and assessment process.

■ PREVALENCE OF LOSS AND LEVEL OF SERVICE

Of all audiologic rehabilitation efforts, those focusing on the child are probably the most frequently applied. While numbers vary depending on the criteria used, it is commonly reported that there are approximately 50,000 youngsters who are deaf in the U.S. educational system (about 1 in every 1,000 children) and that well over 90 percent of them receive special services. There are 20 to 40 in every 1,000 children (2 to 4 percent) who can be considered to be permanently hard of hearing in both ears at levels poorer than 20 dB HL in the speech range, and there is a much poorer rate of service for the hard of hearing as compared to the deaf. This estimate would suggest that 1 million to 2 million school-age youngsters in the United States are seriously hard of hearing; but when we include minimal hearing loss with levels poorer than 15 dB HL (bilateral or unilateral) and high-frequency losses, we add another 3 million children. Conductive or temporary losses add at least another 1.5 million. Inclusion of the younger population (0 to 5 years) could put the total at close to 10 million children with hearing loss (Bess, Dodd-Murphy, & Parker, 1998; Niskar et al., 1998). Slightly higher and lower estimates have been reported, but the above numbers represent a reasonable estimate (ASHA, 2002; Downs, Whitaker, & Schow, 2003).

Study of minimally hard of hearing children in Tennessee shows that they experience excessive grade repetition (Bess et al., 1998). When hearing loss in the Iowa public schools was studied extensively, the rate of mild to moderate sensorineural and mixed losses was relatively constant in school children from grades K to 12. Conductive, temporary losses decreased as the children got older, but high-frequency, noise-induced types of losses increased (Shepard, Davis, Gorga, & Stelmachowicz, 1981). The level of services (the percentage of youngsters receiving rehabilitation help) reported in Iowa for youngsters having sensorineural and mixed losses varies by the degree of loss. Specifically, there was only a 27 percent level of service for the mildest losses, but up to a 92 percent level for the worst losses. Although Iowa was then considered to have exemplary services (70 school audiologists, 500 speech–language pathologists, 100 teachers of the hearing impaired) for its school-age children with hearing impairment, the state was found to be serving only 46 percent of all such youngsters with some kind of special placement or itinerant service. Also, slightly less than 50 percent of the overall sensorineural–mixed group was amplified. These data indicate a clear need to address, in a more comprehensive fashion, the needs of children with hearing impairments of all types and degrees.

■ TERMS AND DEFINITIONS

As noted in Chapter 1, a rigid distinction between habilitation and rehabilitation is not being made in this book. Although some prefer to use the word *habilitation* when dealing with children having prelingual hearing impairments, we use the term *audiologic rehabilitation* because of its generic usage in the profession.

Audiologic rehabilitation for the child may be viewed best as an advocacy, in which the rehabilitation professional works with the parents and the child to identify needs in relation to the hearing loss and subsequently arranges to help meet those needs. Needs resulting from hearing loss are detailed in the chapters on amplification (Chapters 2 and 3), auditory and visual skill development (Chapters 4 and 5), speech–language communication (Chapter 6), and psychosocial (Chapter 7) and school issues (Chapter 8), all of which are contained in the first section of this book. Audiologic rehabilitation (AR) includes both assessment and management (see discussion in Chapter 1). While all these AR needs are important, they should be approached differently for various children, depending, among other variables, upon the degree and time of onset of the hearing loss and the age of the child. Consequently, in order to be meaningful, a discussion of audiologic rehabilitation should be seen in the context of a profile of possible clients. The following section specifically focuses on severity and type of hearing loss, age of child, and other disabilities.

■ PROFILE OF THE CLIENT

Hearing Loss

Deafness categories for children include *congenital* (present at birth), *prelingual* (onset before 3 to 5 years), and *postlingual* (onset at or after age 5). Youngsters with congenital deafness should generally be served through early-intervention programs, which include parent–infant and preschool programs. As soon as the loss is identified (preferably by 3 months of age or before), the parent–infant or individual family service plan (IFSP) should start. Preschool programming typically begins when the child is about 3 years of age and may run concurrently with parent–infant programming. Ideally, children continue with such programs until AR services are provided in connection with school placement. Youngsters with prelingual deafness, with onset after birth, will generally receive similar treatment. Children with postlingual deafness, however, will most likely be served only in the schools.

A variety of children who are hard of hearing also participate in audiologic rehabilitation. Youngsters with milder losses are sometimes identified early and receive AR through early intervention. Other youngsters with slight or mild losses are not identified and/or do not receive assistance until after they start school. Indeed, some losses are progressive and reach significant dimensions only as the child gets older. One type of slight to mild loss involves middle-ear infections, which result in conductive hearing problems. Frequently, such losses are of a transient nature, but in other cases they persist over a long period and require rehabilitation assistance. These conductive problems can have an educational impact on children even if the loss is only on the order of 15 dB HL.

Since many more children are hard of hearing than are deaf, most AR work should be performed with children who are hard of hearing (although audiologic rehabilitation should not be neglected with either group). Involvement with children who are deaf may be more intensive because of the greater problems caused by the severity of the hearing loss. The child with more pronounced hearing loss tends to experience more language, speech, and educational difficulties, and more remedial efforts will, therefore, be necessary (see Table 1.2). In this chapter we describe the various types of rehabilitative efforts, without precisely distinguishing between service models for children who are deaf and those for children who are hard of hearing. Although this approach involves some loss of specificity, it is

Congenital refers to hearing loss present at birth. *Prelingual* refers to the onset of hearing loss prior to the acquisition of spoken language. *Postlingual* refers to the onset of hearing loss after spoken language has been acquired.

The individual family service plan (IFSP) is required by special education law to guide birth to age 3 services. It is developed in collaboration with the family to identify family and child strengths and needs and to outline objectives for the early intervention program.

necessary in order to avoid excessive duplication. There is, naturally, much in common in AR services regardless of the degree of hearing loss or the mode of communication used. Thus, the reader must selectively apply AR techniques consistent with the individual child's needs.

Age

If the assumption is made that children become adults somewhere between 18 and 21 years of age, graduation from high school provides a natural line of demarcation between childhood and adulthood. In that case, we may separate the years from birth to 18 into two basic divisions: those before school years (0 to 5) and the school years themselves (5 to 18). In addition, we may make a number of other subdivisions, including the years of infancy and toddlerhood (0 to 3), the preschool years (3 to 5), and the kindergarten, grade school, junior high, and high school years (5 to 18).

In this chapter, we use the two-way division (0 to 5 and school years), since children who are deaf or hard of hearing generally undergo a major adjustment of rehabilitation services when they enter regular school programming. Before that, audiologic rehabilitation includes parent–infant and preschool programs. When kindergarten begins, the school personnel will generally take over rehabilitation responsibilities from the early-intervention–preschool professional. These age ranges are general; consequently, some children progress through intervention programs more quickly than others. Services are not time locked, but sequential, depending on the child's progress.

Other Disabling Conditions

Youngsters with hearing impairment often have other disabling conditions such as visual impairments, motor disabilities, or mental retardation. The percentage is on the order of 30 to 50 percent, based on data from national surveys of young children with hearing impairment (Watkins, 2004; see also Chapters 6 and 8). Improvements in medical science have resulted in the survival of more children with multiple disabilities. This underscores the need for a multidisciplinary approach to rehabilitation in which important professionals coordinate all services to ensure integrated treatment of the child. (See Chapter 11, Case 1, for an example in working with such a youngster.)

Multidisciplinary approach involves a team of specialists from a variety of disciplines in the child's care.

■ REHABILITATION SETTINGS AND PROVIDERS

AR settings and providers are determined to a great extent by the child's age, the severity of the hearing loss, and the presence of other handicapping conditions. Typically, services start as family-centered programs in the home coordinated by a parent advisor, and progress through preschool programs up through the formal school years. Throughout the rehabilitation process, the services of many professional disciplines are called upon in addition to continued strong parental involvement. Figure 9.1 contains an overview of the AR process as it relates to the roles of clinical audiologists, educators, and medical personnel.

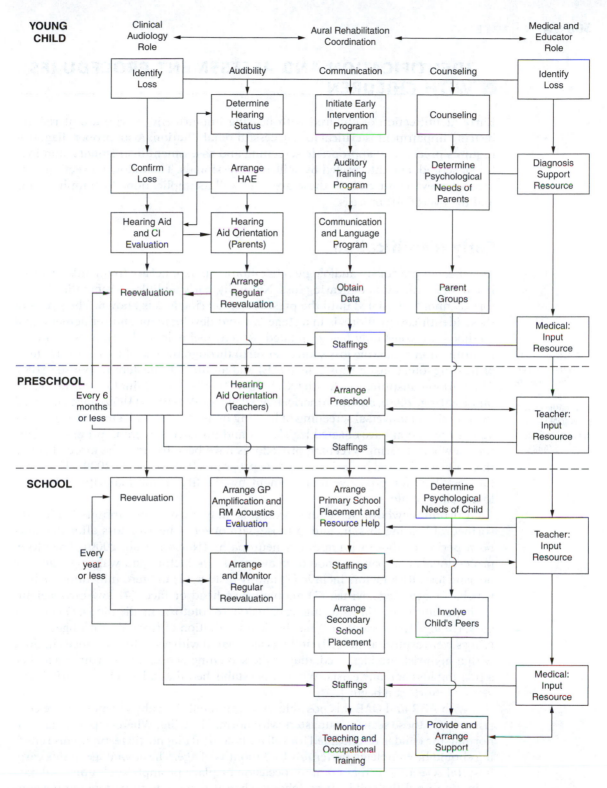

FIGURE 9.1

Overview of the AR process.

307

IDENTIFICATION AND ASSESSMENT PROCEDURES ■ WITH CHILDREN

Early identification of children with hearing impairment or who are at risk for hearing impairment is critical for successful rehabilitation. Also, proper diagnosis requires precise and appropriate screening and assessment instruments, administered, scored, and interpreted by skilled professionals. The following sections will present prevailing trends in these areas as well as implications for amplification and the overall AR process.

Early Identification

As indicated previously, audiologic rehabilitation personnel are frequently involved in early identification of hearing loss. Naturally, early audiologic rehabilitation efforts cannot be initiated until the presence of hearing loss is known. The status of these identification efforts is in a stage of rapid development and refinement, and methods are constantly being updated. Recent technological advances allow for identification of hearing loss soon after birth through the use of two objective tests of hearing, otoacoustic emissions (OAE) and auditory brainstem response (ABR). The National Institutes of Health (NIH-NIDCD) (1993), the Joint Committee on Infant Hearing (2000), and the American Academy of Pediatrics (1999) have endorsed the practice of universal screening of hearing in newborns, and a majority of states across the nation have enacted legislation and initiated screening programs. Current newborn hearing screening procedures have been found to be more effective than previously used high-risk screening programs (Norton et al., 2000). These initiatives allow for proactive management by identifying the majority of hearing losses early in life.

> Two objective tests of hearing used in early identification programs are otoacoustic emissions (OAE) and auditory brainstem response (ABR).

Current newborn screening protocols may miss some infants with sensorineural hearing loss, including those with onset of hearing loss after the newborn period or those with auditory neuropathy (Norton et al., 2000). Therefore, professionals and parents should be aware of risk factors and warning signs for hearing loss. Risk factors include (1) family history, (2) in utero infections such as rubella or cytomegalovirus, (3) anomalies of head or face, (4) low birthweight, (5) hyperbilirubinemia requiring transfusion, (6) ototoxic medications, (7) meningitis, (8) low Apgar scores, (9) mechanical ventilation of five days or longer signifying severe asphyxia, and (10) findings associated with a syndrome. Once children with a high risk are identified, diagnostic screening is used to determine whether a hearing loss actually exists. When it is established that a loss exists, early intervention efforts can begin.

With ABR and OAE it is possible to determine if the baby's responses are consistent with those seen in youngsters with normal hearing. When responses are not normal, the child is rescheduled for full audiological diagnostic testing. This retesting should be completed preferably by 3 months of age. The advantage of this early hospital screening is that no other occasion or place prompts such universal participation until the child enters school, when it is too late to be looking for congenital hearing loss.

Beyond these early screening efforts, some hearing losses in very young children are identified by physicians. Usually such identification is based upon the report of alert parents who notice that their child does not respond appropriately to sound or fails to develop speech and language at the expected time. When organized screening or high-risk programs are not available, attentive physicians and parents are the major sources for hearing-loss identification. The dimensions of the loss can subsequently be established through testing in an audiology clinic.

School Screening

Most children with severe hearing losses and some with milder losses are identified before they enter school. A number of children, however, are not identified until they reach school age. Nearly all schools in the United States conduct a pure-tone hearing screening program beginning with kindergarten children or first-graders. Although the specifics of these programs vary, a good model has been recommended by the American Speech–Language–Hearing Association (ASHA, 1997). Most children identified in school hearing-conservation programs demonstrate conductive hearing loss. The rehabilitation efforts, therefore, involve coordination with parents, medical practitioners, and teachers. Some children with previously unidentified sensorineural losses may also be identified in these school programs. In such cases, medical referral is indicated to clarify the medical aspects of the loss, followed by audiologic rehabilitation assistance provided by educational audiologists or other personnel.

Medical and Audiologic Assessment

Before audiologic rehabilitation is initiated, the child should undergo a medical examination as well as a basic hearing assessment. Complete, definitive results are not always available on very young children. When the child is old enough, results from such assessments should include information on both ears, giving (1) otoscopic findings, (2) degree and configuration of loss, (3) type of loss and cause, (4) speech (clarity of hearing) recognition ability, (5) most comfortable level (MCL), (6) threshold of discomfort (TD), and (7) hearing aid performance and audibility measures. Functional skills in the areas of academic achievement, language, and amplification systems should also be evaluated using questionnaires and audiologic procedures (Anderson & Matkin, 1996; Roush & Matkin, 1994).

Sometimes there is a tendency to omit certain aspects of testing, as, for example, speech recognition on youngsters with severe to profound losses, and sometimes there is a failure to consider hearing aid insertion gain measures at all frequencies and at varying input levels.

Medical clearance becomes necessary when decisions about amplification are made. After initial hearing aid fitting, regular assessments should take place even for children with sensorineural losses, since temporary conductive loss may occur and complicate the hearing situation, especially in young children. Audiologic data should be obtained on a regular basis so that, if necessary, amplification or other dimensions of the rehabilitation program can be changed. In the early and preschool years, children should be seen for audiologic assessment at least every six months. After that they should be clinically tested at least once a year.

School screening is important to identify children when they reach school age.

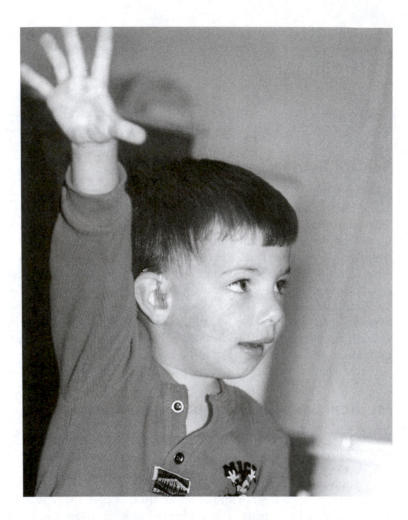

ASPECTS OF AUDIOLOGIC REHABILITATION: EARLY INTERVENTION FOR PARENT–INFANT ■ AND PRESCHOOL

Rehabilitation Assessment: IFSP

With children, the extensive rehabilitative assessments that generally precede management (see model in Chapter 1) are integrated with management more than with adult clients. Thus, we outline here an ongoing assessment approach to the audiologic rehabilitation of the young hearing-impaired child, beginning at the confirmation of the loss and continuing through the child's school years. As suggested in the AR model (Chapter 1), the rehabilitation assessment includes (1) consideration of communication status, (2) overall participation variables, including psychosocial and educational issues, (3) related personal factors, and (4) environmental conditions. An individual family service plan (IFSP), as discussed earlier, is developed using this assessment information.

Management

ENVIRONMENTAL COORDINATION AND PARTICIPATION

FAMILY-CENTERED PRACTICES: AN ASSESSMENT AND INTERVENTION FRAMEWORK. In recent years there has been an increasing appreciation for the central role family relationships play in a child's development. Many professionals contend that the young child cannot be effectively evaluated or instructed apart from the ecological system of the family. There is recognition that developmental influences are bidirectional: The infant's responses affect the family and the family's responses affect the infant. Recognition of the importance of these relationships on the child's development has led to interventions that focus on the child within the family system.

The recognition that social interaction with caregivers exerts powerful influences on infant development has led to an evolution in early intervention practices since the 1990s. Child-focused therapy models have given way to family-centered models, where the focus is on supporting family involvement, reciprocity, and decision making. When an AR clinician works with a family one or two hours a week, one cannot expect this to have a major impact on a child's development. On the other hand, if family members are empowered with the knowledge and skills to promote the infant's development, the impact can be extensive and lasting. Dunst (2001) pointed out that two hours per week is only 2 percent of a toddler's waking hours. However, diapering, feeding, and playing happen at least 2,000 times before the first birthday. If caregivers optimized just 10 interactions per waking hour in everyday activities, a toddler would have more than 36,000 learning opportunities between the ages of 1 and 2 years. This is why early intervention practices have shifted away from child-focused therapy to techniques that support quality relationships and interactions between infants and their family members. Some major principles of family-centered practice include:

1. The primary goal of early intervention is to support care providers in developing competence and confidence in helping the infant learn (Hanft, Rush, & Sheldon, 2004).
2. Family-identified needs should drive the intervention agenda, and professionals should adapt to the unique values, culture, and goals of each family.
3. Family members are recognized as the constant in the child's life and experts on the child's development. Professionals draw on the expertise of the family to address needs.
4. Families are equal team members. Professionals seek to establish balanced partnerships with family members in the intervention process.
5. Professionals respect the decision-making authority of the family.

Consistent with the concept of family-centered practice, federal legislation (Part C of IDEA) also requires the provision of early intervention services in *natural environments*. Although this term has been interpreted in a variety of ways, the intention is that infants and their families should receive services in the home or in routinely accessed community settings, rather than in clinics or center-based programs. The purpose of early intervention is to support and assist families in providing learning opportunities for their infant within the activities, routines, and events of everyday life. Parent advisors are encouraged to integrate their coaching within typical

Family-centered practice includes a focus on family-identified needs, efforts to form partnerships with parents to address child needs, and empowerment of families as the primary decision makers for their child. *Child-centered practice* refers to an intervention that provides direct service for the child, with limited direct involvement of the parent in intervention.

Natural environments are promoted in federal early intervention laws. The term is used to promote the provision of services in the home or in community settings that families routinely access.

routines and settings that comprise daily events for the family. It is believed that infants will have more opportunities to develop requisite skills if parents and other caregivers have been involved in the planning and have learned to incorporate strategies into daily routines using items that are part of their own households.

Family-centered practices and the concept of parent–professional partnerships are valuable tools to implement in response to universal newborn hearing screening programs. As a result of early screening efforts, infants are identified more than two years earlier than they were previously. This requires that the content of early intervention shift to focus on the parent–infant relationship in ways that support parent–infant attachment, bonding, and social reciprocity in communication. The professional works together with the family to promote a nurturing and responsive social and communicative environment. Some professionals prefer the term *early development*, rather than *intervention*, to characterize this work. The concept of *development* captures the joint goals of nurturing infant growth through parent–infant interaction and of supporting the growth of parenting skills. Professionals need to cultivate the skills of being sensitive and responsive to family-identified needs in order to implement such programs.

> Parent–professional partnerships involve family members collaborating with professionals to identify needs and implement strategies to encourage infant development.

EFFECTIVENESS OF EARLY INTERVENTION: FAMILY AND CHILD OUTCOMES. The primary goal of early detection and hearing intervention programs, then, is to maximize sensitive periods for language development in infancy by promoting a responsive social and communicative environment and to support family adjustment to the diagnosis. Studies suggest that several important benefits accrue when families are systematically involved in intervention.

Research has shown that interventions can influence families in the following positive ways:

1. *Reduce familial stress.* Stress can alter the emotional availability of parents and affect the caregiver style, resulting in less than optimum interactions (Bronfenbrenner, 1974). Early intervention programs have been shown to reduce the anxiety and stress parents experience following diagnosis of a child's hearing impairment (Meadow-Orlans, 1995).

2. *Support parental self-confidence.* Parent–professional partnerships, a cornerstone of family-centered practice, are designed to empower parents and build their self-confidence for parenting the child. Social support given in early intervention has significant positive effects on mothers' interaction with children who are deaf (Meadow-Orlans & Steinberg, 1993). These factors are associated with improved long-term outcomes for the child. However, Calderon, Bargones, and Sidman (1998) found that parents who had late access to intervention did not demonstrate high levels of confidence or independent understanding of ways to enhance the child's communication. This finding further supports the need for early family support programs.

3. *Promote or support responsive communicative interactions.* Calderon (2000) demonstrated the positive impact on a child's language, reading, and social skills when mothers developed effective skills for communicating with the child. Some hearing parents of deaf children are able to make intuitive adjustments to their parenting style to enhance communicative interactions with the

child (Lederberg & Prezbindowski, 2000). For others, this aspect of the program has primary importance.

Most professionals are strongly committed to the notion that early intervention is effective and essential for infants with hearing loss. However, in the past, objective documentation of the effectiveness of early intervention has been limited (see Calderon & Greenberg, 1997, for a comprehensive review of past research).

Several recent studies demonstrate that early intervention is effective in preventing or reducing the consequences of hearing loss on child language and literacy development. Some selected primary findings are the following:

1. Children who are identified prior to 6 months of age consistently outperform later-identified children on measures of language, administered through 3 years of age (Yoshinaga-Itano, Sedey, Coulter, & Mehl, 1998). Moeller (2000) found that age of enrollment in intervention was a significant predictor of vocabulary and verbal reasoning skills at 5 years of age. Children enrolled in services early (in this case, below 11 months of age) had better vocabulary and verbal reasoning skills at age 5 than their later identified counterparts.
2. In the Yoshinaga-Itano et al. (1998) study, the early identification advantage was observed regardless of a number of background variables, such as communication mode, degree of hearing loss, or socioeconomic status.
3. Children enrolled in services prior to 6 months of age, on average, showed near normal rates of language development through age 3 years, whereas later identified children showed delayed development (Yoshinaga-Itano et al., 1998).
4. Family involvement was found to be a significant contributor to child outcomes. It was concluded that children will benefit most from early identification that is paired with comprehensive interventions that actively involve families (Moeller, 2000).
5. Age of entry in intervention predicts better short- and long-term language performance, and better language performance is associated with better early reading skills and more positive social–emotional adjustment (Calderon & Naidu, 2000).
6. When mothers become actively involved as strong communication partners with their children, their children demonstrate better language development, early reading skills, and social–emotional development (Calderon, 2000).
7. For the first time ever, not only deaf infants, but children who are hard of hearing can be identified in infancy. This provides a unique research opportunity, being capitalized upon by developmental laboratories across the country. Several state EHDI programs are collaborating with the Marion Downs Center (www.colorado.edu/slhs/mdnc/) in an effort to gather outcome data following early intervention.
8. Furthermore, the advent of new technologies such as cochlear implants in infants has shaped the research agenda. Several studies have documented benefits of early implantation (i.e., 6 to 18 months) on the development of babble, auditory, and language performance (Colletti et al., 2005, Geers, Nicholas, & Sedey, 2003; Schauwers et al., 2004). It is likely that studies in progress will enhance our understanding of the features of intervention that are useful for a diverse array of infants and their families.

The implications of these collective findings are clear. Environmental influences can have a significant impact on the child's development. Alleviation of stress in the family system will contribute to positive interactions and to a healthy language environment. Rehabilitative efforts that facilitate a nurturing interaction style between parent and child are likely to have long-term positive consequences for the child. Child-centered programs that fail to address the needs of the family system are likely to be of limited success.

SHIFTING ROLES AND STRATEGIES IN THE AUDIOLOGIC REHABILITATION PROGRAM. The principles of family-centered practice require reconceptualization of professional roles. AR professionals now work with families who have very young infants; a child-focused model simply does not fit this scenario. There is work to be done to ensure that early intervention is family centered in its focus. Survey studies indicate that many programs lack substantial family participation and tend to implement child-centered approaches (Roush, Harrison, & Palsha, 1991). Furthermore, Brinker, Frazier, and Baxter (1992) stressed the need for programs to examine how family-centered care can best be approached with disadvantaged families. Knowledge of the roles and strategies for building partnerships with families is a first step in addressing these needs.

A team of experienced AR professionals (Stredler-Brown, 2005; Stredler-Brown et al., 2004) contends that there is both an art and a science to early intervention conducted in the home with families. The *science* is the special knowledge of deafness, infancy, and families that the parent-infant educator brings to the task. These skills are critical for cultivating early listening and vocal and visual behaviors in the context of responsive, reciprocal communication. On the other hand, the *art* is the human side. It has to do with how we are joining with families in a manner that conveys respect, builds trust, and establishes effective partnerships. Specialized skills AR clinicians need for serving families in the birth to age 3 period are summarized in Table 9.1 (Stredler-Brown et al., 2004). Further, analysis of the behaviors of skilled providers revealed several roles and techniques that promote collaboration with families on home visits. These were called "tools of the trade" by the authors, and they include the following:

1. *Information resource.* Although this role may be obvious, it takes skill to adapt to the learning needs of individual families, to provide information in objective ways, and to share information-gathering responsibilities, so that families become independent advocates and learners. Professionals work with families to access a variety of sources of information and experiences to build an objective information base (see Figure 9.2). This knowledge base aids families in the decision-making process. The process of timing of the information is also critical. Professionals are sensitive to the overwhelming experience of being a new parent and work to share information in manageable ways.

2. *Coach/partner role.* Coaching in this sense does not mean directing parents in their actions. Rather, it is a mindset for interaction that shifts the focus away from expert-driven ideas toward "learner-focused" techniques (Hanft et al., 2004). Adults (parents and clinicians) are the learners, but parents are in the "driver's seat," and the clinician is literally on the sidelines, providing tips or

TABLE 9.1

Specialized Knowledge and Skills Required of AR Specialists in Early Intervention

SCIENCE: SPECIALIZED KNOWLEDGE AND SKILLS	ART: SKILLS FOR INTERACTION WITH FAMILIES
• Infant development • Family systems, values, and culture • Impact of hearing loss in development • Communication, auditory, speech, and language development, and techniques for enhancing skill of parents and infants in natural contexts • Communication approaches and fluency • Amplification and listening devices • Assistive technology • Appropriate developmental expectations • Infant–family assessment skills	• Creates an atmosphere of trust, experimentation, learning from one another • Active listener who conveys understanding, empathy, acceptance • Responds to feelings, moving away from "what ought to be" • Acts as a nonjudgmental sounding board • Recognizes the role of grief in healthy adjustment • Enhances self direction/independence • Recruits and accepts parents' interpretations, advice, and predictions about infant

Contributors: A. Stredler-Brown, M. P. Moeller, R. Gallegos, P. Pittman, J. Cordwin, M. Condon.

Source: Stredler-Brown et al. (2004).

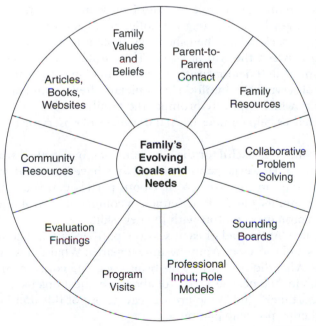

FIGURE 9.2

This model represents some of the experiences and sources of support that can be brought together in partnership with families to facilitate decision making.

guidance that supports the integration of skills by the parent. Coaching provides opportunities for family members to integrate new skills within their typical interactions with the child. The clinician uses skills of observation, well-timed input, and outcome analysis to support and guide the interaction. The box on the following page contrasts a clinician-directed response with a partnership and a coaching-oriented response.

3. *Joint discoverer.* This is a key ingredient in a partnership process. Family members learn that any question can be addressed as an "experiment" (Moeller & Condon, 1994). This prepares families to try techniques with the child and evaluate how they work. It allows clinicians to maintain balance in the relationship. Instead of telling the parent what to do (expert-driven), the idea can be proposed as an experiment (learner-focused). As an example, the clinician might observe that the parent is having trouble getting the baby's auditory attention because there is an attractive mobile captivating her imagination. The clinician can pose an experiment by asking, "I wonder what would happen if you set the mobile to the side and called her name before you start talking. I wonder if that will help her listen." This is a subtle, but important distinction. It is likely that the suggested adaptation will work, but it will be the parents who bring about the success. The role of joint discoverer also means that the AR clinician and the parents are becoming skilled observers of the child's successes and needs. The process of evaluation is integrated in each session, as this becomes the guide or road map for future sessions.

4. *News commentator* (Moeller & Condon, 1994). This technique also promotes partnership and the process of basing decisions upon ongoing evaluation of what works. The news commentator role is one of providing objective, descriptive feedback about key behaviors (e.g., "I notice that each time she vocalizes, you vocalize right back to her. Then she takes another turn. That keeps communication going between the two of you.") This strategy points out to families what is working well. It demonstrates that the clinician is figuring out what to do based on observing the family. The clinician often comments on what the child is doing, which typically prompts the family to give an interpretation. These experiences help families learn the strategy of observing to figure out what works.

5. *Partner in play.* Sometimes it is useful for the clinician to demonstrate a strategy or new skill for parents. However, parents should then have immediate opportunities to "try the skill on for size" so that both parties can see if the technique works in the parents' hands. Practicing in a context of playful interactions with the infant promotes comfort with the new skill.

6. *Joint reflector and planner.* At the end of each session, partners work together to list key observations and successes from the time together. What did we get out of today's session? What did we learn? This brings ongoing concerns into focus, and sets agendas for the next session. Collaborative questions like, "So what should we do next time?" and "Who are we leaving out of this and how will we share it with them?" promote planning.

One of the most dramatic role shifts occurring in audiologic rehabilitation as a result of family-centered practice goals is that decision-making authority is to rest

Advantages of Partnership or Coaching Approach

Clinician-Directed	Partnership Approach	Advantage of Partnership
"When your baby wakes up in the morning, be sure you test the battery, check the hearing aids, and put them in right away."	"Tell me about your early morning routine with the baby. What do you think might work best for putting the hearing aids in?"	Conveys to parents that the clinician recognizes and values their expertise. Best strategies can be negotiated by first considering the parental observations.
Clinician-Directed	**Coaching Approach**	**Advantage of Coaching**
"I need you to pull that toy into her line of vision and then use the name for it."	"What happens when you pull that toy into her line of vision?" "Oh, she looks right at you." "Right, face-to-face communication is a good time to use the word."	The clinician-directed example leaves the professional in the role of expert. In the Coaching example, the same idea is posed as a question or experiment, and the parent is the one who is successful with the technique.

with family members. Professionals are challenged to help parents gain the skills and knowledge to be effective advocates and decision makers for their child. Previously, professionals made many of the decisions regarding the habilitative management of the child. Now professionals are being challenged to work as partners with families in assessment, management, and decision making. So, for example, in the parent advisor–family partnership, the parent advisor relies on family members to direct the thrust of the services. The young child's needs are expressed as part of the family's concerns. Family members know the child's likes, dislikes, time schedules, favorite toys and activities, food preferences, and many other matters that the parent advisor can't be expected to know. One mother stated, "The advisor I worked with was wise enough to know that no one knows my child better than I do. She respected my suggestions and opinions as much as I respected hers" (Glover et al., 1994, p. 323). Being understanding of the family's cultural values and practices enhances the partnership. As the parent advisor–family partnership develops and as respect and trust mature, the parent advisor has the opportunity to help family members explore their feelings, clarify their concerns and desires for the child, and see and appreciate the child's unique skills and strengths. Other examples of collaborative decision making with parents are contained in Chapter 11 (see Case 2).

> Professionals need to shift their traditional roles and ensure that families are placed in the role of primary decision makers for the child.

A second major shift in service delivery influences the teamwork roles of the AR clinician. In order to meet comprehensive family and child needs, professionals must employ transdisciplinary teamwork. No one discipline has all the knowledge and expertise to adequately address the comprehensive nature of most cases. The AR clinician in a parent advisor role has a particularly critical role on the team. Because the parent advisor has frequent contact with the family in their home (e.g., one to two times per week), this professional is often in a good position to gain a full understanding of the family's strengths and priorities, and to work with the parent to

> Transdisciplinary teamwork refers to a process in which team members collaborate and are interdependent. Rather than each member separately working with the child and sharing viewpoints, team members work together and integrate their perspectives.

> ### Parent Perspectives on Early Intervention Teams as Told in SKI-HI Parent Interviews and Team Surveys, 1995–1998
>
> A good team is "a lifesaver if it works right. Team members have training in areas that I need their help in, but I know my child best. . . . I think a team can be a lifeline when you are feeling so helpless for a little while and frightened."
>
> "There needs to be more correlation in services . . . each service provider tends to come in and do their own thing. I could use more help in coordination as it is difficult for a parent to coordinate all of the services."
>
> Asked if parents feel listened to or heard, one parent said, "No! Team members need to ask us as parents what our goals are for our child."
>
> "Usually team members ask me as the parent which would be best for my child and family if there is a difference of opinion. We then proceed in the direction that I think is best."
>
> *Source:* Glover, B. (1999). *Working Together on Early Intervention Teams* (pp. 13–14, 42, 48, 60). Used with permission.

implement strategies to achieve these priorities. The parent advisor may also serve in a role of case coordination with the assistance of a services coordinator.

The parent advisor–AR clinician can and should draw upon the resources of a community-based team of professionals, depending on the needs that present themselves. Parent advisors need to cultivate the skills for collaborative consultation and teamwork in order to effectively serve families. Idol, Paolucci-Whitcomb, and Nevin (1986) state, "Collaborative consultation is an interactive process that enables teams of people with diverse expertise to generate creative solutions to mutually defined problems. The outcome is enhanced and altered from the original solutions that any team member would produce independently" (p. 9).

> *Collaborative consultation comes about when team members contribute diverse expertise to creatively solve intervention problems.*

SUPPORTING FAMILIES IN DECISION MAKING. Newborn hearing screening has brought about a paradigm shift in the ways AR clinicians and educators work with families. In earlier decades, parents may have noted their child's lack of or inconsistent responses to sound. When hearing loss was diagnosed, this news was difficult, but also confirmed the parents' suspicions in many cases. Today, hospital personnel or audiologists are telling parents of newborns, who have no reason to suspect a problem, that there may be a hearing loss. This information is delivered at a time of tremendous personal adjustment (to the birth of a baby). Luterman (2004) states, "This presents a very different counseling paradigm than the parent-initiated model where the audiologist is often seen as an ally confirming that parent's suspicion." He advocates for increased training in counseling in the preparation of audiologists/AR professionals.

Upon diagnosis of hearing loss, families are met with a host of decisions about communicating with the infant, about technologies, about educational programs, and about parenting this baby in the context of the family. At a consensus conference on early intervention for infants who are deaf and hard of hearing (Marge & Marge, 2005), professionals unanimously agreed that parents should have access to objective information about all communication, technological, and educational options for the child. Few would disagree with this notion. However, much is to be learned about best ways to provide this information to families who are in the process of adjusting to the birth of a new baby. In some cases, programs provide written brochures explaining various options. In other cases, families have opportunities to meet with other parents, visit programs, search the Internet, etc. In reality, each family should have an approach that is tailored to its individual needs. This requires of the AR professional both sensitivity and the establishment of effective partnerships with families.

Decision making is not a reading activity—it is a *process*. Within that process, family members (1) get to know their infant as well as the infant's special needs, (2) become skilled at observing the baby and figuring out what strategies are successful for making communication connections in the family, (3) clarify the goals they have for themselves and their child, (4) have opportunities for parent-to-parent contact and support, and (5) and learn about various options in education, technology, and communication. This entire process typically does not happen in the few weeks after diagnosis. For many families, the process unfolds over several months, and opinions about what to do change as the family gains relevant experiences, support, and knowledge. It is important to recognize that the "learning about options part" is one of five steps! It is not sufficient to give parents reading materials and ask that they decide. Instead, families benefit from a variety of supports and experiences as they make decisions for the infant. The role of the AR professionals is to help families clarify which supports may be helpful at different times and to assist families in accessing these. Some possible sources of support and information are visualized in Figure 9.2. This could be thought of as a puzzle. The pieces that will fit

---

Perspectives of Professionals on Early Intervention Teams as Told in SKI-HI Professional Interviews and Team Surveys, 1995–1998

"It is a new concept for some people. But, I think once people participate on a team they will realize how it works to benefit families. On our team we write a group report of the assessment instead of everybody writing a separate report. We gather the information that everybody has, then we take turns writing the report. . . . This makes it a lot easier and less fragmented for family members."

"It was very difficult at first because team members were holding their own ground and not wanting to share information with other team members. It is not like that now. . . ."

"I think that the families I work with are not as overwhelmed as they used to be. Before, there were lots of different service providers coming in at different times to work on different things with their child. Now we are coordinating our goals, and we look at service for the child in a holistic approach with the service coordinator directing the activities that are carried out with the child and family."

Source: Glover, B. (1999). *Working Together on Early Intervention Teams* (pp. 17, 18, 70). Used with permission.

together to make a whole picture will be unique for each individual family. The AR clinician seeks to be a facilitator and sounding board as the family builds its system of supports.

A parent organization in Colorado, called Hands and Voices, provides perspectives and information that are helpful to parents and professionals alike (see www.handsandvoices.org). They acknowledge that making choices for the child is a process that is flexible, ongoing, and changeable. Many families do not make "one choice" on their communication journey with the child. They often adapt and choose a variety of tools and approaches as the child's needs evolve. DesGeorges (2004) published a "wish list" from parents for audiologists that supports many of the points raised so far. Selected excerpts include:

PARENT WISH LIST FOR AUDIOLOGISTS

- Provide us with the information we need to make well-informed decisions.
- If we ask a question and you don't have the answer, help us find the resources where we can find the answer.
- Be connected to community resources.
- As children and parents grow, their choices and need for information grow and change.
- Respect the choices that families make. Let us, the parents, make the final decision. (DesGeorges, 2004)

An aspect of decision making that sometimes gets overlooked concerns the resources within the family system to support the communication or technology approach. Families should not only understand options from an objective viewpoint, they also should consider what the particular approach will require of them as a family. This type of information is covered in program materials from *Beginnings for Families* (www.beginningssvcs.com). Current options for communication are described along with family responsibilities that come along with the approach. Such information is another helpful piece of the puzzle.

IMPLICATIONS OF FAMILY-CENTERED CARE FOR INTERVENTION. Family-centered parent–infant programs, then, focus on family members as the primary interventionists. The audiologic rehabilitation specialist provides guidance and coaching to the family in several key content areas: (1) fitting and adjustment of amplification and assistive devices; (2) auditory learning (use of residual hearing); and (3) techniques for optimizing communicative development (speech, language, signing, cognitive, and preliteracy skills). Another vital content area for the program is helping the family meet its support needs and providing activities that promote psychosocial well-being. Once the child is of preschool age (around 3 years old), services typically shift to center-based models where the child attends a preschool or individual auditory–verbal sessions. These services are commonly provided in a regular preschool setting with support services, a setting that integrates children who are typically developing with those who have hearing loss, or a self-contained preschool for deaf or hard of hearing children. Wherever the service delivery or whatever the model, family-centered practices continue to be vital. Families learn at the parent–infant level to be knowledgeable advocates for their children. They become intricately involved in influencing the child's success. It would be a mistake to "graduate" the child into a center-based program and minimize the contributions family members can make. Instead, programs should continue to address family needs, family support, and family guidance into the preschool years. In the next sections we describe approaches in each of the key content areas at the parent–infant and preschool levels.

AUDIBILITY, AMPLIFICATION, AND ASSISTIVE DEVICE ISSUES

HEARING AID FITTING. Once preliminary medical and audiologic findings are available on the child, the selection of amplification, when appropriate, becomes an early goal in the rehabilitative program. Experts agree that hearing aids are extremely important tools in early-intervention programs in helping children develop their residual hearing and their speech and language abilities. Unfortunately, as previously noted, many youngsters with hearing impairment do not typically use amplification. Consequently, the efforts of the audiologic rehabilitationist may need to be directed toward achieving that goal. The hearing aid fitting will be performed by an audiologist who may also be providing other rehabilitative services (see Figure 9.1). If the AR therapist does not perform the fitting, he or she will want to review its adequacy. In recent years, the focus in fitting children has been to move away from procedures based on threshold to those focusing more on how the amplified speech range fits into the child's usable hearing range. The Desired Sensation Level (DSL) method is an example of this latter approach and is reviewed in Chapter 2. Many important considerations in fitting hearing aids in children are contained in a Pediatric Amplification Protocol (AAA, 2003). Although hearing aid fitting is a first priority, other assistive amplification devices should also be considered.

> Desired sensation level (DSL) is a computer-based method of determining a child's usable hearing with amplification.

Pediatric and school-age amplification should focus on personal amplification devices but not exclude personal or classroom FM systems and other assistive listening devices. Fitting protocols should include ongoing evaluation, verification, and validation of the child's performance with all devices. Evaluation should be used to confirm and monitor actual or fluctuating hearing levels. Verification of the devices' appropriateness can be completed using real ear measures such as real ear to coupler difference and speech mapping. Validation of performance should include measures that document whether the child has access to the speech of others and is able to clearly monitor his or her own speech. All measures should be completed with consideration of the ever-changing auditory needs of preschool and school-age children. Functional assessment measures such as checklists and questionnaires can be used to validate and document individual performance in individual and natural listening environments. Parents and teachers can provide valuable input using some of these instruments, which are designed for use by individuals in the child's life. A review of these tools can be found in the Pediatric Amplification Protocol (AAA, 2003), and specific tools can be accessed on the text website.

> In addition to hearing aids, assistive listening devices like FM systems for use in noisy environments (e.g., classrooms) should be considered.

TYPE AND ARRANGEMENT OF AID. The type of aid and the arrangement (monaural, binaural, or other special fitting, such as a direct input feature or integrated FM capability) need careful attention and review in the AR process. Behind the ear (BTE) aids are used by most children from infancy through the teenage years (Bentler, 1993). Some children, especially teenagers, use in-the-ear or -canal aids. While requiring special adjustment, these are feasible for use by certain individuals. (See a discussion of various hearing aid issues in Chapter 2, which covers hearing aid fitting procedures.) From a rehabilitative standpoint, binaural fittings are nearly always the rule, since children with hearing impairment require every educational advantage possible. Unfortunately, the minority of hearing-impaired children with bilateral losses are using binaural aids. Various reports place this minority at somewhere between 20 and 40 percent (Bentler, 1993). Even after a careful analysis to eliminate the children with bilateral losses who were not candidates for a second aid, Matkin (1984) found that only 38 percent of the children who could use two aids were doing so. In some settings, the use of aids by children is excellent, as in one local school district where 22 of the 23 children are properly fitted. But all settings do not have such excellent services.

> Cochlear implants may be considered for children with deafness who have received limited benefit from hearing aids.

If children are found to have little usable residual hearing or serious progressive loss, cochlear implants may be considered (see Chapter 3). Promising results with children who have been implanted are leading to an increased use of these implants, which have now been used on well over 15,000 U.S. children since the FDA approved such use beginning in June 1990. Implant device surgery is very expensive, and when children are implanted, extensive audiologic rehabilitation follow-up is needed. When needed, implants can be placed by age 1.

HEARING AID FEATURES

1. *Earmold fit and gain setting of aid.* With very young or fast-growing children, the earmold will need to be changed frequently to ensure a well-fitting mold and to provide adequate gain without feedback even though feedback is less of a problem now with the new technology. Turning the gain down will help eliminate the feedback, but it is an unacceptable long-term solution. The therapist should not rely entirely on the clinical audiologist or the dispenser for this assessment, but should personally monitor the earmold condition on each rehabilitation visit. In some situations, the audiologic rehabilitationist is trained to make ear impressions. This can be a valuable asset to the program, especially considering the frequency of mold changes in an adequate program (see Table 9.2).

2. *Real-ear measures.* Precise information on aided results can be obtained with real-ear measures, which provide accurate and complete information (see Chapter 2). They make it possible to evaluate benefit from the aids thoroughly without requiring more than passive cooperation from the the child.

3. *Electroacoustic assessment of aid.* An electroacoustic check of a hearing aid should provide information on the frequency response, the gain, the OSPL, and the distortion of the instrument (see Chapter 2 for a description of this process). These data can help uncover inadequacies in the amplification that can otherwise be devastating to the child's progress in the rehabilitation program. Electroacoustic checks are particularly helpful in the case of distortions, which are not found in the real-ear tests, and when biologic listening checks do not reveal a distortion problem.

4. *Six-sound test of aid.* In connection with hearing-aid adjustment, it may be helpful for the AR therapist to use the six-sound test described by Ling (1989). According to Ling, the sounds /u/, /a/, /i/, /ʃ/, /s/, and /m/ can be used to determine the effectiveness of an aid. With the infant, visually reinforced audiometry can be used

TABLE 9.2

Average Months per Set of Earmolds for Children Whose Molds Were Replaced at the First Evidence of Feedback Difficulty[a]

	Average Months per Mold	
DEGREE OF LOSS (dB)	<2½-YEAR-OLD CHILD (N = 25)	2½- TO 5-YEAR-OLD CHILD (N = 27)
Mild (30–55)	3.0	5.2
Moderate (56–75)	2.7	4.1
Severe (76–90)	2.5	5.6
Profound (91–110)	2.0	4.6

[a]Also included are average loss and gain values for children in total project (N = 52) with properly fitting molds. Mean loss pure-tone average (PTA), 75 dB; mean aided loss, 44 dB; mean gain, 31 dB.

Source: Reprinted by permission: SKI-HI data.

to determine if the child can hear these sounds. Older children can simply indicate they hear the sounds by imitating or giving a detection response.

HEARING INSTRUMENT ORIENTATION. It is helpful for parents, teachers, and other involved professionals to be knowledgeable about hearing aids or cochlear implants so that they can help monitor use. This information can be provided in home visits, in clinic counseling sessions, in parent groups, and through inservice training in the school setting. (See suggestions in Chapters 3 and 10.)

The benefit of these devices may not be readily obvious to parents or teachers, especially in cases where auditory communication is minimal. The purposes of the device may include some or all of the following: verbal communication, signal or warning function, and environmental awareness. Parents must recognize why their child is wearing the device, since with younger children, parents have the major responsibility for maintaining them and ensuring that they are used regularly. If parents understand hearing aids, they will be encouraged to help their child form good habits of use.

These devices will be more acceptable to the child when they function properly, but the procedures for obtaining accessories, repairs, or loaners will vary with local conditions. The AR provider should be aware of these conditions in order to be an effective resource person.

REMEDIATION OF COMMUNICATION ACTIVITY

AUDITORY LEARNING: PARENT–INFANT AND PRESCHOOL LEVELS. There are many natural opportunities in the home setting for exposing the child to sound. Once the child is fitted with appropriate amplification, the parents and clinician work to provide meaningful and frequent auditory experiences to encourage the child to rely on his or her residual hearing. For many children, systematic introduction to sounds during the early years will have a positive impact on language learning. Effective

Auditory learning activities for infants should focus on observing and promoting natural listening opportunities throughout natural daily routines.

stimulation of residual hearing is critical to the development of spoken communication. Early auditory learning training should consist of observing and promoting the child's listening experiences in many meaningful daily activities. As Marlowe (1984) recommended, the clinician should "stress listening to people sounds rather than environmental sounds unless the latter are incorporated in meaningful experiences" (p. 6).

A variety of materials have been developed that describe auditory skill development. Erber (1982) developed a particularly useful model that distinguishes between levels of detection, discrimination, identification, and comprehension (a complete discussion of Erber's model is contained in Chapter 4). In addition, other auditory skills such as hearing at a distance or localization are also part of the child's auditory development. Both of these are important as part of diagnostic/functional assessments and may occasionally be incorporated in AR therapy. These two skills are shown along with the four developmental stages suggested by Erber in Table 9.3.

Koch (1999) applies Erber's classic model in an approach to auditory development that integrates listening, producing speech, and developing language concepts. In each AR session, she includes four basic components of listening therapy: (1) auditory attention, (2) perception/production, (3) sound/object association, and (4) language and listening integration (Table 9.4). The first component (auditory attention) is comparable to Erber's level 1 in Table 9.3. The goal of training at this level is to develop a child's ability to spontaneously alert to the presence of speech and environmental sounds. It also provides the clinician an opportunity to determine if the child is responding to amplification devices in his or her usual manner. Koch's second component (perception/production) involves the child's actively listening through audition alone and imitating the spoken model. Such activities incorporate elements of Erber's concepts of discrimination and identification (levels 4 and 5 in Table 9.3). The goal is to provide systematic and frequent opportunities for a child to discover the connection between speech/phoneme perception and production. The third therapy component (word/object association) incorporates elements covered by item 5 in Table 9.3. The clinician presents closed set listening tasks that are strategically adapted to challenge the child. Factors that are adjusted include content and presentation. For example, the clinician adjusts the content by manipulating: (1) the familiarity of the language (e.g., *cat* vs. *kangaroo*), (2) the set size (three vs. six vs. twelve items), (3) the acoustic contrast (*pea/banana* vs. *pea/bee*), and (4) the number of critical elements of meaning (*hat* vs. *soft striped hat*). Presentation can be adjusted by manipulating the following factors: (1) speaking rate, (2) use of acoustic highlighting (*Can you find the CAR?*), (3) number of repetitions provided, and (4) use of visual cues. Koch's fourth component of each AR session involves embedding the listening skills into natural communication activities to promote carryover of listening and learning in daily routines. This component, called language and listening integration, incorporates Erber's concept of comprehension (level 6 in Table 9.3). Activities are designed to challenge the child's listening in the context of a natural conversation or language lesson. By systematically incorporating all four components, children are challenged to work on perceptual skills and to immediately apply these skills in a conversational context.

TABLE 9.3

Auditory Skill Development Sequence

AUDITORY SKILLS	CHILD'S BEHAVIOR	STIMULATION SKILLS
1. Auditory awareness (detection) and attending	Child learns to spontaneously alert to meaningful environmental sounds and speech; child selectively attends to speech.	Encourage parent to use child's name to get his or her attention. Draw child's attention to meaningful sounds in the environment (e.g., "I hear the phone. . . . Oh listen, that's the microwave. . . . Listen, Daddy is calling your name").
2. Listening from a distance	Child responds to sounds from increasing distance and at various locations.	This skill can be incorporated whenever working on awareness; simply present the meaningful stimulus from greater distance. This helps children strengthen selective attention to auditory signals/speech.
3. Locating	Child searches for or locates sound or vocal sources in the environment. Localization skills help child associate sound sources with their meanings.	Create natural opportunities for child to search for the source of sound. Involve children in "hide-and-seek" games in the home, where mom or dad call the child, and the child searches to find the parent.
4. Discrimination	Child perceives similarities and differences between two or more sounds/words. Child learns to respond when he notices that a sound is different or has changed.	Play peek-a-boo with the family and young child. Encourage child to listen to familiar expressions (Where's Joey? Where's Joey?) and respond only when the sound changes (e.g., "Peek-a-boo"—child pulls blanket down). Encourage parents to play motor games where family members move slowly to a slow stimulus (walk-walk-walk) and rapidly to a fast one (hippity hop). When children are older, same/different tasks can be used to clarify identification or comprehension errors ("Listen, are cat/sat the same or different?").
5. Identification	Child can reliably associate a sound with its source and eventually name it (That's the telephone). Child is able to label words heard by imitating or pointing to objects/pictures.	In early stages, children play games that develop association between high-contrast sounds (beep-beep; uuuuuuuup) with familiar toys (car vs. airplane). As the child's skills develop, clinician and family present finer contrasts in the words presented during naturalistic activities. While sitting in mom's lap, the child finds pictures that she names in the storybook. Dad says familiar nursery rhyme (Itsy Bitsy Spider) and the child uses the associated gestures.
6. Comprehension	Child understands the meaning of spoken language by answering a question, following a direction, making an inference or joining in a conversation.	Family is guided to give children opportunities to listen and respond to cognitively challenging questions (e.g., "The airplane goes up. What else goes up?"). Emphasis is placed on strengthening attention and remembering (e.g., listening to a simple story and being expected to "tell it in your own words" or act it out with toys). Family members help children listen and relate information in books to their own experiences (e.g., "The bumble bee is frustrated. Can you remember a time when you were frustrated?")

Many new curricular guides are available for promoting auditory learning in infants and young children who are deaf or hard of hearing. Although many have been developed to address the needs of children with cochlear implants, the strategies have broad application for children with hearing aids as well. A few excellent examples include the following:

- *Bringing Sound to Life* (Koch, 1999). Videotape and guidebooks for developing an integrated approach listening and language development using auditory–verbal methods (see Table 9.4 for an outline of the therapy components that Koch includes in each AR session to promote an integration of language, speech and listening skills).
- *My Baby and Me: A Book about Teaching Your Child to Talk* (Moog-Brooks, 2002). A family friendly, highly readable guide for families about encouraging development of listening and talking.
- *Listening Games for Littles* (Sindrey, 1997). Specific auditory–verbal activities for developing language-based listening skills in infants and young children.
- *Listen, Learn and Talk* (Cochlear Corp., 2003). Videotapes and guidebook written to encourage parents in their roles of daily auditory and language stimulation for the infant.
- *Auditory Speech and Language (AuSpLan)*. McClatchie and Therres (2004) have developed a manual for professionals working with children who have cochlear implants or amplification. This is a valuable resource for evaluating and guiding auditory progress.
- *SKI-HI Curriculum* (Watkins, 2004). This curriculum has been used for many years by early intervention programs to guide their work in families in a number of developmental areas, including listening. This resource was recently updated and has a wealth of resources for working with families.

Teachers and clinicians in the preschool setting can also take advantage of natural opportunities to encourage the children to rely on their residual hearing. It is common for clinicians in preschool settings to integrate auditory challenges throughout curriculum lessons. Rather than specifying a "listening lesson" or "lis-

---

TABLE 9.4

Four Basic Components of Auditory Rehabilitation Sessions for Children

- **Auditory Attention:** The development of auditory awareness and the ability to attend to various environmental sounds.
- **Syllable Approximation:** The ability to imitate what is heard through the integration of speech perception and speech production.
- **Sound-Object Association:** The development of a connection between what is heard and what it represents.
- **Listening and Language Integration:** The integration of auditory skills as a foundation for understanding and processing new information through spoken language.

Source: Koch (1999).

tening time," clinicians integrate auditory learning as a process that pervades all activities. This can be challenging in a total communication program, where the focus is on visual learning. Clinicians in TC settings need to make a conscious effort to provide realistic auditory challenges to the child that support other communicative goals. Erber's (1982) concept of adaptive auditory skill development is very useful at the preschool level. This concept implies that a clinician constantly is monitoring a child's level of success with a particular auditory contrast or task, and adjusting the task as necessary to bring about successive approximation to the goal.

It is important for AR clinicians to fit auditory skill development within a conceptual model of speech and language learning. For many children with hearing loss, the auditory channel is viable for language learning, given appropriate amplification and stimulation. Boothroyd (1982) and Ling (1976) stress the primacy of the auditory channel for speech and language learning. Throughout the course of development, the AR clinician should closely integrate listening goals with those of speech and language learning. For example, a preschool child learning to discriminate temporal patterns should also be working on production of the appropriate number of syllables in simple word approximations. The child learning to detect sounds should have opportunities to answer in a socially appropriate manner when his or her name is called. A child with residual hearing benefits from auditory-based correction when a speech error is made. Ling (1976) stresses the importance of helping the child establish an auditory feedback loop. That is, auditory skills need to develop to the point where the child can self-monitor his or her speech productions through audition. These goals are realistic for many children with appropriate amplification. Language, audition, and phonological acquisition are intricately related processes, that should be addressed in an integrated fashion. Rather than "auditory training," the notion is "auditory learning" or "auditory communication." For some children, progress toward auditory goals will be slow, due to limitations of residual hearing. Alternative sensory communication devices may be considered by the team in these cases.

Documentation of learning rates in audition is useful in selecting intervention approaches and in ascertaining the need for additional sensory aids. Several tools have been developed to assist AR clinicians in monitoring auditory development in infants and young children. Some selected examples follow.

- *Auditory-Verbal Ages and Stages of Development* (Estabrooks, 1998a)
- *Early Listening Function* (ELF) (Anderson, 2003)
- *Listening Skills Scale for Kids with Cochlear Implants* (Estabrooks, 1998b)
- *Infant-Toddler Meaningful Auditory Integration Scale* (Robbins, Zimmerman-Phillips, & Osberger, 1998)
- *Early Speech Perception Test* (Moog & Geers, 1990)

COMMUNICATION AND LANGUAGE STIMULATION: PARENT–INFANT. At the same time that auditory skill development is being initiated in the home, the clinician helps parents build upon their communication strategies with the child. Effective interaction between parent and child is fundamental to the process of language acquisition. The communicative interaction between the child and family members is a primary focus of parent–infant rehabilitation.

> Adaptive auditory skill development refers to the continual monitoring of a child's responses and adjustment of the level of difficulty of the task to bring about success or further challenge.

When parents and professionals team together in a partnership, intervention can proceed in a fashion of joint discovery (Moeller & Condon, 1994). During home intervention sessions, family members engage the infant in stimulating routines, and the parent and clinician actively monitor the child's responses and adjust techniques as necessary. Family members also receive guidance, information, and support during home visits. Components of a home-based program are shown in Figure 9.3.

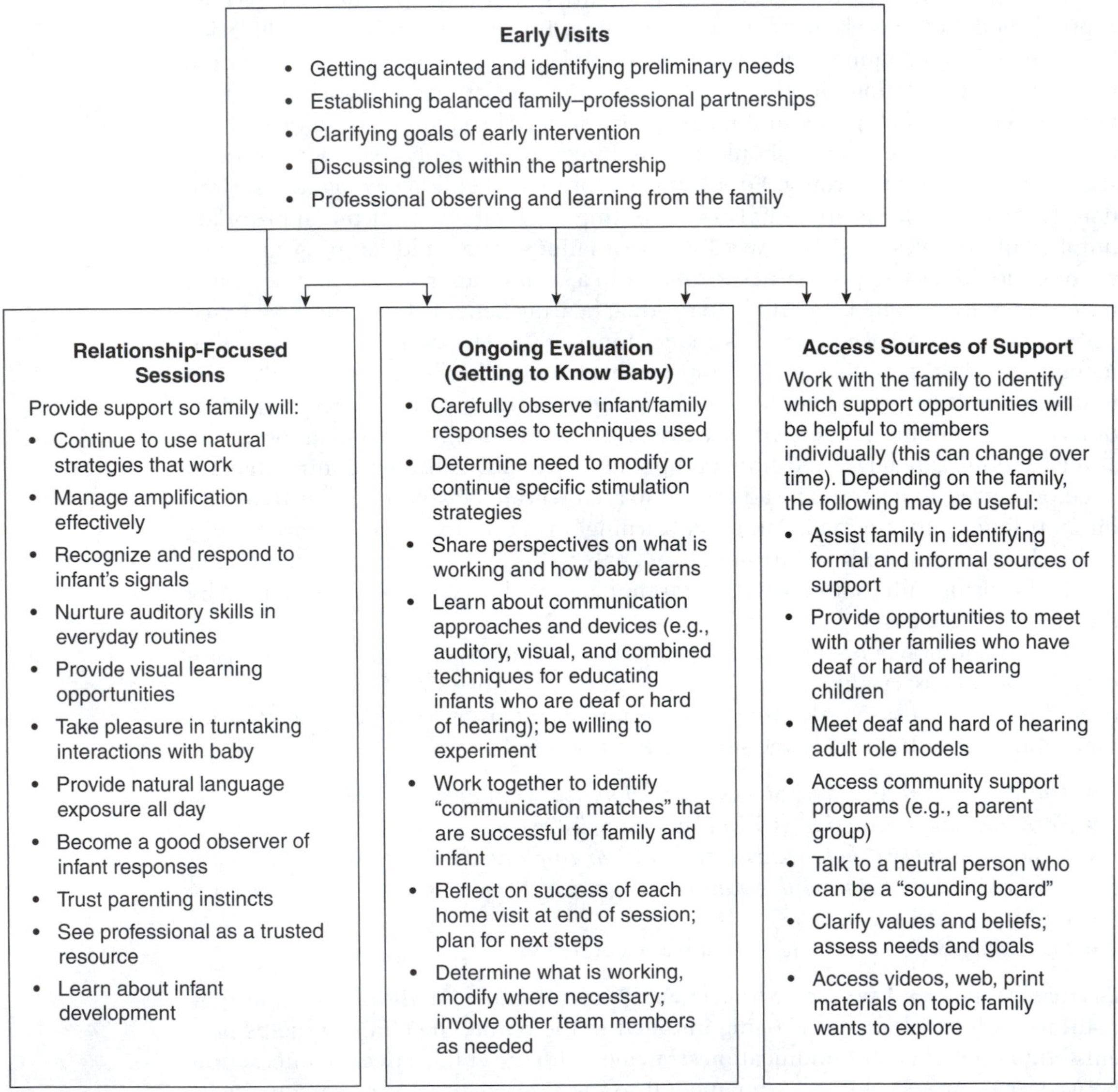

Early Visits
- Getting acquainted and identifying preliminary needs
- Establishing balanced family–professional partnerships
- Clarifying goals of early intervention
- Discussing roles within the partnership
- Professional observing and learning from the family

Relationship-Focused Sessions

Provide support so family will:
- Continue to use natural strategies that work
- Manage amplification effectively
- Recognize and respond to infant's signals
- Nurture auditory skills in everyday routines
- Provide visual learning opportunities
- Take pleasure in turntaking interactions with baby
- Provide natural language exposure all day
- Become a good observer of infant responses
- Trust parenting instincts
- See professional as a trusted resource
- Learn about infant development

Ongoing Evaluation (Getting to Know Baby)
- Carefully observe infant/family responses to techniques used
- Determine need to modify or continue specific stimulation strategies
- Share perspectives on what is working and how baby learns
- Learn about communication approaches and devices (e.g., auditory, visual, and combined techniques for educating infants who are deaf or hard of hearing); be willing to experiment
- Work together to identify "communication matches" that are successful for family and infant
- Reflect on success of each home visit at end of session; plan for next steps
- Determine what is working, modify where necessary; involve other team members as needed

Access Sources of Support

Work with the family to identify which support opportunities will be helpful to members individually (this can change over time). Depending on the family, the following may be useful:
- Assist family in identifying formal and informal sources of support
- Provide opportunities to meet with other families who have deaf or hard of hearing children
- Meet deaf and hard of hearing adult role models
- Access community support programs (e.g., a parent group)
- Talk to a neutral person who can be a "sounding board"
- Clarify values and beliefs; assess needs and goals
- Access videos, web, print materials on topic family wants to explore

FIGURE 9.3

Model showing major components of a home-based early intervention program.

An outstanding curriculum guide for working with families was developed by Karen Rossi, long-time parent–infant educator and Director of the Omaha Hearing School. The program, entitled *Learning to Talk Around the Clock,* is intended to guide the content of home visits conducted in natural settings. Rossi (2003) identified *Signature Behaviors* in language and listening that foster the development of spoken language. Signature behaviors represent a hierarchy of skills parents can master to provide a language-rich environment for the child. The program includes thematically based lesson ideas and educational handouts for parents. Principles of family-centered practice are integrated throughout this developmentally appropriate material. It provides substantive direction for guiding families in a coaching-based approach.

When the home is the primary intervention setting, the parent advisor and parent use the natural environment and daily events as the milieu for teaching. As much as possible, parents, siblings, and other significant persons in the child's life are encouraged to be "in the driver's seat" in the intervention sessions. Instead of bringing an adult-directed lesson plan with demonstration activities, the parent advisor and parent take advantage of natural interaction situations to practice the provision of nurturing input for the child. For example, a parent advisor might take advantage of the siblings' affinity for a "ring around the rosy" game to emphasize the skill of sound detection for the deaf toddler. A toddler's feeding time can become an ideal time for reinforcing prelinguistic communicative signals and strengthening turntaking. Bedtime storybook sharing is one of many natural opportunities to contribute to the infant's or toddler's literacy development (Watkins, 1999). Reinforcing toddler games and toys available in the home can also be introduced to encourage language and thinking, but they should not be the primary focus. Parents are supported when language and auditory intervention schemes can fit into the rhythm and habits of their daily lives. Parents may need help to discover that it is their "all-day-long" routine interactions with the child that build language skills (Simmons-Martin & Rossi, 1990), not structured "sit-down" therapy activities. Language and auditory intervention strategies need to fit within the context of natural positive parenting.

> Language and auditory development techniques need to be incorporated into natural parenting routines.

A primary focus of the intervention program is promoting nurturing and effective interactions between the parents and the infant. Although mothers of children who are deaf have been described as being overly controlling in interactions with their children, there are many examples in clinical practice of parents who interact in highly facilitative ways with their infants who are deaf and hard of hearing. Perhaps family-centered practices will result in different characterizations of maternal and paternal styles. Some parents will need direct guidance to develop facilitative styles with their infants. However, the parent advisor should not assume this to be the case. There may be many strengths that can be built upon in the parent–child interaction.

During home intervention sessions, the parents and parent advisor work together to implement nondirective language stimulation approaches. Some primary techniques include:

1. Ensuring that family members recognize the infant or toddler's prelinguistic communication signals (e.g., gestures, vocalizations, eye gaze, cries, points, etc.).

2. Helping parents interpret communication signals as conversational "turns" and then provide semantically appropriate responses, such as comments or expansions. For example, if the child reaches for the bottle and vocalizes, does the parent recognize that this was a complex signal? How does the parent respond? Optimally, the parent will interpret the child's intention and put the child's idea into words (e.g., "Oh, you want more milk. Here's your bottle.").

3. Facilitating the establishment of conversational turntaking between primary interactants and the child. Are family members following the child's interest and conversational lead? How does the child respond when family members follow his or her lead? What activities promote extended turntaking?

4. Helping parents consider the need to contrive developmentally appropriate opportunities for the child to respond to auditory stimuli in the environment. When the child responds to meaningful sounds, how does the family react? Do they comment on the child's observation and give the sound a name? Do they take the child to the sound and reinforce that it is the source of the sound?

5. Guiding the parents in taking advantage of everyday occurrences to expose the child to relevant language concepts. What language concepts occur naturally and are of interest to the child? What is the child curious about? Primary language targets become evident from observing typical interactions and also from following the child's interest lead.

6. Guiding family members to provide the words for what a child is trying to express. This involves helping family members to be accurate interpreters of the child's message and then providing the verbal model for that message.

7. Helping family members develop positive ways to secure and maintain the child's visual attention. Joint attention on objects is positively correlated with vocabulary acquisition in young children. Some evidence suggests that hearing mothers may not always use the most facilitative strategies for securing joint attention on objects. Deaf mothers of children who are deaf have been observed to implement effective strategies in this regard. Further study of approaches by parents who are deaf would provide useful input for working with parents with normal hearing.

8. Helping family members use parallel talk strategies that describe what the child is doing, seeing, or thinking while experiencing an event.

9. Guiding parents in strategies for encouraging cognitive and sensorimotor play skills within communicative routines. Parents should learn to encourage the early pretend skills of the toddler, mapping language onto these accomplishments.

A comprehensive summary of methods for establishing effective parent–child communication is included in Table 9.5.

In addition to the Rossi (2003) material described above, several resources are useful in helping family members implement an indirect language stimulation approach. One was developed at the Hanen Early Language Resource Centre in Toronto for children with speech and language delay. The program provides inservice training to professionals and distributes a parent guidebook entitled, *It Takes Two to Talk* (Manolson, 1985). This program can be very useful to clinicians in encouraging developmentally appropriate interactions with infants. Curricular materials for guiding parents and professional training are also available from the Infant Hearing

TABLE 9.5	
Some Methods for Parents to Establish Effective Communication with Their Child Who Is Deaf or Hard of Hearing	
Identify the child's early use of signals and respond interactively	Understand the importance of early communication and how babies learn to communicate Identify child's early communication Respond to child's early communication Use interactive turntaking Respond appropriately to child's cry Encourage smiling and laughing in early interactions Give child choices Utilize daily routines for communication
Optimize daily communication in the home	Minimize distracting noises Get close to child and on child's level Establish eye contact and direct conversation to child Provide a safe, stimulating communication environment Communicate frequently with child each day
Optimize parent communication with child in early interactions	Understand how parents communicate to babies and young children Increase the "back and forth" exchanges in turntaking Encourage vocalization in communicative interactions Use touch and gestures in communicative interactions Use facial expressions and intonation in communicative interactions Interact with child about meaningful here-and-now experiences; make an experience book

Source: Watkins, S., et al. (2004). *The SKI-HI model: A resource manual for family-centered home-based programming for infants, toddlers, and pre-school children with hearing impairments* (p. 262). Used with permission.

Resource (Parent/Infant Communication, Schuyler & Sowers, 1998) and from Project SKI-HI (Watkins, Taylor, & Pittman, 2004). Also, Infant Hearing Resource recently published a guidebook with videotapes called "For Families." This material is especially useful and practical for guiding early listening and communication.

Families involved in signing programs often desire and benefit from opportunities to learn about deaf culture. Furthermore, many parents are seeking resources and support for learning American Sign Language (ASL). The SKI-HI Institute has developed and tested Deaf Mentor Programming, which enables family members to learn American Sign Language and to learn about Deaf culture. The program utilizes the services of adults who are deaf as mentors and models of the language and culture of the deaf. These Deaf Mentors make regular visits to the home, interact with the child using ASL, show family members how to use ASL, and help the family understand and appreciate deafness and Deaf culture. Meanwhile, the family continues to receive visits from a parent advisor who focuses on helping the parents promote English acquisition in the young child who is deaf. In this way, the family and child use both English and ASL and participate comfortably in both the hearing and deaf worlds. A variety of Deaf Mentor materials are currently being developed at the

Motherese or *parentese* are terms used to describe the baby talk that parents use when they talk to a young infant. Adults make a number of modifications to their speech (e.g., shorter, simpler ideas with higher pitch and varied intonation), which are believed to support infants' language development.

Shared Reading Project

An innovative and practical program developed by David Schleper (1996) at Gallaudet University has supported hearing parents who want to incorporate ASL and/or visual principles into their communication with young children. The Shared Reading Project (SRP) is designed to support deaf children's literacy development through the provision of fluent models of storytelling. Deaf individuals are trained to go into family homes and coach the parents in visual methods for sharing books with their young children. This innovative program has been implemented through support from Gallaudet in several states across the United States. A most innovative application has been developed in the state of Washington through the efforts of Nancy Hatfield and Howie Seago. In this application, the SRP is brought to families throughout the state through videoconferencing technology. Information on this approach may be found at www.srvop.org.

Fluency of sign refers to the smoothness, accuracy, and flow of movement from one sign to the next. Prosody relates to the ways a signer segments thought units and stresses certain ideas in the message.

SKI-HI Institute, including guides for teaching families ASL, information on Deaf culture, and Deaf Mentor Program operation guides. An array of data has been obtained on the children and families receiving Deaf Mentor Programming. These data were compared with data on children who were not receiving bilingual–bicultural programming. Children receiving this early bilingual–bicultural (bi–bi) Deaf Mentor programming made greater language gains during treatment time, had considerably larger vocabularies, and scored higher on measures of communication, language, and English syntax than the matched children who did not receive this programming (Watkins, Pittman, & Walden, 1998). Data on program operation, service satisfaction from persons involved in the program, and cost-effectiveness also were obtained (Watkins, Pittman, & Walden, 1996).

Hatfield and Humes (1994) also describe a parent–infant program that has incorporated a bilingual–bicultural model, and Busch and Halpin (1994) describe an approach to incorporating Deaf culture into the early-intervention program. Many professionals and Deaf persons stress the importance of considering the natural ways that American Sign Language, a visual-spatial language, is organized and the potential advantages this language organization may have for the young learner who is deaf.

SPEECH STIMULATION: PARENT–INFANT AND PRESCHOOL. We believe that children in parent–infant programs should not receive formal speech training, which typically involves drill and correction. Instead, we believe parents and professionals should be aware of the general sequence in which speech sounds emerge and then provide extensive modeling of speech at a level that encourages children to move to the next stage of development. An excellent source on speech development for children who are deaf or hard of hearing is *Speech and the Hearing Impaired Child* (Ling, 1976). Another useful source, by Cole (1992), is *Listening and Talking: A Guide to Promoting Spoken Language in Young Hearing-Impaired Children.*

Oller (1983) has identified stages in normally developing infants' vocal development that are useful to consider. From birth to 2 months, infants are in a *phonation stage,* where they produce comfort sounds that may be precursors to vowel production. At this stage, syllables with consonants or vowels are rare. Infants

Preschool Language Stimulation Strategies

1. *Children should be regarded as active learners, not passive recipients of information.* Clinicians need to recognize that children bring to tasks past experiences, knowledge, and assumptions that contribute to learning. By exploiting children's background knowledge during lessons, clinicians help children to construct new knowledge in a mentally active manner. This can happen through provision of choices, teacher-guided questioning, and opportunities to solve problems (see Moeller & Carney, 1993, for further discussion).

2. *Children who are deaf or hard of hearing typically benefit from a systematic approach to vocabulary development.* Typically, developing children access word meanings and experiential knowledge through overhearing the conversations of others. Children with hearing loss may have less access to this path for developing word and world knowledge. Therefore, vocabulary development approaches that seek to expand world knowledge and build connections between new and established words are useful with this population. Yoshinaga-Itano and Downey (1986) describe such an approach.

3. *Developmentally appropriate practices should be at the foundation of any program serving preschoolers.* Guidelines from the National Association for the Education of Young Children are included in Table 9.6 (Bredekamp, 1987).

4. *Question asking should be a priority goal with children who are deaf and hard of hearing.* For all children, language serves as a powerful tool for accessing information and making discoveries about the world. One of the most frequent verbalizations of a 4-year-old is "Why?" Children who are deaf or hard of hearing are equally curious. If children with hearing loss are encountering difficulty forming questions, they benefit from supportive contexts, modeling, and multiple opportunities to participate in question asking. Activities and routines that purposely provoke curiosity are ideal.

5. *Question understanding is also a priority so that children benefit from classroom discourse routines that guide thinking.* In quality preschool programs, many teachers use collaborative learning methods within learning centers. During explorative activities, teachers use questions to elicit observations and guide children's thinking and discovery. A useful classroom discourse model for developing children's ability to respond to questions of increasing abstraction was developed by Blank, Rose, and Berlin (1978). Emphasis on answering increasingly abstract questions helps to develop children's verbal reasoning skills.

6. Quality preschool programs recognize that language (whether oral, signed, or written) is a tool for conveying meanings and for communicating purposefully. Language "lessons," then, need to be integrated in pragmatically appropriate contexts that have communicative value.

7. *Thematic or literature-based units can be a useful way to present concepts and vocabulary in an organized manner with relevant topical links.* Themes should be developmentally appropriate, interesting, and relevant to the child's communicative needs.

8. *Opportunities for exploration through play should be provided regularly.* Children learn thinking, language, and social skills through playful exploration. Adults can guide children's learning during play by using thought-provoking questions, by pointing out or instigating problems in need of solution, and by helping the child to make and express choices. Children benefit from a play process that includes (a) opportunities to learn to verbally plan prior to playing, (b) support from adult play partners in the form of descriptive comments,

Children are not passive learners. They actively construct meaning by testing out ideas, manipulating materials, asking questions, and making discoveries.

problem-solving opportunities, and questions, and (c) a period devoted to verbally recall-ing what happened during play (Hohmann, Banet, & Weikart, 1979).

9. Children benefit in many ways from exposure to quality children's literature. Story-telling should be a daily curricular component. Exposure to stories helps children expand upon event knowledge (scripts), develop a notion of story grammar, and prepare for future literacy tasks. There are many indications in the literature that children who are read to with regularity at home become the most literate. Parents should be actively involved in the storytelling program.

10. Children at the preschool level benefit from exposure to early literacy opportuni-ties. These include reading books and being read to, demonstrating knowledge about books (e.g., book handling, reading pictures, recognizing environmental print), beginning to recognize simple print forms, being exposed to functional uses of print, and having oppor-tunities to explore with written symbols.

Marginal babbling develops in the period from 4 to 6 months and occurs when the baby produces simple consonant–vowel (cv) syllables. Canonical babble includes strings of repetitive syllables (e.g., /bababababa/) and emerges between 7 and 10 months of age.

enter a *cooing stage* during the 2- to 3-month period. They produce comfort sounds often articulated in the back of the oral cavity. These are not well-formed, mature syllabic productions. Next is the *expansion stage* (4 to 6 months). Infants at this stage produce various new sound types, like squeals, growls, yells, whispers, and a variety of isolated vowel sounds with occasional vowel tract closure, making sim-ple consonant–vowel syllables, and forming "marginal" babbling. Mature syllables

TABLE 9.6

Guidelines for Developmentally Appropriate Practices

1. The clinician or teacher prepares the learning environment and plans activities to promote discoveries and exploration.
2. Content and strategies presented are age appropriate.
3. Curriculum techniques are adjusted to respond to children's learning style, personality, or cultural background.
4. Child-initiated but adult-supported play is primary vehicle of encouraging developmental growth in all domains.
5. Developmental and learning domains are integrated within the curriculum (e.g., motor, social, language, cognitive, emotional).
6. Learning materials are concrete, real, and relevant to the experiences of young children.
7. Learning materials are presented at various developmental levels to interest and challenge children. They are non-sexist and reflect cultural diversity.
8. Play materials allow for sensorimotor, symbolic, and constructive play.
9. Adults are responsive and comforting. They encourage independence and treat children with respect and dignity.
10. Adults use discipline techniques that guide children to learn self-control, redirect children to use more acceptable behaviors to resolve conflict, and remind children of rules.

Source: Adapted from Bredekamp (1987).

are not yet evident, though. The next stage is considered to be a developmental landmark, and is called the *canonical stage* (7 to 10 months). At this point, infants produce well-formed, reduplicated syllables like /mamama/ or /dadada/. This is considered to be a critical stage, as these syllables function as phonetic building blocks of words. Nonreduplicated canonical utterances (e.g., /bi/, /ada/, /imi/) are also heard frequently at this stage. The period of 11 to 12 months brings about the *variegated babbling stage*. Here, infants systematically produce utterances with differing consonantal or vocalic elements. Useful clinical systems for transcribing and studying infant vocalizations have been described by Stoel-Gammon and Cooper (1984).

In most cases, infants who are deaf or hard of hearing spontaneously produce some vocalizations. Parents should encourage the child to develop an abundance of vocalizations by being responsive to the child's vocal attempts (Ling, 1989). Parents can respond by smiling, moving closer to the child, interpreting the vocal attempt communicatively, and imitating the child (Cole, 1992).

Parents can also encourage the child's initial vocalizations by providing animated models of vocalizing during active play with the child.

> As the child is being gently bounced on the parent's knee, the parent can say /up-up-up/. Vocalizations like /a-boo; a-boo/ would be appropriate during a peek-a-boo game. Parents should be encouraged to respond warmly to reinforce any early accidental vocalizations. At the expansion and canonical babbling stages, parents can reinforce the child's vocal exploration by imitating and modeling interesting auditory patterns. The parent can say, "You said up-up-up! Let's ride horsey up-up-up the hill." For the older infant, new sounds can be imitated and then repeated in syllable chains and then used in simple words ("/ha-ha-ha/— yes, that is HOT!").

Parents should encourage the infant's development of early suprasegmental aspects of speech. Breath control can be developed through playful duration games, where the child is encouraged to vocalize long or short sounds (e.g., vocalizing /u:/ while the sand pours out of a container).

> Intensity and pitch control can be developed in play where the child is encouraged to make soft and loud (e.g., whisper while the baby doll sleeps; make a loud voice to wake her up) and high and low sounds. Speech rhythms can be learned by encouraging the child to participate in play activities in which speech tempos are produced slowly and quickly (e.g., during a horsey-back ride, the movement and the sound can be contrasted from slow to fast repetitions).

At the preschool level, children often benefit from a goal-oriented approach to speech development. This process begins with a comprehensive analysis of the child's speech-production skills to determine appropriate intervention targets. This might include a phonologically based assessment (e.g., *Test of Phonology;* Bankson & Bernthal, 1990), an articulation test, or a procedure specifically designed for deaf and hard of hearing students (Ling, 1976). The decision about which type of assessment to use depends on the diagnostic questions of the clinician and the skill level and residual hearing of the child. For some children who are hard of hearing, for example, a developmental phonological process approach can be very useful. Whatever tools are chosen, the clinician should be well informed about the typical characteristics of speech in children with hearing loss.

> A comprehensive appraisal of speech should include assessment of (1) functional auditory skills; (2) phonetic level skills; (3) phonological skills; (4) suprasegmental and vocal behaviors; (5) stimulability for sound production or emergence of skills; and (6) speech intelligibility.

Often an oral mechanism assessment is valuable. In our opinion, the speech assessment should not rely solely on imitative productions, but should examine spontaneous productions and extent of carryover, as well.

When working on speech, AR clinicians should encourage the child to rely as much as possible on residual hearing.

A thorough discussion of the many speech training approaches is beyond the scope of this chapter. Speech development should always be viewed within the broader context of communication, with emphasis on speech generalization and carryover. See Chapter 6 of this book for a discussion of various speech management approaches.

Too often, speech training materials are presented at a basic level. They require labeling of pictures or creating simple ideas from pictured stimuli. Children may have difficulty with carryover of speech skills when tasks are abstract and demand a lot of their mental attention. Training materials that incorporate increasingly complex cognitive–linguistic demands will help children to generalize. At the same time, the child is working on materials useful for language and cognitive development. When the child is ready, approaches that integrate several levels of goals are both useful and expedient.

A task has complex cognitive and linguistic demands when it challenges the child to think abstractly and to respond by understanding or using complex language forms.

COUNSELING AND PSYCHOSOCIAL ASPECTS. During the early years of the child's life, the psychosocial aspects of the hearing deficit are, for a great part, related to the parents as the primary caregivers and teachers. Parenthood is a great challenge for all fathers and mothers. The added responsibility of having a child with hearing impairment enhances this challenge in various degrees and ways.

NEEDS OF PARENTS. Psychosocial support is vital for the parents of infants with hearing impairment. Mindel and Vernon (1987) wrote that "unless parents' emotional needs are attended to, the programs for young hearing handicapped children have limited benefit" (p. 23).

During the child's early years, the parent advisor is often the key person in enabling families to understand hearing loss and deal creatively and positively with the child. Because over 90 percent of children who are deaf or hard of hearing have parents with normal hearing, these parents typically have had little or no experience with deafness. Although family members may not know much about deafness, they have hopes and dreams for their child, and they have many concerns and questions. Often family members are confused and surprised by the variety of emotions they experience by having a family member who is deaf or hard of hearing. The competent parent advisor is able to listen to family members sensitively

Concepts Common to Recommended Speech Training Approaches for Children with Hearing Impairment

1. The speech training program should exploit the use of residual hearing to the fullest extent possible. Auditory and speech development should be closely integrated in this process.

2. Adult expectations can have a significant impact on a child's development of speech. In the classroom and at home, children benefit from regular encouragement to rely on speech to the best of their abilities. This should not be implemented to the degree that it interferes with communication. However, adults need to recognize the value of regular, brief practice opportunities in natural contexts (Ling, 1976) and the value of high expectations.

3. Many programs find that collaborative consultation models work well for integrating speech into the classroom. The speech–language clinician or AR clinician works closely with the preschool classroom teacher to determine how speech intervention targets can be incorporated naturally in classroom activities. Consultants can assist the teacher in maintaining appropriate and challenging expectations for speech and auditory skill development in the classroom. Although individual speech intervention is often valuable, there may be problems with generalization and carryover if speech is not emphasized in natural routines and contexts. A collaborative team approach can be very effective in accomplishing the goal of generalization of speech skills.

4. Speech development should always be viewed within the broader context of communication. Speech generalization and carryover are critical steps in intervention. Carotta, Carney, and Dettman (1990) discussed a systematic plan for carryover of speech targets that involved the gradual inclusion of the target in increasingly abstract and cognitively demanding contexts. Using the preschool discourse model described earlier (Blank et al., 1978), they proposed a series of activities that took the child through a progression from cognitively simple to cognitively challenging language contexts. For example, if the child was working on a vowel like /au/, the sound would be included in phonologically based activities in the following manner:

    a. Matching perception (simplest level of abstraction)
       Name objects seen in a bag (*cow, mouse, towel*)
    b. Selective analysis of perception
       Name something that is ... (attentive to one or two categorical characteristics).
       Example: Name an animal (*cow, mouse*)
       Example: Name something little and brown (*mouse*)
    c. Reordering perception
       Identify similarities: How are a cow and a mouse the same?
    d. Reasoning about perception
       Forming a solution from another person's perspective
       The man saw a nail sticking out of the house. What should he do? (*pound the nail; sit down and pout*)

and with more care, interact with them, and provide needed support, information, and skills.

One of the most valuable contributions the parent advisor can make to the family is to gently and gradually help the family understand and appreciate deafness. Rather than perceiving deafness as a "pathology," a "problem," or "something to be

When parents have to accept that their child has a hearing loss, it can be helpful if they watch the hearing tests and observe first-hand the sounds their children can hear and cannot hear.

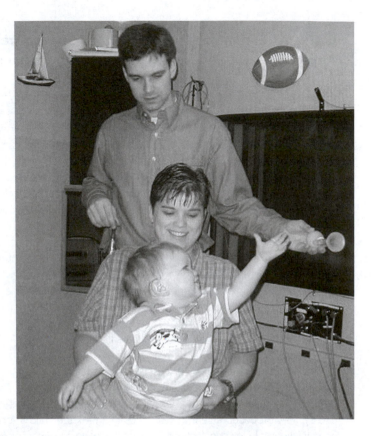

feared," parent advisors can help families to see deafness as a unique human experience that may include linguistic and cultural aspects. Perhaps the very best way for families to understand and appreciate deafness is to interact with deaf persons themselves. The Deaf Mentor Program at the SKI-HI Institute provides the opportunity for families to interact regularly with adults who are deaf (Deaf Mentors).

Of course, the process of understanding and appreciating deafness and the situation of having a child who is deaf is gradual. For most parents with normal hearing the initial reaction to the diagnosis of deafness includes shock, denial, and confusion. Parents have wished for and expected a "normal" child. Now their dreams are shattered, and they feel devastated and helpless. The shock has numbed them into a state of immobility. They may be unable to assimilate what information is given them. Sometimes, after learning the diagnosis for the first time, parents are utterly and literally lost, unable even to locate their cars in the parking lot.

After the initial shock, denial, and confusion stage, some parents experience anger, depression, and guilt: "Why me?" Luterman (1987) noted:

> Anger comes from a violation of expectations. Parents have many expectations about their unborn children, not the least of which is that they will be normal. When they find that the child does not hear normally and cannot be cured, they feel cheated and wonder why they were singled out. (p. 42)

Anger also results from loss of control of personal freedom. Parents may experience a kind of aesthetic disavowal of the child with hearing impairment as they envision the restrictions the child may impose on their plans for the future. Anger also results from not knowing how to help the child. In addition to anger, parents often experience strong guilt feelings, manifested by overindulging the child who has hearing impairment, or placing excessive demands on him. If these findings of guilt and despair are not resolved, parents begin an unending search for a "magic cure" by a doctor who will deny the difficulty or the location of the "best" school.

This period of anger, depression, and guilt can be followed by a time of withdrawal, solitude, and introspection. As parents learn about deafness and interact with persons who are deaf, they come to see that these people reside, work, produce, and lead normal lives in society. Arrival at this stage does not preclude continued problems and adjustments. On the contrary, as new crises surface, as new programs, new medical problems arise, parents may go through additional emotional adjustments.

Gradually, most parents come to see that their child has a future, and they begin to accept the disability. Acceptance of the disability leads the parents back to the feelings they were experiencing toward their child before the diagnosis of deafness. The duration of each stage depends upon the parents. Some stages may pass in a matter of minutes, others may last for months or years, and, as indicated, the parents may reexperience some of the stages later in their lives. Generally, however, parents go through the stages just described. (See Chapter 7 for additional detail. There, this period is divided into four stages: shock, denial, depression, and acceptance.)

SUPPORT FOR PARENTS. It is the responsibility of the parent advisor first and foremost to convey positive attitudes and perceptions about deafness to family members. Deaf adults (mentors) are invaluable in enabling families to understand and appreciate deafness. For parents experiencing the stages of grief described above, the parent advisor will want to sensitively help the parents deal with these stages. The parent advisor will not want to hurry parents through the stages or encourage avoidance of them; rather, parents should be skillfully, but gently, helped to progress from one stage to the next. The following discussion offers some suggestions as to how this may be accomplished. (See also case examples, Chapter 11.)

During the first stage, which is characterized by confusion and denial, the parent advisor–audiologic rehabilitationist establishes contact with the family. This is done immediately after the diagnosis of a hearing loss. The professional's role is to offer emotional support and realistic hope. The parent advisor explains programs that will involve all family members and how these programs will help the child who is deaf or hard of hearing.

During the next stage, anger and depression, the parent advisor may erroneously try to counteract the parents' emotions by helping them feel less depressed. At this period, the parent advisor needs to exhibit genuine understanding and good listening skills rather than attempt to talk the parents out of their feelings (Moses, 1985).

The effective parent advisor contributes greatly to the third stage, that of quietude and introspection. It is during this time that parents usually open up and ask questions about the future of their child, educational considerations, and society's perception of them and of their youngster. Perhaps the most important contribution the parent advisor can make during this stage is to plan with the parents constructive activities for family members that help the child's listening, communicative, and language abilities. When the parents see the child responding, growing, and learning, acceptance occurs. They realize they have a child who can be taught and loved just like any other child.

CONSULTATION BETWEEN PSYCHOLOGIST AND AR THERAPIST. Some parents do not move easily through the stages just outlined. On the way they may have problems: unrealistic expectations for the child, overprotection, rejection, or confusion over conflicting information about educational methods. They may have problems with general childrearing practices, such as discipline and sibling rivalry. The parent advisor may need special help from psychologists or social workers in dealing with these problems. Sessions can be set up between the parent advisor and the psychologist or social worker for this purpose. The psychologist or social worker can offer suggestions that can in turn be tried by the parent advisor in the home or discussed with the family as appropriate. For parents who want psychological counseling, the AR therapist should act as facilitator and ensure such therapy is arranged.

NEEDS OF AND SUPPORT FOR THE CHILD. Successful resolution of parental anxieties, warm acceptance of the child who is deaf, and establishment of communication with the child promote normal psychosocial development. However, the child may also present social, emotional, or psychological problems. Consequently, the therapist must have a knowledge of what to expect from the child with hearing impairment in these developmental areas.

Support Group Meetings

Another invaluable way of giving psychosocial support to parents is to arrange parent group meetings. "There is probably no greater gift that a professional can give to families than to provide them with a support group. Groups are marvelous vehicles for learning and emotional support" (Luterman, 1987, p. 113). Support group meetings are part of many early-intervention programs. Often eight or nine meetings are held, once a week, with a psychologist or social worker in charge. The first part of each meeting often consists of a presentation by a professional. Such topics as Language Development, Communication Methods, Development of Self-Concept, and Making the Home Environment Responsive can be discussed. The last part of each meeting is devoted to group interaction. Luterman (1987) described the benefits of support group interactions: (1) They enable members to recognize the universality of their feelings; members come to appreciate that others in the group have similar feelings; (2) they give participants the opportunity to help one another; and (3) they become a powerful vehicle for imparting information.

Parents are great sources of help and comfort to other parents. In attending support group meetings we have been constantly impressed with the amount of help and moral support parents give each other. Inclusion of adults who are deaf in support groups is highly recommended. Such adults can describe their experiences of being deaf and answer questions about deafness that professionals with normal hearing simply cannot do.

Development scales established by Vincent et al. (1986) and others enable professionals to know what behaviors a child should exhibit at a particular age (see resource website). The audiologic rehabilitationist observes the child's behaviors and determines what age levels they typify. In addition to developmental scales, the therapist should arrange for appropriate developmental and psychosocial assessments for the child. These tests should be administered by competent psychologists who are familiar with hearing-impaired children. According to Davis (1990), this may be difficult since "most psychologists receive little or no training in testing or working with hearing-impaired children" (p. 36).

If the child is lagging in a specific area, the audiologic rehabilitationist can seek help from other professionals such as child development specialists, psychologists, social workers, occupational and physical therapists, pediatricians, and nurses.

ASPECTS OF AUDIOLOGIC REHABILITATION: SCHOOL YEARS

Rehabilitation Assessment: IEP

Public law stipulates that primary and secondary school placements must be based on assessments of the child, which are reviewed in an individualized educational program (IEP) meeting (see Chapter 8). The IEP meetings serve to develop, review, or revise educational program goals for the student. The AR therapist is responsible for completing an appropriate assessment prior to the IEP meeting. The AR therapist working with the school-age student may be an educational audiologist, an educator of the hearing impaired, a speech–language clinician, or some other professional charged with the responsibility of coordinating components of the child's educational support services. Assessment of the school-age child includes the four general areas described in the AR model presented in Chapter 1:

> An individual educational plan (IEP) is a document developed for each student receiving special education services in the schools. Required by law, this document includes specific objectives and progress indicators.

1. Communication status, including audiologic and amplification issues, receptive and expressive language, and social communication skills
2. Overall participation variables of academic achievement, psychosocial adaptation, and prevocational and vocational skills
3. Related personal factors
4. Environmental factors

In many cases, multidisciplinary input is valuable in gaining a comprehensive understanding of student needs. Assessment guidelines are available in Moeller (1988) and Alpiner and McCarthy (2000). Consistent with the goal of ecologically valid assessment practices, it is useful to include a classroom observation and/or teacher questionnaires regarding the student's performance in that setting. As the section on communication rehabilitation stresses, classroom communication behaviors are unique and complex. Many standardized tests do not reflect the kinds of language skills that are required in the classroom setting. Therefore, observations in that setting and teacher impressions offer invaluable insights for the IEP The S.I.F.T.E.R. (Screening Instrument for Targeting Educational Risk; see Chapter 8 and the resource website) is an example of an efficient tool for recruiting teachers' impressions of the student's performance in relation to her peers. A member of the assessment team or a representative of the team who is familiar with the results of the assessment (often the audiologic rehabilitationist) must attend the IEP meeting along with the teacher, parents, and child, as appropriate. Based on the educational recommendations from the child's IEP, the AR therapist proceeds to arrange for or provide the needed services. Excellent guidelines for comprehensive service provision have been published by ASHA (2002).

Management

ENVIRONMENTAL COORDINATION AND PARTICIPATION. As a part of the overall coordination, the therapist is responsible for maximizing the child's learning environment (classroom), assisting in securing ancillary services, promoting development of social skills, teaching hearing conservation and self-advocacy, and arranging for special college preparation or occupational training. If the primary educational programming is delivered by someone other than the AR therapist (e.g., the teacher), the therapist needs to assume a supporting role and assist the teacher in these areas.

CHILD LEARNING ENVIRONMENT (CLASSROOM MANAGEMENT). School placement alternatives are necessary so that the best educational setting can be selected. For the older child, additional placement options are available beyond those listed for the preschool child.

The audiologic rehabilitationist is responsible for informing the child's teachers of the conditions that will optimize learning: that is, seating, lighting, visual aids, and reduction of classroom noises. Helpful guides for teachers who have children with hearing impairment in their classrooms have been written (see also Appendix). In addition, the therapist should ensure that an appropriate student–teacher ratio is maintained.

The AR therapist should also promote home and school coordination. Cooperation can be facilitated by regular conferences between parents and teachers, periodic visits to the home by the teacher, notes, newsletters, and special student work sent home to the parents, telephone conversations, and allowing parents to participate in classroom activities.

ANCILLARY SERVICES. The therapist may also need to help set up ancillary services required for the hearing-impaired child. Services like otologic assessments and treatment; occupational or physical therapy; medical exams and treatment; social

---

Placement Options

The range of options includes (1) integration into public schools with ancillary services like speech therapy; (2) day school or day classes for the hearing impaired; (3) resource rooms where the child with hearing impairment learns communication skills and is integrated into regular classrooms for less language-oriented subjects, such as math and physical education; (4) residential school placement; and (5) team-taught combined classes of normal and hearing-impaired youngsters. (See Chapter 8 on school placement alternatives for a discussion of these options.)

services; and neurologic, ophthalmologic, and psychological services are important components for the welfare of a child with hearing impairment. Finally, secondary students with hearing impairment in public school programs may require the services of notetakers or interpreters.

DEVELOPMENT OF SOCIAL SKILLS. In a study of forty mainstreamed students with hearing impairment, Davis, Effenbein, Schum, and Bentler (1986) found a high incidence of social problems, including peer acceptance difficulties. Over 50 percent of the students with hearing impairment expressed concerns with peer relations, in contrast to 16 percent of similar concerns expressed by hearing students. The authors stressed the need for increased attention by school programs to the development of positive self-esteem and social interactions in students with hearing impairment. The AR clinician should monitor the social adjustment of the student with hearing impairment and make appropriate referrals as needed. The school counselor or other mental health professional can be supportive in addressing the social integration of the student. Refinement of social language skills can also be supportive of this goal area.

HEARING CONSERVATION. School-age children should be educated regarding the importance of protecting their hearing from damage due to noise exposure. Children exposed to excessively loud sounds can experience noise-induced hearing loss. Specific groups of students such as band members, students who use firearms, and students who are exposed to loud agricultural or recreational equipment or who participate in shop or automotive classes may be more at risk to experience noise-induced hearing loss. Bennett and English (1998) summarize the literature regarding the need for hearing conservation programs, including an increasing incidence of hearing loss due to noise exposure among the school-age population and describe the benefits of using a problem-based learning approach compared to a more traditional lecture-based approach for presenting hearing conservation programs. The AR therapist can create activities to stimulate the student's thinking regarding the structure and function of the normal ear, pathways of sound, dangerous levels of sound, and ways to protect individual hearing sensitivity.

SELF-ADVOCACY. The AR therapist should encourage students with hearing loss to develop self-advocacy skills. These skills may include understanding the legal rights associated with the Individuals with Disabilities Education Act and the Americans with Disabilities Act, developing an understanding of individual needs, appropriately expressing communication needs, locating and accessing services within the community, and empowering the individual to take responsibility for meeting his or her unique needs. English (1997) states that potential employers and college instructors may not know the rights of individuals with hearing loss. It is the individual's responsibility to know the law and advocate for individual rights once leaving the school environment.

AUDIBILITY, AMPLIFICATION, AND ASSISTIVE DEVICE ISSUES. If children obtain their hearing aids during the early intervention period and go through the adjustment and orientation steps described earlier in this chapter, they have a good start on dealing with amplification concerns. However, this area requires a continued focus, since new amplification needs or problems may arise when children enter school. Regular hearing aid reassessment at six-month to one-year intervals and daily monitoring of the aid by school personnel should occur. Unfortunately, such regular monitoring is often neglected (Langdon & Blair, 2000). Therefore, audiologic rehabilitation personnel need to be vigilant in this area (see Chapter 8). The major deficit for these children is their impaired hearing. Therefore, the most obvious management is to restore as much of that hearing through amplification devices and excellent acoustic listening conditions as possible. In this manner, we may remove the need for some therapy that would otherwise be required.

Daily hearing aid monitoring is an essential, but often neglected, practice.

HEARING AIDS. Some children with hearing impairment are not identified until they reach school, and some of them receive their first amplification attention at this time. As indicated in the section on early intervention, when children with hearing losses are identified, they should also be evaluated medically and audiologically. After specific assessment information has been obtained, the way is cleared for carefully evaluating the place of amplification in the overall management program. Children with mild or more serious losses in the speech frequencies should proceed with a hearing aid assessment, and additional audiologic rehabilitation can assist them in hearing aid orientation aspects, as described previously.

Children with slight losses, high-frequency losses, or chronic conductive losses present a more difficult problem in terms of amplification. A careful assessment of such children's language and speech status and a report on their ability to function in the classroom will help determine whether they can function successfully without amplification. Preferential seating can provide some help, but this is, at best, an imperfect and perhaps only temporary solution. Some have recommended fitting hearing aids on children with chronic conductive losses and have shown

Successful hearing aid fitting is based on gathering accurate audiologic information, which can be a challenging activity with young children.

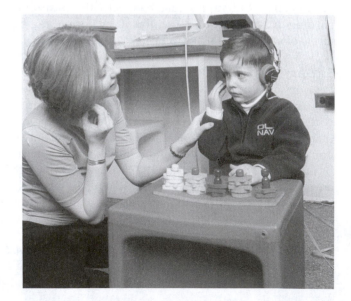

that it is a feasible alternative (Northern & Downs, 2002). Another possible solution is temporary use of FM amplification devices until the hearing problems are resolved. Such units may also be used for children with slight sensorineural losses. However, when a hearing aid can be fitted comfortably, it is generally better to fit children with sensorineural losses with aid(s) while they are younger. As they get older, they tend to become more concerned about the unfortunate social stigma associated with amplification devices. In contrast, children who use amplification from an early age know how much it can help them and are less likely to part company with it as they get older. Nevertheless, getting children to use their hearing aid(s) on a regular basis may be one of the greatest challenges faced by the AR therapist.

Teachers and parents and, later, the child him- or herself can provide information on how regularly the hearing aid is used. The therapist should seek out this information and try to modify behavior when necessary. Young children will often respond to methods like public charting of their daily hearing aid use. The child can be made responsible for the charting. Older children should understand the purpose for amplification. When they are old enough, therefore, they need to receive the same instruction and information about their hearing loss as their parents were given previously. (See Availability, Amplification, and Assistive Device Issues under Early Intervention in this chapter.)

Full-time use of hearing aids is preferable, in part because the child is less likely to forget or lose the instruments. With older children, however, it is sometimes unrealistic. In the case of mild loss, the aids may provide little, if any, benefit in many play or recreational circumstances. The teenager, therefore, may elect not to use the hearing aids during these times. The audiologic rehabilitationist may help the young person identify the situations where the aids should be used.

As the child gets older, he or she can begin to assume the responsibility for the care and management of the hearing aids. At that point, the AR therapist should teach the child about hearing aid function, repair, and use (see Chapter 2 and Chapter 10 including HIO BASICS). Maintenance of children's hearing aids is often neglected, as shown in a series of studies starting with Gaeth and Lounsbury (1966). These writers found that approximately half the hearing aids in their study were not in working order and parents were generally ill-informed about the rudiments of aid care. Unfortunately, that situation has not improved appreciably as reflected in subsequent studies, nearly all of which have shown 50 percent poor function among children's aids (Blair, Wright, & Pollard, 1981). Furthermore, school programs have been similarly negligent about maintaining children's aids, even though some projects have demonstrated that children's aids may be substantially improved by regular maintenance (Langdon & Blair, 2000).

In cases where the child's management skills are deficient due to age or length of experience with the aid, help and instruction should be provided (see Chapter 8 for suggestions).

> Older children can be taught to take full responsibility for the care and maintenance of their amplification devices, including recognizing times when devices are not functioning properly.

COCHLEAR IMPLANT SUPPORT AND ORIENTATION. As the number of children with cochlear implants increases, so does the demand for cochlear implant services. Like hearing aids, cochlear implants must be properly fitted or mapped and their function monitored. The AR therapist should establish communication with the mapping audiologist to develop a relationship. The AR specialist, parent, or other trained person can complete basic monitoring.

Basic monitoring of a cochlear implant may include

1. Checking battery function.
2. Monitoring the child's ongoing ability to detect or discriminate the Ling sounds.
3. Use of a signal check device to monitor if a signal is being transmitted.
4. Checking all cords for shorts or intermittencies.
5. Keeping a supply of extra cords, magnets, and batteries.

The cochlear implant manufacturers provide excellent troubleshooting guides for educators.

Both families and school personnel need thorough orientation to the use of the cochlear implant. Families will usually receive this training at the time of initial stimulation. Each time the cochlear implant recipient works with new school personnel, orientation to the device should be provided. The AR therapist may be the person who is most knowledgeable regarding the function of the cochlear implant and the needs of the recipient.

ASSISTIVE LISTENING DEVICES AND CLASSROOM ACOUSTICS. Other aspects of amplification that become important in the school years include use of classroom amplification systems and the concern for quiet classroom environments. While no knowledgeable person would dispute the importance of quiet conditions for persons with hearing impairment, there has been some controversy about whether school-age youngsters should use educational (FM) auditory systems instead of personal hearing aids.

Personal hearing aids have improved appreciably over the past years so they now provide good fidelity, cosmetic appeal, and often built-in FM systems (see Chapter 2). In addition, they allow good student-to-student communication and self-monitoring by the child, and in small groups they provide satisfactory amplification for teacher-to-student communication purposes.

Chapters 2 and 8 contain a description of the different types of classroom amplification equipment in use. *FM radio-frequency* systems, used almost exclusively now, allow teacher and students more freedom and flexibility than other systems. Personal systems are used in the majority of cases, but increasingly more classrooms are being outfitted with sound field systems wherein between two and four loudspeakers allow all students in the classroom to benefit from an improved auditory signal (Flexer, 1999). These sound field systems have the advantage that they provide improved listening to students with hearing impairment without any stigma, which may be associated with using special equipment that they alone must wear. Personal FM systems may also be integrated within hearing aids or by direct audio hookup and by induction loop transmission. The older forms of classroom amplification, the *standard* or *hard-wire* systems and *induction loop amplification* (ILA) systems, are rarely used. One other device is the *infrared system*, which utilizes light rays for transmission. The infrared system is usable in classes, auditoriums, and public buildings and for personal use and TV watching by some persons with hearing impairment.

The audiologic rehabilitationist must be knowledgeable about the various types of equipment and must be able to instruct others in daily operation and monitoring. Occasionally, AR professionals will also be asked to recommend the best

FM radio-frequency amplification systems are commonly used in classroom settings to control the effects of background noise and distance on understanding of the spoken message.

arrangement for a particular setting. More frequently, they will simply be responsible for regularly evaluating, or getting someone else to evaluate, the function of existing systems. Several sources (DeConde-Johnson et al., 1997; Ross, 1987) contain thorough discussions of factors that should be considered when evaluating amplification equipment. Suffice it to say that attention should be given to (1) electroacoustic considerations, (2) auditory self-monitoring capability of the units, (3) child-to-child communication potential, (4) signal-to-noise ratios, (5) binaural reception, and (6) simplicity and stability of operation.

OTHER ASSISTIVE DEVICES. It is important that the youngster with hearing impairment be introduced to other available accessory devices that can be useful in a variety of situations. Such devices include amplifiers for telephone, television, and radio; decoders for television; signal devices for doorbells and alarm clocks; and so forth. These devices are described in Chapter 2. In addition, therapy materials are available to help in familiarization (Castle, 1984).

SOUND TREATMENT. Well-functioning personal and group amplifying systems will be more effective if used in an acoustically treated environment. In this regard, youngsters with hearing impairment with sensorineural losses will have more serious difficulties than the child with normal hearing when noise is present. When all sounds are amplified, it is important to avoid excessive reverberation in the amplified environment. Reverberation occurs when reflected sound is present and added to the original sound. In an unbounded space (anechoic chamber) there is no reverberation. A sound occurs, moves through space, and is absorbed. However, in the usual listening environment like a classroom, sound hits various hard surfaces as it fans out in all directions, and it is reflected back. Consequently, not only the original unreflected sound, but a variety of reflected versions of the sound are present at once. This results in less distinct signals since signals are "smeared" in the time domain.

Reverberation time (RT) is a measure of how long it takes before a sound is reduced by 60 dB once it is turned off. In an anechoic chamber, RT is near 0 seconds. In a typical classroom, it is around 1.2 seconds. However, in a sound-treated classroom, one with carpets, acoustical tile, and solid-core doors, the RT can be on the order of 0.4 second. Finitzo-Heiber and Tillman (1978) showed the effect of RT and environmental signal-to-noise (S/N) ratio. The S/N ratio is a measure of how loud the desired signal (such as a teacher's voice) might be, compared to other random classroom noise. A +12 dB S/N ratio is considered acceptable for children with hearing impairment while +6 S/N and 0 S/N ratios are more typical of ordinary classrooms. As seen in Table 9.7, the speech identification of both children with normal hearing and children with hearing impairment is adversely affected when S/N ratios are poorer and RTs are increased. The performance of the child who is hard of hearing is more adversely affected by poor conditions than it is for children with normal hearing.

In the ordinary classroom, noise levels tend to be about 60 dBA, but in an open classroom they rise to 70 dBA. Gyms and cafeterias have noise levels of 70 to 90 dBA, with high amounts of reverberation. A carpeted classroom with five students and a teacher generates about 40 to 45 dBA of random noise. According to Finitzo-Heiber (1988), since voices at close range average 60 to 65 dBA, the S/N ratio in sound-treated classrooms may be +20 dB if the listener is close to the teacher. If the listener

Reverberation time is a measure of how long it takes for a sound to be reduced by 60 dB once it is turned off. Signal-to-noise (S/N) ratio measures the level of the teacher's voice in relation to background noise. Both of these characteristics of a room can influence word recognition.

TABLE 9.7

Mean Word Recognition Scores of Normal-Hearing and Hearing-Impaired Children under a High-Fidelity (Loudspeaker) and through an Ear-Level Hearing Aid Condition for Various Combinations of Reverberation and S/N Ratios

REVERBERATION TIME (RT) (SEC)	S/N RATIO (dB)	MEAN WORD RECOGNITION SCORE (%)		
		Normal Group (PTA = 0 to 10 dB) *Loudspeaker*	Hearing Impaired Group (PTA = 35 to 55 dB) *Loudspeaker*	*Hearing Aid*
0.4	+12	83	69	60
	+6	71	55	52
	0	48	29	28
1.2	+12	69	50	41
	+6	54	40	27
	0	30	15	11

Source: Adapted from Finitzo-Heiber, T., & Tillman, T. (1978). Room acoustics' effects on monosyllabic word discrimination ability for normal and hearing impaired children. *Journal of Speech and Hearing Research, 21,* 440–458.

is farther away from the teacher, the signal will get weaker and the S/N ratio will be poorer. In view of poor performance by youngsters who are hard of hearing in noisy conditions (see Table 9.7), it is recommended that class noise levels be 45 dBA for gym and arts and crafts classes, but 30 to 35 dBA in the classrooms where these students spend most of their time. It has also been suggested that noise levels of about 50 dBA may be more feasible. This would allow minimally acceptable S/N ratios of +15 to 20 dB. Reverberation times are easier to reduce than noise levels. Thus, carpeting, acoustical tile, and even commercially available foam sheets may be placed in classrooms to help absorb noise. A feasible goal may be to reduce the RT to 0.3 to 0.4 second. In addition, provisions should be made to keep the child with hearing impairment close to the speaker (teacher). This can be accomplished through use of amplification equipment, when the location of the microphone is, in effect, the position at which listening occurs. Extensive rationale and methods for providing sound treatment are available elsewhere (Berg, 1993; Crandell & Smaldino, 2000).

To summarize, the audiologic rehabilitationist plays a crucial role in providing and encouraging both routine and extensive checks of individual and group amplifying systems and in obtaining adequate sound treatment in the educational setting.

COMMUNICATION AND LANGUAGE STIMULATION: SCHOOL-AGE LEVEL. The goal is for all facets of the child's program to be closely integrated, with the focus of the AR program being on building language skills to support academic success. To accomplish this goal, the AR clinician must be in regular communication with the child's educational team and be aware of the communicative demands of the classroom and the academic curriculum.

School-age students are placed in a variety of educational settings. Yet many students who are deaf and hard of hearing spend some time in inclusive educational

---

Barriers

Two commonplace barriers to successful education of deaf and hard of hearing students in regular education settings are the following:

1. Classroom educators and administrators often underestimate the impact of the child's language problems on academic performance. Because the child who is hard of hearing, for example, may speak well on the surface and carry on conversations effectively, the teacher assumes that the child's language is "intact." Teachers may focus on whether the child can "hear" the instruction rather than whether the child can effectively process and understand the language of instruction. Blair, Peterson, and Viehweg (1985) documented significant lags in achievement of students with mild hearing impairment by the fourth grade when compared to their grade-mates with normal hearing. Teachers need to become aware of common language weaknesses that will interfere with academic development unless addressed.

2. Too often, support services are provided in a fragmented fashion.

---

environments, where the language demands can be complex. Several premises guide quality practices when serving these students.

1. *Intervention goals should be based on a comprehensive evaluation of a student's individual strengths and areas of need in communication and language.* In designing a comprehensive evaluation for an individual school-age student, the AR clinician should consider the language demands of the classroom and curriculum. Questions similar to the following can be helpful in designing a classroom-relevant evaluation process.

- Does the student understand paragraph-length or story-length conversation?
- Can the student recall facts from information presented by the teacher?
- Does the student understand abstract questions related to the curriculum?
- Is the student able to recall past events in well-organized narratives?
- Does the student take the listener's perspective into account when sharing information?
- Is the student able to use complex language functions efficiently (e.g., persuading someone, making comparisons and contrasts, summarizing ideas, justifying an answer, using cause–effect reasoning)?
- Does the student recognize when she or he does not understand? If so, what strategies are used to seek clarification?
- Does the student have strong vocabulary skills, supported by an extensive world knowledge? How does the student go about learning new words?
- Can the student shift the manner of conversation for different partners (e.g., peer versus person in authority)?
- Is the student able to use complex grammatical forms (e.g., embedded, subordinate clauses)?

Although this is not an exhaustive list, it illustrates the process of probing the kinds of language skills that are typically challenged in school environments. Formal tests need to be supplemented with informal procedures and language sampling in order to examine some of these issues.

2. *Intervention should focus on skills that will support the student's functioning in the classroom* (Wallach & Miller, 1988). The following example illustrates this point. For a student who relies on residual hearing, AR often focuses on auditory skill training. Clinicians sometimes present isolated auditory discrimination activities. It is unclear how such training might generalize to the classroom setting. The AR clinician can support classroom functioning by focusing on skills that lead toward *successful classroom listening behaviors*. Examples include

1. Listening for the main idea in a paragraph.
2. Drawing a conclusion from several details.
3. Making comments relevant to the remarks of other students in a discussion.
4. Recognizing when a critical piece of information has been missed and appropriately seeking clarification.

It can be helpful to observe the student in the classroom and/or request input from the teacher on the student's listening habits.

3. *School-age students often need opportunities to expand their world knowledge and link new vocabulary words to existing knowledge.* Delays and gaps in vocabulary and word knowledge are common in students with hearing loss. Vocabulary delays can interfere with reading comprehension and with understanding of academic discussions. It is not sufficient to teach new words in isolation (e.g., sending home a list of unrelated spelling words to be practiced and memorized). Rather, students need support in building networks of associated meanings. As an example, suppose that you heard the word *barracuda* in a conversation. Immediately, you would consider options for what the word might mean (e.g., a fish, a type of car, a song, an aggressive person). Then you hear your friend say, "Oh, I forgot my barracudas this morning." Right away, you revise your hypothesis. In essence, you do a "best of fit analysis." You draw on your knowledge of grammar to help you. The words "*my* barracudas" tip you off that it cannot be any of the word meanings mentioned before and that it is likely a personal item that can be carried. If you knew that your friend was a swimmer and then the friend added, "I prefer my barracudas because they don't leave rings around my eyes," you would conclude that she was talking about goggles. Vocabulary training needs to help students to use their fund of word knowledge and experience to figure out what words mean and to store new words in relation to associated meanings. Some excellent strategies for implementing such an approach are discussed by Yoshinaga-Itano and Downey (1986).

4. *Many students will benefit from opportunities to work on self-expression at the narrative level.* During a school day, students are asked to express themselves in various modes (e.g., giving an explanation, justifying a response, or writing a theme). If a need is identified in this area, the AR clinician can provide practice and support at the narrative level of conversation. Emphasis on the organization of face-to-face narratives may positively influence written language as well. Some narrative functions that are common in school include explaining, describing, debating, negotiat-

Narratives involve the telling of stories in various forms. One commonly used narrative form is a personal narrative through which a student shares a past event with another.

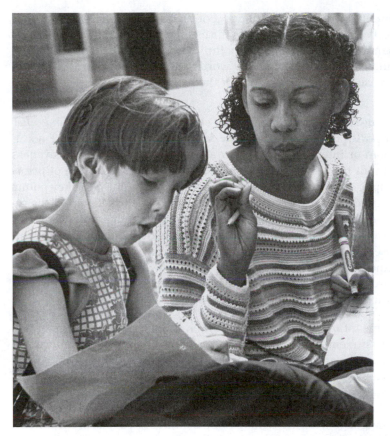

Individual therapy provides an opportunity to focus on the development of specific communication skills.

ing, comparing and contrasting, justifying, summarizing, predicting, and using cause–effect reasoning. AR clinicians can devise activities that address these literate language functions. For example, a student might be encouraged to take an opinion poll related to a recent political event. Functional speech intelligibility can be reinforced while the student asks others for their opinions. He or she can then be asked to draw summary statements and explain them to a peer. Finally, the student could be encouraged to write an article for the school paper about his or her discoveries.

5. *As the school years progress, demands for verbal reasoning increase. Therefore, students may benefit from interventions designed to encourage verbal reasoning skills.* AR clinicians can take advantage of any daily problem to support the student's expansion of problem-solving skills. It is useful to guide the student in analyzing the nature of the problem (e.g., I left my assignment at home and I will get an F if I fail to turn it in) and alternative solutions (e.g., brainstorming ways to get the assignment finished in time). The student can then be guided in evaluating the various alternatives and needed resources, leading to the selection of the best alternative. The student should evaluate both the outcomes and ways to prevent this problem in the future. These strategies can help the student learn useful problem-solving processes that can be implemented when faced with peer conflicts, social pressures, or other everyday problems. It is also useful to discuss the feelings that result from problems and their consequences. Students may have a limited fund of affective vocabulary. Gaining a better understanding of affective words and their relation to problem situations can increase students' awareness of themselves and of the perspectives of others.

6. *Some school-age students will profit from emphasis on study skills and other classroom survival skills.* If at all possible, the AR clinician should observe a student in the classroom or interview the teacher about the student's responsiveness in the classroom. Input from these sources is useful in the identification of priority needs. For example, one student had significant difficulty identifying key points for notetaking. He tried to write down all the points from a class lecture. This resulted in a lack of organization and many missing elements in his notes. The IEP team decided to provide a notetaker to ease the processing demands on the student. The AR clinician used the notetaker's transcripts to illustrate some key points about organizing notes and studying from notes. The student learned about what to attend to in the lecture from this process. Through observation and discussions with the teacher, a priority need was effectively addressed.

This list is not meant to be all-inclusive. Rather, it illustrates examples of priority areas for many students who are of school age. It emphasizes the importance of selecting goals that will support the student to function as well as possible in the learning and social environments at school. This can only come about when the AR clinician works closely with the educational team to identify skills that need to be addressed so that the student can communicate more effectively in the classroom. Sensitivity to the language-learning demands of a student's school program will lead to the selection of relevant interventions.

COUNSELING AND PSYCHOSOCIAL ASPECTS

COUNSELING. The AR therapist needs to be a good listener and information/personal adjustment counselor. Students with hearing loss and their families may need a supportive and knowledgeable person to empathize with the emotional issues associated with hearing loss. The AR therapist should learn to be a good listener and establish a trusting relationship with students so they feel free to communicate needs and feelings. School-age children may experience isolation, need help developing a sense of self-confidence, and need someone with whom they can share their feelings freely. Additionally, families of students with hearing loss may need someone who can listen, provide support, or make referrals for other counseling as needed. The AR therapist should be familiar with local and community resources so referrals for professional counseling can be made when the student or family needs exceed the therapist's expertise or comfort level.

ADJUSTMENTS FOR MILD LOSSES AND AUDITORY PROCESSING PROBLEMS. Children with mild hearing problems (i.e., mild sensorineural loss, conductive loss) and those with central auditory processing disorders (CAPD or APD) may require communication rehabilitation along with children who demonstrate more pronounced losses. Although the language-related problems may be minimized in the case of milder losses, they are apt to be present and require attention. A careful multidisciplinary assessment of the child's difficulties should be conducted consisting of reports from teachers, parents, the child, and others in addition to observation and diagnostic testing (see website and Schow et al., 2000).

Most authorities agree that CAPD involves one of the following:

1. Delay in development
2. Disordered development
3. A specific central lesion

Such difficulties involve a deficit in neural processing of auditory stimuli not due to higher order language or cognitive function (ASHA, 2005). CAPD may occur in isolation, but CAPD often occurs in conjunction with attention deficit hyperactivity disorder (ADHD) and/or learning disorder (LD), Autistic spectrum disorders, reading problems, and/or speech–language deficits.

Auditory processing disorder (APD) involves either a delay in development, a disorder in development, or a specific central lesion. APD often accompanies attention deficits, specific learning disabilities, and/or speech–language delays.

When intelligence and peripheral hearing are within normal limits and the child seems to be showing deficits mainly in hearing tasks, then CAPD, rather than a more general problem, may be the cause, and this is possible with or without these other conditions (ADHD, LD, etc.). In these cases, a rehabilitation evaluation focused on CAPD is indicated. ASHA (2005) has proposed that seven different related symptoms or assessment areas may be evaluated in CAPD, but usually current batteries only assess a more limited number of these. Musiek and Chermak (1994) recommended that the following ASHA areas be assessed: (1) monaural tasks in background competition, (2) auditory pattern recognition, and tasks involving (3) binaural separation and integration. A Multiple Auditory Processing Assessment (MAPA battery) that follows this recommendation has been found to separately measure these tasks and is now available through Auditec of St. Louis, Missouri (Domitz & Schow, 2000; Schow et al., 2000; Schow & Seikel, in press). Electrophysiologic or electroacoustic tests are also recommended, but only rarely are they a key issue in APD diagnosis.

Also, various self-report tools are being used with CAPD, as noted in Chapter 8. The *Scale of Auditory Behaviors (SAB)* follows the recommendations of the Bruton Conference (Jerger & Musiek, 2000) and has gone through a careful process of development and refinement (Schow & Seikel, in press). It is shown in Figure 9.4 and may be used to track common behaviors in these youngsters from the beginning of the rehabilitation process.

The advantage of these developments in assessment is that audiology is emerging from the imprecision of an earlier era in CAPD. Now that ASHA has defined the areas of concern in APD and assessments are being developed to measure these areas of weakness and auditory skills, remediation strategies can be focused specifically on any or all of the three deficit areas and then can be measured again post-therapy to determine improvement. For example, the use of FastForward and Earobics, commercial products used at times in schools (see resource website), may remediate problems in auditory pattern recognition. As data using these and other remediation methods are gathered to test this assumption, more will be learned about ways to help children. Although specific skills remediation may be

SCALE OF AUDITORY BEHAVIORS (SAB)

Please rate each item by circling a number that best fits the behavior of the child you are rating. At the top of the column of numbers there is a term indicating the frequency with which the behavior is observed. Please consider these terms carefully when rating each possible behavior. A child may or may not display one or more of these behaviors. A high or low rating in one or more of the areas does not indicate any particular pattern. If you are undecided about the rating of an item, use your best judgment.

Name: _____ Age: _____ Grade: ____ Today's date: _____

Teacher: _____ School: _____ Score: _____

(Informant)

Freq	Often	Sometimes	Seldom	Never	ITEMS
1. 1	2	3	4	5	Difficulty hearing or understanding in background noise
2. 1	2	3	4	5	Misunderstands, especially with rapid or muffled speech
3. 1	2	3	4	5	Difficulty following oral instructions
4. 1	2	3	4	5	Difficulty in discriminating and identifying speech sounds
5. 1	2	3	4	5	Inconsistent responses to auditory information
6. 1	2	3	4	5	Poor listening skills
7. 1	2	3	4	5	Asks for things to be repeated
8. 1	2	3	4	5	Easily distracted
9. 1	2	3	4	5	Learning or academic difficulties
10. 1	2	3	4	5	Short attention span
11. 1	2	3	4	5	Daydreams, inattentive
12. 1	2	3	4	5	Disorganized

FIGURE 9.4

Scale of auditory behaviors.
Source: Schow & Seikel (in press).

indicated at times, children with CAPD can also be helped with strategies that improve the signal (through improvement of the signal-to-noise ratio), and they may be helped by being taught improved cognitive strategies for learning and remembering. Chermak and Musiek (1992) offered a series of helpful suggestions (see Table 9.8) that address such improved signal and cognitive strategies. These recommendations may be useful to the child regardless of the particular problems. In the future, it appears that audiologic rehabilitation specialists working with school-

---

TABLE 9.8

Management of Central Auditory Processing Disorders

FUNCTIONAL DEFICIT	STRATEGIES	TECHNIQUES
Distractibility and inattention	Increase signal-to-noise ratio	ALD/FM system; acoustic modifications preferential seating
Poor memory	Metalanguage	Chunking, verbal chaining, mnemonics, rehearsal, paraphrasing, summarizing
	Right hemisphere activation	Imagery, drawing
	External aids	Notebooks, calendars
Restricted vocabulary	Improve closure	Contextual derivation of word meaning
Cognitive inflex: predominantly analytic or predominantly conceptual	Diversify cognitive style	Top-down (deductive) and bottom-up (inductive) processing, inferential reasoning, questioning, critical thinking
Poor listening comprehension	Induce formal schema to aid organization, integration, and prediction	Recognize and explain connectives (additives; causal; adversative; temporal) and patterns of parallelism and correlative pairs (not only/but also; neither/nor)
	Maximize visual and auditory summation	Substitutions for notetaking
Reading, spelling, and listening problems	Enhance multisensory integration	Phonemic analysis and segmentation
Maladaptive behaviors (passive, hyperactive, impulsive)	Assertiveness and cognitive behavior modification	Self-control, self-monitoring, self-evaluation, self-instruction, problem solving
Poor motivation	Attribution retraining: internal locus of control	Failure confrontation, attribution to factors under control

Source: Chermak and Musiek (1992).

age children will be equipped with improved methods for evaluating and remediating CAPD.

S U M M A R Y

This chapter has provided an introduction to the process of audiologic rehabilitation at two distinct levels: the early intervention level and school-age service levels. Although services in these settings are provided by a variety of personnel and in various communication modes, one professional—the parent advisor or the AR therapist—often assumes the important roles of coordinating service provision and serving as an advocate for children and families. This chapter has emphasized the critical importance of family-centered practice and the role of the family throughout the child's educational program. After appropriate assessment and selection of intervention priorities, including a communication system, audiologic rehabilitation services throughout the child's life focus on four major areas: (1) environmental coordination and integration of services; (2) audibility, amplification, and assistive device issues; (3) communication activity rehabilitation with a model of language and literacy attainment; and (4) counseling and psychosocial support for the child and family. At the school-age level, the importance of integrated service delivery that considers the unique communicative demands of the classroom setting has been emphasized. Rehabilitation presents challenges to parents, children, and therapists. Nevertheless, if proper attention is given to all of these aspects, prospects for effective management may be very good. If the problems of the child with hearing impairment are underestimated or neglected, the student may experience long-term negative consequences on language, literacy, and social skill attainment. Aggressive and early management of children who are deaf or hard of hearing through audiologic rehabilitation is therefore very important.

SUMMARY POINTS

- Rehabilitative management of children who are deaf and hard of hearing begins with comprehensive, transdisciplinary evaluation. During intervention, ongoing assessment is necessary to document outcomes, make appropriate adjustments to therapy routines, and identify additional intervention priorities.
- Universal newborn hearing screening procedures allow for identification of hearing loss in the neonatal period, much earlier than in the past. To gain maximal benefit, early identification needs to be paired with early intervention programs that seek to involve and support families.
- Most early intervention programs seek to offer family-centered practices. In this approach, families are empowered in their roles as decision makers for the child, professionals seek to form balanced partnerships with parents, and family-identified needs are addressed through collaborative teamwork.
- Families in early intervention programs benefit from full access to information on options to guide decision making. Stress is reduced when informal and formal support systems (e.g., support group meetings) are made available. Parent advisors use coaching methods to support families in providing a nurturing language environment for infants with hearing loss.
- Appropriate management of personal amplification, cochlear implants, and FM systems is a primary step in facilitating a child's use of residual hearing. Children benefit from regular monitoring of amplification, encouragement to wear devices their full waking hours, and opportunities to listen throughout daily routines. Auditory learning can be fostered during natural interactions.
- Preschool-age children benefit from language intervention techniques that stimulate thinking, problem solving, and active learning. Children should be

encouraged to master question–answer routines, because this aspect of language supports them in making discoveries about the world.

- Because children who are deaf and hard of hearing have fewer opportunities to "overhear," they may experience gaps and delays in vocabulary and world knowledge. Both preschool- and school-aged children profit from approaches that help them to build networks of word meanings. They need to learn to tie new information to familiar concepts.

- Speech development programs for children with hearing loss should be structured to maximize the child's reliance on residual hearing. When children strengthen their reliance on listening skills, they often learn to self-monitor, which contributes to the generalization of speech training.

- The AR specialist should be involved as a team member in providing input to the child's IFSP (birth to 3 years) or IEP (3 years on). In the school-age years, AR specialists need to communicate regularly with the educational team so that goals will relate to the student's classroom communicative needs.

- Family members should be involved in the child's AR program throughout the course of the child's education. Furthermore, children with any degree of hearing loss may be candidates for some level of AR service. Team approaches benefit all children, but especially those with multiple disabilities.

RECOMMENDED READING

Alpiner, J. G., & McCarthy, P. A. (2000). *Rehabilitative audiology: Children and adults.* (3rd ed.) Baltimore: Williams & Wilkins.

American Speech–Language–Hearing Association (ASHA). (2002). Guidelines for audiology service provision in and for schools. Rockville, MD: Author.

Cole, E. B. (1992). *Listening and talking: A guide to promoting spoken language in young hearing impaired children.* Washington, DC: Alexander Graham Bell Association for the Deaf.

DeConde-Johnson, C., Benson, P. V., & Seaton, J. B. (1997). *Educational audiology handbook.* San Diego: Singular Publishing Group.

Roeser, R., & Downs, M. (Eds.). (1995). *Auditory disorders in children* (3rd ed.). New York: Thieme.

Roush, J., & Matkin, N. D. (1994). *Infants and toddlers with hearing loss.* Baltimore: York Press.

Watkins, S. (2004). *SKI*HI curriculum. Family-centered programming for infants and young children with hearing loss.* Logan, UT: Hope, Inc.

RECOMMENDED WEBSITES

www.infanthearing.org

www.beginningsvcs.com

www.handsandvoices.com

www.clerccenter.gallaudet.edu

www.boystownhospital.org

www.skihi.org

www.babyhearing.org

REFERENCES

Alpiner, J. G., & McCarthy, P. A. (2000). *Rehabilitative audiology: Children and adults.* (3rd ed.) Baltimore: Williams & Wilkins.

American Academy of Audiology. (2003). *Pediatric amplification protocol.* Accessed May 5, 2006, from http://www.audiology.org

American Academy of Pediatrics. (1999). Newborn and infant hearing loss: Detection and Intervention. Task Force on Newborn and Infant Hearing. *Pediatrics, 103,* 527–530.

Anderson, K. L. (2003). *Early Listening Function* (ELF). www.phonak.com.

Anderson, K., & Matkin, N. (1996). *Screening instrument for targeting educational risk in preschool children* (age 3-kindergarten). www.edaud.org.

American Speech–Language–Hearing Association (ASHA). (1997). Committee on Audiometric Evaluation. *Guidelines for audiologic screening,* 1–60. Rockville, MD: Author.

American Speech-Language-Hearing Association (ASHA). (2002). *Guidelines for audiology service provision in and for schools.* Rockville, MD: Author.

American Speech-Language-Hearing Association (ASHA). (2005a). Central auditory processing: Current status of research and implications for clinical practice. *American Journal of Audiology, 5*(2), 41–54.

American Speech-Language Hearing Association (ASHA). (2005b). *(Central) Auditory processing disorders:* Accessed May 4, 2006, from http://www.asha.org/members/deskref-journals/deskref/default

Bankson, N. W., & Bernthal, J. E. (1990). *Bankson–Bernthal test of phonology.* San Antonio, TX: Special Press.

Bennett, J., & English, K. (1999). Teaching hearing conservation to school children: Comparing the outcomes and efficacy of two pedagogical approaches. *Journal of Educational Audiology, 7,* 29–33.

Bentler, R. A. (1993). Amplification for the hearing-impaired child. In J. G. Alpiner & P. A. McCarthy (Eds.), *Rehabilitative audiology: Children and adults.* Baltimore: Williams & Wilkins.

Berg, F. S. (1993). *Acoustics and sound systems in schools.* San Diego, CA: Singular Publishing Group.

Bess, F. H., Dodd-Murphy, J., & Parker, R. A. (1998). Children with minimal sensorineural hearing loss: Prevalence, educational performance, and functional status. *Ear and Hearing, 19*(5), 339–54.

Blair, J., Petersen, M., & Viehweg, S., (1985). The effects of mild sensorineural hearing loss on academic performance of young school-age children. *Volta Review, 87*(2), 87–93.

Blair, J., Wright, K., & Pollard, G. (1981). Parental understanding of their children's hearing aids. *Volta Review, 83,* 375–382.

Blank, M., Rose, S., & Berlin, L. (1978). *The language of learning: The preschool years* (pp. 8–21). New York: Grune & Stratton.

Boothroyd, A. (1982). *Hearing impairments in young children.* Englewood Cliffs, NJ: Prentice-Hall.

Bredekamp, S. (1987). *Developmentally appropriate practice in early childhood programs serving children from birth through age 8* (expanded ed.). Washington, DC: National Association for the Education of Young Children.

Brinker, R., Frazier, W., & Baxter, A. (1992, Winter). Maintaining involvement of inner city families in EI programs through a program of incentives: Looking beyond family systems to social systems. *OSERS News in Print, 4*(1), 9–19.

Bronfenbrenner, U. (1974). *Is early intervention effective? A report on longitudinal evaluations of preschool programs* (vol. II). (Department of Health, Education and Welfare, Office of Human Development, Office of Child Development, Children's Bureau, Department of Health, Education, and Welfare Publication No. OHD-76-30020). Washington, DC: U.S. Government Printing Office.

Busch, C., & Halpin, K. (1994). Incorporating deaf culture into early intervention. In B. Schick & M. P. Moeller (Eds.), *Proceedings of the Seventh Annual Conference on Issues in Language and Deafness* (pp. 117–125). Omaha, NE: Boys Town National Research Hospital.

Calderon, R. (2000). Parental involvement in deaf children's education programs as a predictor of child's language, early reading, and social–emotional development. *Journal of Deaf Studies and Deaf Education, 5*(2), 140–155.

Calderon, R., Bargones, J., & Sidman, S. (1998). Characteristics of hearing families and their young deaf and hard of hearing children: Early intervention follow-up. *American Annals of the Deaf, 143*(4), 347–362.

Calderon, R., & Greenberg, M. T. (1997). The effectiveness of early intervention for deaf children and children with hearing loss. In M. J. Guralnick (Ed.), *The effectiveness of early invention* (pp. 455–483). Baltimore: Paul H. Brookes.

Calderon, R., & Nadiu, S. (2000). Further support for the benefits of early identification and intervention for children with hearing loss. *Volta Review, 100*(5), 53–84.

Carotta, C., Carney, A. E., & Dettman, D. (1990). Assessment and analysis of speech production in hearing-impaired children. *Asha, 32,* 59(A).

Castle, D. (1984). *Telephone training for hearing-impaired persons: Amplified telephones, TDD's, codes.* Washington, DC: Alexander Graham Bell Association for the Deaf.

Chermak, G. D., & Musiek, F. E. (1992). Managing central auditory processing disorders in children and youth. *American Journal of Audiology,* 61–65.

Cochlear Corporation. (2003). *Listen, learn and talk.* Lane Cove West, NSW, Australia: Author.

Cole, E. B. (1992). *Listening and talking: A guide to promoting spoken language in young hearing impaired children.* Washington, DC: Alexander Graham Bell Association for the Deaf.

Colletti, V., Carner, M., Miorelli, V., Guida, M., Coletti, L., Fiorino, F. (2005, March). Cochlear implantation at under 12 months: Report on 10 patients. *Laryngoscope, 115*(3), 445–449.

Crandell, C., & Smaldino, J. (2000). Classroom acoustics for children with normal hearing and with hearing impairment. *Language, Speech, and Hearing Services in Schools, 31,* 362–370.

Davis, J. (1990). Personnel and service. In J. Davis (Ed.), *Our forgotten children: Hard of hearing pupils in the school* (2nd ed.). Washington, DC: Self Help for the Hard of Hearing.

Davis, J., Effenbein, J., Schum, R., & Bentler, R. (1986). Effects of mild and moderate hearing impairments on language, educational, and psychosocial behavior of children. *Journal of Speech and Hearing Research, 51*(1), 53–63.

DeConde-Johnson, C., Benson, P. V., & Seaton, J. B. (1997). *Educational audiology handbook.* San Diego, CA: Singular Publishing Group.

DesGeorges, J. (2004). *Parent wish list for audiologists.* www.handsandvoices.org.

Domitz, D., & Schow, R. L. (2000). Central auditory processes and test measures: ASHA revisited. *American Journal of Audiology, 9*, 63–68.

Downs, S. K., Whitaker, M. M., & Schow, R. (2003). *Audiological services in school districts that do and do not have an audiologist.* Educational Audiology Association Summer Conference, St. Louis, MO.

Dunst, C. J. (2001). *Parent and community assets as sources of young children's learning opportunities.* Asheville, NC: Winterberry Press.

English, K. (1997). *Self-advocacy for students who are deaf and hard of hearing.* Austin, TX: Pro-Ed.

Erber, N. P. (1982). *Auditory training.* Washington, DC: Alexander Graham Bell Association for the Deaf.

Estabrooks, W. (1998a). Auditory-verbal ages and stages of development. In *Cochlear implants for kids* (pp. 80–88). Washington, DC: Alexander Graham Bell Association for the Deaf.

Estabrooks, W. (1998b). Listening skills for kids with cochlear implants (based on the work of A. L. Phillips, N. Erber, C. Edwards, & W. Estabrooks). In *Cochlear implants for kids* (p. 400). Washington, DC: Alexander Graham Bell Association for the Deaf.

Finitzo-Heiber, T. (1988). Classroom acoustics. In R. Roeser & M. Downs (Eds.), *Auditory disorders in school children* (pp. 221–233). New York: Thieme-Stratton.

Finitzo-Heiber, T., & Tillman, T. (1978). Room acoustics' effects on monosyllabic word discrimination ability for normal and hearing impaired children. *Journal of Speech and Hearing Research, 21*, 440–458.

Flexer, C. (1999). *Facilitated hearing and listening in young children* (2nd ed.). Clifton Park, NY: Singular Publishing Group.

Gaeth, J., & Lounsbury, E. (1966). Hearing aids and children in elementary schools. *Journal of Speech and Hearing Disorders, 31*, 283–289.

Geers, A. E., Nicholas, J. G., & Sedey, A. L. (2003, February). Language skills of children with early cochlear implantation. *Ear and Hearing, 24*(1 Suppl), 46S–58S.

Glover, B. (1999). *Working together on early intervention teams.* Logan, UT: SKI-HI Institute.

Glover, B., Watkins, S., Pittman, P., Johnson, D., & Barringer, D. G. (1994). SKI-HI home intervention for families with infants, toddlers, and preschool children who are deaf or hard of hearing. *Infant–Toddler Intervention: The Transdisciplinary Journal, 4*(4), 319–332.

Hanft, B., Rush, D. D., & Sheldon, M. (2004). *Coaching families and colleagues in early childhood.* Baltimore: Paul H. Brookes.

Harrison, M., & Roush, J. (1996). Age of suspicion, identification and intervention for infants and young children with hearing loss: A national study. *Ear and Hearing, 17*, 55–62.

Hatfield, N., & Humes, K. (1994). Developing a bilingual-bicultural parent-infant program: Challenges, compromises and controversies. In B. Schick & M. P. Moeller (Eds.), *Proceedings of the Seventh Annual Conference on Issues in Language and Deafness.* Omaha, NE: Boys Town National Research Hospital.

Hohmann, M., Banet, B., & Weikart, D. (1979). *Young children in action.* Ypsilanti, MI: High/Scope Press.

Idol, L., Paolucci-Whitcomb, P., & Nevin, A. (1986). *Collaborative consultation.* Rockville, MD: Aspen.

Jerger, J., & Musiek, F. (2000). Report of the consensus conference on the diagnosis of auditory processing disorders in school-age children. *Journal of the American Academy of Audiology, 11*(9), 467–474.

Joint Committee on Infant Hearing (JCIH). (2000). *Position statement.* Accessed May 4, 2006, from http://www.asha.org/about/legislation-advocacy/federal.ehdi

Koch, M. (1999). *Bringing sound to life.* Timonium, MD: York Press.

Langdon, L., & Blair, J. (2000). Can you hear me: A longitudinal study of hearing aid monitoring in the classroom. *Journal of Educational Audiology, 8,* 34–37.

Lederberg, A., & Prezbindowski, A. (2000). Impact of child deafness on mother–toddler interaction: Strengths and weaknesses. In P. Spencer, C. Erting, & M. Marschark (Eds.), *The deaf child in the family and school* (pp. 73–92). Mahwah, NJ: Lawrence Erlbaum.

Ling, D. (1976). *Speech and the hearing impaired child: Theory and practice.* Washington, DC: Alexander Graham Bell Association for the Deaf.

Ling, D. (1989). *Foundations of spoken language in hearing impaired children.* Washington, DC: Alexander Graham Bell Association for the Deaf.

Luterman, D. (1987). *Deafness in the family.* San Diego, CA: College-Hill Press.

Luterman, D. (2004, November 16). Children with hearing loss: Reflections on the past 40 years. *ASHA Leader,* 6–7, 18–21.

Manolson, A., (1985). *It takes two to talk* (2nd ed.). Toronto: Hanen Early Language Resource Centre.

Marge, D. K., & Marge, M. (2005). *Beyond newborn hearing screening: Meeting the educational and healthcare needs of infants and young children.* Report of the National Consensus Conference on Effective Educational and Healthcare Interventions for Infants and Young Children with Hearing Loss, September 10–12, 2004. Syracuse, NY: SUNY Upstate Medical Center.

Marlowe, J. A. (1984). The auditory approach to communication development for the infant with hearing loss. In W. Perkins (Ed.), *Current therapy of communication disorders: Hearing disorders* (pp. 3–9). New York: Thieme-Stratton.

Matkin, N. D. (1984). Wearable amplification: A litany of persisting problems. In J. Jerger (Ed.), *Pediatric audiology: Current trends* (pp. 125–145). San Diego, CA: College-Hill Press.

McClatchie, A., & Therres, M. K. (2004). *Auditory Speech Language (AuSpLan): A manual for professionals working with children who have cochlear implants or amplification.* Accessed May 4, 2006, from http://www.agbell.org

Meadow-Orlans, K. P. (1995). Sources of stress from mothers and fathers of deaf and hard of hearing children. *American Annals of the Deaf, 140,* 352–357.

Meadow-Orlans, K. P., & Steinberg, A. G. (1993). Effects of infant hearing loss and maternal support on mother–infant interaction at 18 months. *Journal of Applied Developmental Psychology, 14,* 407–426.

Mindel, E. D., & Vernon, M. (1987). *They grow in silence: The deaf child and his family* (2nd ed.). Silver Spring, MD: National Association of the Deaf.

Moeller, M. P. (1988). Language assessment strategies [Monograph Supplement]. *Journal of the Academy of Rehabilitative Audiology, 21,* 73–99.

Moeller, M. P. (2000). Early intervention and language outcomes in children who are deaf and hard of hearing. *Pediatrics, 106*(3) 43, 1–9.

Moeller, M. P., & Carney, A. E. (1993). Assessment and intervention with preschool hearing-impaired children. In J. Alpiner & P. McCarthy (Eds.), *Rehabilitative audiology: Children and adults* (2nd ed.; pp. 106–136). Baltimore: Williams & Wilkins.

Moeller, M. P., & Condon, M.-C. (1994). D.E.I.P.: A collaborative problem-solving approach to early intervention. In J. Roush & N. D. Matkin (Eds.), *Infants and toddlers with hearing loss* (pp. 163–194). Baltimore: York Press.

Moog, J., & Geers, A. (1990). *Early Speech Perception Test.* St. Louis: Central Institute for the Deaf.

Moog-Brooks, B. (2002). *My baby and me: A book about teaching your child to talk.* St. Louis, MO: Moog Center for Deaf Education.

Moses, K. L. (1985). Infant deafness and parental grief: Psychosocial early intervention. In F. Powell et al. (Eds.), *Education of the hearing impaired child* (pp. 85–102). San Diego, CA: College-Hill Press.

Musiek, F. E., & Chermak, G. D. (1994). Three commonly asked questions about central auditory processing disorders: Assessment. *American Journal of Audiology, 3,* 23–27.

National Institutes of Health and National Institute on Deafness and Other Communication Disorders (NIH-NIDCD). (1993, March 1–3). *National Institutes of Health Consensus Statement: Early identification of hearing impairment in infants and young children.* Bethesda, MD: Author. http://odp.od.nih.gov/consensus/cons/ 092/092 intro.htm

Niskar, A. S., Kieszak, S. M., Holmes, A., Esteban, E., Rubin, C., & Brody, D. (1998). Prevalence of hearing loss among children 6 to 19 years of age: The Third National Health and Nutrition Examination Survey. *Journal of the American Medical Association, 8,* 279(14), 1071–1075.

Northern, J., & Downs, M. (2002). *Hearing in children* (5th ed.). Baltimore: Williams & Wilkins.

Norton, S. J., Gorga, M. P., Widen, J. E., Folsom, R. C., Sininger, Y., Cone-Wesson, B., Vohr, B., & Fletcher, K. A. (2000). Identification of neonatal hearing impairment: Summary and recommendations. *Ear and Hearing, 21*(5), 529–535.

Oller, D. K. (1983). Infant babbling as a manifestation of the capacity for speech. In S. E. Gerber & G. T. Mencher (Eds.), *The development of auditory behavior* (pp. 221–236). New York: Grune & Stratton.

Oller, D. K., & Eilers, R. E. (1988). The role of audition in infant babbling. *Child Development, 59,* 441–449.

Pugh, G. (1994). *Deaf and hard of hearing students: Educational service guidelines.* Alexandria, VA: NASDSE.

Robbins, A. M., Zimmerman-Phillips, S., & Osberger, M. J. (1998). *Infant-Toddler Meaningful Auditory Integration Scale (IT-MAIS).* Advanced Bionics. http://www. bionicear.com.

Ross, M. (1987). Classroom amplification. In W. Hodgson & P. Skinner (Eds.), *Hearing aid assessment and use in audiologic habilitation* (3rd ed.; pp. 231–265). Baltimore: Williams & Wilkins.

Ross, M., Brackett, D., & Maxon, A. (1991). *Assessment and management of mainstreamed hearing-impaired children: Principles and practices.* Austin, TX: Pro-Ed.

Ross, M., & Tomassetti, C. (1987). Hearing aid selection for preverbal hearing impaired children. In M. C. Pollack (Ed.), *Amplification for the hearing impaired* (3rd ed.; pp. 213–253). New York: Grune & Stratton.

Rossi, K. G. (2003). *Learning to talk around the clock.* Washington, DC: Alexander Graham Bell Association for the Deaf.

Roush, J., Harrison, M., & Palsha, S. (1991). Family-centered early intervention: The perceptions of professionals. *America Annals of the Deaf, 136*(4), 360–366.

Roush, J., & Matkin, N. D. (1994). *Infants and toddlers with hearing loss.* Baltimore: York Press.

Schauwers, K., Gillis, S., Daemers, K., DeBeukelaer, C., & Govaerts, P. (2004, May). *Otology and Neurotology, 25*(3), 263–270.

Schleper, D. (1996). Gallaudet University and Pre-College National Mission programs. *15 principles for reading to deaf children.* Accessed May 5, 2006, http://www.gallaudet.edu/~pcnmplit/literacy/srp/15princ.html

Schow, R. L., & Seikel, J. A. (in press). Screening for (central) auditory processing disorder. In F. Musiek & G. Chermak (Eds.), *Handbook of (central) auditory processing disorder: Volume 1.* San Diego, CA: Plural Publishing.

Schow, R. L., Seikel, J. A., Chermak, G. D., & Berent, M. (2000). Central Auditory processes and test measures: ASHA 1996 revisited. *American Journal of Audiology, 9,* 65–68.

Schuyler, V., & Sowers, N. (1998). *Parent infant habilitation: A comprehensive approach to working with hearing-impaired infants and toddlers and their families.* Portland, OR: HIR Publications.

Shepard, N., Davis, J., Gorga, M., & Stelmachowicz, P. (1981). Characteristics of hearing impaired children in the public schools: Part I. Demographic data. *Journal of Speech and Hearing Disorders, 46,* 123–129.

Simmons-Martin, A. A., & Rossi, K. G. (1990). *Parents and teachers: Partners in language development.* Washington, DC: Alexander Graham Bell Association for the Deaf.

Sinclair, J. S., & Freeman, B. A. (1981). The status of classroom amplification in American education. In F. Bess et al. (Eds.), *Amplification in education.* Washington, DC: Alexander Graham Bell Association for the Deaf.

Sindrey, D. (1997). *Listening games for littles.* London, Ontario: Word Play Publications.

SKI-HI Institute. (1994). *SKI-HI 1992–1993 national data report.* Logan UT: Utah State University, SKI-HI Institute.

Stoel-Gammon, C., & Cooper, J. A. (1984). Patterns of early lexical and phonological development. *Journal of Child Language, 11,* 247–271.

Stredler-Brown, A. (2005, January 18). The art and science of home visits. *ASHA Leader,* pp. 6–7, 15.

Stredler-Brown, A., Moeller, M. P., Gallegos, R., Cordwin, J., & Pittman, P. (2004). *The art and science of home visits* (DVD). Omaha, NE: Boys Town Press.

Vincent, L., Davis, J., Brown, P., Broome, K., Funkhouser, K., Miller, J., & Gruenewald, L. (1986). *Parent inventory of child development in nonschool environment.* Madison: University of Wisconsin, Department of Rehabilitation Psychology and Special Education.

Wallach, G., & Miller, L. (1988). *Language intervention and academic success.* Boston: College-Hill Press.

Watkins, S. (1999). *The gift of early literacy for young children who are deaf or hard of hearing and their families.* Logan, UT: SKI-HI Institute.

Watkins, S. (2004). *SKI*HI curriculum: Family-centered programming for infants and young children with hearing loss.* Logan, UT: Hope, Inc.

Watkins, S., & Clark, T. C. (1993). *SKI*HI resource manual: Family-centered, home-based programming for infants, toddlers, and preschool-aged children with hearing impairment.* Logan, UT: Hope, Inc.

Watkins, S., Pittman, P., & Walden, B. (1996). *Bilingual-bicultural enhancement for infants, toddlers, and preschoolers who are deaf through deaf mentors in family-centered early home-based programming (The Deaf Mentor Project).* Final Report to U.S. Department of Education, Office of Special Education Programs. Logan, UT: SKI-HI Institute.

Watkins, S., Pittman, P., & Walden, B. (1998). The deaf mentor experimental project for young children who are deaf and their families. *American Annals of the Deaf, (29).*

Watkins, S., Taylor, D. J., & Pittman, P. (Eds.). (2004). SKI*HI resource manual: Family-centered programming for infants and young children with hearing loss. Logan, UT: Hope, Inc.

White, K. R., Maxon, A. B., & Behrens, T. R. (1992). Neonatal hearing screening using evoked otoacoustic emissions: The Rhode Island Hearing Assessment Project. In F. H. Bess & J. W. Hall (Eds.), *Screening children for auditory function* (pp. 207–214). Nashville, TN: Bill Wilkerson Center Press.

Yoshinaga-Itano, C., & Downey, D. (1986). A hearing-impaired child's acquisition of schemata: Something's missing. *Topics in Language Disorders, 7*(1), 45–57.

Yoshinaga-Itano, C., Sedey, A. L., Coulter, B. A., & Mehl, A. L. (1998). Language of early and later-identified children with hearing loss. *Pediatrics, 102*(5), 1168–1171.

APPENDIX

GENERAL SUGGESTIONS FOR THE CHILD WITH HEARING IMPAIRMENT IN THE REGULAR CLASSROOM

1. The child with hearing impairment should be encouraged to watch the teacher whenever he or she is talking to the class.
2. The teacher should use natural gestures when he or she complements, not substitutes for speech.
3. Whenever reports are given or during class meetings, have children stand in the front of the class so the child who is hard of hearing can see lips.
4. During class discussions, let the child who is hard of hearing turn around and face the class so he or she can see the lips of the reciter.
5. To help the child follow instructions accurately, assignments should be written on the board so he or she can copy them in a notebook.
6. Like other children with sensory defects, the child with impaired hearing needs individual attention. The teacher must be alert to every opportunity to provide individual help to fill gaps stemming from the child's hearing defect.
7. Ask the child with hearing impairment if he or she understands after an extensive explanation of arithmetic problems or class discussion. Write key words of an idea or lesson on the chalkboard or slip of paper.
8. Enlist class cooperation in understanding the problem of the child with hearing impairment. Designate a student to be the helper in assignments, someone who notes that he or she is on the right page and doing the right exercise. However, do not let the child with hearing impairment become too dependent on the "helper."
9. The child with impaired hearing should be seated no further than five to eight feet from the teacher. He or she should be allowed to shift his or her seat in or-

der to follow the change in routine. This position will enable him or her to see the teacher's face and to hear his or her voice more easily.

10. If the child's hearing impairment involves only one ear or if the impairment is greater in one ear than the other, seat the child in the front with the poorer ear toward the noisy classroom and the better ear turned to the teacher or primary signal. When both ears have the same loss, center placement is recommended.

11. Seat the child with hearing impairment away from the heating/cooling systems, hallways, playground noise, etc.

12. If a choice of teachers is possible, the child with a hearing loss should be placed with the teacher who enunciates clearly. Distinct articulation is more helpful than a raised voice.

13. The child with hearing impairment should be carefully watched to be sure he or she is not withdrawing from the group or is not suffering a personality change as a result of his or her hearing impairment. Make all students feel like "one of the gang."

14. Be natural with the child who is hard of hearing. The child will appreciate it if he or she knows you are considerate of his or her disability.

15. In the lower grades, watch particularly that the student with hearing impairment does his or her part and is not favored or babied.

16. Use visual aids in your presentation of lessons. Visual aids provide the hearing impaired with the association necessary for learning new things.

17. Encourage the child with hearing impairment to accept his or her disability and inspire him or her to make the most of it. Maintain the child's confidence in you so he or she will report any difficulty.

18. Parents should know the truth about their children's achievement. If marking is lenient because of the disability, the parents should know that the child is not necessarily equaling the achievement of a child with normal hearing.

19. Students with hearing impairment need special encouragement when they pass from elementary to junior high school and later into senior high. The pace is swifter. There is much more discussion. Pupils report to five or more teachers instead of one.

20. As the youngster with hearing impairment approaches the age of 16, be especially watchful. She may want to give up. Explain that she needs much preparation to enjoy a life of success and happiness.

HOW TO HELP A CHILD WITH HEARING IMPAIRMENT USE SPEECHREADING SKILLS MORE EFFECTIVELY

1. Don't stand with your back to the window while talking (shadow and glare make it difficult to see your lips).

2. Stand still and in a place with a normal amount of light on your face while speaking.

3. Keep your hand and books down from your face while speaking.

4. Don't talk while writing on the chalkboard.

5. Be sure you have the child's attention before you give assignments or announcements.

6. Speak naturally. Do not exaggerate or overemphasize. It is to be expected that it will be more difficult to hold the attention of the child who is hard of hearing. Never forget that the hearing impaired get fatigued sooner than other children because they not only have to use their eyes on all written and printed work, but also have to watch the lips.

7. Particular care must be used in dictating spelling. Use the words in sentences to show which of two similar words is meant (i.e., "Meet me after school" and "Give the dog some meat"). Thirteen words look like *meat* when spoken, such as *been, bead,* and *beet.* The word *king* shows little or no lip movement. Context of the sentence gives the child the clue to the right word. Have the child who is hard of hearing say the words to him- or herself before a mirror while studying spelling lesson.

8. If the child who is hard of hearing misunderstands, restate the question in a different way. Chances are you are using words with visual images that are difficult to speechread. Be patient and never skip these students. Be sure that things are understood before you move ahead.

CHAPTER 10

Audiologic Rehabilitation for Adults and Elderly Adults

Assessment and Management

Kathy Pichora-Fuller
Ronald L. Schow

CONTENTS

■ INTRODUCTION

Some individuals who lived with hearing loss as children or teenagers continue to experience hearing loss as adults. Some adults become late-deafened. Some experience sudden hearing loss. Some undergo medical or surgical treatments ranging from middle ear reconstruction, to removal of acoustic neuroma, to cochlear implantation. For many, exposure to hazardous levels of recreational or occupational noise over extended periods of time results in permanent sensorineural hearing loss. Hearing conservation programs to prevent hearing loss and identify early signs of hearing loss may be considered as an early type of hearing care along a continuum of care for adults who, sooner or later, will need various forms of audiologic rehabilitation (AR). Overall, the etiology of hearing loss is well known for some adults, but the vast majority of adults experience very gradual age-related declines in hearing for which there may be no obvious cause or explanation other than just aging.

Some adults lose their hearing suddenly but most lose it very gradually.

The provision of services for adults who are hard of hearing has always been challenging, but with an ever expanding elderly population and with new technology increasingly available, this challenge is larger than ever. More needs to be done, and more can be done. Senior adults continue to live longer and maintain more active lifestyles. It is striking that the segment of the population over the age of 85 years is increasing in numbers faster than any other age group. A major ingredient for maintaining and enhancing quality of life is to maintain communication skills. Most individuals experiencing hearing loss will retain some residual hearing, but what they lose will erode their ability to hear others effectively, and *communication activity* will become compromised. Hearing loss will gradually reduce their *participation* in many rewarding activities of life. Both *personal* and *environmental factors* will interact to complicate these changes.

■ PROFILE OF THE ADULT CLIENT

Hearing Loss over the Lifespan

The prevalence of hearing loss increases with advancing age, as reflected by Table 10.1 and Figure 10.1. These numbers suggest that hearing problems increase gradually throughout life, but note that there are substantial numbers of younger adults who have hearing loss too. Table 10.1 gives an estimate of impairment or hearing loss based on interview data; Figure 10.1 shows disability or communication activity data based on hearing and understanding speech. The numbers are slightly different, but in both cases we see that hearing problems increase for young and middle-aged adults but increase more dramatically for people in the retirement years. By age 75, about half of the general adult population and the vast majority of those living in residential care facilities have a clinically significant degree of threshold hearing loss. But many listeners first notice problems hearing in everyday life much earlier. Difficulties often begin in the fourth decade, especially in challenging listening conditions, such as when there is background noise or reverberation, even though there may be no real problems in more ideal quiet surroundings (CHABA, 1988).

Hearing loss affects adults of all ages but it increases dramatically as we grow older.

TABLE 10.1		
Prevalence Rates of Hearing Impairment, per 100 Persons, in the Civilian, Noninstitutionalized Population of the United States		
AGE GROUP IN YEARS	NUMBER	PREVALENCE RATE (%)
3–17	968,000	1.8
8–24	650,000	2.6
25–34	1,659,000	3.4
35–44	2,380,000	6.3
45–54	2,634,000	10.3
55–64	3,275,000	15.4
65–74	4,267,000	23.4
75+	4,462,000	37.7
All	20,295,000	8.6

Note: Rates are based on 1990–1991 interview data from the National Center for Health Statistics (Ries, 1994).

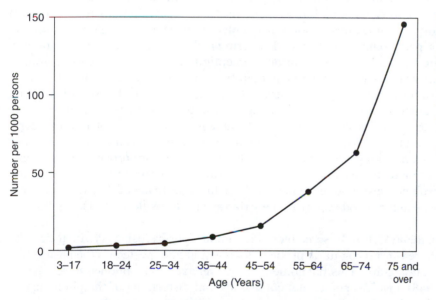

FIGURE 10.1

Average annual age-specific number of persons 3 years of age and over who cannot hear and understand normal speech per 1000 persons: United States, 1990–1991.

Source: Ries (1994).

Inevitably, loss of hearing leads to misunderstandings and stress for individuals, their families, and close associates. After first realizing that hearing has become difficult, adults often need time to accept that they have a hearing loss and that they should get help. It is common for adults to delay seeking help for hearing problems by years and sometimes even decades. Eventually, it is common for family, friends, or the stress associated with hearing loss to convince the individual to have his or her hearing screened or tested, leading to a firm identification of the loss. Rather than dismissing adults in the early stages of hearing loss as poorly motivated or "not yet ready for a hearing aid," innovative audiologists around the world are discovering how to use health education or health promotion approaches to prepare

After noticing a hearing problem, it takes time for adults to seek help from an audiologist.

adults for the eventuality of other forms of AR. Recent research on help seeking and adjustment to hearing loss should help rehabilitative audiologists develop new management approaches for adults living with hearing loss whose abilities, needs, and aspirations change over time and with life circumstances (Noble, 1998; Worrall & Hickson, 2003).

■ PROFILE OF THE ELDERLY CLIENT

We will deal with the elderly somewhat separately from younger adults, because the majority of those who have hearing problems and the great bulk of those who need hearing rehabilitation are elderly. As a group, the elderly are similar in many ways, but the needs of each person will need to be considered on an individual basis.

Hearing Loss

PRESBYCUSIS. Willott (1991) defines *presbycusis* as "the decline in hearing associated with various types of auditory system dysfunction (peripheral and/or central) that accompany aging and cannot be accounted for by extraordinary ototraumatic, genetic, or pathological conditions. The term *presbycusis* implies deficits not only in absolute thresholds but in auditory perception, as well." In its most common form, presbycusis is characterized as high-frequency sensorineural loss that progresses gradually. It is usually assumed that this elevation of thresholds in the higher frequencies is the result of damage in the cochlea. To the extent that age-related hearing loss involves outer hair cell damage, the hearing problems of elderly clients should be very similar to those of younger adults who have similar audiograms. However, aging adults are also likely to have auditory processing problems that are not predictable from the audiogram. Other common causes of age-related hearing problems are thought to involve dysnchronous firing of the auditory nerve and changes in the blood supply to the stria vascularis (Willott, 1991).

> Older adults with a good audiogram may notice problems hearing in noisy everyday situations, even though they have no problem hearing in quiet situations.

PHONEMIC REGRESSION. In some older individuals, presbycusis is characterized by a more severe word recognition problem than would be expected on the basis of the pure-tone audiogram. This phenomenon, first referred to as phonemic regression (Gaeth, 1948), involves perceptual confusions and distortions of the phonetic elements of speech and may not be overcome by amplification alone. Increasing the intensity of speech is not always helpful, because phonemic regression is generally attributed to a central auditory processing disorder (CAPD or APD). Individuals with CAPD perceive a greater hearing problem than those without CAPD (Jerger, Oliver, & Pirozzolo, 1990). Alternative AR approaches beyond just fitting hearing aids may be needed to address the communication problems of the many older adults who have CAPD with or without significant audiometric threshold elevations.

To further complicate matters, an older listener's peripheral and/or central auditory processing difficulties may interact with age-related changes in other senses, motor skills, and cognition. The complexities of age-related hearing loss and how it interacts with other areas of ability require the audiologist to consider many facets of the client's life as a communicator (Kiessling et al., 2003). Over the last decade, much has been learned about age-related changes in perception, and in emotional, social, cognitive, and linguistic performance (Craik & Salthouse, 2000). Nonauditory changes no doubt have a bearing on adjustment to hearing loss in adulthood (Kricos, 2002), as well as on communication competence in general. In trying to understand how adults experience hearing loss, it helps to consider the lifespan changes they experience, especially changes that alter real or perceived communicative competence.

Physical and Mental Health and the Aging Process

An increasing number of lifestyle changes in late adulthood results in a more heterogeneous population than that of any other age group. It is therefore impossible to assess accurately the effect of aging based solely on a person's chronological age. Not all individuals of the same age experience aging in the same way. Some people appear youthful well into their 80s, while others manifest old age behaviors by their early 40s.

> Some people appear youthful well into their 80s, whereas others manifest old-age behaviors by their early 40s.

Most elderly persons are in relatively good health, but as reported by the U.S. Bureau of the Census (1990), approximately 9 percent of adults 65 to 69 years old need assistance with their everyday activities, and this increases to 45 percent for those 85 and over. To some degree, most senior adults are eventually required to adjust to a certain amount of physical disability and reduced activity level. As each new physical problem becomes apparent and deterioration continues, the consequences of aging can significantly affect an individual's attitude toward self-fulfillment. This is why it is difficult to discuss the physical and mental factors contributing to the aging process separately. The interaction between the two is symbiotic, with changes in one almost certainly influencing the other. As senior adults confront lifestyle changes, not all adapt readily. Concomitant declines in sensory and motor skills and increased risk of illness and injury may create an actual and/or a perceived loss of independence and personal control.

Behaviors described as "senile" (e.g., inattentiveness, inappropriate responding) may result from clinically significant cognitive impairments, or they may only be apparent cognitive problems that in reality result from depression or psychological stress related to coping with biological changes or even to age-related reductions in sensory abilities. Experimental research has shown that when healthy young and old adults perform cognitive tasks such as remembering and comprehending spoken speech, there seem to be age-related differences in cognitive performance, but these age-related differences are minimized when the test conditions are adjusted so that perceptual difficulty is equal for all listeners (Schneider, Daneman, & Pichora-Fuller, 2002). It follows that, if older people have more trouble hearing incoming information, they in turn become disadvantaged when performing cognitive tasks such as comprehending or remembering to rely on information that has been heard. In fact, studies have shown that hearing loss can have an adverse effect on quality of life and on emotional, behavioral, and social well-being. Bess et al. (1989) found a systematic relationship between hearing loss and functional-psychosocial status in 153 elderly subjects and determined that hearing loss accounted for a significant amount of the variation when they controlled for demographic variables like age, number of illnesses, and medication amounts. The importance of social, psychological, and environmental issues in adjustment to

> Adjustment to hearing loss interacts with age-related changes in physical, cognitive, emotional, and social function.

hearing loss has received increasing attention in the last decade (Borg, 1998; Ross, 1997). On the one hand, unmanaged hearing loss may have an adverse effect on the physical, cognitive, emotional, behavioral, and social functions of aging adults; on the other hand, the participation of adults with hearing loss may not be restricted so long as rehabilitation, including optimization of social and physical supports, enables them to fulfill their personal and social goals in everyday life. Whereas the causal direction of the link between hearing loss and personal or social adjustment and cognitive performance may be open to debate, the eventual establishment of the link between them for most aging adults is evident. The nature of these links needs to be better understood and incorporated into rehabilitative approaches (Pichora-Fuller & Carson, 2000).

Personal and Environmental Factors

The audiologist must consider the resources or supports that are available to aging clients as they try to adjust to hearing loss. Some older individuals may find it easier than younger adults to adjust to hearing loss because they are able to apply a lifetime of other experiences and generalize lessons they have learned about how to cope with other health problems. Nevertheless, others may be less fortunate and face greater challenges than would a younger adult adjusting to hearing loss. With age, the frequency and severity of significant lifestyle changes continue to increase, as described by Ronch and Van Zanten (1992) and summarized next. Although most aging persons undergo a certain degree of change in every area listed, their capacity to adapt to these changes is highly individualized, depending on genetic inheritance, life experiences, traditional ways of dealing with life, and past and present environmental factors.

1. *Physical condition:* Loss of youth; changes in physiological and biological aspects of the body cause poor health and its emotional consequences.
2. *Emotional and sexual life:* Loss of significant others through death, separation, and reduction in sexual activity due to societal expectations, health, personal preference, or death of partner.
3. *Members of the family of origin:* Parents, brothers, and sisters become ill or die.
4. *Marital relationship:* Strain due to death or illness of spouse, estrangement due to empty-nest syndrome, pressures due to retirement.
5. *Peer group:* Friends die or become separated by geographical relocation for health, family, or retirement reasons.
6. *Occupation:* Many older people retire.
7. *Recreation:* Becomes scarce due to physical limitation or unavailability of opportunities.
8. *Economics:* Income is reduced by retirement; limited income is tapped by inflation or medical costs not covered by insurance.

Economic Status and Retirement

Retirement is perhaps the primary factor for change in the senior adult's economic status. Loss of employment may not only alter financial security, but may also reduce social interaction and erode self-esteem. Adjustments to radical lifestyle changes are easier when economic factors are not a concern. A higher income allows greater mobility to seek better health care and to continue supportive social contacts. The affluent, socially active older person is more inclined to compensate for the detrimental effects of age by purchasing necessary medications, eyeglasses, dentures, or hearing aids. Note that they may have many options, and sometimes they may prefer to try to compensate for the effects of hearing loss in their life by using alternatives to hearing aids. Low-income persons, on the other hand, have fewer options. Women are particularly vulnerable to economic stresses, especially if they have not been in the work force. Because husbands were often the wage earners, widows often have no or limited savings, and they may have had more limited opportunities to develop social supports outside of the home.

Although most older individuals are not considered poor, many live on fixed incomes and have their prime financial asset tied up in the equity of their home. The financial benefit of selling the house is frequently offset by the emotional stress produced by the subsequent loss of neighborhood, territorial familiarity, security, and environmental surroundings. The economic status of senior citizens who live in long-term extended-care facilities is usually lower than that of their counterparts who reside in privately owned homes.

Living Environments

Older adults may live independently, with family members, or in some type of health care facility. Most live in their own residence, while only 15 percent live with a relative other than their spouse or a nonrelative. Many frail elderly adults are confined to their homes due to financial and health considerations and are often cared for by their spouses or children. Just over 50 percent of the aging population lives with a spouse. The number living alone rapidly increases with advancing age until 47 percent are doing so when they are 85 years or over (Taeuber, 1992). On average, women live longer than men so it follows that most of the elderly who live on their own are women. Of course, a person who spends most of their time at home alone will have reduced opportunities for communication. Even though elderly individuals living on their own may have less frequent need to hear conversation, hearing may become extremely important from a safety perspective because they must be able to hear fire alarms, doorbells, and phone rings and to respond appropriately in emergency situations without the help of others.

Older individuals may require professional health care beyond the capabilities of the family environment. For some, this may necessitate only limited assisted care, but health care facilities most often associated with the aging population are nursing homes that provide long-term care. About 52 percent of women versus 33 percent of men will use a nursing home before they die. In addition, 70 percent of women who die at 90 have lived in a nursing home. Those in nursing homes represent an older segment of the geriatric population with generally more advanced physical and mental deterioration. Furthermore, they are more socially isolated, with about half having no nearby relatives. Families frequently use nursing homes for those near death, and most admissions are short term (three-quarters are for less than a year) (Taeuber, 1992). In the past, nursing homes were often operated

Just over 50 percent of the elderly live with a spouse.

Assistive living options are creating new settings for AR.

following a hospital model. Recently, with the graying of the baby boomers, there is a rapidly growing number of seniors with ample financial resources who are seeking high-quality assisted living options that are more like home. This demand has fueled the development of the businesses specialized in "retirement living" residences that provide resort-style accommodation and meals, along with in-house recreational, nursing, and other supportive services that can be phased in as needed. For those in the highest level of care, these facilities often feature special "reminiscence" areas specialized for the care of people with dementia, including those who need a living space with secured entry and exit because they are at risk of wandering and becoming lost. These new settings open up a new option with great opportunities for audiologists to provide AR.

As more recreation-oriented programming in retirement living and assisted living facilities offers more opportunities for social interaction for those living in such residences, the importance of preserving hearing function will only become more important in the future. For nursing home residents and the hospitalized elderly, hearing loss is very common. Schow and Nerbonne (1980) evaluated 202 nursing home residents from five facilities and found that 82 percent of their sample demonstrated pure-tone threshold averages (PTAs) of 26 dB HL or greater, with 48 percent exhibiting PTAs of at least 40 dB HL.

Palliative nursing care occurs in the final stages of a person's life.

Palliative care occurs when saving a life drops in priority and patients are being nursed through the final stages of life. In our experience, nurses doing such care may make audiology referrals because they want to communicate with people at this stage, even though this may have been less important when the nurses earlier were preoccupied with other forms of care. We should not assume that it is unimportant to work with very ill people who have little time to live.

■ MODEL FOR REHABILITATION

In Chapter 1 and in Schow (2001) a model and flowchart were presented to provide an overall framework for AR. The flowchart is shown in Figure 10.2 to provide a frame of reference as we describe rehabilitation for adults. As noted there, this work is divided into rehabilitative assessment and the treatment itself, and it includes an outcome measurement feedback loop. Our model is highly compatible with other current models even though there may be slight differences in terminology. An international consensus paper, including the model shown in Figure 10.3, was recently published by a working group, including many of the world's leading rehabilitative audiologists who met to consider the rehabilitative needs of older adults (Kiessling et al., 2003). The main components of our model, assessment and treatment with feedback from outcome measurement, parallel the main components of the model proposed by the international consensus group who label the components respectively as evaluation and intervention, with ongoing surveillance and maintenance. In both our model and the model of the international consensus group, the core concerns within the assessment (or evaluation) and management (or intervention) components derive from the anchor points provided by the WHO concepts of activity and participation as explained in Chapter 1. Included in both models also are personal and environmental factors.

The main components of our model are like those in a recent international model: assessment (or evaluation) and treatment (or intervention), with feedback from outcome measurement (or surveillance and maintenance).

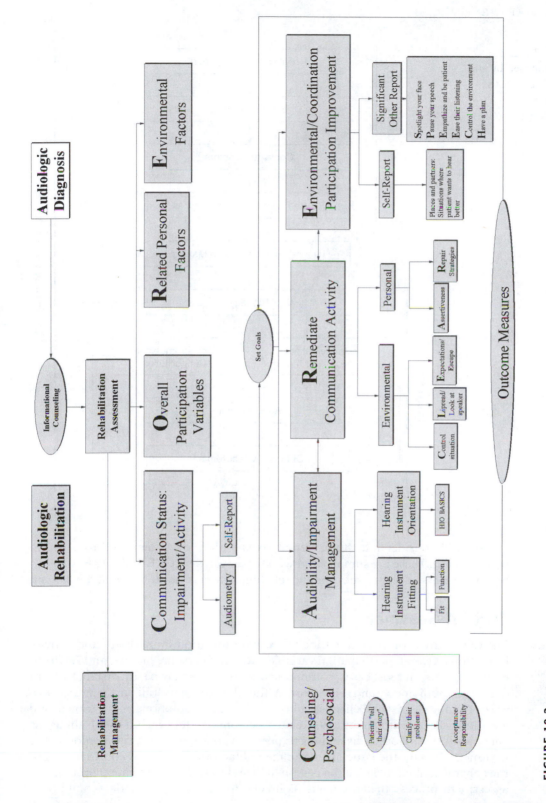

FIGURE 10.2

Model for audiologic rehabilitation.

FIGURE 10.3

AR model proposed by an international consensus working group.
Source: Kiessling et al. (2003).

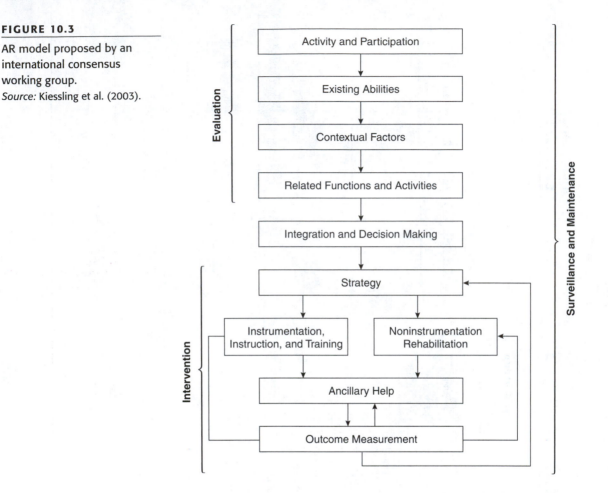

We will consider four fundamental areas within assessment and four within management. These are summarized with the acronyms CORE and CARE, suggesting the core assessment issues and the rehabilitative care needed to treat the patient.

CORE Assessment

The traditional case history is actually a form of self-report, but more formal self-report procedures are also available.

The CORE areas of assessment include **C**ommunication impairment and activity limitations, **O**verall participation variables, **R**elated personal factors, and **E**nvironmental factors. In most cases, communication findings may be drawn chiefly from diagnostic audiometry and self-report. Within the area of overall participation variables, the audiologist and client should consider social, emotional, educational, and vocational issues, among others. Related personal factors include such things as client attitude and other disabilities or personal conditions that may confound the treatment. Finally, the issue of environmental factors encourages consideration of the general context in which the person lives and must communicate. Through this assessment process the audiologist is invited to consider the fundamental issues that bear on rehabilitation. This need not be an extended process, because a good case history and a focused self-report often help us to address these issues. Nevertheless, we need to see these four matters as comprising a rehabilitation battery, and none of these important elements should be neglected.

CARE Management

On the treatment side we see the four aspects summarized by the acronym CARE. **C**ounseling, **A**udibility–amplification, **R**emediation for communication activities, and **E**nvironmental coordination and participation improvement are the focus here. *Counseling* should include information dispensed to the client based on our assessment findings, and through an interactive process, it should allow the client to help set goals for what he or she would like to accomplish in treatment. Treatment goals will fall into three areas: *audibility, activity,* and *participation.*

Audibility treatment usually involves amplification. In many current cases this is the only focus of treatment. But through the current model we propose not only a more precise understanding of the elements within audibility management, but a broader focus to treatment that includes activity and participation issues as proposed by the WHO model. Hearing instrument and audibility treatment involve the fit and function of the instrument, plus hearing instrument orientation (HIO). *Fit* has to do with matters like the style of the aid or the specific assistive device preferred by the client, plus issues like obtaining a suitable mold impression. *Function* has reference to matters such as whether audibility is accomplished through digital or other aids. These matters of *fit and function* have been thoroughly discussed in Chapter 2. *Hearing instrument orientation (HIO)* should cover some fundamental topics. The typical dispensing audiologist may use a handout to cover the basics when this part of the audibility management is performed.

> For many adults treatment must go beyond amplification alone.

Communication activity issues should be addressed by all those fitting hearing aids and others involved in hearing rehabilitation. One approach in this area involves asking the client to consider at least five important communication concepts: (1) control the situation, (2) lipread, (3) realistic expectations or escape, (4) assertiveness, and (5) repair strategies. As noted in the model, these matters involve both personal and environmental factors. A small handout also can be used to help reinforce these concepts, which would be explained by the audiologist and reinforced throughout the entire dispensing process. More advanced communication work may be used to follow up and provide more intensive help.

The final area of treatment involves *environmental and participation* issues. We recommend, for most audiologists dispensing hearing aids, that this concern can be most easily addressed through the use of self-report. When clients select a few areas of major concern wherein they have serious communication difficulties, as they do within appropriate self-report approaches, these generally translate into goals whereby the clients would like to improve his or her communication activities and participation possibilities. If the dispensing audiologist helps the client select at least one unique area of concern, then outcome measures can be used to measure improvement. When self-report questionnaires contain standard situations in which persons with hearing difficulties experience problems, standardized data are available that allow comparison with the client being treated.

Feedback Based on Outcome Measures

Following initial assessment and treatment, it will be essential to use outcome measures to determine if the treatment worked. If the treatment has not addressed the initial needs of the client or if new needs have emerged since the initial assessment, then new rehabilitation plans must be developed and implemented. Follow-up using outcome measures can be thought of as a kind of reassessment. In effect, the process of assessment and treatment cycle repeatedly over time, and changes are introduced based on the results obtained using outcome measures. Three main categories of outcome measures concern how well the person performs, how much use he or she makes of the treatment, and how satisfied he or she is with it. Performance and use measures may be objective or subjective, but to measure benefit and satisfaction the most informative outcome measures are obtained by self-report. Self-report is used in outcome measures with prefitting and postfitting scores that address a variety of participation areas.

Conceptual Framework

The WHO model helps to standardize approaches to AR.

The model described in this textbook is based on the concepts of the WHO (2001) and provides a relatively simple protocol for AR with the hope that more precision and unanimity might be obtained in this work. We believe that this AR model will be helpful for those doing the most common form of AR: hearing instrument fitting and follow-up for adults. It is broader, however, than the narrow rehabilitation concerns surrounding amplification. Sadly, the simple reality is that most persons who undergo assessment for their hearing problems are not evaluated as thoroughly as we recommend, and many adults receive only a semblance of the idealized treatment that we summarize in this chapter. For most adults, hearing aids, and sometimes ALDs, along with pre- and post-purchase counseling and orientation tailored to the life circumstances of the individual, will be the key components of AR. But hearing aid dispensing on its own, with no goal other than making a sale, will be woefully inadequate. Unfortunately, such narrow, sale-focused hearing aid counseling and orientation are often provided in a terribly abbreviated fashion (see the survey of rehabilitation procedures on the website provided with this text).

Some rehabilitation-oriented audiologists have proposed methods of counseling and orientation that will be simple and readily used by more practitioners (e.g., Gagné, 2000). In most cases, counseling and orientation need not be complicated nor go on interminably. Client-centered efforts that focus on real needs and problem solving will allow us to achieve effective rehabilitation as soon as the problems are solved. These efforts will also take into consideration the life context of the person, including many nonauditory age-related changes in abilities, needs, and aspirations. The main challenge facing rehabilitative audiologists today is to find approaches based on a deeper understanding of adults with hearing loss and how different forms of rehabilitation can be combined to achieve solutions tailored to meet their specific abilities, needs, and aspirations in a timely and effective fashion (Dillon & So, 2000; Stephens, Jones, & Gianopoulos, 2000). Montgomery (1994) recommended a simple protocol based on the acronym WATCH, which he hoped would inspire more audiologists to standardize their approach to rehabilitation at the time of hearing aid fitting. Others (e.g., Gagné & Jennings, 2000; Goldstein & Stephens, 1981; Stephens, 1996a) have also proposed models to help us better understand the rehabilitation process, but none of these previous efforts has incorporated the WHO model. By laying out a recommended protocol for those involved in dispensing and by providing supportive materials to facilitate the adoption of a newer approach based on the WHO concepts, as is done in this chapter and elsewhere, we hope to move toward the acceptance of a more standardized procedure in rehabilitation (Schow, 2001; Schow et al., 2005). With this broader focus and grounding within WHO, we are hopeful that the acronyms from this model will simplify the concepts and help the student to somewhat standardize rehabilitative work.

■ REHABILITATION SETTINGS

Traditionally, rehabilitative care for hearing has been delivered in a variety of settings. These include university speech and hearing clinics, community hearing centers, hospitals, otologic clinics, senior citizen centers, vocational rehabilitation offices, audiology private practices, and hearing aid sales offices.

University Programs

Early adult AR centers were provided in university training programs that served World War II veterans with hearing loss. The focus was directed toward improvement of the adult's communication skills through the use of appropriate amplification and communication training, with counseling and education of adults with hearing impairment, their families, and significant others.

This early approach continues to influence present-day programs. At the Idaho State University Hearing Clinic, for example, faculty and students provide a comprehensive program of hearing care (see Brockett & Schow, 2001; Schow, 2001). After diagnostic audiology, rehabilitation assessment, and counseling, consideration is given to solving audibility deficits through the use of personal amplification systems used alone or in conjunction with assistive listening devices. After the devices are fit, the client is given hearing instrument orientation through a process called HIO BASICS, and the client is given a handout (Figure 10.4) to facilitate this process. Communication activities are routinely treated through the use of a program called CLEAR, and this has a handout also (Figure 10.5). Self-report information is used to assess aspects of participation that the client is concerned about and chooses to address. In addition, a handout called SPEECH (Figure 10.6) is provided for family members and for friends to teach them some basic concepts about communication. In this manner, rehabilitation addresses these broad concerns in working to solve impairment problems through improved audibility, communication activity is targeted with common useful remedies, and participation issues are chosen by the client that, when solved, will improve his or her quality of life. Usually, the approach is individual. Occasionally, clients choose to attend four 2-hour group sessions. Significant others, usually spouses, may be included in AR sessions.

HIO BASICS

Hearing expectations. Even the most advanced hearing aid technology will not give you normal hearing. Also, remember that even people with normal hearing do not understand everything all the time. Some situations will be difficult. Properly fitted hearing aids will allow you to hear soft sounds better while keeping loud sounds appropriately loud. You may find, however, that sounds such as water running, crackling newspaper, wind blowing, crying babies, or dishes in a restaurant will sound different. This difference may be annoying, but with continued use and adjustment to the hearing aids it should become acceptable.

Instrument operation. Be sure that you understand the controls on your hearing aid. What controls are on your aid: volume control, T-coil switch, memory button, directional microphone switch, others? Review each control and be sure that you can adjust it. Ask for help if you need to go over the controls again. Practice and patience will help while you are learning. Experiment to find the best way to use the telephone, but remember not to hold it too close to your hearing aid and that tilting it slightly to the side can prevent feedback. Assistive devices for telephone use are available if you continue to have difficulty.

Occlusion effect. The occlusion effect is an echo that you may hear that can make your voice sound more hollow. If you notice this bothering you, bring it to the attention of your hearing care professional.

Batteries. These come in different sizes. Write your correct size and number here _____. Batteries usually last 1 to 2 weeks depending on how much you wear your hearing aids. Be sure you know how to obtain replacements. The battery has to be inserted with the shiny side facing up. If you cannot change your battery, be sure to ask for help. Keep batteries away from children because they are dangerous if swallowed or placed inside the nose or ear.

Acoustic feedback. Feedback is the squealing sound that your hearing aids sometimes make. It happens when the amplified sound gets into the microphone. If you hear it when you hold the hearing aid in your hand, you know that your hearing aid is turned on. If you hear it when the hearing aid is in your ear, you know that the earmold is not snug or the volume is too high. If you cannot wear your hearing aids at the best loudness level without feedback, ask your hearing care professional for help.

System troubleshooting. If your hearing aid is not working, first check the battery. Then check if there is wax in the microphone or receiver opening. Remove the wax using the simple tools that come with your hearing aids. If you still have problems, ask your hearing care professional for help.

Insertion and removal. It is very important to learn how to insert and remove your hearing aids properly because, if you find it difficult or uncomfortable to do this, you won't want to use the aid. Practice regularly to improve and maintain your skill. Ask if you need more help.

Cleaning and maintenance. Wax or other debris can block the opening on the microphone or receiver. Learn how to use tissues, brushes, and wax loops to keep your hearing aids clean. Clean your hearing aids every day and not just when there is a problem.

Service. Knowing where and how to get service on the hearing aid is important. Read your warranty to be sure you understand it. Take advantage of the regular follow-up appointments that the hearing care professional will schedule for you. The usual life of hearing aids is four to five years if they are well cared for, but one day you will need new hearing aids even if your hearing stays the same.

FIGURE 10.4

Handout of suggestions for Hearing Instrument Orientation (HIO).

Source: Schow (2001); Brockett & Schow (2001).

CLEAR

Control your communication situations. Maximize what you are trying to listen to and minimize anything that gets in the way of what you are trying to hear. Position yourself so that you can see the talker well and hear him or her most clearly and with the least interference from others. Turn on some lights or move your conversation to an area that is better lit. Move conversations away from noisy areas. If the talker is too far away or the interference from others is too bothersome, you can mic that person with an assistive device. In short, whenever you can, be sure to control the lighting or your position in the room and favor your better ear if you have one.

Look at and/or lipread the talker to ease the strain of listening. Watch the person so you can read body language, facial expressions, and lip movements to clarify information that is hard to hear. Remember that much of the information that is hard to hear is easy to see. Lipreading is easier if you face the person directly, but you can also get useful information from the side. In general, the closer the better, but 5 to 10 feet away is ideal.

Expectations need to be realistic. When the situation is just too difficult, you can use communication escape strategies to help you to reduce frustration. If you are realistic about how well you can hear, you may decide that some situations are unreasonably difficult. Anticipate the fact that you will likely have difficulty, and plan options for dealing with a breakdown in communication. For example, if a restaurant is a difficult listening situation, rather than staying at home, agree to have another person in your party explain the specials to you or do the ordering. This is called an anticipatory strategy.

Assertiveness can help others understand your hearing difficulties. Let others in your conversation know that you have difficulty hearing and encourage them to get your attention before talking and to look at you when they speak. Let them know that short, uncomplicated sentences are easier to understand than longer, complicated ones. Being timid will not serve you well; you must speak up and be assertive in order to move the conversation away from a noisy area or ask the talker to slow down or talk louder. Be pleasantly assertive and let your needs be known. Most people will want to be helpful in these circumstances.

Repair strategies for communication breakdown can help you and the talker. If you miss important information and you don't understand enough of what is being said, repeat back what you did hear and ask others to clarify what you missed. You can ask others to speak more loudly or slowly or distinctly. You can ask them to spell a word or even write it down. Counting on your fingers may help with numbers. Develop different ways to repair a conversation, and do it in an interesting way or with a sense of humor if possible. Saying "I'm going to listen the best I can now, so please say that once more" as you face and watch the person is a more pleasant way to ask for repetition than simply saying "What?" You can also reduce the need for repairs by being the one who begins a conversation or by being sure you know what the topic is before you enter into a conversation.

FIGURE 10.5

Handout of communication suggestions to help the person with hearing loss.
Source: Schow (2001); Brockett & Schow (2001).

Community Centers and Agencies

Community medical centers and hearing societies, such as those in New York City and a few other large cities, provide rehabilitation settings and classes where participants are usually highly motivated and well directed toward management of their problems. Vocational rehabilitation offices provide adults whose hearing is impaired with access to networks of assessment and management services that are

SPEECH

S*potlight* your face and keep it visible. Keep your hands away from your mouth so that the hearing-impaired person can get all the visual cues possible. Be sure to face the speaker when you are talking and be at a good distance. Avoid gum, cigarettes, and other distractions when possible. And be sure not to talk from another room and expect to be heard.

P*ause* slightly between the content portions of sentences. Slow, exaggerated speech is as difficult to understand as fast speech. However, speech at a moderate pace with slight pauses between phrases and sentences can allow the person who is hard of hearing to process the information in chunks. This procedure is sometimes called CLEAR SPEECH.

E*mpathize* and be patient with the hearing-impaired person. Try plugging both ears and listen for a short while to something soft that you want to hear in an environment that is distracting and noisy. This may help you to appreciate the challenge of being hard of hearing, and it should help you to be patient if the responses seem slow. Rephrase if necessary to clarify a point and remember, empathy, patience, empathy!!!

E*ase* the person's listening. Get the listener's attention before you speak and make sure that you are being helpful in the way you speak. Ask how you can facilitate communication. The listener may want you to speak more loudly or more softly, more slowly or faster, or announce the subject of discussion, or signal when the topic of conversation shifts. Be compliant and helpful and encourage the listener to give you feedback so you can make it as easy as possible for him or her.

C*ontrol* the circumstances and the listening conditions in the environment. Maximize communication by getting closer to the person. If you can be 5 to 10 feet away, that is ideal. Also, move away from background noise and maintain good lighting. Avoid dark restaurants and windows behind you that blind someone watching you.

H*ave* a plan. When anticipating difficult listening situations, set strategies for communication in advance and implement them as necessary. This might mean that at a restaurant you carry on the communication with a server instead of having your hard of hearing family member or friend do so.

FIGURE 10.6

Handout of communication suggestions to help the person to communicate with someone who has a hearing loss.
Source: Schow (2001); Brockett & Schow (2001).

often important for optimizing their potential for gainful employment and for helping them function as contributing members of a community.

Military

Various AR programs are available for current and former military personnel in military and Veterans Administration medical centers. Programs range from one-time, 1-hour hearing instrument orientation sessions after hearing aid fitting to comprehensive programs meeting over an intense 3-day period. Generally, the sessions are individual, but some group sessions may be conducted, such as at Walter Reed Army Medical Center in Washington, DC, and Bethesda, Maryland. Rehabilitation covered may include counseling, self-assessment inventories, orientation, communication, and assertiveness training.

Consumer Groups

An important hearing rehabilitation source may by found in such groups as the Hearing Loss Association of America (SHHH) (see the resource website). SHHH has existed since 1979 and has a nationwide network of support groups for all persons who are hard of hearing. SHHH can be described as a self-help, social, outreach, and advocacy group. SHHH publishes a periodical and sponsors an annual convention. Local chapters hold monthly social activities and informative meetings. Consumer groups provide a vehicle by which adults with hearing impairment can improve their ability to self-manage their problems. They promote installation of group amplification systems in theaters, churches, lecture halls, and other public meeting places. But the involvement of informed hearing specialists is important if these groups are to do the most good.

Hospitals, Medical Offices, Private Practice Audiologists, and Hearing Instrument Specialists

It is estimated that well over 90 percent of all hearing rehabilitation services are offered by audiologists or other dispensers in private practice or by those affiliated with hospital or medical groups. These services do not necessarily extend beyond the fitting of a hearing aid, orientation to its use, and counseling regarding management of hearing problems. For most adults with hearing impairment, this service appears to satisfy their rehabilitative needs. But in many cases, the hearing aid does not resolve their major communication difficulties. Nor do such limited services begin to meet the needs of those few clients who have very complex rehabilitation issues. Audiologists comprise about half of those dispensing hearing aids, while the remainder are hearing instrument specialists in sales offices (Skafte, 2000). Hearing instrument specialists also tend to provide only limited help with hearing aids and associated devices and assist in initial adjustment to hearing aid use. Few of these specialists are trained to provide extensive rehabilitative services. In the future, given the great advances in hearing aid technology that have taken place over the last decade and given the increasing importance of the connection between the quality of service and customer satisfaction, it is predicted that practice may shift by putting less emphasis on the device and more emphasis on the provision of comprehensive AR services.

AR will become even more important in the future.

■ REHABILITATION ASSESSMENT

As explained in Chapter 1, the overall effect of hearing loss is called *disability* by the World Health Organization (WHO, 2001). One part of disability can be measured audiometrically as hearing loss (called *impairment* by the WHO), and another part, communication activity limitation, can be measured most readily by self-report. A loss of hearing is measured easily in terms of decibels on an audiometric grid or percent correct on a word recognition test, thereby yielding numerical indicators of the amount of hearing impairment. Unfortunately, these numbers are not necessarily indicators of the day-to-day experiences of the person with the hearing impairment. We know from experience, for example, that two individuals with the same numerical hearing loss may encounter entirely different problems in their everyday lives.

Assessment of the consequences of hearing loss is important in the AR process for several reasons. First, there is a need to obtain information that will help us to understand the hearing loss and communication consequences of hearing impairment. We have extensive, well-established methods for measuring impairment and communication. Second, an assessment of the psychosocial consequences of the hearing loss is needed. Emotional and psychological problems may be more detrimental to the well-being of the individual in a way that goes beyond the organics of the loss and the effect on communication. Client input is helpful in dealing with this aspect of AR. Self-report procedures can be used to evaluate communication function and emotional, social, and vocational well-being. Knowledge of the value of self-report techniques to measure not only impairment but also its primary and secondary consequences has advanced greatly over the last decade or two (e.g., Newman & Jacobsen, 1993; Noble, 1998; Schow & Smedley, 1990). The need to combine audiometric measures with self-report assessment for determining hearing impairment and its consequences continues to be a priority for clinicians and researchers involved in hearing loss management. Fortunately, audiologists in the United States are giving greater attention to these self-report instruments. Schow et al. (1993) reported that self-assessment use by ASHA audiologists had increased from 18 percent in 1980 to 37 percent by 1990. By 2000, use of self-report had increased further to 58 percent (Millington, 2001).

Third, the final piece of the assessment puzzle is finding out what listening environments are encountered by clients as they engage in activities and participate in everyday life. The specific nature of the individual's listening environments must be known so that the right technology can be selected and fitted and so that the right non-instrumental rehabilitation can be designed. Very recently, new technology to log data about the acoustics of the listening environments of clients has begun to offer an important source of information about the acoustical environments that challenge listening in the client's everyday life. This powerful combination of assessment tools, audiometric performance measures, self-report, and data logging, provides the most complete approach to understanding the abilities and needs of our clients.

The majority of audiologists now use self-report measures.

Assessing Impairment

The audiometric assessment assists in two areas: (1) diagnosis and (2) rehabilitation. The basic diagnostic test battery consists of pure-tone air and bone conduction audiometry, speech threshold tests, word recognition tests, immittance, and measures of uncomfortable level (UCL). The basic audiometric battery results indicate whether a hearing loss exists, the degree and type of loss, and if the loss is likely to be remedied medically or surgically, or compensated for through amplification. A variety of test procedures may be added to the standard assessment battery to differentiate cochlear from retrocochlear problems, determine vestibular function, assess middle ear function, and measure central auditory processing ability.

Basic speech audiometry involving the repetition of simple words heard monaurally in quiet is part of the typical audiometric test battery. More ecologically valid tests of ability to understand speech have become increasingly popular among rehabilitative audiologists who are interested in obtaining speech performance measures that are more representative of everyday listening. Newer tests such as *Quick Speech-in-Noise Test* (*Quick SIN;* Killion et al., 2004) or the *Hearing in Noise Test* (*HINT*; Nilsson, Soli, & Sullivan, 1994) can be used to measure how well a person can hear speech in different amounts of background noise and whether he or she is able to take advantage of spatial separation between the target speech and the source(s) of background noise.

Impairment can be measured with an audiogram, and data logging can record information about the listening environment, but activity and participation issues require self-report.

Assessing Activity and Participation

The information gathered in the standard diagnostic battery is necessary for hearing aid fitting. However, there is a need to go further and develop relevant goals and treatments for improving communication skills and addressing the implications of the hearing loss for activity and participation by the person in his or her everyday life situations. Audiologists usually work in offices and clinics where they assess the rehabilitative needs of people in highly artificial conditions. Most clinical tests are conducted in a sound attenuating booth using standardized materials presented under earphones or over one or two loudspeakers. Many of the most challenging social and physical dimensions that confront listeners in everyday life are difficult if not impossible to assess directly in typical clinical settings. For example, even though the concerns of family members often motivate first visits to the audiologist, the problems plaguing the communicative interactions between the person with hearing loss and family members are infrequently appraised, either indirectly or directly (Hétu, Jones, & Getty, 1993). We should extend the assessment to include identification of those circumstances under which clients experience their greatest communication difficulties and tailor treatment to improve their functioning as they select places where, or persons who, they want to hear better. The case history, self-report questionnaires, and data logging provide a powerful combination of tools to complete the AR assessment. These same types of pre-treatment assessment tools can be used as post-treatment outcome measures.

The case history, self-report questionnaires, and data logging provide a powerful combination of tools to complete the activity and participation aspects of an AR assessment.

CASE HISTORY. A case history interview is actually a form of self-report and is one way of obtaining information on the day-to-day activity limitations resulting from a hearing deficit. The history, along with the audiogram, provides the clinician with an initial impression of the client. The case history usually includes a list of predetermined questions to elicit specific answers (e.g., "Have you ever had ear surgery?"). By including some open-ended questions (e.g., "What brings you here today?"), clients are given an opportunity to tell their own stories and explain their own needs in their own words (Carson, 2005).

SELF-REPORT QUESTIONNAIRES. Within the past forty years, significant efforts have been made to assess the consequences of hearing loss using tools to extend the traditional case history. Approaches used for assessment are discussed in the section that follows, and their role in AR is explained. Most of the instruments involve self-report by questionnaire. Such questionnaires have been used in an abbreviated form for screening purposes to select rehabilitation candidates, in longer versions to explore a small number of consequences resulting from a hearing problem, or in very comprehensive instruments that explore multiple dimensions of hearing loss.

In a valuable review paper, Schow and Gatehouse (1990) provided a summary of a variety of fundamental concerns related to self-report methods (including the need to consider different hearing domains such as impairment and disability in test design and use), a list of about twenty instruments used in self-report of hearing, a review of specific applications for which self-report may be used, and a discussion of a variety of psychometric issues that need careful attention. More recently, Noble (1998) has further underscored the importance of self-report in a thorough update on these methods. Self-report instruments are easy and inexpensive to use. They can be used for a wide variety of purposes and with different populations and are noninvasive and nonthreatening. These factors account for their wide popularity for hearing and other concerns. By assessing the psychosocial and other consequences of hearing loss using self-report, AR clinicians can much more adequately address AR. They can measure not only communication difficulties that may require amplification but also other concerns like tinnitus and dizziness. In a survey of ASHA audiologists (see Table 10.2), the self-report tools most used in the United States were identified. Details about these procedures may be found in the website resource list and also in other sources (Alpiner & Schow, 2000).

It is also interesting to note that the quest for new and better self-report instruments continues as we seek to understand the needs of hard of hearing adults. For example, unlike the artificial world inside a soundbooth, in the real world, multiple sound sources surround the listener, and these sources are altered by room acoustics. The listener must attend to wanted sounds and concentrate on a goal

TABLE 10.2

Use of Various Adult Self-Assessment Questionnaires

QUESTIONNAIRES	2000 N = 218[a]	
	N	%
APHAB	58	27
COSI	53	24
HHIE	36	17
HHS	21	10
SAC/SOAC	9	4
GHABP	6	3
Other	26[b]	12

[a]Of responding clinically active ASHA audiologists, these 127 (58%) were the only ones who reported use of such adult questionaires.

[b]Four of these were unique, informal, or in-house forms.

Source: Millington (2000).

while ignoring extraneous sounds and distractions posed by competing tasks (e.g., a mother trying to have a conversation with her husband while a child is demanding help). One of the most promising new instruments is the *Speech, Spatial and Qualities of Hearing Scale (SSQ)* developed by Gatehouse and Noble (2004). The *SSQ* provides a new window into how people use their hearing in realistic complex environments and how their hearing loss impacts ease of listening and abilities such as localizing and attending to sounds. More information and a copy of the *SSQ* can be downloaded from the website of the Institute of Hearing Research in Glasgow.

ACOUSTIC ENVIRONMENT AND HEARING AID USE DATA LOGGING. New data-logging options built into digital hearing aids now enable audiologists to gain new insights into the acoustic ecologies of their clients by recording information about the sound environments in which the hearing aid is used. Some hearing aid manufacturers have also developed a pre-fitting data logger that can be worn by a person for a period of time prior to his or her first appointment to discuss hearing aids. Self-report by clients about their experiences in the everyday listening situations that are sampled by the new data-logging technology should enable the audiologist to improve the fitting of devices and to provide more tailored noninstrumental rehabilitation to complement and/or augment the fitting of devices.

OUTCOME MEASURES. Performance measures (e.g., speech tests), self-report instruments, and data logging provide information in three different domains that are very useful for initial assessment, and they can also guide reassessment and promote systematic follow-up. In fact, based on an analysis of many measures collected in a large sample of older adults over a period of years, Humes (2003, 2004, 2005) concluded that three different types of measures are important in assessing the overall outcome of hearing aid fittings: (1) speech recognition performance largely based on hearing loss patterns, (2) satisfaction and benefit, and (3) hearing aid usage. A standardized set of outcome measures that cover these three important domains should be used to determine whether hearing aids are adequate and/or if other rehabilitation efforts have been successful (Schow et al., 2005). Speech performance measures provide information about how much the person can hear with the hearing aid, and data logging provides information about how much and in what acoustical environments the client is using the hearing aid. But self-report measures are essential to understanding how well the person is functioning. Self-report measures may be the most important measures in the cycle of assessment and treatment and then reassessment based on feedback gathered using outcome measures.

Speech performance measures, self-reports of benefit and satisfaction, and hearing aid usage provide the essential trio of outcome measures.

Many self-report instruments have been used to measure the effects of hearing aid use, and there are a great number of self-report options that may be used for any number of rehabilitation purposes. A comprehensive list of these is available in a number of sources (Alpiner & Schow, 2000; Noble, 1998). Also, the text website contains a number of self-report forms and links to others.

In this chapter, because the great majority of rehabilitation is being done in dispenser settings, we will describe several highly recommended self-report tools that lend themselves to use by those fitting hearing aids (Nemes, 2003). Copies of these questionnaires are provided to facilitate their use (see Figures 10.7, 10.8, and 10.9), and they can also be found on the text website. These tools include the companion

Self-Assessment of Communication (SAC)

Name: _____ Date: _____

Instructions: The purpose of this form is to identify the problems your hearing loss may be causing you. If you wear hearing aids, answer the questions according to how you communicate *when the hearing aids are NOT in use.*

One of the five descriptions on the right should be assigned to each of the statements below.

Select a number from 1 to 5 next to each statement (please *do not* answer with yes or no, and pick only one answer for each question.)

(1) Almost never (or never)

(2) Occasionally (about ¼ of the time

(3) About ½ of the time

(4) Frequently (about ¾ of the time)

(5) Practically always (or always)

(1) Do you experience communication difficulties in situations when speaking with one other person? (at home, at work, in a social situation, with a waitress, a store clerk, with a spouse, boss, etc.)

| 1 | 2 | 3 | 4 | 5 |

(2) Do you experience communication difficulties while watching TV and in various types of entertainment? (movies, radio, plays, night clubs, musical entertainment, etc.)

| 1 | 2 | 3 | 4 | 5 |

(3) Do you experience communication difficulties in situations when conversing with a small group of several persons? (with friends or families, co-workers, in meetings or casual conversations, over dinner or while playing cards, etc.)

| 1 | 2 | 3 | 4 | 5 |

(4) Do you experience communication difficulties when you are in an unfavorable listening environment? (at a noisy party, where there is background music, when riding in an auto or bus, when someone whispers or talks from across the room, etc.)

| 1 | 2 | 3 | 4 | 5 |

(5) How often do you experience communication difficulties in the situation where you most want to hear better?
Situation _____

| 1 | 2 | 3 | 4 | 5 |

(6) Do you feel that any difficulty with your hearing negatively affects or hampers your personal or social life?

| 1 | 2 | 3 | 4 | 5 |

(7) Does any problem or difficulty with your hearing worry, annoy or upset you?

| 1 | 2 | 3 | 4 | 5 |

(8) How often do others seem to be concerned or annoyed or suggest that you have a hearing problem?

| 1 | 2 | 3 | 4 | 5 |

(9) How often does your hearing negatively affect your enjoyment of life?

| 1 | 2 | 3 | 4 | 5 |

10) If you are using a hearing aid: On an average day, how many hours did you use your hearing aids?

hours_____/16=_____%

Please rate your overall satisfaction with your hearing aids.

1 ☐ *not at all satisfied (0%)*   2 ☐ *slightly satisfied (25%)*   3 ☐ *moderately satisfied (50%)* _____%
4 ☐ *mostly satisfied (75%)*   5 ☐ *very satisfied (100%)*

FOR OFFICE USE ONLY
☐ Pre-Assessment
☐ Post-Assessment
☐ Not currently using Hearing Aid
☐ Current Hearing Aid User

FOR OFFICE USE ONLY
   Score: (Q1-9) _____ (/9) _____ -1 _____ × 25 = _____%
   Score (Q1-5)/5 = _____ (Q6-8)/3 = _____ Q9 = _____
   -1×25 =   D _____%   H _____%   Q _____%

FIGURE 10.7

Self-Assessment of Communication (SAC).

HearX version adapted from Schow & Nerbonne (1982).

Significant Other Assessment of Communication (SOAC)

Name: _____ **Date:** _____

Name or Person Completing Assignment: _____ **Relationship:** _____

Instructions: The purpose of this form is to identify the problems a hearing loss may be causing your significant other. If the patient has a hearing aid, please fill out the form according to how he/she communicates *when the hearing aids are NOT in use.*

(1) Almost never (or never)

(2) Occasionally (about ¼ of the time

(3) About ½ of the time

(4) Frequently (about ¾ of the time)

(5) Practically always (or always)

One of the five descriptions on the right should be assigned to each of the statements below.

Select a number from 1 to 5 next to each statement (please _do not_ answer with yes or no, and pick only one answer for each question.)

(1) Do he/she experience communication difficulties in situations when speaking with one other person? (at home, at work, in a social situation, with a waitress, a store clerk, with a spouse, boss, etc.)

1	2	3	4	5

(2) Does he/she experience communication difficulties while watching TV and in various types of entertainment? (movies, radio, plays, night clubs, musical entertainment, etc.)

1	2	3	4	5

(3) Does he/she experience communication difficulties in situations when conversing with a small group of several persons? (with friends or families, co-workers, in meetings or casual conversations, over dinner or while playing cards, etc.)

1	2	3	4	5

(4) Does he/she experience communication difficulties when you are in an unfavorable listening environment? (at a noisy party, where there is background music, when riding in an auto or bus, when someone whispers or talks from across the room, etc.)

1	2	3	4	5

(5) How often does he/she experience communication difficulties in the situation where he/she most wants to hear better?

Situation _____

1	2	3	4	5

(6) Do you feel that any difficulty with hearing negatively affects or hampers his/her personal or social life?

1	2	3	4	5

(7) Do you feel that any problem or difficulty with your hearing worries, annoys or upsets him/her?

1	2	3	4	5

(8) Do you or others seem to be concerned or annoyed that he/she has a hearing problem?

1	2	3	4	5

(9) How often does hearing loss negatively affect his/her enjoyment of life?

1	2	3	4	5

(10) If he/she is using a hearing aid: On an average day, how many hours will he/she use the hearing aids?

hours_____/16=_____%

Please rate what you feel is his/her overall satisfaction with the hearing aids.

1 ☐ *not at all satisfied (0%)*   *2* ☐ *slightly satisfied (25%)*   *3* ☐ *moderately satisfied (50%)*   _____%
4 ☐ *mostly satisfied (75%)*   *5* ☐ *very satisfied (100%)*

FOR OFFICE USE ONLY

☐ Pre-Assessment
☐ Post-Assessment
☐ Not currently using Hearing Aid
☐ Current Hearing Aid User

FOR OFFICE USE ONLY

Score: (Q1-9) _____ (/9) _____ -1 _____ × 25 = _____%

Score (Q1-5)/5 = _____ (Q6-8)/3 = _____ Q9 = _____
-1×25 =   D _____%   H _____%   Q _____%

FIGURE 10.7   *(Continued)*

Significant Other Assessment of Communication (SOAC).
HearX version adapted from Schow & Nerbonne (1982).

Client Oriented Scale of Improvement (COSI)

Name: _____   Category: New _____   Degree of Change

Audiologist: _____   Return _____

Date: 1. Needs Established _____

2. Outcome Assessed _____

Final Ability
(with hearing aid)

Person can hear

10% 25% 50% 75% 95%

SPECIFIC NEEDS

Indicate Order of Significance

		Worse	No Difference	Slightly Better	Better	Much Better	CATEGORY	Hardly Ever	Occasionally	Half the Time	Most of Time	Almost Always
☐	....											
☐	....											
☐	....											
☐	....											
☐	....											

NATIONAL ACOUSTIC LABORATORIES

Categories
1. Conversation with 1 or 2 in quiet
2. Conversation with 1 or 2 in noise
3. Conversation with group in quiet
4. Conversation with group in noise
5. Television or Radio @ normal volume
6. Familiar speaker on phone
7. Unfamiliar speaker on phone
8. Hearing phone ring from another room
9. Hear front door bell or knock
10. Hear traffic
11. Increased social contact
12. Feel embarrassed or stupid
13. Feeling left out
14. Feeling upset or angry
15. Church or meeting
16. Other

FIGURE 10.8

Client Oriented Scale of Improvement.

SAC/SOAC (Schow & Nerbonne, 1982), the *Client Oriented Scale of Improvement* (*COSI;* Dillon, James, & Ginis, 1997), and the *International Outcome Inventory-Hearing Aids* (IOI-HA; Cox et al., 2000). There is some overlap among these tools since the HearX revised version of *SAC/SOAC* contains an open-ended item similar to *COSI* and also covers the seven items on the IOI-HA; however, some audiologists use more than one tool in order to obtain more complete data on a client and, in the case of IOI-HA, to allow international comparisons using the same wording.

International Outcome Inventory for Hearing Aids (IOI-HA)

1. Think about how much you used your present hearing aid(s) over the past two weeks. On an average day, how many hours did you use the hearing aid(s)?

none	less than 1 hour a day	1 to 4 hours a day	4 to 8 hours a day	more than 8 hours a day
☐	☐	☐	☐	☐

2. Think about the situation where you most wanted to hear better, before you got your present hearing aid(s). Over the past two weeks, how much has the hearing aid helped in that situation?

helped not at all	helped slightly	helped moderately	helped quite a lot	helped very much
☐	☐	☐	☐	☐

3. Think again about the situation where you most wanted to hear better. When you use your present hearing aid(s), how much difficulty do you STILL have in that situation?

very much difficulty	quite a lot of difficulty	moderate difficulty	slight difficulty	no difficulty
☐	☐	☐	☐	☐

4. Considering everything, do you think your present hearing aid(s) is worth the trouble?

not at all worth it	slightly worth it	moderately worth it	quite a lot worth it	very much worth it
☐	☐	☐	☐	☐

5. Over the past two weeks, with your present hearing aid(s), how much have your hearing difficulties affected the things you can do?

affected very much	affected quite a lot	affected moderately	affected slightly	affected not at all
☐	☐	☐	☐	☐

6. Over the past two weeks, with your present hearing aid(s), how much do you think other people were bothered by your hearing difficulties?

bothered very much	bothered quite a lot	bothered moderately	bothered slightly	bothered not at all
☐	☐	☐	☐	☐

7. Considering everything, how much has your present hearing aid(s) changed your enjoyment of life?

worse	no change	slightly better	quite a lot better	very much better
☐	☐	☐	☐	☐

FIGURE 10.9

International Outcome Inventory for Hearing Aids (IOI-HA).

The *SAC/SOAC* is an extremely practical tool for hearing aid fitting and was recently picked by the USA HEARX company as their first choice out of twenty different self-report outcome measures it tried (Nemes, 2003). Both the hearing-impaired person and a significant other person respond to questions with reference to four standard situations (listening to TV, speaking one on one, speaking in a small group, and speaking with someone under noisy conditions) plus an open-ended item described by the client. In this way we can measure activity limitation (disability), while three other questions lead to a measure of participation restriction (handicap). These can be measured in the unaided condition.

Once a hearing aid is fitted, then residual disability, residual handicap, derived benefit, use time, and satisfaction are measured with reference to these same situations. Percentage scores are derived in all seven areas (two unaided and five aided). We think this comprehensive measurement is important and helpful in checking outcomes in hearing aid fitting. The text website shows that such measures are useful in comparing benefit, use, and satisfaction from those with different patterns of hearing loss. The site also compares findings for different outcome measures, including the *Glasgow Hearing Aid Benefit Profile (GHABP)* by Gatehouse (1999), which has a similar design to *SAC/SOAC*, and the site has links or other self-report tools including HHIE and HHIA.

The *COSI* method is also very useful as an outcome measure and is designed to meet individual needs. It encourages the client to pick up to five situations in which help with hearing is desired, or where he or she wants to hear better. After the hearing aid is fitted, the client is asked to rate on a 5-point scale how much improvement or change the hearing aid has provided and how well he or she now hears in those situations with the hearing aid in place. It is a very simple and straightforward scale, but it has been shown to be as valid as much longer scales. It does not, however, have a set of standard situations.

The *IOI-HA* is the newest tool, and it was designed to be very simple and generic so that it could be used to compare rehabilitation treatments across programs and countries (Cox et al., 2000; see text website for the *IOI-HA* in English and many other languages). The questions can be interpreted by clients in terms of their own life situations, but the *IOI-HA* does not specifically gather information about the nature of those situations. In contrast, the *SAC/SOAC* and *COSI* help the audiologist to understand more about the specific situations relevant to the individual client. The *SAC/SOAC* use some general questions as a framework, but the client also replies with reference to his or her own life situation so these tools can be adapted nicely for any individual or unique purpose. *COSI* is more individualized, but does not include a set of general questions like *SAC/SOAC* and *IOI-HA* (e.g., TV listening, one-on-one situations, etc).

To recap, outcome measures provide feedback and continue the cycle of assessment and treatment. Self-report questionnaires are especially useful because they enable the audiologist to look at use, benefit, and satisfaction with interventions, and they can be used to help document the effectiveness of programs (Cox et al., 2000), while goal-specific outcome measures can be helpful in determining the progress of individuals (Gagné, McDuff, & Getty, 1999). The *IOI-HA* is short and can be used to compare results across different programs and countries. The *SAC/SOAC* and *COSI* gather rich client-specific profiles and can be used to evaluate hearing aid delivery programs and/or individuals (plus significant others of those) fitted with devices. In addition to self-report, there are other measures that can be used to measure the outcomes of rehabilitation. Indeed, as will be noted later, outcome measures based on measures such as daily use of hearing aids have been used to demonstrate how programs can dramatically improve our efforts at rehabilitating hearing aid users (Brooks, 1989). Novel outcome measures have also been developed and used to demonstrate the value of ALDs (Lewsen & Cashman, 1997; Pichora-Fuller & Robertson, 1997), communication therapies (Erber, 1988, 1996; Robertson et al., 1997), and interventions involving modification of the social and physical environment (Pichora-Fuller & Carson, 2000).

The recently developed *IOI-HA* is now being adapted and used to assess other interventions besides hearing aids and to gather information from the perspective of the significant other as well as from the client (e.g., Hickson, Worrall, & Scarinci, 2006). Nevertheless, further development of outcome measures can be expected, especially as the rehabilitative toolkit expands, and objectives shift from an emphasis on impairment and audibility to a greater emphasis on participation in everyday life (Noble, 2002; Wilkerson, 2000; Worrall & Hickson, 2003). Given the increasingly wide range of choices of outcome measures, audiologists need to know which suit their particular purposes in planning individual treatments or group programs (Beck, 2000; Stephens et al., 2000) and in evaluating the results of rehabilitation (Bentler & Kramer, 2000; Gatehouse, 2000). The research of Humes (2003, 2004, 2005) strongly suggests that a combination of three measures tapping speech/audibility issues, usage, and satisfaction combined with benefit are the essential trio of outcome measures. Such evidence is extremely important if audiologists are to continue to improve service delivery. There are many disbelievers among those who need our services, and favorable outcome findings are increasingly needed for documentation to those who pay for services.

CORE Assessment Summary

Audiologic testing and self-report are the fundamental tools for assessment, but a continuing need exists for assessment protocols that present a broader, meaningful profile of the adult with hearing impairment. The new data logging technology is one example of how progress is ongoing. Loss of hearing sensitivity is only one aspect of a complex set of interacting variables, both personal and environmental, that cumulatively interact and affect the hearing problem. The need for such a comprehensive view of audiologic rehabilitation has been championed recently by an international consensus of experts on rehabilitation for older adults (Kiessling et al., 2003). Therefore, it cannot be stressed enough how the assessment process should focus widely, and all four assessment aspects in the model used throughout this book need to be considered.

1. *Communication status* assessment should include both impairment and activity limitations. Once audiologic testing and self-report are completed, there should be reasonably thorough information in these areas.

2. *Overall participation variables* include concerns about social, psychological, educational, and vocational issues. Self-report procedures like *SAC/SOAC* provide useful information about the social and emotional-psychic dimension of the loss, because they ask about three different social/emotional issues. Vocational and educational issues may also be identified by the client as specific situations. Open-ended items on self-reports are valuable for teasing out participation concerns, but a follow-up interview may help uncover other areas of concern, and an effort should be made to touch on any aspect of a person's life that may have special relevance.

3. *Related personal factors* that interact with hearing loss include, among others, health status, activity level, and manual dexterity. Attitude and motivation also are key issues, but for older persons changes in health status have perhaps the most significant effect on an individual's ability to participate actively in remediation. Difficulties with motor coordination, vision, memory, or general health may prohibit an aging person from initiating or sustaining interest in the intervention process. The older person may not be enthusiastic about involvement in audiologic rehabilitation when other disabilities, unrelated to the hearing loss, are life threatening and cause greater concern.

4. *Environmental factors* include not only where a person lives and the social circumstances in which he or she chooses to participate, but they also include all aspects of the environment that may facilitate or impede adjustment to and improvement from the effects of the loss. The acoustic environment can be assessed with the help of data logging. Social environmental assessment includes information about the community and support systems of the client. Environmental factors can often be modified, but first we have to know and understand how they contribute to the problem.

■ REHABILITATION MANAGEMENT

Following assessment, various forms of AR can be undertaken. A common set of management principles applies to most cases, and a large number of adults have similar auditory abilities and quality-of-life issues. Nevertheless, the specific form of rehabilitation will vary between individuals and over time because of the personal and dynamic nature of adjustment to hearing loss in adulthood. In the management process, the rehabilitative audiologist works together with the individual with hearing loss and his or her communication partners to find a combination of solutions that will enable listening goals to be attained and maintained in a wide range of life circumstances. The audiologic management process coherently integrates specific forms of rehabilitation consistent with CARE (Figure 10.2):

1. *Counseling,* which focuses on identifying, understanding, and shaping the attitudes and goals that influence help seeking, decision making, and action taking, with an emphasis on the factors that predispose, enable, and reinforce individuals in their adjustment to hearing difficulties and associated stresses. The audiologist gives the client information based on the results of the assessment and, through an interactive process with the client, goals are set to address needs at three levels: audibility, activity, and participation.

2. *Audibility and instrumental interventions*, in which hearing aids, cochlear implants, and/or a variety of assistive listening devices (ALDs) are discussed, selected, and fitted, with provision of appropriate pre- and posttrial education to ensure the effective use of these technologies. This level of intervention addresses amplification issues in terms of the fit and function of devices and orientation to them.

3. *Remediation for communication activities*, which focuses on changing behaviors that will contribute to enhancing the communication performance of listeners with their communication partners in hearing-demanding activities and environments, including when and how to use devices and other strategies.

4. *Environmental coordination and participation improvement*, with an emphasis on the social and physical supports (in the health care system, the community, and in occupational, educational, and/or family contexts) required to ensure that rehabilitation achieves the individual's goals for participation in everyday life, especially in the priority situations that are targeted in the client-specific goals for rehabilitation.

Issues	Imperatives
Why don't more hard of hearing adults seek and benefit from audiologic rehabilitation?	Audiologists must tailor rehabilitation to the changing needs of individuals over the adult lifespan, because adjustment to hearing loss is a dynamic process.
What role do the nonaudiometric characteristics of the individual play in adjustment to hearing loss?	Audiologists must cultivate their role in facilitating adjustment to hearing loss in terms of how the adult preserves communicative competence and constructs an identity as a hard of hearing person, because there are powerful links between hearing, communicative competence, and identity.
How could more effective solutions be achieved in the everyday lives of hard of hearing adults by combining various forms of rehabilitation?	Audiologists must extend interventions to the individual's communication partners and physical environment, because the social and physical contexts have a profound impact on the individual's experience of hearing loss.

Most rehabilitation programs combine several important components. These components are consistent with the CARE management model used in this text (see Chapter 1 and Figure 10.2). First, the audiologist counsels the hard of hearing adult about hearing loss, explores its significance in the particular life circumstances of the individual, and determines the needs and goals of the person and significant

Two clients being familiarized
with ALDs.

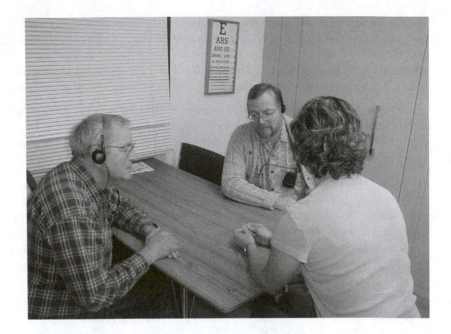

others. This step is crucial insofar as it culminates in the statement of prioritized objectives for rehabilitation. Treatment goals fall into three main areas to be improved:
audibility, activity, and participation. Depending on the objectives that have been set,
a customized combination of interventions can be initiated and continued contingent on ongoing reevaluation. To improve audibility, the client will likely be familiarized with instruments, usually hearing aids and/or ALDs. Activity-specific
communication skills may be improved through training in visual attentiveness, use
of repair strategies or communication tactics, conversational management, and enhancement of goal-directed decision making and assertiveness. Participation may be
improved by involving key communication partners, such as family members, other
professionals, or caregivers, in therapy and/or by modifying the physical environment, including the use of ALDs in public places.

Counseling and Psychosocial Considerations

Counseling builds
the bridge between
the client's lived
experience of hear-
ing loss and the
audiologist's pro-
fessional and scien-
tific knowledge
about hearing.

The varying degrees of adjustment to hearing loss within the adult population reflect the heterogeneity of the group. Lifestyles, hearing-related demands, and experiences of hearing loss vary widely. In counseling, the rehabilitative audiologist
needs to begin by listening to the client so that the person's attitudes toward hearing loss and his or her goals in seeking help for hearing loss can be identified and
understood. Not surprisingly, the way in which the client experiences hearing loss
and expresses issues and concerns about these experiences is unlikely to be cast in
scientific terms such as decibels and Hertz or hair cell counts. By listening to the
client, the audiologist begins to build a bridge between the client's lived experience
of hearing loss and their own professional understanding of the results of the formal audiologic and self-report assessment. Building the bridge between these kinds

of knowledge sets the stage for the important relationship that must develop between the client and clinician if rehabilitation is to succeed (Clark, 1996).

The comments made to audiologists by adults who are hard of hearing provide rich insights into how they experience communication situations in everyday life. The sample of quotes in the box illuminates various obstacles to communication and how the causes and consequences of hearing problems may be manifested. These words also suggest areas to be addressed in rehabilitation. In counseling, the audiologist must be alert to such comments because of their value in guiding rehabilitation planning and because they provide insight into the problems of the client as well as the resources and supports that are available to the client. Furthermore, as a communication expert, the audiologist is uniquely positioned to provide a positive communication experience for the client, thereby demonstrating that solutions to the problems that they describe can be achieved. It is especially important that the audiologist rise above ageist stereotypes when interacting with older adults.

Hearing Loss

These comments provide insights into some of the ways that hearing loss affects people:

Mary: I can appreciate young children being considered inattentive or disruptive in school from this lack of hearing and assimilation and not comprehending why because they don't know that they can't hear. It's not that I don't understand but rather that it is so tiring to listen.

Tom: Jokes aren't funny if you have to ask for a repetition.

Patricia: It's hard to be intimate with my partner when whispers can't be heard and the lights have to be on for lipreading.

Henry: There's no privacy in this home for the aged—no one would hear a knock on the door so people just barge into rooms to find a resident; conversations are never quiet.

These comments suggest helpful tactics that could be addressed in conversational therapy:

Marjorie: By completely sounding each word, the speaker goes more slowly and it gives me time to translate the sounds to meaning. Most TV or radio speakers are too fast, and while I am trying to make sense of the first statement, they are away on to the third or fourth sentence, so I soon have to drop out and so lose interest. Asking for repetition seems to be a way of giving the brain cells time to put sounds into meaning.

Mike: In a group, when someone new begins talking, by the time I figure out who it is, I have lost the thread of the conversation. When I know the topic, I have no problem, but when the topic changes I get lost.

Counseling can then turn to reflection on these attitudes and goals, as well as to a consideration of possible courses of rehabilitative action. Decision making may be guided by discussing factors specific to the life circumstances of the client that have or will predispose or impede taking rehabilitative action (e.g., the positive or negative reaction of a husband to his wife's new hearing aid), factors that will

The client will suc-
ceed in taking and
maintaining reha-
bilitative action if
the factors that pre-
dispose, enable,
and reinforce
change are
optimized.

enable taking a rehabilitative step (e.g., providing a college student with written information about FM systems to give to the professors who will be asked to wear a
transmitter in class), and factors that will reinforce the continuation of the rehabilitative action (e.g., joining a hard of hearing peer support group). It should be
abundantly clear that, although two clients may have the same audiogram and
hearing aid, the personal and environmental factors that influence their decision
making and action taking may be quite different. It is also important to note that
the role of the audiologist is itself one of the factors to be considered (e.g., a routine schedule of follow-up appointments may be critical to the client's success).

COMMUNICATION GOALS AND STYLE. Communication is never perfect; even people
with normal hearing experience miscommunication and vary in their communication behaviors and styles (Coupland, Wiemann, & Giles, 1991). Differences between
communicators will influence how hearing loss affects communication. Com-
pounding the effects of hearing loss on communication, individual differences and
age-related changes in emotional, social, cognitive, perceptual, and linguistic status are likely to influence the process of adjustment and readiness for AR. Two main
functions of communication are *exchange of information* and *social interaction*.
Both functions contribute to communication, but their relative importance varies
depending on the communicators and their roles in a situation (Pichora-Fuller,
Johnson, & Roodenburg, 1998). As people age, emotional aspects of social interaction, especially with close friends and family, tend to become increasingly important, but acquiring new knowledge or exchanging information tends to become
relatively less important (Isaacowitz, Charles, & Carstensen, 2000). Even mild hearing loss can interfere with information exchange (e.g., when a college student listens to the details of instructions in the classroom, phonemes must be perceived
with a high degree of accuracy and new vocabulary must be learned); in contrast,
social interaction may remain well preserved in the early stages of hearing loss (e.g.,
when an elderly spouse judges a partner's emotions, prosodic or visual cues may be
adequate) (Villaume, Brown, & Darling, 1994). In setting rehabilitative goals, it is
important to understand the kind of communicator that the person has been in the
past and to determine his or her current and anticipated priorities for communication in the context of specific relationships and roles.

Communication
goals may empha-
size information
exchange or social
interaction.

One adult may be a well-educated professional who has always been socially
active and a leader in the community. Such a person may be an exceptionally skilled
communicator who is motivated to listen carefully and to draw from nonverbal
cues during difficult information-intense communicative situations (e.g., public
meetings). Although participation in such situations may be restricted by a mild
hearing loss, the person may be well prepared and motivated to embark on rehabilitation to resolve communication problems. Another adult with the same hearing loss may not have been so socially outgoing or adept at adjusting to new
situations and may be concerned primarily about being able to communicate with
close family members, especially a spouse, in the confines of the familiar surroundings of his or her home. The same hearing loss may pose less of a threat to
participation for this individual, partly because the spouse is able and willing to
manage communication breakdowns and partly because unfamiliar and challenging communication situations are avoided; however, the individual may be far less

able to overcome communicative obstacles when it becomes necessary to do so (e.g., when admitted to hospital). It is noteworthy that gender differences in adult adjustment to hearing loss have only fairly recently been recognized as important, and evidence continues to mount showing that hearing loss may take a greater toll on women than men, partly because of the centrality of communication in the roles of wife and mother and partly because women receive less social support from others in adjusting to hearing loss (Hallberg & Jansson, 1996; Hétu et al., 1993). There is still much more to learn about the functional significance of hearing and hearing loss to everyday communication.

The hard of hearing adult may hear well enough to participate appropriately in many communication situations, yet struggle in other communication situations.

STEREOTYPES AND ADJUSTMENT. Even the ageist stereotypes held by family members and professional caregivers can influence an individual's success in adjusting to hearing loss, because such stereotypes can have a profound effect on actual behavior over the long term (Ryan et al., 1986). In challenging situations, verbal messages are likely to be misinterpreted and inappropriate responses may result. Family and friends may be confused by the inconsistency in the person's apparent communicative ability, and they may attribute the person's moments of seeming inattentiveness and lack of appropriate social interaction to a number of causes, ranging from indifference to senility, any of which may lead to less and less social interaction between the aging individual and various communication partners. When deprived of social interaction, due to either a hearing loss and/or the stereotyped attitudes of those around them, older persons become frustrated and may increasingly avoid situations in which difficulties are encountered (i.e., family gatherings, church, movies, and other social activities that they enjoyed previously). Such a loss in close interpersonal communication can lead to decreased stimulation, resulting in depression and self-deprecation. The stereotyped expectations become a self-fulfilled prophecy in what has been called the "communication predicament of aging" (Figure 10.10).

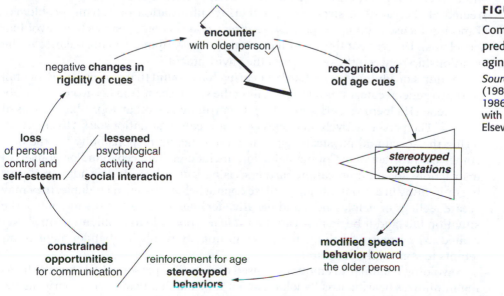

FIGURE 10.10

Communication predicament of aging.

Source: Ryan et al. (1986). Copyright 1986. Reprinted with permission of Elsevier Science.

Ageist stereotypes and geriapathy may make hearing problems more difficult to overcome.

Ultimately, many older persons with hearing impairment exhibit what has been described clinically as the "geriapathy syndrome" (Maurer, 1976, p. 72),

The individual feels disengaged from group interaction and apathy ensues, the product of the fatigue which sets in from the relentless effort of straining to hear. Frustration, kindled by begging too many pardons, gives way to subterfuges that disguise misunderstandings. The head nods in agreement with a conversation only vaguely interpreted. The voice registers approval of words often void of meaning. The ear strives for some redundancy that will make the message clearer. Finally, acquiescing to fatigue and frustration, thoughts stray from the conversation to mental imageries that are unburdened by the defective hearing mechanism.

Geriapathy

The pattern described by clinicians as geriapathy has also been expressed by older adults themselves, as demonstrated in the following comment written by an older woman at a meeting of the Canadian Hard of Hearing Association: "When you are hard of hearing, you struggle to hear; when you struggle to hear, you get tired; when you get tired, you get frustrated; when you get frustrated, you get bored; when you get bored, you quit.—I didn't quit today."

Hard of hearing adults cope by avoiding and/or controlling the situation.

COPING. To deal with obstacles to communication and the stresses associated with hearing loss, the effortfulness of listening, and frequent miscommunications, adults adopt coping behaviors. Rehabilitation planning requires that the audiologist appreciate how persons experience stress and how they cope with it. Lazarus and Folkman (1984) proposed a model of stress and coping that can be readily applied to the situations of adults who are hard of hearing. In their model, the person and the environment are considered to be in a dynamic, bidirectional relationship. Stress entails the constant appraisal of this relationship. When the relationship is perceived to pose a threat, challenge, or harm to the person, then it becomes stressful and a coping response is required. Problem-focused coping responses are directed at the cause of stress (e.g., gathering information or solving problems).

Coping responses can be problem focused or emotion focused.

Emotion-focused coping responses are directed at regulating stress (e.g., avoiding problems). Distress continues until coping is successful in restoring balance in the relationship between the person and the environment.

Studies of adults who are hard of hearing have found that coping behaviors fall into two general categories: (1) controlling the social scene and (2) avoiding the social scene (Hallberg & Carlsson, 1991). Controlling is similar to problem-focused coping. The person actively manages communication situations assertively by altering the social and physical environment and taking responsibility for the outcomes of these actions. Coping behaviors include giving verbal and/or nonverbal instructions to communication partners, using technology, and/or adjusting seating or lighting in a room. Although these coping behaviors seem laudable, they may create feelings of helplessness and negative feelings when attempts to control the situation fail, and it begins to seem that it is not possible to maintain control. Repeated experiences of helplessness may ultimately result in abandonment of attempts to control the situation.

The relationship between *personal factors* and *environmental factors* and the ensuing stress lead to coping responses.

Avoiding is similar to emotion-focused coping. The person who is hard of hearing minimizes hearing loss by joking about it or making positive comparisons between the self and others. The person may avoid challenging communication situations and choose not to use conspicuous hearing technologies. Rather than disclose the hearing problem or the need for accommodation, strategies such as lipreading, positioning oneself near a talker, pretending to understand, or remaining silent may be used to camouflage hearing problems (Jaworski & Stephens, 1998). Avoiding behaviors seem maladaptive, but they may be essential during some phases of adjustment when the person's self-esteem is vulnerable or the person has too little energy to solve problems. It is intriguing to consider that such avoidance may be a key factor in the limited use of hearing aids by those with hearing loss. However, prolonged avoiding may result in social isolation or redefinition of the self as less competent.

Everyone encountering stress engages in a mixture of coping behaviors, and it is important to reexamine these adjustment methods as they relate to hearing impairment in adulthood. What works for one person may not work for another, and what works for a given person at one time may not work at another time, with success necessarily depending on the nature of the person, the environment, and the person-environment relationship at a given time. There is no universally correct form of coping and no stock recipe for managing hearing loss.

Others may influence how well a person copes and adjusts.

Trade-Offs

An example of the trade-offs between controlling and avoiding are demonstrated in the following example. A middle-aged man, attending a peer support group for the hard of hearing, proudly explained to the group how he and his wife had decided to manage the "going to a restaurant for dinner scene." The couple were united in their conviction that the most important part of going out for dinner was for them to enjoy each other's company. By comparison, the man was clear in his mind that he had no interest in social interaction with the restaurant staff. Furthermore, the man did not feel that his masculinity was threatened in any way if his wife did the talking with the restaurant staff, and his wife did not have any hesitation about taking on the responsibility for the required information exchange with these strangers. Both members of the couple were prepared to use an audio input extension microphone to increase the privacy and reduce the stress of their conversation throughout the dinner. After clearly defining what was important, or not, to them in the situation, they agreed on solutions that accomplished their goals, without jeopardizing their roles and relationships. On the one hand, the scenario demonstrates control insofar as action was taken to address important needs (enjoying each other's company); on the other hand, avoiding was a reasonable choice to minimize stress associated with unimportant aspects of the situation (who communicated with the staff). Deciding what is important and what is not is crucial to goal setting and sets the stage for developing an action plan for coping.

Coping styles learned in childhood continue to be utilized throughout one's lifetime to deal with the normal stresses of living, but the ways in which aging adults cope with communicative challenges are also influenced and modified by their interactions with others who may or may not support particular coping behaviors. Given the strong influence of family and caregivers on communicative behavior in older adults, it is helpful to the audiologist to consider how the adjustment of the client may be predisposed or reinforced not only by the client's own behaviors, but also by the behaviors of significant others. In the model of learned dependency, two main patterns of interactions between older people and their social partners in everyday activities in private dwellings and in residential care facilities were described as the *dependence-support script* and the *independence-ignore script* (Baltes & Wahl, 1996). These scripts highlight how older adults maintain and develop dependent and independent behaviors. In the dependence-support script, the dominant pattern was one in which older people engaging in dependent behaviors were immediately attended to and given positive reinforcement. For example, when a man who is hard of hearing waits for his wife to answer the phone, she reinforces his avoidance of the phone by answering it herself, and, in the ensuing phone conversation with a mutual friend, she makes decisions for her husband without passing the phone to him or even consulting with him. After many such events, he begins to doubt his ability to manage conversations on the phone to the extent that he doesn't answer it at all, even when he is alone, thereby eventually losing independence. The less common independence-ignore script was one in which older people engaging in independent behaviors were ignored or discouraged. For example, if a woman tried to put on her own hearing aid (an independent act), her husband might say, "I told you I would help you with that; you never get it in right" (a dependence-supportive act). Sadly, in the study, constructively engaged or proactive social behaviors (e.g., talking to another person) were reinforced only 25 percent of the time, and more frequently, such independent behaviors were discouraged. Ultimately, the older person surrenders independence and complies with the expectations of dependence.

On a positive note, the communication enhancement model in Figure 10.11 suggests how to counteract the communication predicament of aging (Ryan et al., 1995). Accordingly, the audiologist should encourage family and caregivers to use independence-supporting behaviors. A daughter can make comments like "It is so great to get your input on this decision" when the hearing aid is worn or a conversational repair strategy is used, thereby encouraging her mother to take an active role in family discussions. A nurse can use a personal amplifier to ease a resident's communication effort. Successful communication experiences will predispose, enable, and/or reinforce the behavior changes targeted as goals for the client.

> The communication enhancement model illustrates how to counteract the effects of stereotypes on communication.

SETTING OBJECTIVES. In counseling, the audiologist and client explore the complex backdrop against which the rehabilitation plan will be enacted, including the client's attitudes, activity and participation goals, coping and communication styles, coexisting health issues, the influence of family and caregivers, and the personal and environmental factors that have and will support or impede adjustment to hearing loss. Counseling culminates in setting objectives. Objectives should be clearly stated and specify *who* will do *what, how much*, by *when*. Objectives can target behavioral or environmental changes to be adopted by the person who is hard of hearing or by significant others. Examples of a priority rating of objectives developed from an analysis of complaints for a particular client are provided in Table 10.3 (explained in more detail later). Over time, evaluation of whether goals have been achieved will become an important topic of discussion between the audiologist and the client and significant others as they go on to make new decisions and set new rehabilitative goals to meet new or changing needs.

> Goals must state who will do what, how much, by when.

FIGURE 10.11

Communication en-
hancement model.
Source: Ryan et al.
(1995).

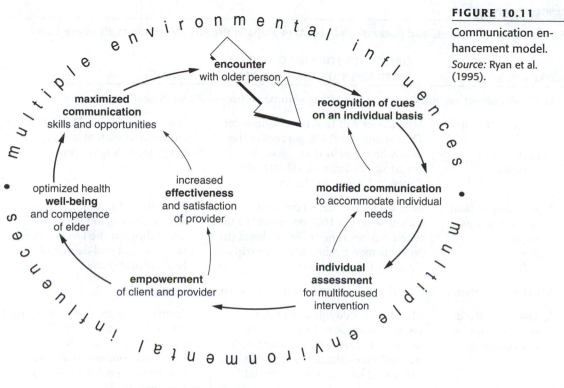

Effective Communication Strategies

Why?

Enhance the interaction
Increase adherence to the rehabilitation plan
Facilitate successful aging

Key Features

Be "inspiring" *vs.* "dispiriting"
Convey high expectations
Facilitate communication skills of older client
Seek feedback about how communicating
Affirm personhood by listening
Recognize individual life goals and strategies
Assess collaboratively
Assess and build on strengths
Negotiate treatment plan

Amplification and Instrumental Interventions to Achieve Audibility

Amplification is the most common form of rehabilitation. First, the audiologist must determine if the client is ready for a hearing aid or ALD. A decision to go ahead with instrumental rehabilitation will depend on the nature and degree of the client's hearing loss, the nature of the client's activity and participation needs, and the client's willingness to trade the potential benefits against the burdens of using

TABLE 10.3

Complaints, Objectives, and Recommended Action Steps in Priority Order for an Example Case

INITIAL COMPLAINT	OBJECTIVES FOR END OF THE THIRD WEEK OF THE TRIAL PERIOD	ACTION
A. Audibility objectives addressed by practicing volume control skills with hearing aid		
1. Turning TV up too loud (daughter's complaint)	Mrs. Carter will find her comfortable TV listening level 100 percent of the time when watching the news by adjusting her hearing aid after the daughter has preset the level.	Practice adjusting TV and hearing aid volume with Mrs. Carter and daughter in a quiet room.
2. Inability to hear whispers, soft sounds	Mrs. Carter will detect car turn indicator sound 100 percent of the time when driving in her neighborhood (to be confirmed by daughter on a trip at the end of the 3 weeks).	Explain and practice how to adjust hearing aid volume depending on the level of the target signal and degree of background noise.
B. Activity objectives addressed by conversational therapy with client and partner		
3. Daughter tired of repeating conversation	Mrs. Carter's daughter will reduce needed repetitions in a 10-minute sample of daily conversation by 50 percent from the amount needed on samples taken on 3 days pretrial.	Instruct daughter to turn off background sounds (e.g., radio, TV), make eye contact before talking, state and confirm topic changes, and slow speech rate during conversation).
4. Difficulty understanding conversation with friends in the dining room	Mrs. Carter will understand the gist of 90 percent of conversations with her friend Mrs. Brown during lunch in the dining room at their facility (to be self-assessed by Mrs. Carter).	Explain benefits of visual attention to the talker and how to select a seat away from noise sources and discuss when two preferred repair strategies could help.
C. Participation objectives addressed by use of ALD (FM system)		
5. Confusion at church services	Mrs. Carter will demonstrate to her daughter that she understood 100 percent of the announcements made at the Sunday service of the third week.	Explain and try new hearing aid with existing FM system at her church.
6. Frustration on Senior Adult Center bus outings	Mrs. Carter will increase her understanding of messages from the driver by 75 percent as demonstrated to the recreation staff who accompany the seniors on outings.	FM system and its use with the hearing aid to be explained to the bus driver and the recreation staff and to be used on the bus.

an instrument. Having decided to go ahead with instrumental rehabilitation, the next steps for the audiologist are to fit an appropriate device, ensure that it functions as expected, and counsel and orient the client to its use and care. Of course, follow-up post fitting is essential to confirm that a successful fitting has been achieved and that no further rehabilitative issues have emerged.

IS THE CLIENT READY FOR AN INSTRUMENT? Sensorineural hearing loss is not medically treatable at the present time, but the alternative choice, wearing amplification, is not highly regarded among adults of any age. Hearing loss is stigmatizing (Hétu, 1996). By putting on a hearing aid for the first time, the hard of hearing person discloses to the world that he or she has a hearing loss and is not "normal." Hearing aids are considered to be ugly, unkind associations are made between deafness and intelligence, and uncharitable jokes about deafness and aging are prevalent. In addition to the social costs, wearing a hearing aid also has other costs: the initial high financial costs of hearing aids, ongoing costs for batteries and maintenance, continued lack of knowledge and confusion about the service delivery system, and transportation costs and time needed for visits to clinics and hearing aid offices. Ideally, these costs are balanced by the acoustic benefits of amplification. Nevertheless, sometimes the acoustical benefits may fall short, because even the latest digital hearing aids continue to be of limited benefit in adverse noisy or reverberant acoustical environments. In a survey of members of the hard of hearing association in the United Kingdom, the first priority was to improve hearing aids (endorsed by 100 percent), and the second priority (endorsed by 95 percent) was to educate the general public about hearing loss (Stephens, 1996b). It is essential for further progress that there be a combination of improved and appropriately fitted technology, along with reduction of stigma by changing societal attitudes toward hearing, hearing loss, and increasing hearing accessibility. Put another way, balancing the benefits and costs of wearing a hearing aid can be accomplished by increasing benefit and/or reducing costs.

> Wearing a hearing aid increases the audibility of sound, but it is often stigmatizing.

A client may not be ready to purchase a hearing aid for a number of reasons. Results of a questionnaire interview survey conducted almost thirty years ago among a random sample of 153 elderly individuals who had not purchased hearing aids pointed to a number of obstacles. Responding to the question, "What prevents older persons with hearing difficulties from getting help?", 47 percent of the respondents cited the high cost of aids as the prime reason, 15 percent indicated lack of knowledge concerning where to go for assistance and what services were available, 11 percent attributed lack of transportation as the main problem, and 7 percent cited pride and vanity as the primary reasons for not seeking help. The remaining 20 percent described a variety of other problems, including fear of doctors and hearing aid dealers, lack of awareness of a hearing difficulty, projected determination to get by without assistance despite the handicap, and unfavorable reports about hearing aids from relatives and friends (Lundberg, 1979). Despite advances in technology, studies over the intervening decades have found similar results (Holmes, 1995).

Reasons for seeking help are also varied. Studies have repeatedly found that help seeking for hearing loss depends more on perceived disability (activity limitation) and handicap (participation restriction) than on measured impairment (audibility reduction), with those who feel themselves to be more handicapped seeking help sooner. Older persons who accept hearing loss as a "normal part of aging," tend to report less handicap and tolerate greater impairment than younger persons before seeking audiologic assistance for their problems. While social pressure, especially from family members, who themselves may experience handicap, is a major incentive for help seeking for hearing loss, lack of referral from primary care physicians is a major disincentive. Of course, it is possible that hearing impairment

Social pressure from others is a common reason for seeking help, and lack of referral from primary care physicians is a common reason for delaying help seeking for hearing loss.

has less effect on many older adults because of their particular life circumstances, including their greater social expertise and less demanding communication goals. In keeping with the communication enhancement model, the audiologist will need to explore the participation goals of each person as an individual in his or her own person-environment relationships. Readiness for a hearing aid or ALD must be appraised within this context.

Acknowledging the need for amplification represents considerably more than simply admitting to a sensory deficit within this age group. It is inevitably linked to recognition of the reality of aging, an acknowledgment that another bodily system is failing, and that control in life situations is at risk. As one woman emphatically stated during a hearing aid counseling session, "Well, I suppose this thing will go along with my dentures, glasses, and support brace. It's getting so it takes me half the morning to make myself *whole!*" Nonetheless, most older persons can benefit from appropriately fitted hearing aids and/or ALDs if the predisposing, enabling, and reinforcing conditions are optimized.

FIT AND FUNCTION OF THE INSTRUMENT. Although amplification is worn by individuals of all ages, most people who wear aids are beyond the sixth decade of life (Holmes, 1995). This trend has been obvious for many years, and it is only likely to increase as the population ages, especially as the number over 85 years increases to unprecedented proportions. Over the last two decades, hearing aids have become increasingly miniaturized, and at the same time there have been advances such as greater sophistication in hearing aid selection and fitting techniques, programmable technology, better consumer protection through FDA regulations, and increased professional awareness of the need for adequate rehabilitative follow-up. Nevertheless, hearing aid users still express serious concerns, which can be instructive in helping avoid certain pitfalls. Smedley and Schow (1990) summarized a large number of these complaints based on their survey of 490 elderly users. Most complaints fell into four categories: (1) the negative effects of background noise (28 percent); (2) fitting, comfort, and mechanical problems (25 percent); (3) concerns that the aid provides too little benefit (18 percent); and (4) feelings that the cost of aids, batteries, and repairs is excessive (17 percent).

Follow-up post fitting is crucial.

ALDs may be used with or instead of a hearing aid.

Some solutions will come from further improvements in digital signal processing and other technological advances. Other solutions will come from improvements in and wider use of ALDs. A seemingly endless number of products and devices are now available for assisting adults in a variety of situations. The hearing aid may be looked on as a general purpose device, while ALDs serve a variety of special listening needs, such as telephone listening, TV listening, or listening in large meeting rooms where the listener is some distance from the talker. A number of other listening and speaking devices are available, ranging from simple hardwire amplification systems for use in automobiles to infrared and FM systems for use in nursing homes, churches, and auditoriums (see Chapter 2 for a complete listing of devices; see also Lubinski & Higginbotham, 1997). Some ALDs are used instead of conventional hearing aids, while others are used in conjunction with them. ALDs may be preferred over hearing aids by younger adults in the early stages of hearing loss who have very specific needs (e.g., hearing on the telephone or in an auditorium). They may also be the device of choice for very old adults whose co-occur-

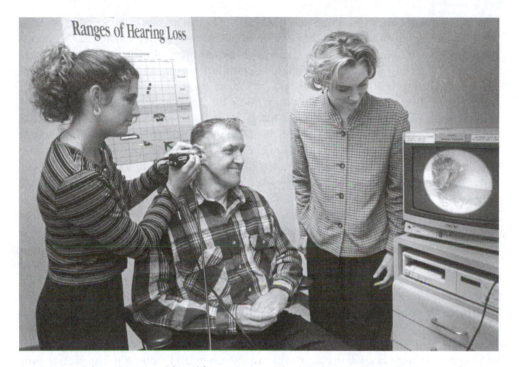

Inspection of the outer ear with a video-otoscope prior to taking an ear impression can be helpful in hearing aid fitting.

ring cognitive, vision, or dexterity problems increase the difficulty of using conventional hearing aids.

MODIFYING PROCEDURES. For some older adults, it may be necessary to modify the conventional techniques used to determine the fit and function of instruments as described in Chapter 2. First, the length and number of appointments may need to be modified. Susceptibility to fatigue, lengthened reaction time, and a lower frustration threshold may mandate shorter sessions and the need for return visits to complete the evaluation. Although this recourse is often not desirable because of transportation problems, it may be necessary in view of other factors, including variability in performance scores (some of which may be associated with time of day or other health issues), necessity for additional assessment, and, perhaps most crucial, the need for concurrent counseling and ongoing support and assistance to enable and reinforce use of the hearing aid.

Conventional techniques used to determine the fit and function of instruments may need to be modified for older adults.

Second, different tests may need to be selected. Conventional word lists, sound field procedures, real-ear measurements, and programmable adjustments may need to be altered or expanded to capture pertinent auditory processing abilities, even though at the same time it may be necessary to abbreviate testing due to the older patient's diminishing alertness and susceptibility to fatigue. Depending on the environments in which the person will be using the hearing aid or ALD, tests for sentence comprehension in cafeteria noise or with competing speech (intelligible background conversation) may provide a more valid estimation than monosyllabic word lists in quiet surroundings. Some excellent tests of performance in noise have become popular, including the *HINT* and *QuickSIN* that were suggested earlier in this chapter as more ecological measures of speech performance. Matthies, Bilger, & Roezchowski (1983) found that the age-related decrement in speech intelligibility in noise tended to disappear over a ninety-day period as their subjects gained experience wearing amplification in noise, although others have reported that older hearing aid users do not show the same benefits from *acclimatization* as do younger adults (Cox et al., 1996; Humes, 2003), presumably because of central processing problems that are not remedied by amplification (Chmiel & Jerger, 1996). Recent ground-breaking research also suggests that even for healthy older adults, individual differences in cognitive performance are significantly related to benefit from complex digital signal processing hearing aids; those with higher cognitive performance are able to take advantage of faster processing schemes, whereas those with lower cognitive performance are less able to do so (Gatehouse, Naylor, & Elberling, 2003; Lunner, 2003). At the present time there are no audiologic clinical tests of cognition, but it has been recognized that there is the need to develop and incorporate such tests in the hearing aid fitting test battery (Pichora-Fuller, 2003). Research is needed to determine how early hearing aid experience relates to brain reorganization and how brain plasticity may be affected by training in individuals with different cognitive processing abilities (Pichora-Fuller & Singh, 2006). Care should be taken to assess use, benefit, and satisfaction from a hearing aid after a period of acclimatization following 6 to 12 weeks of hearing aid use because the degree of improvement in listening performance over time may vary from person to person as they become more adept and comfortable using amplification in their everyday lives and improve in handling the device.

Third, hearing aid selection may be highly influenced by nonauditory considerations. The number of hearing aid choices may be restricted by the individual's lack of management skills or by firmly entrenched attitudes as to what type of instrument will and will not be tolerated. Fourth, additional types of appointments may need to be planned. The biologically aging segment of the population often requires more extensive follow-up for a variety of possible reasons, including counseling, supervised orientation, hearing aid earmold modifications, and consultation with caregivers, communication partners, and/or other health care professionals. It may be necessary to discuss expected and actual benefit from the hearing aid in different situations once the person has been able to use it in his or her everyday life.

Adjustment to amplification needs to be reviewed over time.

Benefits of binaural fitting must be considered for each individual.

BINAURAL FITTING. The question of whether aging persons should wear one hearing aid or binaural amplification is an individual one, depending on the degree of central processing deficit in binaural hearing, and to a great extent on prosthesis management and financial capabilities, which should be weighed against perceived gains in social receptive skills. An added variable is the attitudinal difference between wearing one instrument as opposed to two. Thus, it is not uncommon to hear an elderly person comment, "I don't need two of these, do I? I'm not deaf!" Apparently, if one hearing aid represents a milestone in adjustment to sensorineural aging, two become a millstone! Nevertheless, life satisfaction generally is greater for those who can adjust to appropriately fitted binaural amplification, and this is likely to increase as newer technologies implement more sophisticated binaural signal processing schemes that may offset some kinds of central auditory processing deficits. Birk-

Nielsen (1974) noted in comparing monaural versus binaural amplification that two aids reduced the amount of social hearing handicap among older persons. This two-ear advantage includes better speech perception in noise, reduced localized autophony (voice resonance), improved spatial balance and localization, and improved sound quality. Recent research using the *SSQ* suggests that segregation of sounds in complex environments is perhaps the most important possible benefit of wearing two hearing aids (Noble, in press). Among those who have physical, financial, or cosmetic limitations, or whose quiescent lifestyles fail to support the need for two instruments, the choice of which ear to fit becomes an issue. Considerations that enter into this decision among older adults include (1) earedness for social communication gain in quiet and in noise, (2) severity of arthritic or other physical involvement in the arms and hands as related to prosthesis manipulation, (3) handedness, (4) accustomed ear for telephone use, and (5) lifestyle factors affecting sidedness, such as driving a car or location of bed in a convalescent home.

SPECIAL DEVICE FEATURES. On the one hand, newer signal processing hearing aids with built-in automatic controls have provided relief for some whose dexterity problems would make manipulations such as adjusting the volume control difficult. On the other hand, some advanced hearing aid features may be inappropriate for the frail elderly with co-occurring cognitive, vision, and dexterity problems. In particular, the success of hearing aids depends to a great extent upon the individual's ability to handle and maintain the prosthesis. Some hearing aid companies have developed special features to accommodate the physical limitations of older persons by offering oversize or touch-type volume controls, foolproof battery compartments, attachments to reduce risk of loss, and fingernail slots or removal handles for easier removal of in the ear hearing aids. A few hearing aid manufacturers have grown concerned about the special needs of elderly persons in nursing homes and convalescent hospitals, persons whose dexterity and visual, tactile, neuromuscular, and memory difficulties contraindicate conventional forms of amplification. Therefore, Frye Electronics, for example, designed an inexpensive rechargeable body-type amplifier that features a large, red volume control and accommodates a variety of hearing loss candidates. The visibility of a body aid may benefit nursing home residents with poor management skills and visual limitations. There is also less risk that a large device will become lost. Similarly, when earmold insertion becomes prohibitively challenging, headset-style ALDs are often preferred because they are easier to put on, but also because they can be removed without assistance, thereby supporting independence. A set of helpful tips concerning hearing aid and earmold choices for the specific challenges posed by frail elderly clients with co-occurring cognitive, vision, and dexterity problems is listed on the text website (Fairholm, 2001).

> Dexterity and memory may be important factors in selecting a device.

BEYOND THE HEARING AID. Older adults with physical and cognitive limitations require special accommodations, and it is often even more important to include family and/or professional caregivers in the rehabilitation plan for such individuals. Furthermore, those with central auditory processing problems may derive less benefit from hearing aids because increased audibility of the amplified signal does not overcome their need for better signal-to-noise conditions. Such central auditory processing deficits, usually involving declines in temporal and binaural processing,

> Rehabilitation can be successful even for the most challenging situations if the appropriate supports are in place.

may not be apparent from the results of a conventional hearing test, but may be revealed during a comprehensive audiologic assessment including speech-in-noise tests. Kricos et al. (1987) endorsed the need to counsel patients with central auditory processing deficits (CAPD) about the benefits and limitations of amplification. Hearing aids may not produce significantly improved speech recognition scores, but may allow centrally impaired persons to maintain what these investigators describe as "more natural auditory contact with the world" (p. 341). Stach (1990) has shown that ALDs may provide some help for these CAPD cases because they are designed specifically to overcome adverse signal-to-noise conditions. When the rehabilitation program incorporates appropriate supports, it has been shown that even those living in residential care are able to benefit from ALDs (Lewsen & Cashman, 1997; Pichora-Fuller & Robertson, 1997). Certainly, the recommendation for amplification should not be ignored or contraindicated because of central impairments without a quantitative assessment of potential benefits during a reasonable trial period with different devices. A consideration of contextual factors will guide decision making.

> Benefits from rehabilitation for frail elderly can be observed in context.

Assessing benefits in the actual real-world context may be easier for frail clients and may provide crucial information about the nature of the social and physical environment and the supports that are available to the person. This information will guide the choice of technology best suited to the participation needs of the individual. Greater opportunity for communication will provide motivation for using a hearing aid (Lubinsky, 1984). Peer support may inspire a new hearing aid user to try and continue use of a hearing aid (Carson, 1997; Dahl, 1997). If caregivers or volunteers are willing to assist with the hearing aid and their involvement becomes part of the rehabilitation plan, a hearing aid may be an option for a person with cognitive impairment who would not be able to manage the device independently (Hoek et al., 1997). If a participation priority of the person is attending group activities (e.g., bingo in the cafeteria), an FM system may provide a vital improvement in signal-to-noise ratio that would not be achieved with a personal hearing aid. If telephone conversations with family in another city are a participation priority, a telephone amplifier may be sufficient, cheaper, and easier to manage than a hearing aid with a T-switch. The hearing aid evaluation process among the elderly may encompass the entire thirty- to sixty-day trial period offered by the dispenser, often taxing the patience of those whose primary interest is sale closure. However, the clinical audiologist must remain steadfast in terms of ethical responsibilities toward even the slowest clients and must remain open to alternative or complementary solutions.

Several methods are available for measuring the perceived benefit of amplification and, indeed, self-report has been shown to be useful in dealing with acclimatization issues (see Chapter 2). Smedley and Schow (1992) used benefit, use, and satisfaction measures, including *SAC/SOAC* and a simple seven-point scale, and showed how these may help provide feedback from users of new devices, such as the newer programmable hearing aids. Brooks (1989) used a relatively simple self-report tool of 39 items, the *Hearing Assessment Questionnaire* (along with measurements of hearing aid use time), to evaluate 758 newly fitted patients seen over one year. The data produced in this extremely valuable study clearly demonstrate the importance of extensive counseling and hearing aid orientation (see Figure 10.12). Brooks's work carefully controlled for age and hearing loss of the clients, and it may be noted that hearing aid use time for those who are extensively counseled improved dramatically

(a) Distribution of 758 subjects fitted with NHS BTE hearing aids according to age and hearing loss, and whether (EC) or not (NEC) extra counseling was provided.

		Age (Years)							
		≤60		61–70		71–80		≥81	
		EC	NEC	EC	NEC	EC	NEC	EC	NEC
	≤41	39	68	53	60	43	57	7	11
Hearing	41–50	19	16	23	30	34	49	28	32
Loss (dB)	51–60	9	8	7	11	19	25	27	22
	61–70	2	4	2	6	7	11	10	19

(b) Average daily use time for patients having NHS aids supplied without extra counseling, as a function of degree of hearing loss and age when fitted.

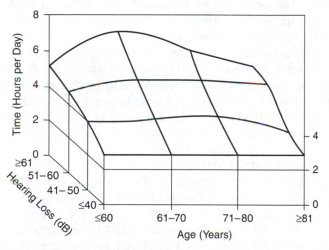

(c) Average daily time use for patients having NHS aids supplies with extra counseling, as a function of degree of hearing loss and age when fitted.

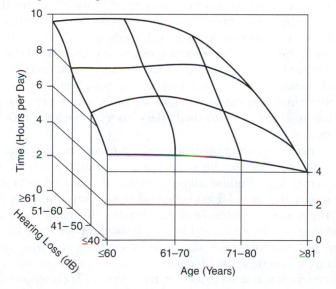

FIGURE 10.12

Data from Brooks (1989) based on United Kingdom National Health Service (NHS) provision of hearing aids.

(in some cases by a factor of two) as compared to those who did not receive extra counseling. Other orientation activities involving reading or group rehabilitation have demonstrated reduced return rate and clearly show the importance of thorough rehabilitation services (Beyers & Northern, 2000; Kochkin, 1999). Diligent follow-up is perhaps even more important for the frail elderly because their needs and abilities may change unexpectedly. When appropriate supports are in place for this special population, regular use and benefit from amplification can be maintained by experienced hearing aid wearers, even though a first-time user of a hearing aid would be unlikely to succeed (Hoek et al., 1997; Parving & Phillip, 1991; Pichora-Fuller & Robertson, 1997). Use or benefit or satisfaction may be useful measures for those who are still participating in activities; for those who have stopped participating in activities and have already become more socially isolated, increases in the number of activities in which the individual participants may provide a telling outcome measure (Pichora-Fuller & Robertson, 1994). For those with a significant degree of cognitive impairment, questionnaires are too difficult, but benefit from amplification has been demonstrated by other kinds of outcome measures, such as staff observations of reductions in behavioral problems (Palmer et al., 1999). Clearly, counseling and ongoing support and follow-up are necessary for success in many cases.

Observation of behavior may be used to evaluate benefit for those who have cognitive impairment.

ORIENTATION TO INSTRUMENTS. Initial experiences with the hearing aid or an ALD, especially in the first few weeks, are critical. The audiologist should be ready for any problem that might occur among the client, the instrument, and the environment. Counseling, whether face to face, by telephone, or on the Internet, is a continuing commitment that is based on the adjustment needs of the individuals and their partners. As pointed out earlier, the reasons for rejection of devices are infinite, ranging from simple management difficulties to complex attitude adjustment problems. The clinician must allow these reasons to surface early in the trial period before rejection becomes ingrained. An important concept to be aware of during counseling is that rejection often works in tandem with other age-related deficits that undermine appropriate use of the device. For example, rejection and reduced short-term memory may combine to become counterproductive, as summed up in the statement of an 89-year-old woman who, during a moment of exasperation, announced, "I can never remember which way the battery goes in, and I hear better without this thing, anyway!" Needless to say, she had the battery inserted backward. Other problems may be less obvious.

Improvement may be reported by the person with the new hearing aid or by a significant other.

Even if the person wearing the hearing aid does not notice much benefit from amplification, it is possible that his or her communication partner does notice improvement in terms of not finding talking so stressful: "Harry doesn't think my voice is any easier to hear, but now I don't have to shout at him so it really makes my life a lot easier!" The primary complaints of the client, family members, and friends during the preintervention phase should be readdressed during the trial period. Information from an example case illustrates the utility of this approach. The preintervention counseling session included the list of complaints and associated objectives to be reviewed at follow-up as shown in Table 10.3. Consequently, audiologic surveillance in the first two weeks was aimed not only at use of the hearing aid, but also at taking appropriate measures to reduce or eliminate each complaint. Two additional strategies for addressing the complaints were an introduction to conversational therapy for the client and her daughter and familiarization with the use of an FM system in challenging acoustical conditions. The conversational therapy targeted the frustration of the daughter during conversation with her mother, and it also targeted communication with a close friend in the dining hall at the residence of the client. An FM system was already available in the client's church, and its use in conjunction with the hearing aid was practiced with both client and daughter. Furthermore, the use of an FM system would enable listening to the bus driver on group outings, and the driver and recreational staff were involved in implementing this solution. Considered separately from the environment, the hearing aid would have been doomed to failure given the person's usual seating choices, the high level of reverberation in the church, and the high level of noise on the bus. Similarly, the overloud TV volume control was corrected by allowing the daughter to adjust the loudness to a "comfortable" level while the client was seated in her customary chair with her aids turned to half-gain. This listening level was subsequently marked on the TV volume control with an easily visible fingernail polish. Had this solution failed to meet the objectives, the next step would have been to consider using a television device providing FM transmission of the signal directly to the hearing aid wearer. Setting clear and measurable objectives helped to clarify that the rehabilitation plan was on track during the follow-up appointment during the trial period.

INDIVIDUAL ORIENTATION. The majority of hearing aid and ALD users receive help within an individual rather than a group orientation structure (Millington, 2001; Schow et al., 1993). Although group sessions have certain advantages that will be discussed later, many people are unable to meet regularly in the group environment. Individual sessions permit rehabilitation to focus more on accomplishing the specific goals of the individual. Whenever possible, it is important to have significant other persons in attendance during therapy sessions or even to conduct sessions on site in locations where the target activities take place (e.g., at the chapel or in the dining hall of a care facility), one reason being to facilitate carryover to the person's everyday participation in real-world environments.

Frequently, individual device orientation focuses on developing competence in using the device. A prerequisite to achieving audibility is for the clients and/or their caregiver to become skilled at handling, operating, and caring for the hearing aid or ALD. These skills are difficult for older adults to acquire, but even middle-aged adults may need more help than is routinely provided, as suggested by a study of working-aged adults in which it was found that one in four new hearing aid owners had problems operating his or her aid at the one-month post-fitting follow-up appointment (Alberti et al., 1984). Common problems for users of all ages are improper placement of the aid, insertion of the mold, operation of the controls, and battery insertion. Even if the new wearer has mastered the skills necessary to operate the hearing aid, it may take him or her more time to become proficient in taking advantage of the advanced features of a hearing aid, such as multiple memory options. All clients should be given instruction in both the essential and the advanced skills needed to take full advantage of the hearing aid, as well as being given written information that they can continue to refer to over time. An example handout for clients is HIO BASICS (see Figure 10.4). Handouts may need to be translated into foreign languages or produced in large print for those with vision problems. For

The necessary skills in operating and caring for hearing aids and assistive devices should be checked to be sure that no further training is needed.

those requiring more intensive instruction, it will help to focus on specific skills and to use step-by-step training to improve each skill (Maurer, 1979). In such training, the skill to be acquired (e.g., inserting the earmold) is broken down into discrete steps that are repeated until each is mastered. At each step, encouraging comments are provided by the audiologist as successes are achieved. It is also crucial for the client to learn how to judge if he or she has been successful or not, often on the basis of tactile and visual cues regarding how the earmold looks and "feels in the ear" when it is properly seated, how it "feels to the fingers" when it is properly seated, and how it "feels to the fingers" when it is grasped properly. Such programs may be completed in a single session or over multiple sessions. Caregivers may be trained to prompt, assist, and/or check that the person is using the skills on an ongoing basis. Skills should always be reevaluated at follow-up to ensure that they have been maintained and to further reinforce and refine them. An example of this is as follows.

> Mrs. Andrew's chief complaint about her new hearing aid was lack of battery life.
>
> "Are you opening the battery case at night when you're not using the instrument?" the audiologist inquired.
>
> "Heavens, no. You didn't tell me to do that!"
>
> "Yes, she did, mother," the daughter chimed in. "Don't you remember? It's even stated in that booklet in your purse."
>
> "Well, this is the first time I've *heard* about it," the older woman retorted.

ORIENTATION IN GROUPS. Some persons may fit into a group training structure rather than, or in addition to, individual sessions. This will not be feasible for everyone, however, because all do not have attitudes or cultural beliefs that favor group interaction with strangers; they may prefer meeting times that do not coincide with the group meeting time; or they may simply prefer or need the individual attention created by a one-on-one situation. But when group sessions are feasible, they can be very helpful. Aging individuals may become socially isolated. As noted earlier, their nu-

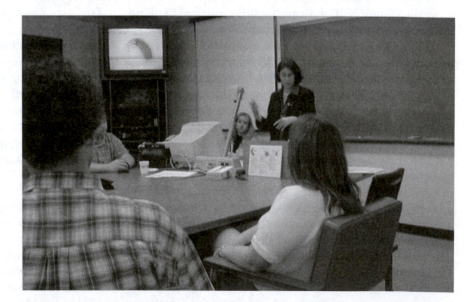

Group AR activities can help clients learn about hearing aids.

cleus of peers is smaller than in previous years, and the opportunity to participate in a group experience is often welcomed. An important aspect of a small group is the opportunity to share information. In addition to the benefits to those receiving information, sharing information is often a positive experience for the information giver. In such meetings, the audiologist takes the position of group leader and facilitates discussions by (1) bringing out those persons who are reluctant to share their experiences, (2) inhibiting those few who might dominate the group, (3) permitting the discussion topics to surface from the group rather than from the clinician, (4) acting as a resource person when expertise is needed, and, most importantly, (5) acting as a good listener. Achieving homogeneous grouping (i.e., bringing together persons who have similar perceived communication problems, as revealed in self-assessment profiles), when feasible, may be desirable. It may also be advantageous to mix more expert, experienced hearing aid users with beginners so that peer teaching and modeling can be incorporated into group sessions.

> It is important for the audiologist to be a good listener.

Like individual orientation sessions, group sessions also tend to focus mostly on the use of hearing aids, with lesser amounts of attention on communication strategies, auditory training, ALDs, and speechreading (Schow et al., 1993). In addition to the ideas on hearing aid orientation listed in Chapter 2 and in the HIO BASICS, a good group meeting is one that (1) is primarily success rather than problem oriented, (2) provides an element of entertainment, (3) focuses on no more than three learning objectives, (4) incorporates sharing of ideas in a counseling medium, and (5) culminates with a clear understanding of how each member can take charge of his or her newly acquired learning through carryover activities. The clinician may improve group cohesiveness by asking members to contact each other by telephone between sessions; for example, the objective of a homework assignment might be for the person called to guess who the "mystery caller" is and report on the experience at the next group meeting. Additional help in planning group meetings can be found in the text website.

THE SIGNIFICANT OTHER. The significant other person should understand the prosthetic device, its main components, and the conditions under which it should be worn; should possess information regarding basic troubleshooting, warranty, and repair; and should be proficient at inserting and removing the instrument. It is helpful to provide a written description of this information and resources for obtaining further information on particular topics. Resource information always includes the audiologist's phone number, as well as information such as the following: the location and telephone number of a local drugstore providing low-cost batteries, suppliers of special alerting, wake-up, or other communication devices; information on captioned films for television; lists of local facilities with hearing accessibility options (e.g., loops or FM systems); a schedule for planned hearing aid checks; notices of AR meetings, and call-back for annual audiologic assessment. Furthermore, in addition to learning new information and communication skills so that they can help the person with the hearing loss, significant others themselves must adjust to living with a person with hearing loss; they may benefit as much as the client from group discussions with peers in which information and common experiences may be shared (see Figure 10.6).

ADVOCACY IN RESTRICTIVE ENVIRONMENTS. Just as it is important to set objectives that address the goals of individuals, at the institutional level, the best method for securing the participation of the administration and staff of convalescent hospitals, nursing homes, high-rise facilities for the aging, senior adult centers, or assistive living facilities is to find out what client and staff needs the organization leaders perceive can be addressed by the AR program. Unfortunately, they may perceive the hearing problems of their clientele to rank low in priority when compared to the sleeping, eating, cleaning, entertainment, and other health needs within the facility. Most staff lack knowledge of hearing loss and hearing aids, and they may not perceive hearing help to fall within their job description. Sometimes it is difficult to gain entry into a restrictive environment on the basis of one client who has a hearing impairment and needs carryover assistance. A workable strategy for overcoming staff resistance is to seek out the staff member who is most likely to appreciate the communication and listening needs of the person (e.g., the activities director) and explain that you are working with the client and his or her family. Sometimes housekeeping or nutrition staff spend more time communicating with residents than do nurses. Offer to provide services that will help all staff involved in the case to work more easily with the client. Another possibility is to offer a more general information session on hearing and aging as an inservice activity aimed at helping the staff understand and manage all clientele with hearing difficulties. A stimulating, solution-oriented inservice presentation nearly always produces advocates among residents, family, volunteers, and staff members, individuals who later may become allies in the rehabilitation plan. Once allies are made, interest is maintained through a recognized need for further education as well as an open communication line to the audiologist's office. Leaving a designated staff member with this public service gesture and a copy of your professional credentials removes much of the suspicion frequently associated with the doorstep intervention tactics of some commercial vendors.

Elsewhere we have reported a variety of experiences in providing hearing services for nursing homes (Hoek et al., 1997; Pichora-Fuller & Robertson, 1997; Schow, 1992). In a number of such homes where hearing was tested, we found that only about 10 percent of potential hearing aid candidates were using amplification, whereas another 20 percent responded that they had hearing aids but were not using them. Importantly, rehabilitation has been shown to be valuable in maintaining the use of devices by those in residential care. Therefore, the need for rehabilitation is apparent, and residents will be at a disadvantage if it is not provided. A multistep program is proposed as an effective plan for ensuring that hearing services are available in these facilities (see Table 10.4).

ALTERNATIVE MEDIA. Face-to-face interactions between the rehabilitative audiologist and those in residential facilities will be crucial, but in some situations other media, ranging from posters and videotapes to the Internet, may augment face-to-face interactions. Hurvitz and colleagues (1987) demonstrated an effective self-paced computer AR program designed to provide communication training to a nursing home population. Their software program covers content related to (1) mechanism of the ear, (2) audiograms, (3) management of the hearing problem, (4) speechreading, (5) hearing aids, and (6) communication skills training. Short in-

TABLE 10.4

Multistep Program for Those in Residential Care

1. Screening of hearing, as required by federal law, with pure tones, visual inspection (including determination of need for removal of cerumen), and self- and staff members' assessment of hearing (e.g., Nursing Home Hearing Handicap Index).
2. Cerumen management as indicated, followed by thorough diagnostic testing for those who fail screening, along with charting and informing staff of results and arranging for referrals as needed.
3. Consultation with communication partners if appropriate to identify objectives of staff, family, or significant others.
4. Identification of objectives for rehabilitation for individuals and subgroups of residents who share particular interests or activities (e.g., attending services in chapel, going on bus outings).
5. Selection of candidates for devices, trials with hearing aids or ALDs in context, and thorough orientation for those who are reestablishing use or becoming new users of devices.
6. Inservices to staff, including instruction on the auditory mechanism, explanation of the causes and effects of hearing loss in the elderly, discussion of the role of the audiologist and facility staff in hearing health care, development of skills in using and caring for amplification devices, and guidance on how to encourage independent communication behaviors and an environment that facilitates positive interpersonal relationships among residents and staff.
7. Recommend changes to routines and physical environment that will enable best use of amplification and assistive technology.
8. Implement method for ongoing monitoring of and help for all amplification users and key communication partners, including family, staff, peers, and volunteers.

formational paragraphs are presented followed by multiple-choice questions in a user-friendly format. Patients trained with this program showed more knowledge gains than in a conventional group classroom approach. At present, use of the Internet by older adults in our society is rapidly increasing; about 1 in 10 seniors had Internet access at home in 1999, but by 2003 almost 1 in 4 did. Health information on the Internet has growing appeal to many adults who want to find or review information on health topics at a time and place of their own choosing. In the future, Internet connection will no doubt be used to facilitate more immediate communication between the audiologist and staff, family, or residents at different locations that are geographically distributed.

Remediation for Communication Activities

Traditionally, communication rehabilitation has focused on auditory and visual communication training, with an emphasis on speechreading and auditory training. Typically, it was provided when counseling and instrumental interventions proved insufficient. In light of the growing understanding of the lengthy but important process of adjusting to hearing loss, many rehabilitative audiologists today offer communication rehabilitation to a broader segment of the population and in more varied forms that target more specific activity goals. All clients should be familiarized with the principles of communication rehabilitation in discussion with the audiologist, and written materials should be provided for the client to refer to later or share with significant others. An example of such a handout is **CLEAR** (see Figure 10.5). In addition to introducing these general principles to clients, their specific activity goals can also be addressed by individual or group communication remediation tailored to their needs.

Rehabilitative training is being rejuvenated in new programs that emphasize listening.

As in the past, audiovisual communication rehabilitation may be provided to those whose needs have not been met adequately by amplification. The analytic and synthetic approaches to speechreading and auditory training have been encompassed into a more holistic conversation-based approach to communication rehabilitation, and this form of rehabilitation has targeted people who are hard of hearing and their communication partners (Erber, 1988, 1996; Tye-Murray, 1997). New computer-based programs such as *Listening and Communication Enhancement* (*LACE;* Sweetow & Henderson-Sabes, 2004) have been designed to enable clients to practice listening to more realistic speech materials in signal-to-noise conditions that are adjusted to the performance level of the new hearing aid wearer. In addition to communication remediation for those using amplification, communication training is now being provided to assist individuals in the process of adjusting to hearing loss who may not yet be ready to try a hearing aid. Other exciting new programs use a health promotion approach in programs for older adults with no known clinically significant hearing loss so that they will be better prepared for taking action when they do begin to experience hearing problems (Hickson et al., in press; Worrall et al., 1998).

"Bridge" Therapy

Individual speechreading instruction was deemed appropriate for a 62-year-old woman who had suffered loss of hearing in one ear due to Ménière's disease. Socially active in the community and reluctant to disclose her impairment to others, the woman preferred the privacy of individual therapy. She was an avid bridge player, and participation in her bridge club was of utmost importance to her. To address her single goal of retaining excellent ability to participate in bridge games, individual therapy activities were chosen that satisfied the same five ingredients described earlier for a good group meeting. One such therapy activity consisted of "playing" bridge through a two-way mirror with only visual cues for statements, such as "I bid three spades," "I pass," and so forth. The woman improved her ability to speechread the language of her favorite game. This proved fortuitous, since the signs of Ménière's syndrome (roaring tinnitus, vertigo, and nausea) signaled the eventual loss of hearing in her good ear. As her hearing loss deteriorated further, additional goals were formulated and therapy activities undertaken.

CONVERSATIONAL THERAPY AND TACTICS. The critical implication of hearing loss for an aging individual is that it affects the lenses through which the client views reality. Thus, when the speech signal and content of messages are altered, the older person comes to distrust what others say as well as his or her own interpretation of communicative events. Restoring control and trust in communication may become an objective for communication rehabilitation that is accomplished in conversational therapy. When communication needs become apparent in a wider range of everyday life situations, and when reduced communicative competence comes to have far-reaching effects on the person's well-being, a broader approach to communication training becomes essential. Conversation-based communication training has been promoted for nearly two decades by Erber (1988, 1996) and is explained in Chapters 4 and 5. Just as in face-to-face communication, conversation-based therapy necessarily engages the person in auditory and visual perception of speech. However, the therapy stresses how the person can take advantage of and manipulate many of the redundant sources of information that are available in the communicative interaction, including many aspects of the person–environment relationship. Whereas some sources of information come from the external world (e.g., seeing the waitress approach a table in a restaurant), others come from internally stored knowledge of the world (e.g., knowledge that the restaurant script for ordering food often begins by the waitress asking the customers if they are ready to order). During therapy, clients learn how they can optimize the usefulness of available information, especially by using conversational strategies. For example, miscommunication resulting from mis-perceived speech sounds can be overcome if conversational strategies are used to establish the topic. A peripheral high-frequency hearing loss alters coding of the speech signal, thereby affecting comprehension of the content of the message and even influencing the ongoing response to the message:

> Mr. Jacobson was helping his grandson paint the family shed. "Gramps," the younger person said, "let's quit for awhile and go get some thinner."
> The older man stared in amazement at his grandson, "Go get some dinner? Son, we just had lunch!"

The confusion arising from the *thinner-dinner* misperception would have been repaired more gracefully if the grandfather had been more cautious and asked, "What do you want to get?" before jumping to a conclusion that he actually recognized to be inconsistent with the situation. For AR to be successful for the older person, positive change must be brought about in the entire social-communicative milieu.

Conversation-based therapy cultivates the communication skills pertaining to the four elements in any communication situation: listener, talker, message, and environment. The client develops skills in each area: (1) listening (and watching) to comprehend, (2) coaching talkers to produce more easily understood speech and language (e.g., by suggesting helpful accommodations such as "Could you keep your hand away from your face and speak slower?"), (3) using linguistic and world knowledge to interpret the meaning of the message, and (4) altering the acoustical and lighting properties of the situation to improve the signal and reduce interference from extraneous sources. The communication partner also develops corresponding skills pertaining to each of the skill areas. Both the client and the communication partner develop methods that are effective for them in their relationship with each other. These methods may be different for spouses who have lived together for fifty years than for a college student and his new professor or for a 90-year-old with dementia and the nurse providing her with care in a hospice. The audiologist–counselor, acting in the multiple roles of diagnostician, hearing aid specialist, AR specialist, and gerontologist, becomes an integral part of the client's milieu.

PARTNER COMMUNICATION. It is worth noting that hearing loss in one communication partner may coexist with hearing loss in the other partner. It is also common

The communication issues of the partner may need to be addressed, too.

for one or both partners to have another communication disorder. Spouses may develop vocal pathology as a result of chronically raising their voice to be heard by their hard of hearing partners. Spouses may have trouble hearing the poorly intelligible or soft voices of partners with Parkinson's. Most individuals who have had total laryngectomy surgery are within the senior adult age group and have hearing difficulties. Furthermore, since esophageal speech generally has reduced intensity and less well-defined vowel formants, persons with laryngectomies are less intelligible to peers, who are also likely to be aging and hard of hearing. Withdrawal from social situations may result from the combination of hearing and speaking difficulties and may affect the relationship between spouses and friends. Communicative rehabilitation often entails using visual cues to improve speech perception; however, this may not be an option for the many older adults with vision loss. In one home for the aged, the audiologist was surprised when a woman who was blind asked to join the lipreading class until the woman explained that she wanted to learn how to talk more clearly so that her roommate who was hard of hearing would be able to lipread her better. It may become necessary to address the other communication issues of the client or even the communication issues of the spouse in order to achieve a solution in communication rehabilitation.

SIMULATIONS AND ROLE PLAYING. The counselor–audiologist is positioned between the aging client and reality, because the counselor's own communication skills and knowledge are called into play to assist the older person in restructuring the client's lifestyle to ameliorate or compensate for the hearing impairment to achieve participation. The audiologist may even play the role of the client when the communication partner is receiving conversational training or the role of the communication partner when the client is being trained. The ability to re-create these roles is enhanced by the use of Erber's HELOS (hearing loss simulator), which can be used to introduce the effects of hearing impairment into the signal heard by a person with normal hearing (Erber, 1988), but the therapy can also be done without HELOS. Importantly, such role playing enables the audiologist to model more effective communication strategies, and it also promotes empathy, mutual respect and consideration, and sharing of experiences with and between the client and his or her communication partner(s).

EMPATHY AND LISTENING. During communication rehabilitation, as in all stages of AR, the empathy achieved through listening will have great effect on the outcome of the rehabilitation program. Slower in adapting to change and more fixed in their attitudes than younger persons with hearing impairment, elderly patients demand more professional time for their feelings to surface. In some instances, the audiologist can bring about positive changes by simply *permitting the client to register complaints,* thereby achieving a more favorable outlook in decision making. Listening helps the audiologist appreciate the delicate balance between the client's enjoyment of hearing and the perceived nuisances of the new device. Listening also helps the audiologist learn from the ingenuity of clients who find their own novel solutions to problems. The many personal preferences, attitudes, and beliefs of clients will guide the setting of objectives and the selection of an action plan for rehabilitation that can be reevaluated over time (see Figure 10.6).

> ### Allowing the Client to Register Complaints
>
> *Client:* My voice is so difficult with these aids on. [Shakes head.] I don't think I can get used to them.
>
> *Audiologist:* Uh-huh.
>
> *Client:* Do I sound like this to others? My voice sounds so gravelly.
>
> *Audiologist:* Hmm.
>
> *Client:* I wonder if I've been talking too loud to people . . . before I got these, I mean. [Eyes brighten.] Well, I certainly keep my voice down now.
>
> *Audiologist:* Uh-huh.
>
> *Client:* I can hear a whisper now . . . in a quiet room. But . . . Oh, the racket when I'm doing dishes! I took them off and put them on the window sill.
>
> *Audiologist:* Uh-huh.
>
> *Client:* I could hear the clerk in the checkout line yesterday. Heard everything he said. . . .
>
> *Audiologist:* Hmm.
>
> *Client:* I suppose it's a matter of . . . getting used to them. [Nods head.] They help . . . they really do.

Environmental Coordination and Participation Improvement

As demonstrated so far in this chapter, a well-coordinated rehabilitation program for adults requires an organized body of knowledge about the clientele. This includes clinical sensitivity toward persons in general who are at various lifespan stages, a thorough understanding of the individual in question, and prioritization of this information into a meaningful rehabilitative plan. Directive, informational counseling that includes "laundry lists" of questions, often constructed on the basis of stereotypes, is not well advised. Although such an approach may be useful for some purposes, the salience of the information sampled in this noninteractive, narrow manner may be lost in the undertow of real needs and feelings that surface when the clinician simply listens to the client. In too many instances, failure or rejection of hearing amplification or other treatment during the intervention process is due either to lack of clinical sensitivity toward the individual client's needs, feelings, and goals or to insensitivity toward the subpopulation of adults to which the individual belongs. Adults are heterogeneous, and their particular needs must be determined by the audiologist. The elderly segment of the world population of persons with hearing impairment has a wealth of life experiences that may influence their course of rehabilitation both positively and negatively. There is also variability among younger adults, including young adults completing their education and vocational training, adults raising young families, adults caring for aging parents, working adults in

A profile of the client focuses on the person's lifestyle and listening needs.

> ### Client Profile
>
> Areas of intake information that provide context for the overall coordination of the program:
>
> - Hearing status, including history, duration, and potential site(s) of lesion, as well as self-assessment of the hearing problems and assessments by significant other persons.
>   - What problems are the most important to this person and his or her partners?
>   - What are the past, present, and desired activities of this person?
> - Previous help seeking and medical or prosthetic intervention.
>   - What factors contributed to the success or failure of previous rehabilitative action?
> - Associated health issues, such as arthritis, neuromuscular limitations, visual problems, tinnitus, and memory difficulties.
>   - To what extent do physical, mental, social, or economic conditions make this individual dependent on others?
> - Personal and environmental factors that will predispose, enable, and reinforce decision making and action taking.
>   - What kinds of social or environmental supports would be needed by the individual in his or her activities?
>   - What costs and benefits might influence rehabilitative choices?

stressful senior positions, and adults with unusual health or occupational challenges. For older and younger adults alike, their need for audiologic services may range from minimal to extreme. Each case must be appreciated in a dynamic context.

The pervading question is whether the rehabilitation program will make a significant, positive impact on the life satisfaction of this person. A well-developed client profile, based on both formal assessment measures and informal information gathering during counseling, substantially increases the probability of successful AR. Thus, the profile permits an educated focus on current aspects of the person's lifestyle. It addresses client needs, rather than those of the clinic or the practitioner. It delineates whether the individual is a candidate for intervention, the particular plan that should be tailored to meet the person's needs, the hypothetical objectives and terminal goals that might be accomplished, significant other persons who should be involved, environmental modifications that will be needed to achieve a solution for the person, and where, when, and under whose auspices the program should be carried out. The individual's adjustment to hearing loss and preparedness for taking rehabilitative action is foremost in the rehabilitative agenda, but rehabilitation may fall short of meeting the individual's goals if the importance of social and physical environmental supports is overlooked.

PARTICIPATION IN SITUATIONS AND RELATIONSHIPS. Most of the complaints of adults about their hearing difficulties, for example, are about participation in a specific situation or role: "I can't hear in church," "I can't understand the lecturer when my classmates are talking," "I don't watch the news on television because the announcer talks too fast," "I feel like I'm letting my teenage son down because I can't have conversation with him without making him repeat all the time." Knowledge about such concerns provides for a practical, operational baseline from which positive rehabilitative changes can be measured. Self-assessment measures such as the *SAC* and *COSI* are useful for identifying the needs of the individual and documenting changes with respect to these needs. New tools such as data logging can be used to discover more about the communication environments encountered by the client in everyday life. More informal information gathering during counseling, however, is still necessary if the audiologist is to fully appreciate how personal, social, and physical environmental factors should best be tackled to achieve a successful rehabilitative solution.

SOCIAL ENVIRONMENTAL SUPPORTS. The key to whether significant other persons should be included in the plan and subsequent coordination of the rehabilitation program is the extent of their present and potential contribution toward the elderly individual's life satisfaction and the achievement of the client's top priority goals. Observing interactions between the client and others may reveal the kind of support that they will provide and whether they will be allies during intervention. Perhaps one of the paramount questions that the clinician should ask on an intuitive level is whether significant others' support is based on a valid concern for the individual or whether it is irregular or counterproductive, or independence or dependence supporting. Relatives, friends, and staff members in the geriatric environment can constitute important links in the rehabilitative chain and can be helped by review of a handout like the one shown in Figure 10.6. Others who may act in concert with the audiologist to facilitate adjustive behaviors include members of the professional community who have knowledge about the client and his or her family support system, culture, and lifestyle. Relevant parties may include members of the clergy, physicians, welfare workers, and administrators or leaders of organizations and clubs in which the client holds membership.

Relatives, friends, and professionals can be important partners in AR.

PHYSICAL ENVIRONMENTAL SUPPORTS. The physical environment may also be crucial to the client's ability to participate fully. Environmental supports can be optimized by selecting favorable environments or modifying unfavorable environments. The client may need to investigate which restaurants are quiet and well lit and learn how to pick the best table and seat. Where choices are not possible, modifications may be required. Noise and reverberation may need to be reduced by interior decorating (e.g., carpeting, upholstery, drapes) or architectural changes to increase sound absorption by room surfaces. Electromagnetic interference can also interfere with participation by people who are hard of hearing. For example, when a department head in a large company moved into her new office, she was horrified to discover that she was unable to use her T-switch for the telephone or with ALDs in the conference room. To the embarrassment of the architect, the acoustical consultant who was hired to assess the problem determined that the problem was caused by the high level of electromagnetic interference produced in a machine room located directly below the new offices. A large insulating panel was installed by the employer to eliminate the problem. The nature of the client's problem and the method for solving it eluded the audiologist, whose clinical measures showed that there was no change in the client's hearing and that her devices were working properly. The cooperation of the employer and the expertise of the architect and acoustical consultant were vital to achieving the environmental piece of the solution. Greater involvement of

Acoustical consultants may help with architectural solutions.

professionals and policymakers responsible for the built environment will likely be seen as AR catches up with other rehabilitative fields in which accessibility adaptations (e.g., ramps for wheelchairs) have long been accepted as societal obligations, especially in workplaces or public educational, health, and law facilities.

Further Illustration of CORE and CARE

The approach recommended in this chapter suggests that the rehabilitation of hearing loss should be based on the strategy suggested by CORE and CARE (see Figure 10.2). We further note that most of the rehabilitation done by audiologists is done in connection with hearing aid fitting. We know that in a certain number of special cases, such as with a cochlear implant client, that rehabilitation may be much more involved, but these special cases will be the exception. Therefore, we want to provide a clear emphasis on hearing aid fitting. Before concluding this chapter we would like to describe a hearing aid client recently seen in our clinic to illustrate how this rehabilitation procedure plays out in real life. This individual, John, was a male, age 54, who had been experiencing hearing problems for the past few years, which finally prompted him to have his hearing tested with the idea he might need hearing aids. In the C (communication) assessment phase, we tested hearing by audiometry and self-report. The audiogram revealed equal results in both ears, so the thresholds were 1K Hz = 35 dB HL, 2K Hz = 40 dB HL, 4K Hz = 45 dB HL (Figure 10.13). The loss was sensorineural and, based on better ear thresholds and the sys-

FIGURE 10.13

John, age 54, initial audiogram.

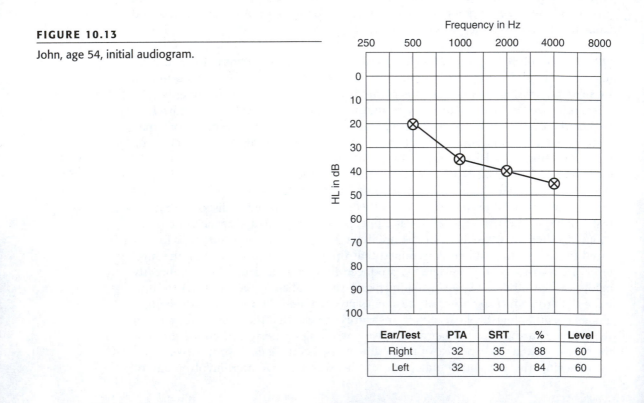

Ear/Test	PTA	SRT	%	Level
Right	32	35	88	60
Left	32	30	84	60

tem used in this text for sorting hearing loss into exclusive groups, the loss was in the category F1 (see Chapter 1 and text website).

We also had John complete a *GHABP.* At an initial interview and before any decision was made about hearing aids, the *GHABP* allowed us to measure the initial disability or communication activity limitation. This score is based on four standard listening situations and up to four situations supplied by the client that are of concern. John provided two areas of hearing concern beyond the four standard ones, and his *GHABP* results for the relevant six items are shown in Figure 10.14. The percentage disability score (*activity limitation*) obtained on the *GHABP* for John was 60 percent. Scoring procedures and practice in scoring for the *GHABP* can be accessed on the website that goes with this text.

In terms of O (overall) participation, we considered vocational, social, and emotional issues. John said his work as a janitor was not affected by his hearing, but his major concerns were in social activities and some emotional problems related to these social activities. Again the *GHABP* was helpful in measuring this handicap or *participation restriction,* because it measured how much his hearing problems cause him to be worried, annoyed, or upset in the six situations. This score was 45 percent.

We have gathered and published scores on over 800 clients sorted into exclusive hearing categories, and when we compared John's two scores (60 percent and 45 percent) with others who have hearing losses in the same category as his, we found he was within one standard deviation of the mean for all clients with such a hearing loss (see data in Chapter 1 and on the text website). However, his scores were located toward the upper end of that mid range, showing he has more than average *activity limitation* and *participation restrictions.* We also explored R (related personal) and E (environmental) factors that had a bearing on John's hearing loss. We found his attitude about improving his hearing was excellent (a type I) and that he was an extrovert who would like to get out more if his hearing were better. In terms of environmental issues, his wife also wanted him to socialize more and

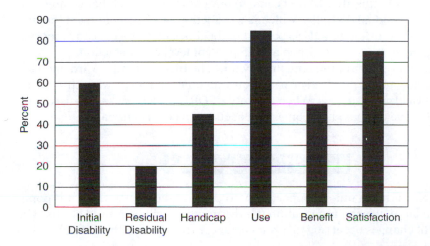

FIGURE 10.14

Glasgow (GHABP) findings for John. Pre-hearing aid results are initial disability and handicap. Post-fitting results are residual disability, use, benefit, and satisfaction.

encouraged him to obtain hearing aids. She filled out a *GHABP* also, modified for use by a significant other person. Thus we considered all four of the CORE issues.

As John told us his story during the C (counseling) phase of the treatment, goals were determined based on input from him. These goals were set in the areas of A (audibility), R (remediation of communication activities), and E (environmental or participation goals). By counseling and setting goals in these three areas, we recommended a reasonably standardized procedure in rehabilitation (CARE) much as audiologists do in diagnostic audiology (Schow, 2001). After John decided to obtain hearing aids, the necessary decisions were made about fit and function of the aid, and ear impressions were made. When he came back to pick up his hearing aids, we used the HIO BASICS handout (Figure 10.4) in a 45-minute session for hearing instrument orientation. A week later in a second 45-minute follow-up session the remediation of communication issues was addressed with the CLEAR handout (see Figure 10.5). This provided John with some help in fundamental areas of concern surrounding communication. Had John been interested in getting more help in these areas, we would have recommended our four sessions of group therapy, which are provided each semester, but John did not elect to enroll for these sessions, which are provided free with all of our hearing aid fittings.

John did elect to focus his efforts in the next two 45-minute follow-up sessions on the two environmental participation issues that he had identified as a major concern on his *GHABP*. John was concerned that he could not hear his grandchildren when they came for their weekly visit. Also, he was concerned about hearing TV when his wife is watching, and he cannot turn the volume as loud as he would like it. We spent a full follow-up session with John talking about ways that he could improve communication with his granddaughter, age 10, and his grandson, age 8. We went over the SPEECH handout (Figure 10.6) with his wife to help her communications with him and urged her to review these communication improvement suggestions with the two grandchildren. He and his wife decided to control the environment by turning off the TV when he is visiting with these children, and by getting them to sit closer and watching their lips, he could improve his success in communication. Also, in another follow-up session we helped him obtain a listening device for his TV that was successful for use when his wife watched TV with him. We sent a *GHABP* scale to John six months after he first came to our clinic and found that he now had only 20 percent residual disability, which is a reduction of 40 percent from the first assessment. He was using the aids 85 percent of the time and receiving good reported benefit (50 percent) and was satisfied at a 75 percent level of satisfaction.

Certainly, all rehabilitation outcomes will not be this straightforward and successful. But new goals may be set based on outcome measures when the initial plans do not yield good success. When the entire CORE–CARE package is used with clients, we believe that good outcomes can occur on a consistent basis.

SUMMARY

The AR specialist has a unique opportunity to provide services to the adult population over a large lifespan range, although the majority will be retired adults. The complexity of changes occurring in advanced age, together with the difficulties encountered due to auditory deficits, requires that the audiologist become resourceful and willing to modify established techniques and protocols. The audiologist can contribute to a positive future for aging persons who are hard of hearing—a future that is of higher quality, more productive, and/or less isolated. Better communication skills may help lessen the stress caused by other disabilities, as well as facilitating ongoing social interaction between older adults and their environments.

The need for specialized training in adult lifespan changes and gerontology among graduate students specializing in speech and hearing sciences becomes increasingly apparent as longevity increases and the population ages (Kricos & Lesner, 1995). The last decade has seen a substantial growth in our knowledge of aging in general and auditory aging in particular. Following on these advances in research, it is now time for a greater commitment to training in gerontology among graduate programs so that audiologists can take on a leadership role in the care of aging persons who are hard of hearing. Addressing the problems of adults who are hard of hearing is a professional challenge that we must all face together.

SUMMARY POINTS

- Adults acquire hearing loss due to illness, accident, noise exposure, and aging, but most lose their hearing through the aging process.
- Hearing loss leads to misunderstandings and stress for the individual, family, and friends.
- A number of personal and environmental factors may complicate the situation for elderly persons with hearing loss.
- Presbycusis is the name for age-related hearing loss.
- Phonemic regression is a common presbycusic problem wherein there is a more severe word recognition problem than would be expected on the basis of hearing thresholds.
- Speech in noise tests such as the *HINT* or *QuickSIN* are more representative of listening ability in the conditions encountered in everyday life.
- It is not uncommon for over 80 percent of a nursing home population to have hearing loss.
- The CORE and CARE model of rehabilitation employed throughout this text provides the framework for rehabilitation assessment and management.
- Rehabilitation settings include university speech and hearing clinics, military facilities, community centers, medical clinics, and private practice offices of dispensers.
- Assessment begins with audiometry and self-report and progresses to concerns about participation, personal, and environmental factors.
- Three self-report measures, the *IOI-HA*, *COSI*, and *SAC/SOAC*, are included here as used in assessment and are also extremely valuable later as outcome measures. Other tools like *GHABP* are also useful.
- Data logging enables the audiologist to track how much and in what kinds of acoustical environments the hearing aid has been used.
- Rehabilitative goals must be set by considering the current audibility, activity, and participation needs of the individual.

- The personal, social, and physical environmental factors supporting or impeding decision making and action taking must be considered when goals are set.
- Goals should clearly state and specify *WHO* will do *WHAT, HOW MUCH,* and by *WHEN.*
- Goals must be reevaluated and reset as needed at the time of follow-up, a crucial step in the rehabilitative cycle.
- An essential trio of outcome measures should include speech performance tests, hearing aid usage, and self-reported benefit and satisfaction.
- Rehabilitation involves change on the part of the individual who is deaf or hard of hearing, but may also involve his or her communication partners or necessitate changes in the physical environment.
- More people will seek and benefit from rehabilitation as technology improves, but it will also be crucial for stigma to be reduced by social change.
- Even individuals who do not use amplification might benefit from other forms of audiologic rehabilitation.
- Adjustment to hearing loss is a dynamic process that we do not yet fully understand.

RECOMMENDED READING

Craik, F. I. M., & Salthouse, T. A. (Eds.). (2000). *The handbook of aging and cognition* (2nd ed.). Mahwah, NJ: Lawrence Erlbaum.

Erber, N. P. (1996). *Communication therapy for adults with sensory loss* (2nd ed.). Melbourne, Australia: Clavis Publishing.

Kiessling, J., Pichora-Fuller, M. K., Gatehouse, S., Stephens, D., Arlinger, S., Chisolm, T., Davis, A. C., Erber, N. P., Hickson, L., Holmes, A., Rosenhall, U., & von Wedel, H. (2003). Candidature for and delivery of audiological services: Special needs of older people. *International Journal of Audiology, 42,* Suppl 2, 2S92–2S101.

Kricos, P. B., & Lesner, S. A. (Eds.). (1995). *Hearing care for the older adult: Audiologic rehabilitation.* Boston: Butterworth-Heinemann.

Lubinski, R., & Higginbotham, J. (Eds.). (1997). *Communication technologies for the elderly: Vision, hearing, and speech.* San Diego, CA: Singular Publishing Group.

Noble, W. (1998). *Self-assessment of hearing and related functions.* London: Whurr.

Tye-Murray, N. (1997). *Communication training for older teenagers and adults: Listening, speechreading and using conversation strategies.* Austin, TX: Pro-Ed.

Willott, J. F. (1991). *Aging and the auditory system: Anatomy, physiology, and psychophysics.* San Diego, CA: Singular Publishing Group.

Worrall, L., & Hickson, L. (2003). *Communication disability in aging: Prevention and intervention.* San Diego, CA: Singular Publishing Group.

RECOMMENDED WEBSITES

World Health Organization International Classification of functioning, disability, and health:
www.who.int/icidh/

American Academy of Audiology:
www.audiology.org/professional/positions/

American Speech-Language-Hearing Association:
www.asha.org

Perry Hanavan's site that defines AR and includes about 30 links:
www.augie.edu/perry/ear/ardefine.htm

By far the most comprehensive AR site available. It is very stable and has been there for years with regular updating. It has over 100 sites that are AR related. http://ctl.augie.edu/perry/ar/ar.htm

Gatehouse website for GHABP and SSQ:
www.ihr.gla.ac.uk/products/index.php

Outcome measurement from ISU site:
www.isu.edu/csed/profile

IOI in English and other languages:
www.icra.nu

REFERENCES

Alberti, P. W., Pichora-Fuller, M. K., Corbin, H., & Riko, K. (1984). Aural rehabilitation in a teaching hospital: Evaluation and results. *Annals of Otology, Rhinology and Laryngology, 93*(6), 589–594.

Alpiner, J. G., & Schow, R. L. (2000). Rehabilitative evaluation of hearing-impaired adults. In J. Alpiner & P. McCarthy (Eds.), *Rehabilitative audiology: Children and adults* (3rd ed.). Baltimore: Williams & Williams.

Baltes, M. M., & Wahl, H-W. (1996). Patterns of communication in old age: The dependence-support and independence-ignore script. *Health Communication, 8*(3), 217–231.

Beck, L. (2000). The role of outcomes data in health-care resource allocation. *Ear and Hearing, 21*(4) Supp., 89S–96S.

Bentler, R. A., & Kramer, S. (2000). Guidelines for choosing a self-report outcome measure. *Ear and Hearing, 21*(4) Supp., 37S–49S.

Bess, F., Lichtenstein, M. J., Logan, S. A., Burger, M. C., & Nelson, E. (1989). Hearing impairment as a determinant of function in the elderly. *Journal of the American Geriatric Society, 37,* 123–128.

Beyers, C. M., & Northern, J. L. (2000). Audiologic rehabilitation support program: A network model. *Seminars in Hearing, 21*(3), 257–265.

Birk-Nielsen, H. (1974). Effect of monaural versus binaural hearing and treatment. *Scandinavian Audiology, 3,* 183–187.

Borg, E. (1998). Audiology in an ecological perspective—development of a conceptual framework. *Scandinavian Audiology, 27,* Supp. 49, 132–139.

Brockett, J., & Schow, R. L. (2001). Web site profiles common hearing loss patterns. *Hearing Journal, 54*(8).

Brooks, D. (1989). The effect of attitude on benefit obtained from hearing aids. *British Journal of Audiology, 23,* 3–11.

Carson, A. J. (1997). Evaluation of the "To Hear Again" program. *Journal of Speech–Language Pathology and Audiology, 21,* 160–166.

Carson, A. J., (2005). "What brings you here today?" The role of self-assessment in help-seeking for age-related hearing loss. *Journal of Aging Studies, 19,* 185–200.

CHABA: Committee on Hearing, Bioacoustics, and Biomechanics. (1988). Speech understanding and aging. *Journal of the Acoustical Association of America, 83,* 859–895.

Chmiel, R., & Jerger, J. (1996). Hearing aid use, central auditory disorder, and hearing handicap in elderly persons. *Journal of the American Academy of Audiology, 7,* 190–202.

Clark, P. G. (1996). Communication between provider and patient: Values, biography, and empowerment in clinical practice. *Aging and Society, 16,* 747–774.

Coupland, N., Wiemann, J. M., & Giles, H. (1991). Talk as "Problem" and communication as "Miscommunication": An integrative analysis. In N. Coupland, H. Giles, & J. M. Wiemann (Eds.), *"Miscommunication" and problematic talk* (pp. 1–17). Newbury Park, CA: Sage.

Cox, R., Alexander, G. C., Taylor, I. M., & Gray, G. A. (1996). Benefit acclimatization in elderly hearing aid users. *Journal of the American Academy of Audiology, 7,* 428–441.

Cox, R., Hyde, M., Gatehouse, S., Noble, W., Dillon, H., Bentler, R., Stephens, D., Arlinger, S., Beck, L., Wilkerson, D., Kramer, S., Kricos, P., Gagne, J., Bess, F., & Hallberg, L. (2000). Optimal outcome measures, research priorities, and international cooperation. *Ear and Hearing, 21*(4) Supp., 106S–115S.

Dahl, M. (1997). To Hear Again: A volunteer program in hearing health care for hard-of-hearing seniors. *Journal of Speech–Language Pathology and Audiology, 21,* 153–159.

Dillon, H., James, A., & Ginis, J. (1997). Client oriented scale of improvement (COSI) and its relationship to several other measures of benefit and satisfaction provided by hearing aids. *Journal of American Academy of Audiology, 8,* 27–43.

Dillon, H., & So, M. (2000). Incentives and obstacles to the routine use of outcome measures by clinicians. *Ear and Hearing, 21*(4) Supp., 2S–6S.

Erber, N. P. (1988). *Communication therapy for hearing-impaired adults.* Victoria, Australia: Clavis Publishing.

Erber, N. P. (1996). *Communication therapy for adults with sensory loss* (2nd ed.). Melbourne, Australia: Clavis Publishing.

Erber, N. P., et al. (1999, June). Caregiver communication training program. *Speech Pathology Australia,* 12–14.

Fairholm, D. (2001). Vancouver/Richmond Health Board Community Audiology Centre Outreach to Hard of Hearing Seniors Program, personal communication.

Gaeth, J. (1948). *A study of phonemic regression associated with hearing loss.* Unpublished doctoral dissertation, Northwestern University.

Gagné, J.-P. (2000). What is treatment evaluation research? What is its relationship to the goals of audiologic rehabilitation? Who are the stakeholders of this type of research? *Ear and Hearing, 21*(4) Supp., 60S–73S.

Gagné, J.-P., & Jennings, M. B. (2000). Audiological rehabilitation intervention services for adults with acquired hearing impairment. In M. Valente, H. Hosford-Dunn, & R. Roesor (Eds.), *Audiology treatment.* New York: Theme.

Gagné J.-P., McDuff, S., & Getty, L. (1999). Some limitations of evaluative investigations based solely on normed outcome measures. *Journal of the American Academy of Audiology, 10,* 46–62.

Gatehouse, S. (1999). Glasgow hearing aid benefit profile: Derivation and validation of a client-centered outcome measure for hearing-aid services. *Journal of American Academy of Audiology, 10,* 80–103.

Gatehouse, S. (2000). The impact of measurement goals on the design specification for outcome measures. *Ear and Hearing, 21*(4) Supp., 100S–105S.

Gatehouse, S., Naylor, G., & Elberling, C. (2003). Benefits from hearing aids in relation to the interaction between the user and the environment. *International Journal of Audiology, 42,* 1S77–1S86.

Gatehouse, S., & Noble, W. (2004). The Speech, Spatial and Qualities of Hearing Scale (SSQ). *International Journal of Audiology, 43*(2), 85–89.

Goldstein, D. P., & Stephens, S. D. G. (1981). Audiological rehabilitation: Management model I. *Audiology, 20,* 432–452.

Hallberg, L., & Carlsson, S. (1991). A qualitative study of strategies for managing a hearing impairment. *British Journal of Audiology, 25,* 201–211.

Hallberg, L., & Jansson, G. (1996). Women with noise-induced hearing loss: An invisible group? *British Journal of Audiology, 30,* 340–345.

Hétu, R. (1996). The stigma attached to hearing impairment. *Scandinavian Audiology, 25,* Supp. 43, 12–24.

Hétu, R., Jones, L., & Getty, L. (1993). The impact of acquired hearing impairment on intimate relationships: Implications for rehabilitation. *Audiology, 32,* 363–381.

Hickson, L., & Worrall, L. (2003). Beyond hearing aid fitting: Improving communication for older adults. *International Journal of Audiology, 42,* Suppl 2, 2S84–91.

Hickson, L., Worrall, L., & Scarinci, N. (2006). Measuring outcomes of a communication program for older people with hearing impairment using the International Outcome Inventory. *International Journal of Audiology, 45*(4), 238–246.

Hoek, D., Pichora-Fuller, M. K., Paccioretti, D., MacDonald, M. A., & Shyng, G. (1997). Community outreach to hard-of-hearing seniors. *Journal of Speech–Language Pathology and Audiology, 21,* 199–208.

Holmes, A. (1995). Hearing aids and the older adult. In P. B. Kricos & S. A. Lesner (Eds.), *Hearing care for the older adult: Audiologic rehabilitation* (pp. 59–74). Boston: Butterworth-Heinemann.

Humes, L. E. (2003). Modeling and predicting hearing-aid outcome. *Trends in Amplification, 7*(2), 41–75.

Humes, L. E. (2004). Factors affecting long-term hearing aid use. *Seminars in Hearing, 25,* 63–72

Humes, L. E. (2005). Processing in the elderly. *Ear and Hearing, 26*(2), 109–119.

Humes, L. E., & Wilson, D. L. (2003). An examination of changes in hearing-aid performance and benefit in the elderly over a 3-year period of hearing-aid use. *Journal of Speech, Language, and Hearing Research, 46,* 137–145.

Hurvitz, J., & Goldojarb, M. (1987, November). *Comparison of two aural rehabilitation methods in a nursing home.* Paper presented at the ASHA National Convention, New Orleans.

Isaacowitz, D. M., Charles, S. T., & Carstensen, L. L. (2000). Emotion and cognition. In F. I. M. Craik & T. A. Salthouse (Eds.), *The handbook of aging and cognition* (2nd ed.; pp. 593–632). Mahwah, NJ: Lawrence Erlbaum.

Jaworski, A., & Stephens, D. (1998). Self-reports on silence as a face-saving strategy by people with hearing impairment. *International Journal of Applied Linguistics, 8,* 61–80.

Jerger, J., Oliver, T., & Pirozzolo, F. (1990). Speech understanding in the elderly. *Journal of the American Academy of Audiology, 1,* 17–81.

Kiessling, J., Pichora-Fuller, M. K., Gatehouse, S., Stephens, D., Arlinger, S., Chisolm, T., Davis, A. C., Erber, N. P., Hickson, L., Holmes, A., Rosenhall, U., & von Wedel, H. (2003). Candidature for and delivery of audiological services: Special needs of older people. *International Journal of Audiology, 42,* Suppl 2, S292–2S101.

Killion, M. C., Niquette, P. A., Gudmundsen, G. I., Revit, L. J., & Nanerjee, S. (2004). Development of a quick speech-in-noise test for measuring signal-to-noise ratio loss in normal-hearing and hearing-impaired listeners. *Journal of the Acoustical Society of America, 116,* 2395–2405.

Kochkin, S. (1999). Reducing hearing instrument returns with consumer education. *The Hearing Review, 6*(10), 18, 20.

Kricos, P. (2006). Audiologic management of older adults with hearing loss and compromised cognitive/psychoacoustic auditory processing capabilities. *Trends in Amplification, 10,* 1–28.

Kricos, P., Lesner, S., Sandridge, S., & Yanke, R. (1987). Perceived benefits from amplification as a function of central auditory status in the elderly. *Ear and Hearing, 8,* 337–342.

Lazarus, R. S., & Folkman, S. (1984). *Stress, appraisal and coping.* New York: Springer.

Lewsen, B. J., & Cashman, M. (1997). Hearing aids and assistive listening devices in long-term care. *Journal of Speech–Language Pathology and Audiology, 21,* 3, 149–152.

Lubinski, R. (1984). The environmental role in communication skills and opportunities of older people. In C. Wilder & B. Weinstein (Eds.), *Aging and communication: Problems in management* (pp. 47–57). New York: Haworth.

Lubinski, R., & Higginbotham, J. (Eds.), *Communication technologies for the elderly: Vision, hearing, and speech.* San Diego, CA: Singular Publishing Group.

Lundberg, R. (1979). *Research survey.* Unpublished manuscript, Portland State University.

Lunner, T. (2003). Cognitive function in relation to hearing aid use. *International Journal of Audiology, 42,* S49-S58.

Matthies, M., Bilger, R., & Roezchowski, C. (1983). SPIN as a predictor of hearing aid use. *Asha, 25*(10), 61.

Maurer, J. E. (1976). Auditory impairment and aging. In B. Jacobs (Ed.), *Working with the impaired elderly* (pp. 72). Washington, DC: National Council on the Aging.

Maurer, J. E. (1979). Aural rehabilitation for the aging. In L. J. Bradford & W. G. Hardy (Eds.), *Hearing and hearing impairment* (pp. 319–338). New York: Grune & Stratton.

Millington, D. (2001) *Audiologic rehabilitation practices of ASHA audiologists: Survey 2000.* Unpublished masters thesis, Idaho State University.

Montgomery, A. A. (1994). WATCH: A practical approach to brief auditory rehabilitation. *Hearing Journal, 47*(10), 10, 53–55.

Nemes, J. (2003). Despite benefits of outcomes measures, advocates say they're underused. *Hearing Journal, 8,* 19–25.

Newman, C. W., & Jacobsen G. P. (1993). Self-assessment of hearing. *Seminars in Hearing, 14*(4), 299–384.

Nilsson, M., Soli, S. D., & Sullivan, J. A. (1994). Development of the Hearing in Noise Test for the measurement of speech reception thresholds in quiet and in noise. *Journal of the Acoustical Society of America, 95,* 1085–1099.

Noble, W. (1998). *Self-assessment of hearing and related functions.* London: Whurr.

Noble, W. (2002). Extending the IOI to significant others and to non-hearing-aid based interventions. *International Journal of Audiology, 41,* 27–29.

Noble, W. (in press). One or two hearing aids. *International Journal of Audiology.*

Palmer, C. V., Adams, S. W., Bourgeois, M., Durrant, J., & Rossi, M. (1999). Reduction in caregiver-identified problem behaviors in patients with Alzheimer disease post-hearing-aid fitting. *Journal of Speech and Hearing Research, 42,* 312–328.

Parving, A., & Phillip, B. (1991). Use and benefit of hearing aids in the tenth decade—and beyond. *Audiology, 30,* 61–69.

Pichora-Fuller, M. K. (2003). Cognitive aging and auditory information processing. *International Journal of Audiology, 42* (Supplement 2), S26–S32.

Pichora-Fuller, M. K., & Carson, A. J. (2000). Hearing health and the listening experiences of older communicators. In M. L. Hummert & J. Nussbaum (Eds.), *Aging, communication, and health: Linking research and practice for successful aging* (pp. 43–74). Mahwah, NJ: Lawrence Erlbaum.

Pichora-Fuller, M. K., Johnson, C., & Roodenburg, K. (1998). The discrepancy between hearing impairment and handicap in the elderly: Balancing transaction and interaction in conversation, *Journal of Applied Communication Research, 25,* 99–119.

Pichora-Fuller, M. K., & Robertson, L. F. (1994). Hard of hearing residents in a home for the aged. *Journal of Speech–Language Pathology and Audiology, 18,* 278–288.

Pichora-Fuller, M. K., & Robertson, L. (1997). Planning and evaluation of a hearing rehabilitation program in a home-for-the-aged: Use of hearing aids and assistive listening devices. *Journal of Speech–Language Pathology and Audiology, 21,* 174–186.

Pichora-Fuller, M.K., & Singh, G. (2006). Effects of age on auditory and cognitive processing: Implications for hearing aid fitting and audiological rehabilitation. *Trends in Amplification, 10,* 29–59.

Ries, P. W. (1994, March). Prevalence and characteristics of persons with hearing troubles United States, 1990–91. *Vital Health Statistics, 10*(188), 1–75.

Robertson, L., et al. (1997). The effect of an aural rehabilitation program on responses to scenarios depicting communication breakdown. *Journal of Speech–Language Pathology and Audiology, 21,* 187–198.

Ronch, J. L., & Van Zanten, L. (1992). Who are these aging persons? In R. Hull (Ed.), *Rehabilitative audiology* (pp. 185–213). New York: Grune & Stratton.

Ross, M. (1997). A retrospective look at the future of aural rehabilitation. *Journal of the Academy of Rehabilitative Audiology, 30,* 11–28.

Ryan, E. B., Giles, H., Bartolucci, G., & Henwood, K. (1986). Psycholinguistic and social psychological components of communication by and with the elderly. *Language and Communication, 6,* 1–24.

Ryan, E. B., Meredith, S. D., Maclean, M. J., & Orange, J. B. (1995). Changing the way we talk with elders: Promoting health using the Communication Enhancement Model. *International Journal of Aging and Human Development, 41,* 89–107.

Schneider, B. A., Daneman, M., & Pichora-Fuller, M. K. (2002). Listening in aging adults: From discourse comprehension to psychoacoustics. *Canadian Journal of Experimental Psychology, 56,* 139–152.

Schow, R. L. (1992). Hearing assessment and treatment in nursing homes. *Hearing Instruments, 43*(7), 7–11.

Schow, R. L. (2001). A standardized AR battery for dispensers. *Hearing Journal, 54*(8) 10–20.

Schow, R. L., Balsara, N., Smedley, T. C., & Whitcomb, C. J. (1993). Aural rehabilitation by ASHA audiologists; 1980–1990. *American Journal of Audiology, 2*(3), 28–37.

Schow, R., Brockett, J., Bishop, R., Whitaker, M., & Horlacki, G. (2005). *Standardization of outcome measures in hearing aid fitting.* International Collegium of Rehabilitative Audiology Conference, Florida.

Schow, R. L., & Gatehouse, S. (1990). Fundamental issues to self-assessment of hearing. *Ear and Hearing, 11*(5), Suppl., 6–16.

Schow, R. L., & Nerbonne, M. A. (1980). Hearing levels among Elderly nursing home residents. *Journal of Speech and Hearing Disorders, 45*(I), 124–132.

Schow, R. L., & Nerbonne, M. A. (1982). Communication screening profile: Use with elderly clients. *Ear and Hearing, 3*(3), 133–147.

Schow, R. L., & Smedley, T. C. (1990). Self-assessment of hearing. *Ear and Hearing, 11*(5), Suppl./Special Issue.

Skafte, M. D. (2000). The 1999 hearing instrument market—the dispensers' perspective. *Hearing Review, 7*(6), 8–40.

Smedley, T. C., & Schow, R. L. (1990). Frustrations with hearing aid use: Candid observations from the elderly. *Hearing Journal, 43*(6), 21–27.

Smedley, T. C., & Schow, R. L. (1992). Satisfaction/disability rating for programmable vs. conventional aids. *Hearing Instruments 43*(11), 34–35.

Stach, B. (1990). Hearing aid amplification and central processing disorder. In R. E. Sandlin (Ed.), *Handbook of hearing aid amplification,* Vol. 2 (pp. 87–111). Boston: College-Hill Press.

Stephens, S. D. G. (1996a). Hearing rehabilitation in a psychosocial framework. *Scandinavian Audiology, 25,* Supp. 43, 57–66.

Stephens, S. D. G. (1996b). Evaluating the problems of the hearing impaired. *Audiology, 19,* 105–220.

Stephens, S. D. G., Jones, G., & Gianopoulos, I. (2000). The use of outcome measures to formulate intervention strategies. *Ear and Hearing, 21*(4) Supp., 15S–23S.

Sweetow, R. W. (2005). Training the adult brain to listen. *Hearing Journal, 58*(6), 10–16.

Sweetow, R. W., & Henderson-Sabes, J. (2004). The case for LACE (Listening and Communication Enhancement). *Hearing Journal, 57*(3), 32–40.

Taeuber, C. (1992). *Sixty-five plus in America.* Washington, DC: U.S. Department of Commerce, Economics and Statistics Administration, Bureau of the Census.

U.S. Bureau of the Census. (1990). *The need for personal assistance with everyday activities: Recipients and caregivers, current population reports,* Series P-70, No. 19, Table B. Washington, DC: U.S. Government Printing Office.

Villaume, W. A., Brown, M. H., & Darling, R. (1994). Presbycusis, communication, and older adults. In M. L. Hummert, J. M. Wiemann, & J. F. Nussbaum (Eds.), *Interpersonal communication in older adulthood: Interdisciplinary theory and research* (pp. 83–106). Thousand Oaks, CA: Sage.

Wilkerson, D. (2000). Current issues in rehabilitation outcome measurement: Implications for audiological rehabilitation. *Ear and Hearing, 21*(4) Supp., 80S–88S.

World Health Organization (WHO). (2001). *International Classification of Functioning, Disability and Health (ICF).* Geneva: WHO. http://www3.who.int/icf/icftemplate.cfm

Worrall, L. E., & Hickson, L. M. (2003). *Communication disability in aging: From prevention to intervention.* Clifton Park, NY: Thomson Delmar Learning.

Worrall, L., Hickson, L., Barnett, H., & Yiu, E. (1998). An evaluation of the *Keep on Talking* program for maintaining communication skills into old age. *Educational Gerontology, 24,* 129–140.

PART

III

Implementing Audiologic Rehabilitation: Case Studies

CHAPTER 11

Case Studies: Children

Mary Pat Moeller

CONTENTS

■ INTRODUCTION

Each child with hearing loss presents with a unique constellation of abilities and needs. An individualized approach to diagnostics and case management is essential.

Children with hearing loss represent a heterogeneous group, with highly individual characteristics and needs. Differences in degree of hearing loss, family constellation and resources, medical history, language abilities, school support, and styles of learning contribute to each child's unique profile. The five case examples that follow describe individualized approaches to case management, with process-oriented strategies for problem solution. In each of the cases that follow, two concepts are central to the intervention: (1) Clinicians must ascertain intervention priorities through differential diagnosis and careful determination of a child and family's primary needs, and (2) individualized management requires a process of clinical decision making and objective monitoring of the efficacy of intervention (see Chapter 9).

The process of pediatric audiologic rehabilitation is complex and challenging. Parents and clinicians face numerous management decisions early in the course of audiologic rehabilitation. Should the child's rehabilitation focus on auditory–oral development or is a visually oriented approach needed? What type of amplification will best meet this child's needs? Should a cochlear implant be considered? Will the child's needs be met in an inclusive educational setting, or will a specialized setting better serve this child? Answers to these and other management questions are rarely simple and rarely without controversy. Parents face many of these questions at a time when they are trying to cope with parenting a newborn and the diagnosis of hearing loss. They deserve objective guidance that is based on thoughtful examination of the child's needs and abilities in light of the options available.

Parents should have access to information about all communication options and guidance based on thoughtful evaluation of the child and the family's needs.

AR service delivery for children is further complicated by the increasing incidence of children with hearing loss who have significant secondary disabilities. These children require sophisticated assessment and management through a team approach. Federal mandates require that early intervention be provided in a family-centered manner (Roush & Matkin, 1994). This has brought about a reconceptualization of the professional's role in the decision making and management process. The goal of empowering family members in the management of the child's needs also requires a diverse and individualized approach, given the wide range of family systems represented in the clinician's caseload. Each of these factors dictates the need for objective, individually tailored approaches and flexible, innovative service delivery models.

The case studies that follow represent five unique concerns that influenced the course of rehabilitative management:

1. Family-centered intervention for a child with multiple disabilities
2. Clinical decision making: a student's decision to receive a cochlear implant
3. Issues affecting educational placement decisions
4. Late identification in a child who was hard of hearing: auditory–linguistic considerations
5. Differential diagnosis through professional teamwork: a tool for solving complex intervention problems

In each of the following cases, multidisciplinary service delivery was necessary and advantageous. No one discipline has all the skills and expertise to address the complex nature of the problems that often present themselves. The audiologic rehabilitation specialist needs to cultivate the skills of working as a team member, joining in collaborative consultation with allied professionals and parents. Multidisciplinary perspectives contribute to a holistic understanding of the child's and family's needs.

Although the cases described are based on real persons, names and other biographical facts have been changed to maintain patient confidentiality.

CASE 1   JOEY: FAMILY-CENTERED INTERVENTION: MULTIPLE DISABILITIES

AR specialists working at the parent/infant level are meeting new professional challenges, including the opportunity to work with very young infants in the context of the family system (see Chapter 8). It has been estimated that 33 to 38 percent of infants with hearing loss have complex developmental needs resulting from secondary disabilities (Schildroth & Hotto, 1993; Moeller, Coufal, & Hixson, 1990). This case illustrates the importance of transdisciplinary approaches to case management. Overall coordination among various professionals and families is essential in meeting the needs of deaf infants with additional disabilities (Moeller et al., 1990).

> It has been estimated that between 33 and 38 percent of children with hearing loss have educationally significant secondary disabilities.

Background Information

Joey's profound bilateral sensorineural hearing loss was diagnosed through auditory brainstem response testing when he was 10 months of age. Subsequent behavioral testing demonstrated no response to speech or tonal stimuli at the limits of the equipment. Birth history records revealed that an emergency C-section was done at 36 weeks gestation due to fetal distress. Joey required oxygen and remained in the neonatal intensive care unit (NICU) for five days following birth. Neonatal complications included hyperbilirubinemia and cardiac and respiratory difficulties. Joey was on a heart monitor for the first seven months of his life. Joey also has a medical history of dizziness and balance problems, poor coordination, and hypotonia.

Joey was delayed in achieving developmental milestones. He sat unsupported at 10 months and walked at 18 months. At 4 years of age, Joey is not yet toilet trained. The parents began signing to Joey immediately after diagnosis of the hearing loss, and he produced his first sign at 13 months of age. The mother reported that Joey was producing signed phrases up until about 16 to 18 months. At that time, he discontinued use of many of the signs he knew and did not combine signs. Regression in both social and language behaviors was noted by the family.

> Significant regression in language behaviors in toddlers may be associated with autism.

Previous Rehabilitation

Joey had been served since infancy by a homebound early-intervention program. At 2 years of age, he was placed in a self-contained toddler and preschool program, where he was served by an educator of the deaf, a speech–language pathologist, and an occupational and physical therapist (OT/PT). Although Joey was learning to cooperate with the routine of his preschool classroom, he demonstrated little evidence of learning from the group setting. He rarely initiated interactions or conversations with others. Although he knew over 100 signs, he rarely used them for functional communication. His attention to communication from others was

ABR and OAE testing are valuable in identifying hearing loss in a young child like Joey.

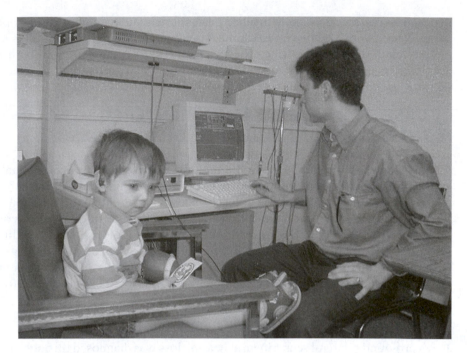

Fleeting visual attention, reduced functionality of communication, and self-stimulatory behaviors are not typical of a child who has hearing loss alone.

fleeting. He demonstrated stereotypical and self-stimulatory behaviors. At 3½ years of age, Joey's family relocated and he was placed in a self-contained public school program for deaf students with support services in speech–language pathology and OT/PT, similar to those of his previous program. Joey's social, behavioral, and attentional difficulties continued in the new school environment. Joey's educational team and parents requested consultation from an AR team due to concerns for his inattention, slow language learning, and atypical behaviors.

A comprehensive, multidisciplinary assessment was initiated in response to the expressed concerns. The communication portion of the evaluation was conducted by a team of AR specialists, who relied on valid instruments relevant to the child's environment and informal observations to analyze Joey's needs. The assessment began with parent interviews. The mother expressed a primary concern that her son may have autism. The mother had read extensively on the subject and was an excellent reporter of her son's unique constellation of behaviors. She indicated that he had extreme fixations with lights and electronic equipment with switches. If left to his own devices, Joey would spend an entire day running and staring at lights or turning a VCR off and on. Although the parents had purchased numerous developmentally appropriate toys, these items did not hold Joey's attention. The mother indicated that Joey did not seem to know how to play with toys.

Joey's mother aptly described her son as socially isolated, preferring to be "in his own world." The family had learned to sign fluently to their son, but few rewards for this effort were forthcoming. Joey's communication remained extremely delayed in comparison to that of his deaf peers at school. The parents faithfully implemented full-time hearing aid use, which they reported resulted in exacerbation of negative behaviors and self-stimulatory vocalizations. During the initial parent interview, Joey was allowed to play in an attractive playroom with numerous developmentally appropriate toys. Joey spent the entire period fixating on the lights in the room and did not become involved with toys or individuals present.

Formal, structured language testing is often inappropriate with a youngster who has fragile social interactions. The AR specialist found it necessary to identify ecologically valid assessment tools that would provide insights on Joey's communicative skills in a variety of environments. The *Communication and Symbolic Behaviors Scales (CSBS)* (Wetherby & Prizant, 1993) was an ideal selection in that it makes use of observational contexts that place few demands on the young child. Symbolic play skills and communicative means can be explored with this tool during semistructured play activities. In addition, the *MacArthur Communicative Development Inventory* (Dale & Thal, 1993), which is a parent report scale, gave the clinician valuable information on Joey's sign vocabulary used in the home. Results indicated that Joey used signs and gestures to communicate a small range of language functions (behavioral regulation, rejecting, and answering). His receptive sign vocabulary of 192 words was roughly equivalent to a 21-month developmental level. He presented as a curious and highly independent youngster. Rather than requesting help with a mechanical toy, for example, he would persist in trying to discover how to operate it.

Joey's warm and supportive home environment was a strength. The family had already learned through discovery various strategies to structure Joey's behavior and attention. They described the need to "Joey-proof" their home. In fact, the parents had become experts in helping their son succeed through environmental structuring. Many family strengths that could be incorporated in the individual family services plan (IFSP) were noted. The family was able to identify many primary needs. Foremost among them was the need for a definitive diagnosis so that appropriate management strategies and expectations could be implemented with Joey. In essence, the parents were "doing all the right things," yet watched as their child remained very delayed and became more difficult to manage. The parents expressed the need for a team to integrate perspectives and to understand their child in the holistic context of the family.

Joey was severely delayed in his symbolic skills, including play. His symbolic play skills at age 4 were commensurate with a 19- to 22-month level. His constructional play skills were well in advance of his symbolic play skills. He exhibited difficulty integrating various sensorial inputs. For example, if Joey's hands were involved in sensory exploration activities, he was not able to attend to any other input. Activities in his classroom frequently seemed to cause a "sensory overload" for Joey. When this occurred, he would "tune into" lights or the feel of his shirt and "tune out" the language input around him.

Typically developing deaf children usually perform well on tests of symbolic play. Children with autism often have relative strengths in constructional play with deficits in symbolic play.

Environmental Coordination and Participation

Team members from various disciplines made multiple observations of Joey in an effort to make a differential diagnosis and understand his needs. Transdisciplinary team discussion centered on the constellation of major findings of (1) serious delays in symbolic language use (in spite of positive opportunities for language acquisition in the home), (2) history of regression in language and social behaviors, (3) limited social interaction, (4) significant delays in symbolic play with strengths in constructional play, (5) tendencies for obsessions with lights and mechanical objects, and (6) self-stimulatory behaviors. Based on these findings, it was the team consensus that Joey was exhibiting the characteristics of childhood autism in addition to profound deafness. This diagnosis had important implications for Joey's intervention program. The team psychologist was able to offer many insights into the impact of the two disabilities on behavior, learning, and daily living. He assisted the family in implementing a consistent behavior management program at home.

Communication Rehabilitation Adjustment

Joey's program, which was designed to meet the needs of young children who are deaf, required adaptation in view of Joey's complex needs. AR team members had the opportunity to observe Joey in his school placement and to problem solve with the school-based intervention team. Observations and the adaptations and recommended strategies included the following:

An integrated team approach is required to effectively meet the complex needs of a child with multiple disabilities.

1. Joey presented with developmental needs across several domains (e.g., cognition, symbolic play, language, fine and gross motor, and social and sensory integration). This complex set of needs was difficult to address in a traditional deaf education classroom. It was determined that his needs would be better served in a special education preschool classroom, with teamwork between a teacher specializing in children with autism and a teacher of the deaf. The special educator had signing skills and was able to provide Joey with a range of developmental activities in a highly structured and predictable classroom routine. Services were also provided by occupational and physical therapists.

2. Joey's special education team worked together to incorporate highly functional learning activities with regular opportunities to communicate through sign. Emphasis was placed on individualized lessons and increasing one-on-one time.

3. Assistance from a behavioral specialist was implemented at home and at school. Emphasis was placed on reducing time spent with fixations and reducing aggressive behaviors.

4. Joey's parents were motivated to implement full-time hearing aid use, and they had accomplished this goal early in the rehabilitation program. However, behavior problems and inappropriate vocalizing escalated greatly when he wore amplification. The team and the parents agreed to remove amplification until other behaviors were brought under control. Amplification would be tried again in the future in the context of the overall behavior program. Although a medical team had suggested a cochlear implant, the parents recognized that there were many contraindications to the recommendation.

5. A priority for Joey's program was to strengthen the social foundation for language learning. He required indirect playful approaches, where he was motivated to remain in interaction with others and engage in turntaking. Strategies from Greenspan's (1990) *Floor Time* program were useful in addressing this goal. This program focuses on goals such as engagement, two-way communication, establishing shared meanings, and developing emotional thinking. Through this program, adults learn a variety of strategies for following the child's lead and building communication circles through such behaviors as a slow and calm approach, gentle looks, supportive postures, and nonintrusive ways of supporting the child's themes and communicative attempts.

6. As Joey's parents found, structuring the environment was instrumental in helping him succeed. He needed boundaries in wide-open spaces. He learned better in rooms without access to switches. He responded well when his limits were clearly defined and he could be actively engaged in lessons.

> Engagement refers to the ability of an infant to share an experience with a parent or caregiver, such as looking at objects together and smiling or laughing in response to an interaction with the object.

Psychosocial and Counseling Aspects

It was critical for the educational and AR teams to consider family needs. In talking with the parents, it was clear that living with Joey 24 hours a day brought many challenges. Sleep disruption was common; going out in public was nearly impossible; controlling driven obsessions was a full-time job. Joey's parents did everything they could to help him. Even so, their rewards came very slowly and in unpredictable ways. It helped for the team to make recommendations that gave consideration to the impact on home life. The parents needed the team to address behavioral issues in a comprehensive and ongoing manner. They also needed a chance to talk to other parents of children like Joey. The family appreciated practical direction to allow them to cope with today and to be hopeful about tomorrow. Respite care opportunities and support from the extended family gave the parents needed breaks.

> Emotional thinking relates to a child's growing ability to understand what they themselves and others are feeling or wanting and how that affects their behavior.

CASE 2   MIKE: DECISION MAKING BY A ■ STUDENT RELATED TO COCHLEAR IMPLANTS

In some cases, successful rehabilitation depends on the willingness of the family, the client, and the AR specialist to explore different options. When students are older, as in this case, they need to have access to the full range of information in order to take an active role in decision making. This case study illustrates the process a preteenager went through in making his decision to receive a cochlear implant and in adjusting to the device. The case illustrates how the AR program was modified as a result of implantation.

> Older students need to take an active role in decision making. In support of this process, they need access to the full range of available information.

Background Information

Mike was diagnosed with a severe-to-profound, bilateral sensorineural hearing loss when he was 15 months of age. Pregnancy and birth history were unremarkable, and the etiology of hearing loss was unknown. Mike had a history of recurrent otitis media, for which he received medical treatment. He achieved developmental milestones as expected for age, with the exception of speech and language skills.

Mike's family lived in a small Midwestern community that provided limited early intervention services locally at the time. The parents enrolled him in the local parent–infant program and sought additional consultative guidance from agencies experienced with deaf infants. This provided them contact with other parents and

Prosodic character-
istics of speech
include such fea-
tures as duration,
pitch control, stress,
and intonation.

support for decision making. The parents elected to implement a total communication approach with a strong emphasis on learning spoken communication. They
focused on the integration of listening into daily routines and supported Mike in
making rapid adjustment to full-time binaural hearing aid use. As Mike grew older,
the parents exposed him to a rich variety of opportunities, including auditory experiences, such as instrumental music lessons.

Mike demonstrated a strong learning rate throughout the preschool years. He
was a curious and eager learner. By 5 years of age, he demonstrated sign and oral
language skills that were age appropriate. He relied on sign for information reception, but expressed himself primarily through oral means. His speech production
skills were progressing, but conversational intelligibility was reduced. The prosodic
characteristics of his speech were significantly affected by his hearing loss. He was
successful in auditory recognition tasks with closed set materials, but had poor
open set discrimination skills. Mike was enrolled in an individualized aural rehabilitation program that focused on (1) improving auditory identification and comprehension of linguistic messages, (2) reducing tendency to elongate and distort
vowels, (3) reducing hypernasal resonance, (4) strengthening self-monitoring for
the production of fricatives and affricates (often produced as stops), and (5) improving speech intelligibility in conversation. Throughout elementary school, this
student was placed in regular classrooms with support services from an educational
interpreter, a teacher of the deaf, and a speech–language pathologist. He utilized
FM amplification in the classroom setting. Mike's socialization with hearing peers
was affected by reduced speech intelligibility.

Hypernasal speech
results when vocal
sounds resonate
through the nasal
rather than the oral
cavity. This is a
common error in
speech in students
with limited resid-
ual hearing.

Aural Rehabilitation Plan: Preimplant

As the school years progressed, Mike became an avid reader and a strong student. His
curiosity was evident each time he visited the audiologist and discussed ways that
hearing aid circuitry might be improved. It was not surprising to the team, then, when
he began to explore the topic of cochlear implants on the Internet at age 10½. Mike
spent many months researching the topic. He was reluctant to undergo surgery, but
considered the possibility that the device would provide him with better functional
auditory skills than his conventional hearing aids. He asked to communicate with
other students near his age who had received implants. He was interested in questioning students with both positive and limited outcomes from the device. He contacted several students by email and interviewed them. He discussed his impressions
with his parents and then requested a cochlear implant orientation. The results of
baseline and candidacy evaluations indicated that Mike had good closed set auditory
identification abilities, but very limited open set word identification abilities (score
of 4 percent on the PB-K test). Once it was determined that he was a candidate, Mike
was scheduled to meet with a counselor, who discussed his expectations, reservations,
and questions related to the device. He was judged to have a realistic view of what the
implant would provide and was minimally concerned about appearance issues.

During his decision-
making process,
Mike questioned
other students who
had both positive
and negative expe-
riences with coch-
lear implants. This
helped him to
develop balanced
expectations.

Mike underwent surgical implantation in the right ear just after his twelfth
birthday. Following hookup and programming of the speech processor, Mike began
his adjustment to the device. His AR program was modified to support this process.

Aural Rehabilitation Plan: Postimplant

In the first few months following implantation, Mike expressed some frustration in his attempts to understand the signal he was receiving. However, he was extremely motivated to resolve these issues and refused to switch back to his hearing aid. He wore his implant device full waking hours and devoted time to practicing listening lessons during daily routines. His parents reported a sense of disappointment. They noted that even though they had been cautioned against optimism they had hoped for their son to respond well immediately.

However, as Mike worked at listening, he began to report significant progress in his recognition of what he was hearing. He noted that many previously unheard environmental sounds were now audible to him and that he had begun to recognize them when he heard them. He began to realize that the implant was providing access to a much wider range of sounds than he experienced with hearing aids.

It was critical to shift the emphasis of Mike's therapy program in light of this increased audibility and his access to a wider range of speech sounds, including fricatives. The therapist began with auditory closure (fill in the blank) activities to take advantage of his strong knowledge base, which helped him to predict the meaning of the unknown word presented through audition alone. As his confidence and closure skills strengthened, larger units of information were presented through audition alone. If Mike struggled, speechreading cues were added; however, with time this was less necessary. Listening skills were embedded in all aspects of the intervention program. Because of Mike's age, he was asked to be responsible for identifying what he wanted to work on in therapy. Some of these areas and strategies that were relevant to his overall goals were the following:

1. Mike was eager to strengthen his oral conversational understanding beyond the single utterance level. Discourse tracking activities were implemented with high-interest materials (e.g., tips for improving a tennis backhand; humorous materials like how to cheat at golf).

2. Mike wanted support to increase his social skills. Auditory-based role play activities were included to practice ways to (a) initiate and sustain innocuous, friendly topics of interest to peers, (b) respond appropriately to remarks of others, (c) detect sarcasm in the voice (e.g., for humor recognition), and (d) tell good jokes with appropriate benign reactions.

3. Mike progressed to the point where he did not need interpreter support for face-to-face peer communication. However, group conversations and noisy contexts were challenging. Emphasis was placed on ways to manage such discourse situations, repair strategies, and listen in noise.

4. Mike did not believe that he was capable of conversing on the telephone. Utilitarian activities, like calling the golf course to get a tee time or ordering pizza, were practiced on a set of phones. Mike discovered that he was able to understand these predictable conversations fairly well, but being understood by the other party was a challenge. He learned ways to shape his intended message to heighten his intelligibility. He began to contact familiar peers to set up social activities.

Mike and his parents were disappointed with the outcome from the device immediately after hookup. It is not unusual for a student with this history to require a lengthy adjustment period.

Discourse tracking refers to a method by which students listen to utterances related to a topic and repeat verbatim the messages that they hear.

Mike needed to learn strategies for managing noisy settings and for maximizing his speech intelligibility over the telephone.

5. Mike wanted support to continue to refine his speech production skills. Focus was placed on auditory self-monitoring for production of fricatives, affricates, and ending sounds. He made more rapid progress than in the past due to increased audibility of these phonemes. In addition, emphasis was placed on more natural prosody, also enhanced by increased audibility. Opportunities for self-expression at the conversational level were incorporated in all the activities described above. Emphasis was placed on conveying meaning accurately and on self-evaluation.

6. Because open set word recognition was challenging, the clinician incorporated analytic training, using minimally paired contrasts that were increasingly challenging.

Intervention Outcomes

Two years following implantation, Mike continues to make progress in his auditory, speechreading, and spoken language skills. His scores on closed set auditory tests ranged from 90 percent to 100 percent at 24 months post-implantation. Figure 11.1 illustrates his scores over time on open set auditory recognition tasks. His best performance was in response to holistic messages, such as the Common Phrases tests, where he scored at 100 percent in getting the meaning and 90 percent in understanding of specific words. His prepost scores show steady improvement in the PB-K phoneme score, with slow but steady growth in the PB-K word discrimination scores.

As face-to-face conversation became more fluent, Mike's social opportunities greatly increased. This had an impact on his satisfaction with the device.

Mike's oral conversational proficiency has been markedly strengthened by his use of the cochlear implant. His open set word discrimination scores tell little about the ease with which he is now able to participate in face-to-face conversation. Mike reports that his opportunities to socialize with peers have markedly increased in the past year. He is now able to participate in extended oral discourse through listening and speechreading. Spontaneous use of frication in his speech is observed over 75 percent of the time. Mike feels highly satisfied with his decision to receive a

FIGURE 11.1

Changes in open set auditory skills over time following implantation.

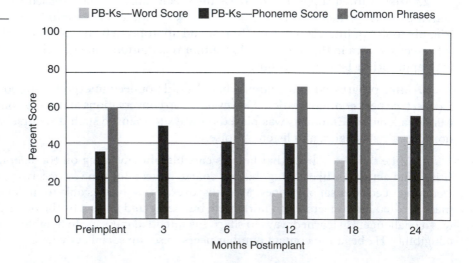

cochlear implant and recognizes many ways in which the device has supported his socialization and extended his communication opportunities.

Summary

Mike was an active participant in steering the course of his audiologic rehabilitation program as he entered the teenage years. His case illustrates the importance of clear delineation of goals that are relevant to the client and persistence in working toward them. Mike and his family were initially disillusioned about his response to the cochlear implant. Mike needed support to leave his comfort zone to rely on new auditory capabilities provided by the implant. Over time, the family discovered that his efforts to adjust yielded many benefits. The ease of social communication was the most clear benefit, which greatly facilitated peer interaction and socialization in his school environment.

CASE 3   AMBER: ISSUES AFFECTING ■ EDUCATIONAL PLACEMENT

Audiologic rehabilitative management frequently includes provision of input to a child's IEP team related to educational placement. This case illustrates the importance of considering audiological, language, academic, and social factors in such decisions.

Background Information

Amber was referred for a multidisciplinary evaluation by the AR team when she was 6 years, 7 months of age. She was born in Korea and spent the first year of her life with a Korean foster family. Birth records indicated a normal, full-term delivery. An American family adopted Amber when she was 14 months of age. Amber walked at 14 months, was toilet trained at 4 to 5 years of age, and had few words at 3 years of age.

A serial audiogram is used when progression is suspected. It logs the thresholds over time for ease of comparison.

At 30 months of age, a bilateral, sensorineural hearing loss was identified. Audiological records indicated that the loss was progressive in nature, as shown in the serial audiogram in Figure 11.2. At the time of her first MDT evaluation, Amber's hearing loss was borderline normal sloping to profound bilaterally (see Figure 11.3A). She received hearing aids at 3 years of age and was reported to have progressed well orally once she received amplification. Amber wore glasses for correction of visual acuity problems. She had a history of otitis media and tube insertion. Amber's parents requested a team evaluation during her first-grade year to gain input on their daughter's progress and to determine if she was ready to access a regular classroom full time. At the point of evaluation, Amber was attending a self-contained classroom for hard of hearing children in the mornings and a regular first grade in the afternoons. The only concern raised by the school was Amber's tendency to "shut down" and avoid responding following some adult requests at school.

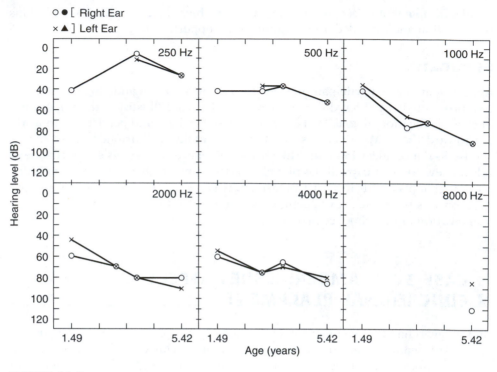

FIGURE 11.2

Case 3: Amber's serial audiogram.

Assessment Findings

A profile can be a useful way to integrate results across disciplines in order to get a "total child" view.

The profile in Figure 11.3B summarizes the results of multidisciplinary findings in the areas of psychology, language, and communication. Filled circles represent the first evaluation; the ×s represent a one-year follow-up evaluation. In the first evaluation Amber's language and academic skills were very delayed in comparison to the hearing peers with whom she was competing in class. Considering that she had limited language at age 3, however, the results were suggestive of a strong learning rate. Although there were errors in speech typical of a child with limited high-frequency audibility, her speech was developing well and was intelligible to unfamiliar listeners. She demonstrated receptive language abilities in the low average range for her age. Amber was imaginative in art and symbolic play. She had an engaging sense of humor and highly supportive home and school environments.

Language formulation difficulties refer to problems that a child encounters in organization of ideas for self-expression.

The primary concern identified during the evaluation was Amber's difficulties in self-expression. Extensive language sample analysis revealed expressive language formulation difficulties that were affecting her social skills in the mainstream environment. Amber's personal narratives were disorganized and reduced in complexity. For example, she attempted to explain to the examiner why she did not like witches in the following narrative. "I don't like witches. That . . . I have . . . my

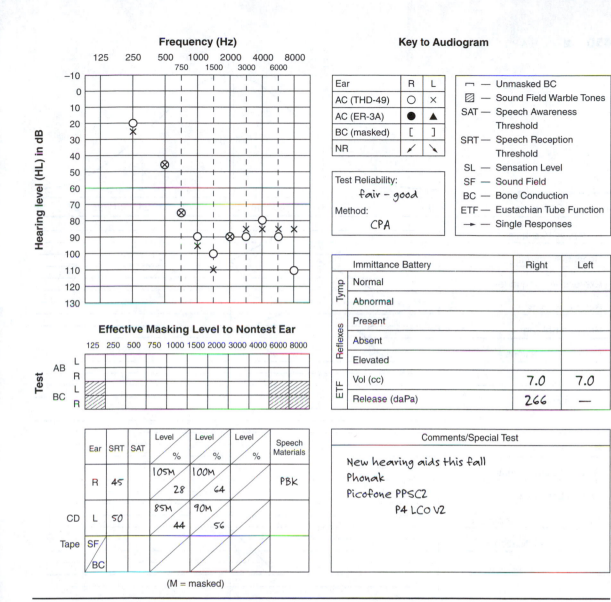

Frequency (Hz)

Key to Audiogram

Ear	R	L
AC (THD-49)	○	×
AC (ER-3A)	●	▲
BC (masked)	[	]
NR	⤢	⤡

Test Reliability: *fair – good*

Method: *CPA*

- ⌐ — Unmasked BC
- ▨ — Sound Field Warble Tones
- SAT — Speech Awareness Threshold
- SRT — Speech Reception Threshold
- SL — Sensation Level
- SF — Sound Field
- BC — Bone Conduction
- ETF — Eustachian Tube Function
- → — Single Responses

Effective Masking Level to Nontest Ear

Immittance Battery		Right	Left
Tymp	Normal		
	Abnormal		
Reflexes	Present		
	Absent		
	Elevated		
ETF	Vol (cc)	7.0	7.0
	Release (daPa)	266	—

Ear	SRT	SAT	Level %	Level %	Level %	Speech Materials
CD R	45		105M / 28	100M / 64		PBK
CD L	50		85M / 44	90M / 56		
Tape SF/BC						

(M = masked)

Comments/Special Test

New hearing aids this fall
Phonak
Picofone PPSC2
   P4 LCO V2

Audiologic Impression:

Borderline normal sloping to profound bilateral symmetrical (at most frequencies) loss w/tm perfs and previous progression

Recommendations:

1. Monitor hearing 3 mos
2. Aided testing w/aided threshold or probe mis tests and with aided word recognition
3. Monitor hearing aid function

Audiological Retest
3 mos locally

FIGURE 11.3A

Case 3: Amber's initial audiogram.

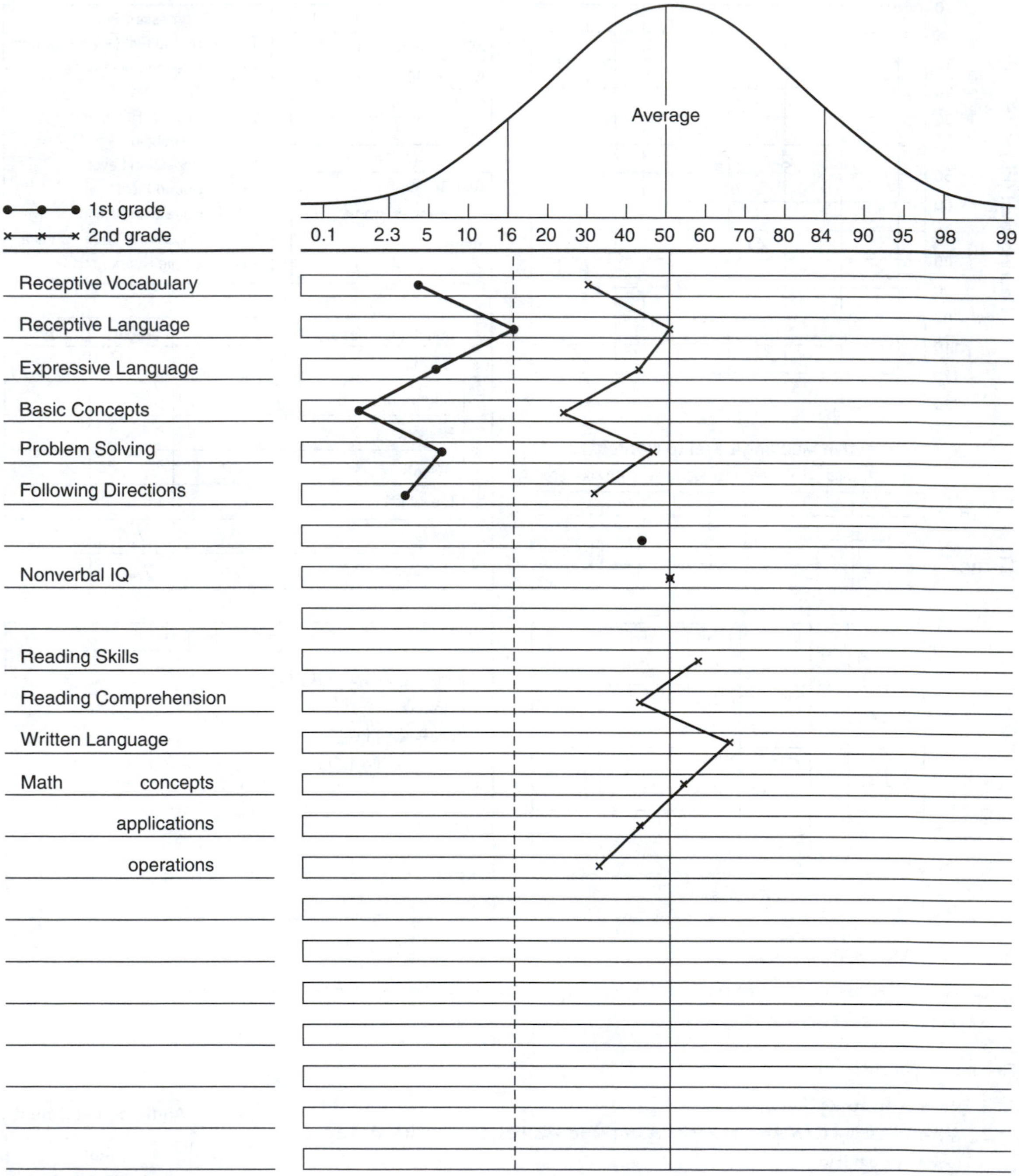

FIGURE 11.3B

Amber's profile of multidisciplinary findings.

grandma have that one (pointing to a picture of a witch). It clap (demonstrates with her hands). And I have one. It's down in the basement . . . in my freezer (she means it is stored beside the freezer). Her clap (gestures). I don't like him. He say heehee-hee." Grammatical errors appeared to be related to audibility. Formulation difficulties were observed in her tendency to produce false starts, her reliance on nonspecific references, semantic errors, and reliance on gestures to help carry the message. These expressive language challenges were affecting her participation in class and her socialization with peers. When she was unsure how to express her idea, she would "shut down," as the school had observed. Her mother described several examples at school when Amber cried in order to solve a verbal problem instead of expressing herself. For example, another student inadvertently picked up Amber's materials and got in line. Amber responded by saying "Hey" and grabbing at the books. When the books were not returned to her, she began to cry.

False starts are instances when a speaker begins a phrase, but stops and revises it. Use of *nonspecific references* means the tendency to use indefinite words, like *it, that, thing,* instead of the specific name for items.

Recommendations for Management

Based on academic performance in the classroom, the parents were eager to fully mainstream their daughter for her second-grade year. It was important to keep two points in mind when counseling the parents on this issue. First, the language demands of the first-grade curriculum are fairly well controlled. Performance on first-grade tasks may not be predictive of Amber's performance in the next few grades, in which demands for verbal reasoning and processing with less context support escalate. Second, Amber has a history of a strong learning rate. She was responsive to language stimulation techniques tried in diagnostic teaching. She appeared to have a good prognosis for improvement and would benefit from some additional language support, particularly in the area of expressive language formulation and social language use.

Amber had a team of highly skilled professionals at her school. After reviewing the findings with the parents and the school team, it was determined that continuing the half-day of self-contained placement and half-day of regular classroom placement was advisable. The teaching team selected the following priorities for her support program: (1) strengthen expressive language formulation through daily opportunities to narrate with support from the team; particular emphasis to be placed on school language functions (e.g., problem solving, reasoning, describing, explaining, sharing personal stories), (2) building vocabulary and using specific references, (3) reducing semantic errors, particularly those based in limited audibility (e.g., pronouns and prepositions), (4) strengthening emotive vocabulary, and (5) role playing to practice verbal social interactions with peers.

Follow-up Assessment

The parent and school team requested a follow-up assessment one year later as a way of monitoring their progress toward the established goals and reconsidering the parental goal of increasing mainstreaming opportunities. Audiological testing revealed that Amber's hearing thresholds had remained stable over the past year and that she was receiving good benefit from her amplification and FM systems. Language and academic retesting demonstrated significant progress in all areas of language and literacy. As illustrated by the ×s on the profile in Figure 11.3B, Amber's language and academic scores were falling within the average range for her age and grade placement. Although Amber was still working through some formulation struggles at times, her personal narratives were better organized and contained few errors. She was able to express her ideas fluently much of the time. The school reported that Amber was getting along better with her peers and solving problems using verbal means. As a result of the positive findings, the parents and educators made a decision to mainstream Amber in the third grade with support services. This case illustrates that social–emotional and communication factors needed to be considered in the decision-making process. Academic test results, especially in the earliest grades, can be misleading in determining readiness for mainstreaming. Amber benefited greatly from an additional year of support, which resulted in stronger linguistic and social preparation for full integration.

CASE 4   GREG: LATE IDENTIFICATION ■ OF A HARD OF HEARING CHILD

Prior to newborn screening, the average age of identification of hearing loss in the United States was 18 months for deaf children and even older for hard of hearing children (Carney & Moeller, 1998). Since the advent of newborn hearing screening, many hard of hearing infants and families have the combined advantage of early and consistent amplification and early intervention services. Many of these children are able to achieve language skills close to their peers with normal hearing (Moeller, 2000; Yoshinaga-Itano, Sedey, Coulter, & Mehl, 1998) and are able to be successfully educated in mainstreamed settings. This proactive approach to management is ideal. Some children still slip through system cracks; others develop later onset hearing loss. This means that professionals and parents must continue to be vigilant and refer for audiological evaluation if there are concerns for speech, language, or hearing. The following case describes a child who was late-identified prior to the implementation of newborn hearing screening. Inconsistency in his responses to sound led to delays in referral for hearing evaluation. This case illustrates the importance of audibility in the formation of language rules by a child who is hard of hearing. In this case, the child needed to learn new ways of gaining meaning from messages around him. His auditory training program needed to focus on helping him develop productive listening and comprehension behaviors.

Background Information

Greg's parents first began to express concerns about his hearing to their pediatrician when he was 2 years old. He was demonstrating inconsistent responses to sound and delayed speech and language development at that time. Results of audiologic testing at a community hospital suggested borderline normal hearing sensitivity in response to speech and narrowband stimuli. One and one-half years later, the parents continued to express concern for Greg's hearing, and testing revealed at least a mild to moderate sensorineural hearing loss in the better ear. However, the audiologist reported questionable test reliability, and Greg was referred for auditory brainstem response testing. Results suggested the probability of a moderate to severe sensorineural hearing loss in at least the higher frequencies, with the right ear more involved than the left. Greg was then referred to a pediatric audiologic team. A severe rising to mild hearing loss in the right ear was confirmed through behavioral testing. Left ear testing revealed responses in the mild hearing loss range, rising to within normal limits at 1 kHz, steeply sloping to the severe hearing loss range at 2 kHz, and then rising to the mild hearing loss range in the higher frequencies. Given the unusual configuration of Greg's hearing loss (see Figure 11.4A), it was not surprising that he passed a screening evaluation that used speech and narrow bands of noise in sound field. Unfortunately, the referral for more definitive testing was delayed by the findings of the screening assessment. Medical–genetic evaluation revealed a family history of hearing loss, but etiology could not be confirmed.

Hearing aid fitting was complex, given the unusual audiometric configuration in the left ear. However, a binaural fitting was selected, with capability for direct audio input for FM amplification. Greg was immediately referred to an AR program for the purposes of evaluating his individual communication needs and determining considerations for educational placement.

Communication Activity Assessment

Greg demonstrated an unusual communication profile at 4 years of age. On standardized tests of language, his receptive language skills approximated a 2½-year level, and his expressive language skills were equivalent to a 3-year level. On many tests, his expressive performance was stronger than comprehension. Analysis of conversational interactions was useful in understanding the complexity of his receptive and expressive language problems. It was evident from the outset that Greg was having serious difficulty understanding those around him. Table 11.1 contains a segment from an interactive language sample, where Greg was conversing with an audiologic rehabilitation clinician.

> Greg's comprehension difficulties were evident in the finding that expressive language was stronger than receptive.

A number of interesting patterns were reflected in Greg's spontaneous speech. Although most of his words were intelligible to the listener, it was difficult to understand Greg due to numerous semantic and grammatical errors in his spontaneous productions. It was suspected that Greg's unusual audiometric configuration had contributed to his formulation of unusual language rules. Spectral information he was receiving may have provided inconsistent cues about grammatical or semantic categories. For example, he frequently marked nouns with /s/, even when a morpheme was not required. He rarely inflected verbs. He was aware that words were marked with morphemes like /s/, but had no consistent basis for application of this rule. Lack of audibility of portions of the speech spectrum may have also led to semantic confusions. Greg confused gender (*girl* vs. *boy*; *man* vs. *lady*), used nouns as verbs, used pronoun forms randomly (with confusion of *I*, *you*, *be*, *she*, and *we*), and had significant difficulty providing the appropriate semantic content in response to questions. Collectively, these errors appeared to be language "differences," rather than simple delays.

> Semantic errors refer to errors in the meaning of the message. For example, referring to a *girl* as a *boy* is an error of meaning.

To understand better the nature of Greg's language problems, the AR clinician constructed probes to examine Greg's language processing strategies. For example,

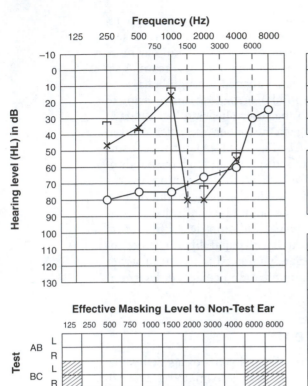

Key to Audiogram

Ear	Air	Bone
AC (THD-49)	○	×
AC (ER-3A)	●	▲
BC (masked)	[	]
NR	↙	↘

⌐ — Unmasked BC
▨ — Sound Field Warble Tones
SAT — Speech Awareness Threshold
SRT — Speech Reception Threshold
SL — Sensation Level
SF — Sound Field
BC — Bone Conduction
ETF — Eustachian Tube Function
+ — Single Responses

Test Reliability: Good
Method: CPA

Immittance Battery		Right	Left
Tymp	Normal	X	X
	Abnormal		
Reflexes	Present		
	Absent	X	X
	Elevated		
ETF	Vol (cc)		
	Release (daPa)		

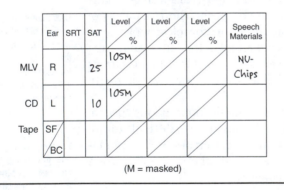

	Ear	SRT	SAT	Level %	Level %	Level %	Speech Materials
MLV	R		25	105M			NU-Chips
CD	L		10	105M			
Tape	SF/BC						

(M = masked)

Comments/Special Test
Discrim scores 6/15-R, 5/15-L
Result of discrim testing may have been effected by vocab and attention

Audiologic Impression:

Recommendations:

FIGURE 11.4A

Case 4: Greg's initial audiogram.

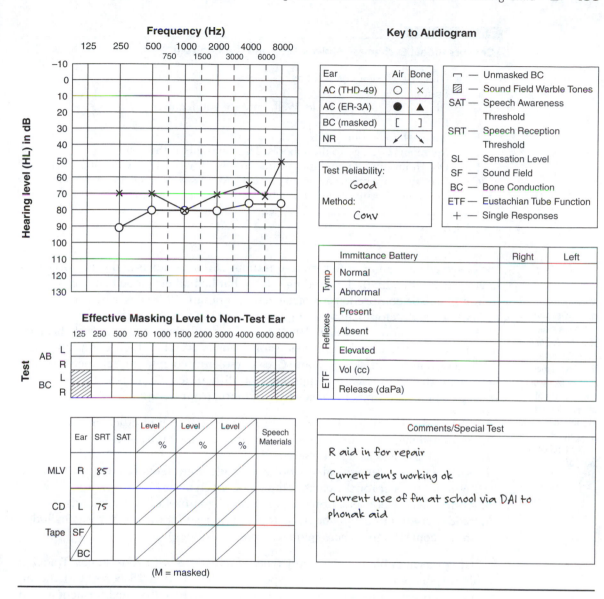

Frequency (Hz)

Key to Audiogram

Ear	Air	Bone
AC (THD-49)	○	×
AC (ER-3A)	●	▲
BC (masked)	[	]
NR	↙	↘

⌐ — Unmasked BC
▨ — Sound Field Warble Tones
SAT — Speech Awareness
        Threshold
SRT — Speech Reception
        Threshold
SL — Sensation Level
SF — Sound Field
BC — Bone Conduction
ETF — Eustachian Tube Function
+ — Single Responses

Test Reliability:
Good
Method:
Conv

Immittance Battery	Right	Left
Tymp — Normal		
Abnormal		
Reflexes — Present		
Absent		
Elevated		
ETF — Vol (cc)		
Release (daPa)		

Effective Masking Level to Non-Test Ear

125 250 500 750 1000 1500 2000 3000 4000 6000 8000

Test
AB L
     R
BC L
     R

	Ear	SRT	SAT	Level %	Level %	Level %	Speech Materials
MLV	R	85					
CD	L	75					
Tape	SF / BC						

(M = masked)

Comments/Special Test

R aid in for repair

Current em's working ok

Current use of fm at school via DAI to phonak aid

Audiologic Impression:

Recommendations:

FIGURE 11.4B

Case 4: Greg's recent audiogram (following progression).

TABLE 11.1

Conversational Exchange between Greg and the Clinician

E	Hi, Greg. How are you today?
C	Fours.
E	Oh, you are four years old. Well, how are you feeling?
C	Fine.
E	Greg, where's your mom?
C	My moms Greg go to the schools. The mom talk it the boats.
E	Oh. Hmmmm, you and mom came to school. Wow, I see you got a star!
C	I got stars my mom say no go outsides. Mom say do suns no go outside. Mom the all raining go put the backs the watch all raining.

C = child; *E* = examiner.

Nonlinguistic comprehension strategies refer to a child's use of cues other than the spoken message to figure out the meaning of a phrase. For example, the child might use context cues to understand what was said.

she observed his responses to various questions across contexts and tasks. Greg was having such difficulty understanding others that he had developed an overreliance on nonlinguistic comprehension strategies. Chapman (1978) described young children's normal developmental use of comprehension strategies in the face of complex linguistic input. Moeller (1988) has observed that students with hearing impairment may use such comprehension "shortcuts" when their comprehension is taxed well into their school years. Greg demonstrated extreme reliance on these behaviors, due to pervasive comprehension difficulties. Greg used the following strategies in his attempts to make sense of input around him:

1. Attended to key words in the message to the exclusion of other information
2. Predicted message intention based on situational context cues
3. Nodded his head as if he understood
4. Selected a key, recognizable word and made comments related to that topic (without respect for the current topic of conversation)
5. Controlled the conversational topic to avoid comprehension demands
6. Said everything known about the topic in hopes that the answer was included in the content somewhere (global response strategy)

Greg was not able to answer any types of questions with consistency. Tracking of his responses revealed correct responses in fewer than 25 percent of the instances. In response to commands, he failed to recognize the need for action, and would instead imitate the command or nod his head. Greg's reliance on nonlinguistic strategies is evident in the discourse example provided in Table 11.2.

In this example, Greg showed his overdependence on context for determining what questions mean. He also demonstrated his tendency to use a global response strategy, and his assumption that "if she asks me the question again, my first response must have been wrong." The clinician observed similar behaviors from Greg in his preschool class setting. He had a "panicked" expression on his face much of the time. Greg did not appear to expect to understand. Rather, he expected to have to guess. In the classroom, he frequently produced long, confused narratives. His teacher, in an effort to be supportive, would abandon her communication agenda and follow Greg's

TABLE 11.2

Greg's Replies to Questions about Simple Objects

E	(*holding a boy doll*) Who is this?
C	Boy.
E	(*puts boy in helicopter*) Who is this?
C	Boy the helicopter.
E	(*holds up a mom doll*) Who is this?
C	Mom boy the helicopter.

C = child; *E* = examiner.

topic to any degree possible. This was problematic, however, in that Greg needed to learn to understand and respond with semantic accuracy to classroom discourse.

Management

REMEDIATION OF COMMUNICATION ACTIVITY: AUDITORY AND LINGUISTIC TRAINING. Once amplification was fitted, Greg was enrolled in a multifaceted audiologic rehabilitation program. Individual auditory language therapy focused on development of productive comprehension strategies and reduction of semantic confusion through attention to appropriate auditory linguistic cues. A parent program was included, with focus on teaching the family natural ways to support Greg's comprehension. Greg had a tendency to imitate each message he heard, which interfered with processing and responding. The parents and therapist agreed to reduce emphasis on imitation and expression until success in comprehension could be increased. Further, the AR specialist provided collaborative consultation to Greg's classroom teacher. The school district provided Greg a diagnostic placement in a Language Intervention Preschool. His teacher was a speech–language pathologist. The teacher and AR specialist developed a scheme for helping Greg repair comprehension breakdowns and for helping him respond accurately in the classroom. Table 11.3 illustrates the type of teaching interaction that was implemented to scaffold or support Greg's emerging comprehension.

> Because imitation interfered with processing, clinicians needed to reduce the emphasis on requests for speech imitation. Focus was placed on listening and comprehending.

These classroom adaptations were successful in helping Greg begin to focus on the content of what he was hearing. As his auditory–linguistic behaviors strengthened, he began to revise language and discourse rules. His auditory language program focused specifically on helping him discriminate among linguistic elements that marked important semantic or syntactic distinctions. For example, he worked with the AR clinician in learning to distinguish pronoun forms (e.g., *I* vs. *you*), various morphological structures, and the meaning of various question forms. All intervention was incorporated in communicatively based activities to ensure the development of pragmatically appropriate conversational skills.

The AR clinician and teacher worked collaboratively to gradually shape in Greg productive listening and comprehension strategies. This was an essential step in helping Greg revise his expressive language behaviors. He needed to develop the confidence that he could understand and that his responses needed to be related to

TABLE 11.3	
Classroom Interaction Designed to Support Greg's Emerging Discourse Skills	

E	Good morning, Greg. Where's your mommy?
C	Mom Greg go go the school. My moms say Greg no go the school the rain. . . .
E	Just a minute, Greg. *Listen* to the question (*focusing prompt*).
E	Where *is* mom? (*highlighting prompt*) At home? In the car? Here at school? (*multiple-choice prompt*).
C	Mom right there. At school! (*points to his mother in the hall—on her way in to be room mother today*).
E	Good, Greg! You answered my question! I asked, "Where's mom?" You told me . . . right there! There she is!

C = child; *E* = examiner.

Source: Moeller, Osberger, & Eccarius (1986).

the conversational topic. Adjustment of Greg's approach to comprehension was necessary to prepare him for learning in a classroom environment.

Intervention Outcomes

Greg was responsive to the auditory–linguistic training program and to the supportive techniques used in the classroom to strengthen language processing. Greg continued to receive a team approach to his rehabilitation and education into his early elementary years. Although the ultimate objective was to enable him to profit from education in a regular classroom, the initial approach was conservative with emphasis on specialty services to help him develop the language foundation necessary for academic success. In this case, the conservative approach was especially fortuitous because Greg experienced progression in his sensorineural hearing loss during his early elementary years. The audiograms in Figures 11.4A and B illustrate the progression in thresholds that occurred, with the initial audiogram on the left and the final audiogram on the right. Hearing thresholds finally stabilized at a severe hearing loss level, with a bilaterally symmetrical configuration. Fortunately, optimal hearing aid fittings have been achieved (see Figure 11.5). Real-ear measures indicate that much of the speech spectrum is audible to Greg with properly fitted personal and FM amplification.

A language assessment was completed when Greg was 10 years of age. All language test scores fell solidly within the average range for his age in comparison to hearing peers. Previous comprehension and discourse problems were no longer present. In the context of a storytelling task, Greg produced complex utterances like "The boy says that the frog should stay on the land while the rest of them sail off on a raft." Greg's expressive language was semantically and grammatically appropriate for his age. Provision of support services will continue to be important for Greg, in spite of his strong language performance. When asked if he was having any problems in school, Greg reported, "Well, it is hard sometimes because you have to be quiet to hear the teacher, but the hearing kids keep talking. Then I always have to watch what everybody's doing, and then I'll know what I'm supposed to be doing."

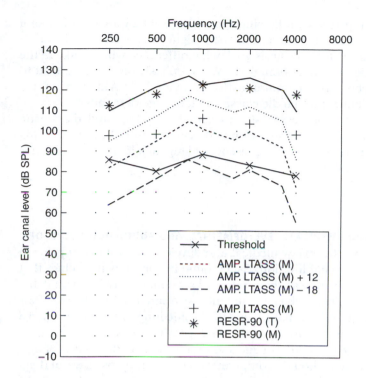

Frequency (Hz)

FIGURE 11.5

Results of real-ear measures illustrating audibility in relation to the long-term average speech spectrum.

Legend:
- ✕— Threshold
- AMP. LTASS (M)
- AMP. LTASS (M) + 12
- AMP. LTASS (M) − 18
- + AMP. LTASS (M)
- ✳ RESR-90 (T)
- —— RESR-90 (M)

Summary

This case has illustrated the critical importance that audibility plays in a child's language rule formation. It also underscores the importance of teamwork to address concerns in all the child's significant learning environments. With aggressive and continuous AR support, a child who is hard of hearing has an opportunity to overcome early delays. Appropriate management of amplification and auditory learning opportunities play a key role in this process.

CASE 5   SAM: DIFFERENTIAL DIAGNOSIS THROUGH PROFESSIONAL TEAMWORK: A TOOL ■ FOR SOLVING COMPLEX INTERVENTION PROBLEMS

Fundamental to the process of audiologic rehabilitation is the need to obtain a comprehensive understanding of a child's strengths and areas of need. This requires accurate and thorough differential diagnosis, best accomplished within the context of a transdisciplinary team. Some children present with a complex array of developmental needs. Unless these are well understood, barriers to progress may not be identified, strengths may not be utilized to the child's advantage, and intervention priorities may be misaligned. Children with language processing difficulties in addition to hearing loss may present with a host of communicative needs. One of the "arts" to audiologic rehabilitation is the ability to prioritize treatment goals so that the impact of intervention on the child as a communicator may be maximized. The selection of intervention priorities following thorough problem analysis is like a craft, requiring skill, theoretical preparation, and insight. It is useful for the clinician to ask the following: (1) If I select this goal, what difference will it make in the child's overall communicative functioning? (2) Will emphasis on this goal lead to generalization or impact on other communicative behaviors? (3) Will work on this goal better prepare the student to handle classroom language demands?

This case illustrates the processes of differential diagnosis and diagnostic teaching leading to appropriate goal selection and prioritization. In the following example, strategies used to determine the presence of language-learning disabilities in addition to deafness are illustrated.

It is important for the clinician to consider the impact that work on a certain goal will have on the student's overall communicative function.

Assessment

BACKGROUND INFORMATION: MEDICAL, DEVELOPMENTAL, AND AUDIOLOGICAL HISTORY. It is essential for clinicians to review medical and developmental history prior to engaging in evaluation and rehabilitation. Background history may hold clues that focus the diagnostic effort. Sam was the product of a premature twin birth, delivered by C-section. He remained in the neonatal intensive care unit for the first four months of his life. He required ventilation due to chronic lung problems. He had a history of feeding difficulties, seizures, poor balance, poor vision, and motor delays. He first sat unsupported at 18 months of age and first walked at 30 months of age. This background information should prompt an AR clinician to pose several diagnostic questions: (1) Has a psychological evaluation been completed in recent years? (2) Has the student been followed for occupational therapy? (3) Are there concerns for sensory integration? (4) Has he been free of seizures in recent years? (5) Is he taking medications for seizures?

Developmental and medical history information helps the AR clinician form diagnostic questions that guide evaluation and further referrals.

This 9-year-old boy had a history of profound, bilateral hearing loss, identified in infancy. He underwent cochlear implant surgery at 2 years of age. He currently uses a HiResolution (HiRes) speech coding strategy.

EDUCATIONAL/REHABILITATIVE HISTORY AND CONCERNS. Sam and his family participated in regular early intervention services in the birth-to-3 period. At age 3, he attended a public school preschool program for children with special needs and then entered a mainstream educational setting. Due to persistent problems with speech and language skills, Sam repeated his kindergarten year. At the time of referral, he was mainstreamed in a first-grade class with support services from an itinerant teacher of the deaf, a speech–language pathologist, a physical therapist, and an educational interpreter. He relied on both speech and signs for communication. The parents and the school sought support from an audiologic rehabilitation team due to concerns for (1) behavioral difficulties and limited motivation in the academic setting, (2) lack of clear benefit from the cochlear implant, (3) poor retention of information, (4) limited generalization of concepts taught, (5) limited use of his interpreter, (6) concerns for integration of sensory information, (7) slow progress, and (8) difficulties socializing with peers.

PSYCHOSOCIAL AND COMMUNICATION FINDINGS. Psychological evaluation revealed that Sam's nonverbal intellectual abilities were in the low average range. Observations of verbal cognitive abilities revealed significant difficulty with categorization, making connections between words and reasoning. He struggled on tasks that required him to use multiple skills simultaneously or to manipulate information in his head without visual cues (i.e., How are an apple and bread alike?). These results have important implications for rehabilitative planning and need to be considered as the diagnostic story unfolds.

On formal language measures, Sam performed well below age expectations receptively and showed marked delays in expressive language. Observations of him in language learning lessons and in the classroom provided important insights about language processing skills. It is challenging to determine if a student has language learning difficulties beyond what can be explained by the hearing loss. Comparison of behaviors to typically developing deaf children can be useful in making this judgment. Table 11.4 summarizes language-learning behaviors exhibited by Sam that are not usual for children with deafness.

Analysis of Sam's spontaneous conversational language supported the impression of language formulation (planning) difficulties. Table 11.5 contains an excerpt from his language sample, along with diagnostic impressions of the language behaviors.

FUNCTIONAL AUDITORY AND SPEECH PRODUCTION SKILLS. Sam relied primarily on oral communication for self-expression, but at times used both speech and sign. His speech intelligibility was reduced, which led the school to question the benefit he was receiving from his cochlear implant device. Given their concerns, formal and informal measures of functional auditory skills were administered. He demonstrated a high degree of accuracy in closed set word and phrase recognition, and his scores had steadily improved over a two-year period. Word lists were created and tested to ensure that they were within his vocabulary. These were then presented auditory-only in an open set context, and he was asked to repeat the words. Sam recognized 88 percent of those words, with most errors accounted for by place of articulation (e.g., *cat* vs. *hat*). Further, Sam was able to follow basic commands and to correct speech production errors when given auditory-only input. It was the impression of the AR team that Sam was making good progress with his cochlear implant. It did not appear that auditory skills were creating a barrier for speech production. This led to the next diagnostic question, "Are other issues affecting spoken word production?" Given that fine motor sequencing issues were observed, it is possible that oral motor execution and planning may be challenging for Sam.

Sam was seen by a speech–language pathologist, who determined that motor difficulties were complicating speech production. An oral motor evaluation revealed that Sam had problems separating head and tongue movements, needed greater strength and mobility in tongue movements, and exhibited difficulties sequencing speech sounds as rate increased. This information is essential for interpreting the cochlear implant results. His benefit from the implant simply could not be judged by his spoken language performance, because it was affected by language processing and motor planning difficulties. Functional auditory evaluation revealed strength and helped the teaching team recognize a key area in which they had facilitated Sam's learning. Interestingly, Sam's teaching team had experienced only two children with cochlear implants. The other child had outstanding outcomes,

The psychologist identified low average nonverbal cognitive skills. Combined with other disabilities, cognition must be considered as a possible limiting factor in Sam's learning.

It is important to consider if the presenting behaviors are "typical" for students who are deaf or hard of hearing.

TABLE 11.4

Atypical Language Behaviors Demonstrated by Sam

RECEPTIVE LANGUAGE CONCERNS	EXPRESSIVE LANGUAGE CONCERNS
• Recognizes concepts, but cannot manipulate them (i.e., can identify a knife and scissors, but cannot answer how they are "alike"). • Relies on contextual cues (e.g., pictures, other student responses) for understanding, instead of processing the language, resulting in misunderstanding and confusion. • Difficulty redirecting his focus after he misunderstood something. • Easily overwhelmed by multiple sources of information (e.g., teacher talking, objects presented, interpreter signing, children answering). Tended to "shut down." • Sometimes distracted by visual support materials. • Difficulties with visual-spatial organization. • Able to answer only basic questions; inordinate difficulty with abstraction.	• Qualitative concerns with vocabulary development; poor skills in word associations and classification, resulting in disorganized word storage. This contributes to problems recalling words. • Word retrieval difficulties seen in misnaming of common words, frustration when naming, misnaming rote concepts (i.e., confusing boy/girl). • Difficulty planning, sequencing, and executing fine motor movements. • Imprecise signed movements, related to poor trunk stability, difficulties with bilateral coordination of movements, and sequencing problems. • Significant difficulty responding to nonconcrete questions. • Language formulation difficulties (start, stop, revise, try again)

Motor sequencing or planning difficulties (e.g., praxis) are not typical in deaf and hard of hearing students. Speech training approaches need to be modified in light of this diagnosis.

leading teachers to conclude that Sam's outcomes were less than satisfactory. Clearly, findings must be interpreted with reference to the child's entire constellation of abilities. For Sam, with his multiple language and learning challenges, the cochlear implant was leading to positive outcomes.

Management

DIAGNOSTIC TEACHING: FINDING STRENGTHS AND EFFECTIVE STRATEGIES. Several sessions were conducted to identify Sam's learning strengths as well as strategies to address his priority needs. Diagnostic teaching is a process whereby the clinician creates learning tasks and objectively analyzes their effectiveness with the child, modifying the approach as necessary to bring about success. The cyclical nature of this process is illustrated in Figure 11.6.

An obvious priority for Sam was to build stronger classification and vocabulary skills so that words could be retained and generalized. Six new words were introduced to Sam during diagnostic teaching activities (e.g., tinker toy construction barrier game; drawing and creating stories) to identify methods that support word learning. Receptively, he learned all six target words introduced to him. He also learned to express these words, but he primarily retained the signed symbol, suggesting that he needed more trials/opportunities to learn the spoken form. In general, Sam showed enhanced retention of novel words when the learning activity contained

TABLE 11.5

Conversational Sample Showing Language Processing Difficulties

	IMPRESSIONS
Clinician: Does dad drive a truck? *Sam:* drive a truck . . . truck. a brown truck. Yeah it have a trailer . . . white trailer.	Sam imitates a phrase from the question asked, perhaps to give him time to process the meaning or organize his response. He then answers and adds a relevant comment, which includes pauses and revisions.
Sam: a box. Dad put on trailer many many all.	He attempts to continue his turn on the topic, but does not give enough information for his partner to understand.
Clinician: Does dad have a tractor?	
Sam: tractor and wagon and combine.	Appropriate response.
Clinician: What do you do with a combine?	
Sam: a corn. The corn have wagon in. In the wagon . . . corn in the wagon.	Takes three tries to produce the phrase he intends.
Clinician: How do you get up in the combine?	
Sam: It tall very wheel like that. Climb wheel. I climb in that.	Language organizational issues apparent as he tries to answer.

- Experiential components (i.e., hands-on materials, active engagement, problems to solve). Drill and practice in isolation was not effective.
- Contrasts in the purposes of tool used (e.g., knowing the purpose of the tinker toy parts made it easier to retain distinctive words for those parts). Pictures alone were ineffective in exploring characteristics of words (such as functions of their parts).
- Recognition to recall opportunities (e.g., place all the word cards out in front of him and give several trials of "find the X" before asking him to "name X.")
- Functional expression (i.e., provide opportunities for him to use the target words in pragmatically appropriate ways).
- Chaining of inputs. Instead of working on all modalities at once, he needed trials where he can: hear it, then say it, then sign it, then read it, then fingerspell it. It was found that simultaneous use of multiple modes was overwhelming. Chaining separate modes was effective. Inclusion of signs aided longer term recall.
- Extra learning opportunities that focus on oral skills (practice in saying and recalling the target words).

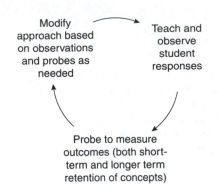

FIGURE 11.6

Model of cycles of diagnostic teaching in audiological rehabilitation.

As another illustration of this process, the **AR** clinicians teamed with an academic specialist to conduct a diagnostic teaching activity related to classification, a priority goal for Sam. To explore ways to blend language and academic objectives, they chose the content area of money, an area in mathematics that was causing Sam some difficulties. The goal of the activity was to help Sam attend to characteristics of money that would help him to compare, contrast, and group bills and coins and eventually help him to problem solve which bill or coin(s) he would need in a given functional situation. Listing characteristics took place in a parallel comparison chart. Two paper bills (a $5 bill and a $20 bill) were placed each at the head of a column on a small whiteboard. A clinician elicited anything that Sam knew about the first bill and wrote the characteristics in a column under the bill:

FIVE-DOLLAR BILL	TWENTY-DOLLAR BILL
$5	$20
money	money

Then, the clinician used guided questions to elicit additional information:

FIVE-DOLLAR BILL	TWENTY-DOLLAR BILL
$5	$20
money	money
made of paper	made of paper
green	green

Finally, the clinician placed new items, one at a time, encouraging Sam to look at the previous examples to help him describe the new items. The contrastive example of the nickel allowed Sam to begin to recognize how things could be similar in one characteristic while different in others.

FIVE-DOLLAR BILL	TWENTY-DOLLAR BILL	TEN-DOLLAR BILL	ONE-DOLLAR BILL	NICKEL
$5	$20	$10	$1	5 cents
money	money	money	money	money
made of paper	made of paper	made of paper	made of paper	made of metal
green	green	green	green	silver

Sam did not automatically make use of the columns and rows to cue himself about important characteristics. With visual structuring, however, he became more independent as the activity progressed. The resulting matrix could be used in the future to build language elements such as "They are all . . . ," "these are made of paper, but this one is made of metal," "the dollar and the nickel are different colors."

The amount of complexity of the language would depend on Sam's response. Eventually, this same matrix could be used for problem solving about how much would be necessary to make a purchase, what the money was worth, and so on. His teachers indicated that he had just learned the names of coins and was having difficulty retaining previously learned information about their value. A similar matrix would help him to differentiate between the questions: "What is the name of this coin?" and "What is this coin worth?"

A QUARTER COIN	A DIME	A NICKEL	A PENNY
quarter	dime	nickel	penny
25 cents	10 cents	5 cents	1 cent

At the end of the activity, Sam successfully sorted the paper money into one group and the coins into another group, starting with one item in each group and placing one additional item at a time into the correct set. This would be the foundation for using language to answer "Why do they go together? What is the same?" Or to summarize, "They are all . . . " Sam benefited from language mediation paired with appropriate (but not overwhelming) visual supports.

Sam also demonstrated strengths in episodic memory. In other words, he was able to remember a paragraph-length story better if it was presented in a script with dialogue. The AR clinicians were able to prompt improved narratives by involving Sam in role-play scenarios and story-retell activities.

PUTTING IT ALL TOGETHER: ADAPTING THE EDUCATIONAL ENVIRONMENT. Sam's dedicated teachers had been experiencing frustration at his lack of motivation and retention difficulties. Many of the findings from the AR sessions helped the teachers understand Sam's progress in a new light. A main point was the need to adjust the lens when interpreting progress. Sam was a student with learning disabilities in addition to deafness. Therefore, the best comparison was Sam to himself over time. Another key point was that Sam was persistent, engaged, and motivated, *when the language of the task was manageable for him.* Sam was inherently motivated; he was simply unable to process the multiple inputs in the classroom (explaining why he was not watching the interpreter). This led to behavioral responses, such as shutting out all input. The evaluation process clarified the strengths in auditory learning with the cochlear implant and ability to profit from script-based learning and selected visual tools. These results were used to make adjustment in the classroom curriculum to accommodate Sam's individual language and learning needs. Motor planning issues needed to be considered in speech therapy, in interpreting cochlear implant outcomes, and in working on written language (keyboarding was recommended, for example). Increased support in the classroom was recommended along with ongoing task analysis during learning activities (e.g., What is Sam doing right now to attempt to complete this task? Is that helping or interfering? Does this activity begin with one of Sam's strengths? How much information is new, and is at least part of the activity familiar? Is the task meaningful for Sam and is he functionally involved?) These "on-line" strategies help teachers identify paths to success with a student like Sam.

Summary

The results of this case underscore the importance of professional collaboration in solving complex intervention puzzles. The case further illustrates the value in implementing a diagnostic teaching approach that assists in identifying priorities and useful solutions to address them. In this process, questions are continually modified to bring about positive results.

REFERENCES AND RECOMMENDED READING

Carney, A. E., & Moeller, M. P. (1998). Treatment efficacy: Hearing loss in children. *Journal of Speech, Language, and Hearing Research, 41,* S61–S84.

Chapman, R. (1978). Comprehension strategies in children. In J. Kavanagh & P. Strange (Eds.), *Language and speech in the laboratory, school and clinic.* Cambridge, MA: MIT Press.

Dale, P., & Thal, D. (1993). *MacArthur Communicative Development Inventory* (Infant and Toddler Scales used). San Diego, CA: Center for Research in Language, UCSD.

Greenspan, S. (1990). *Floor time.* New York: Scholastic.

Moeller, M. P. (1988). Combining formal and informal strategies for language assessment of hearing-impaired children [monograph]. In R. R. Kretschmer Jr. & L. W. Kretschmer (Eds.), Communication assessment of hearing impaired children: From conversation to classroom. *Journal of the Academy of Rehabilitative Audiology, 21,* Suppl., 73–101.

Moeller, M. P. (2000). Early intervention and language development in children who are deaf and hard of hearing. *Pediatrics, 106*(3), 1–9.

Moeller, M. P., Coufal, K., & Hixson, P. (1990). The efficacy of speech–language intervention: Hearing impaired children. *Seminars in Speech and Language, 11*(4), 227–241.

Moeller, M. P., Osberger, M. J., & Eccarius, M. (1986). Cognitively based strategies for use with hearing-impaired students with comprehension deficits. *Topics in Learning Disabilities, 6*(4), 37–50.

Roush, J., & Matkin, N. D. (1994). *Infants and toddlers with hearing loss.* Baltimore: York Press.

Schildroth, A. M., & Hotto, S. A. (1993). Annual survey of hearing impaired children and youth: 1991–92 school year. *American Annals of the Deaf, 138*(2), 163–171.

Schuyler, V., & Sowers, J. (1998). *Parent–infant communication* (4th ed.). Portland, OR: Hearing and Speech Institute, Infant Hearing Resources.

Wetherby, A., & Prizant, B. (1993). *Communication and symbolic behavior scales.* Chicago: Special Press.

Yoshinaga-Itano, C., Sedey, A. L., Coulter, B. A., & Mehl, A. L. (1998). Language of early- and later-identified children with hearing loss. *Pediatrics, 102*(5), 1168–1171.

RECOMMENDED WEBSITE

www.raisingdeafkids.org/special/
For information on working with deaf and hard of hearing children who have additional disabilities.

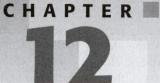

C H A P T E R
12

Case Studies:
Adults and Elderly Adults

Michael A. Nerbonne
Jeff E. Brockett
Alice E. Holmes

C O N T E N T S

◼ INTRODUCTION

The five adult and elderly cases focusing on audiologic rehabilitation described in this chapter involve a wide range of clients with hearing impairment, in terms of both age and communication-related difficulties. While special adjustments must be considered with some elderly patients, such as those found in nursing homes, in general, both adult and elderly persons will most often demonstrate the same kinds of communication problems and, therefore, be candidates for similar rehabilitation strategies. Thus, we have grouped these younger and older cases together and presented them in the same chapter. Although references are made to group therapy (as in Case 1), the major emphasis with each case is on addressing the specific, unique problems that each of these individuals is experiencing. Some of these problems relate as much to psychosocial influences as to auditory effects. Such influences need to be acknowledged in AR approaches.

Although a major goal for each case was to reduce communication-related difficulties, the specific audiologic strategies varied for each client depending on individual needs and motivation. The sampling of cases presented here ranges from involvement in hearing aid selection and orientation and counseling to traditional and more recently developed forms of individual and group communication rehabilitation. In addition, the pre- and postimplantation AR process for a challenging cochlear implant recipient is presented.

In the course of performing audiologic rehabilitation, the audiologist may encounter the wide range of cases described here. We hope that these cases will give some insights into the challenges and possibilities of this work. In general, the model followed here is the one detailed in the introductory chapter of this text (see Figure 1.2), which was inspired by the WHO (2001) classification scheme associated with rehabilitation. The model involves both assessment and remediation phases as part of the total audiologic rehabilitation process.

A variety of pre- and post-AR tests were used in an attempt to objectify the status of the clients during the assessment and management phases of therapy. Self-assessment tools are receiving increased emphasis in AR, and several different communication assessment instruments have been used here, including both screening and diagnostic tools. Also, real-ear (probe tube microphone) measures are used with some cases, demonstrating the utility of this tool in the rehabilitation process. No single test battery is recommended; nor is it implied that one is best for all purposes. Instead, clinicians must select the tests that will be useful for determining the exact needs of the client, assisting in specific therapy strategies, and providing relevant outcome measures to assess the results of management. In addition to the tests and procedures used in this chapter, the reader may refer to numerous other chapters throughout the book for other relevant test and resource materials that may be useful in AR.

Even though all cases included here are based directly on real persons, minor adjustments have been made in the names used and the material presented in order to maintain the anonymity of the clients.

■ CASE 1 DR. M.: PROGRESSIVE HEARING LOSS

Case History

Dr. M. was a 69-year-old man who had retired four years earlier after a forty-year career as a college professor. He reported experiencing frequent difficulties in hear-

ing, particularly at church, social functions, and plays that he and his spouse attended at the university's theater. Dr. M. had noted being aware of hearing difficulties for some time, including the last several years of his teaching career. The onset
of his impairment was reportedly gradual and seemed to affect both ears equally.

Audiologic Rehabilitation Assessment

Figure 12.1 contains the audiometric results obtained with Dr. M. In general, he
was found to possess a mild-to-moderate sensorineural hearing loss bilaterally. The
results of speech audiometry were consistent with the pure-tone findings and indicated that Dr. M. was experiencing significant difficulty in speech perception, especially if speech stimuli were presented at a typical conversation level (50 dB HL).

The *Self-Assessment of Communication (SAC)* and *Significant Other Assessment
of Communication (SOAC)* (Schow & Nerbonne, 1982) screening inventories were
administered to Dr. M. and his spouse to gather further information concerning the
degree of perceived hearing handicap resulting from Dr. M.'s hearing loss. Using
both of these measures provides valuable information about how hearing impaired
persons view their hearing problems, as well as potentially valuable insights from
the person who is communicating with the individual on a regular basis. Scores of
50 and 60 percent (raw scores: 30, 34) on SAC and SOAC tests presented a consistent pattern that, when evaluated according to research (see Table 12.1), provided
further evidence that Dr. M. was experiencing considerable hearing-related difficulties (Schow et al., 1989).

Interestingly, some
people with hearing
impairment that is
similar to Dr. M's
will report much
different (less or
more) hearing
disability. This
important dimen-
sion obviously is
quite individualized.

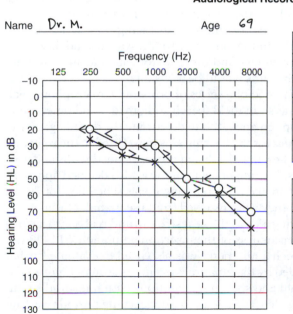

FIGURE 12.1

Case 1: Audiometric results for Dr. M.

TABLE 12.1		
Categories and Associated Scores for Classifying Primary and Secondary Effects of Hearing Loss (Hearing Disability or Handicap) When Using the SAC and SOAC		
CATEGORY	RAW SCORES	PERCENTAGE SCORES
No disability or handicap	10–18	0–20
Slight hearing disability or handicap	19–26	21–40
Mild to moderate hearing disability or handicap	27–38	41–70
Severe hearing disability or handicap	39–50	71–100

Source: Adapted from Schow, R., & Tannahill, C. (1977). Hearing handicap scores and categories for subjects with normal and impaired hearing sensitivity. *Journal of the American Audiological Society, 3,* 134–139. Also from Sturmak, M. J. (1987). *Communication handicap score interpretation for various populations and degrees of hearing impairment.* Master's thesis, Idaho State University; and Schow et al. (1989).

On the basis of these test results and the patient's comments, a hearing aid evaluation was recommended and scheduled.

Management

HEARING AID EVALUATION AND ADJUSTMENT. Prior to any testing associated with hearing aids, Dr. M. was advised about the option of utilizing a behind-the-ear or an in-the-ear style of hearing aid. Like most individuals facing this choice, Dr. M. expressed a clear preference for the in-the-ear style. Dr. M. was also advised that, because of the severity of his hearing loss and other factors such as improved localization abilities, binaural hearing aids would be advisable.

Care must be taken to get accurate and complete ear impressions. No matter how state of the art the circuitry of a hearing aid may be, if it doesn't fit well and feel comfortable the patient probably will not use it.

The hearing aid evaluation consisted of a series of probe-tube microphone real-ear measures with each ear, as well as soundfield speech audiometry. Audiometic data were applied to an existing prescription approach to determine the desired gain, frequency response, and SSPL-90 values for the hearing aids to be fitted in the right and left ears. This resulted in two ITE hearing aids being recommended with moderate gain and high-frequency emphasis. Venting of each unit was also deemed appropriate. Earmold impressions were taken and an appointment was scheduled for Dr. M. to be fitted with his new aids once they were received from the manufacturer.

Dr. M. was fitted with his hearing aids at the next session, and real-ear measures were taken to confirm the appropriateness of the insertion gain and OSPL-90 values for each unit. Soundfield speech audiometry was also used to evaluate further the degree of improvement provided by the binaural system. As seen in Figure 12.1, Dr. M.'s speech reception threshold and speech recognition score improved significantly with the in-the-ear hearing aids. His comments concerning the aids were favorable, and no further adjustments were made with either hearing aid. Following a thorough orientation to the operation and care of his new aids, Dr. M. was advised to return for subsequent follow-up appointments.

Dr. M.'s experience with his new hearing aids was, for the most part, positive. While still noting some problems hearing in group situations and at the theater, he definitely felt that the hearing aids were assisting him. Further discussion with Dr. M. regarding his hearing difficulties at the theater revealed that he had not yet tried the facility's infrared listening system. Encouraging him to do so, the audiologist explained the manner in which the system functions, as well as how Dr. M. could use the infrared receiver either with his hearing aids or as a stand-alone unit. Subsequent contact with Dr. M. revealed that he found the assistive listening device to be remarkably helpful.

While Dr. M. had adjusted well to his hearing aids and received substantial improvement as a result of their use, he did note some persistent communication difficulties. Because of this and his motivation for improvement, Dr. M. agreed to enroll in a short-term group audiologic rehabilitation program for adults.

COMMUNICATION TRAINING. Dr. M. was one of eight adults with hearing impairment who participated in the weekly group sessions. Although the activities and areas of emphasis varied somewhat as a result of the interests and needs of each group of participants, the main components of the program generally followed those outlined in Recent Trends in Speechreading—Adults, found in Chapter 5. The individuals participating with Dr. M. were new hearing aid users with mild-to-moderate hearing losses. Consequently, emphasis was placed on the effective use of hearing aids, care and maintenance of the systems, and the way hearing aids can be supplemented by one or more types of assistive listening devices. Attention was also given to developing more effective listening skills and capitalizing on the visual information available in most communication situations. Interaction among the group participants was encouraged, and valuable information on a variety of topics, including the use of conversation strategies and clear speech, was shared at each session.

> Successful audiologic rehabilitation done with groups of adults will involve both structured content and informal information sharing among the participants. They can learn as much from each other as from the group facilitator.

Following the final session, Dr. M. stated that the sessions had been helpful to him. In addition to the practical information provided, such as where to buy batteries for his hearing aids and the use of hearing aids with the telephone, Dr. M. felt that a number of the communication strategies covered had been of benefit to him. The net result was that he felt much more confident when communicating with others.

Summary

It was clear from the start that Dr. M. had accepted his hearing problem and was motivated to seek out whatever assistance was available to him. His positive and cooperative behaviors, which would be categorized by Goldstein and Stephens (1981) as an example of a Type I attitude (see Chapter 10), facilitated the audiologic rehabilitation process and positively affected Dr. M.'s overall communication abilities. Motivation should be recognized as a key ingredient in successful audiologic rehabilitation with any individual with hearing impairment.

CASE 2 ■ MR. B.: HEARING LOSS, DEPRESSION, AND SUCCESSFUL HEARING AID USE

Mr. B. is a 70-year-old male who was brought in by his neighbor. Mr. B's wife of nearly fifty years passed away one year prior to this visit. His neighbor was concerned that Mr. B. was becoming depressed and a shut-in because of his difficulty in hearing. Mr. B. reported having hearing problems for a very long time and that he had tried at least three different sets of hearing aids over the last twenty years. His newest set was approximately seven years old and was not working. Even when these instruments were new, they reportedly "did him no good." When asked what he didn't like about his current hearing aids (when they were working), he said that "everything was too noisy and loud" and that he "was constantly fiddling with the hearing aids to try and hear better."

Informational Counseling

Following a complete evaluation, the test findings were explained to Mr. B. in such a way that he could understand why he had so many communication difficulties. The audiologic rehabilitation process was described to him, but he seemed somewhat reluctant to proceed.

Rehabilitation Assessment

COMMUNICATION STATUS: IMPAIRMENT ACTIVITY LIMITATIONS

AUDIOMETRY AND COMMUNICATION ASSESSMENT. The results of a complete audiologic evaluation (see Figure 12.2) showed a moderate, symmetrical sensorineural hearing loss with a gradually sloping configuration. This is an F2 category (see website). His word recognition scores at a comfortable presentation level were 76 percent correct in the left ear and 84 percent correct in the right ear, using the CID W-22 word lists.

Mr. B.'s dynamic range was mapped at 500 and 4000 Hz. Results showed a dynamic range of 40 dB at 500 Hz and a significantly reduced dynamic range of 20 dB at 4000 Hz.

Mr. B.'s perception of his communication difficulty was assessed using the *Self-Assessment of Communication (SAC)* (Schow & Nerbonne, 1982). A raw score of 22 indicated only a mild degree of perceived difficulty. His neighbor was given the *Significant Other Assessment of Communication (SOAC)* to get an estimate of how others perceived Mr. B.'s communication difficulty. A raw score of 30 was computed, indicating a higher perception of communication difficulty.

The *Glasgow Hearing Aid Benefit Profile* (Gatehouse, 1999) was used to provide additional information about Mr. B.'s perceived disability and handicap. Scoring the unaided portion resulted in an initial disability of 72 percent and an initial handicap of 59 percent.

OVERALL PARTICIPATION VARIABLES. Based on his report, Mr. B. had little demand on his hearing. He lived alone and did not participate in any social activities. His family was distant and did not keep in touch with him very much. He avoided us-

> Persons routinely engaging in only a limited amount of communication on a day-to-day basis sometimes tend not to report as much hearing disability as another person who does more communicating.

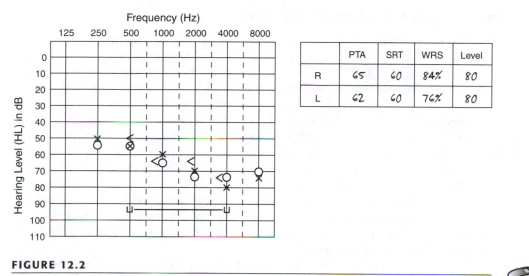

FIGURE 12.2

Case 2: Audiogram for Mr. B., plus loudness discomfort levels at 500 and 4000 Hz.

ing the phone unless absolutely necessary. His neighbor thought that if Mr. B. could hear better he would start to become more active and enjoy life more.

RELATED PERSONAL FACTORS. Mr. B. seemed very quiet, and, although he did not resist being at the evaluation, he did not appear motivated to do anything about his hearing loss. His neighbor mentioned the word "depressed" several times in describing Mr. B.'s behavior.

ENVIRONMENTAL FACTORS. Because Mr. B. lived alone, his communication environment was very restricted. In other words, aside from his neighbor and an occasional trip to the grocery store, he had little communication demand. When he was at home he watched TV and was able to turn the TV up loud enough to hear.

Rehabilitation Management

COUNSELING AND PSYCHOSOCIAL ISSUES. Mr. B. did not have any problem believing and admitting that he had a hearing problem. It was difficult, however, for him to identify what bothered him the most about his hearing difficulty. Because he could manage his communication environment at home by avoiding the telephone and turning up the TV, his perception of "difficulty" was somewhat distorted.

After some discussion, Mr. B. was asked if there were any situations that he would participate more in if he could hear better. He reported that he would like to hear on the telephone so that he could visit with his family and he wanted to hear well in a "group" situation.

It was clear that Mr. B. had some reservations about proceeding, probably due to a combination of three unsuccessful hearing aid fittings in the past and low communication demands. However, getting him to hear better on the telephone and in group environments seemed like appropriate goals.

AUDIBILITY AND IMPAIRMENT MANAGEMENT

AMPLIFICATION (MODIFYING AUDIBILITY). New technology in amplification was discussed, particularly the ability of hearing aids to address how he needs to hear different levels of sound. When it was explained that hearing aids could be adjusted so that he could receive more gain for soft sounds, less gain for average sounds, and even less for loud sounds, he seemed very interested in pursuing a trial period. He was comfortable with the full-shell ITE style and, because his dynamic range across frequencies was different, two-channel, programmable instruments were considered in the design. Because the circuitry could manage the gain for different input levels, the hearing aids were ordered without a user-operated volume control.

When the hearing aids arrived, Mr. B.'s threshold and supra threshold information was entered and the Desired Sensation Level (DSL) I/O fitting formula (Seewald, 1992, 2000) was followed to preset the initial program for the hearing aids. Predicted insertion gain response curves matched the target gain curves for soft, average, and loud inputs reasonably well.

When Mr. B. arrived for his hearing aid fitting and orientation, he seemed excited and anxious to hear the new sound. The hearing aids were placed in his ears and the actual fit of the hearing aids was inspected. The aids slipped in easily and seemed stable once in place. Mr. B. said that the hearing aids felt comfortable. The program was activated, and he had an immediate positive reaction.

An informal, functional assessment was performed using a CD containing different types of speech and environmental sounds presented in a sound field. Using this method, gain levels for soft (<45 dB), average (45 to 65 dB), and strong (>65 dB) inputs were programmed in the hearing aid. The compression ratio in the channel assigned to the high frequencies, where Mr. B. had a narrower dynamic range, was adjusted further to reduce loud sound amplification. Mr. B. reported that soft sounds seemed "distant" but he could still identify the sound. Average sounds were reported to be comfortable, and higher level inputs seemed loud but were not uncomfortable.

Newer hearing aids with multiple channels allow for greater flexibility in meeting the specific needs that a given individual may have.

As an objective measure, probe microphone measurements using modified DSL targets were used to evaluate insertion gain. Results showed good approximation of target in the low and mid frequencies, but the insertion response for soft, high-frequency sounds did not meet target gain values in the 3000 to 4000 Hz range. Gain in the channel assigned to the higher frequencies was increased to better address soft, high-frequency sounds; however, Mr. B. then reported that speech was too "lispy." The hearing aids were returned to the previous setting.

Finally, a formal functional assessment was performed under unaided and aided listening conditions using CID W-22 word lists presented in a sound field at 50 dB HL. Mr. B. was unable to correctly identify any of the words in the unaided condition, but scored 88 percent in the aided condition.

HEARING AID ORIENTATION. Even though Mr. B. was an experienced user, basic hearing instrument orientation, HIO BASICS, was discussed in detail. These topics included the following:

Hearing expectations: Realistic ones

Instrument operation: On/off, telecoil, telephone use

Occlusion effect: User's voice with hearing aids in place

Batteries: Tabs, how long they will last, removal, replacement, dangers

Acoustic feedback: What causes it; when is it OK, not OK?

System troubleshooting: What to do when there are problems?

Insertion and removal: Identifying left, right, insertion, and removal

Cleaning and maintenance: Wax and debris cleaning, hair spray, excessive heat, etc.

Service, warranty, repairs, follow-up process, etc.

Mr. B. was encouraged to maintain a journal of his experiences, both good and bad, so that appropriate adjustments to his hearing aids could be made.

Mr. B. returned for his two-week follow-up, and it was apparent from his attitude that his experience had been favorable. Mr. B. reported that he was so pleased about how he was hearing that the night following his fitting he decided to go to a fiftieth wedding anniversary gathering. As expected, it was "too much, too soon," and he had to remove the hearing aids before the end of the evening.

Mr. B.'s journal included positive comments about how much "clearer" the TV sounded and that one-on-one conversations were much easier for him to hear. On the negative side, he felt that in situations where there was "a lot going on" (background noise) he could actually hear better with the hearing aids removed. He also commented that using the telephone was difficult because it sounded too soft. A combination of reducing gain and increasing the compression kneepoint for both channels was used to address his concerns about background noise. However, when he tried the telephone in our clinic, the volume still seemed too soft. Gain for the telephone coil circuit was increased, and he reported that it was much better. He was scheduled for a one-month follow-up appointment.

His one-month follow-up visit was very positive. Competing noise situations were much better, and he also reported doing much better on the telephone.

> Mr. B.'s overall speech perception was improved dramatically when listening to speech presented at a normal conversational level.

REMEDIATE COMMUNICATION ACTIVITY. At each of his follow-up visits, Mr. B. was given additional information about how to maximize his communication ability. The information included the following items from our CLEAR handout:

Control communication situations by avoiding noisy areas, poorly lit areas, and the like.

Look at speaker: Visual cues from speakers are important and help make up for lost information.

Escape and expectations: Be realistic about situations where it will be easy or difficult to hear. Plan strategies for dealing with unfavorable listening situations.

Assertiveness: Let others know that you have difficulty hearing and encourage them to gain your attention before speaking and to look at you when they are talking.

Repair strategies: If a breakdown occurs in communication, repeat back to the speaker what you *did* hear and then ask him or her to clarify what you *did not* hear.

ENVIRONMENT AND COORDINATION: PARTICIPATION IMPROVEMENT. On Mr. B.'s three-month follow-up, his neighbor (who initially referred him to our clinic) accompanied him. Both were extremely appreciative of what the hearing aids had done to improve his quality of life. Mr. B. reported that he is attending more group functions (group communication goal), has kept in better touch with his family through the telephone (telephone goal), and is less intimidated by difficult communication situations. His neighbor reported that Mr. B. seemed much more outgoing and positive about himself and had been praising the effects of his new instruments to others.

Scoring of the aided portion of the Glasgow profile resulted in scores that supported Mr. B and his neighbor's comments. In the Hearing Aid Use category he scored an 80 percent, indicating a high level of hearing aid use. In the Hearing Aid Benefit category he scored 39 percent, indicating only a moderate amount of perceived benefit. For the Residual Disability category he scored 52 percent, indicating a reduced perception of disability (unaided initial disability was 72 percent). Finally, in the Satisfaction category his mean score was 91 percent, indicating a very high level of satisfaction with his hearing aids.

Summary

This is a classic case because it contains two very common issues in audiologic rehabilitation. The first issue relates to the amplification (modifying audibility) component of audiologic rehabilitation. Mr. B. had a dynamic range problem, and his previous three sets of hearing aids did not manage differing input levels appropriately. He would turn the hearing aids up to hear soft sounds and then loud sounds would be too loud. When he was exposed to loud sounds, he would have to turn the hearing aids down. After a few weeks of use, he would just set the hearing aids to where loud sounds were comfortable and the result was inadequate gain for soft and average inputs. Current multichannel technology has the ability to address differences in dynamic range associated with hearing loss more effectively. Mr. B.'s new hearing aids were programmed to help to manage his problems related to loudness. This capability contributed much toward enabling Mr. B. to be a successful hearing aid user this time around.

The second issue is that hearing loss often results in communication problems that can be perceived as depressionlike symptoms and can ultimately affect one's emotional well-being. Providing amplification can go a long way to relieving some of these problems, but effective rehabilitation should also address other appropriate aspects of communication. For example, effective use of communication strategies, establishing patient-based goals, the inclusion of the communication partner in rehabilitative efforts, and consideration of environmental situations all help to increase communication competence.

Synergy is a process in which the whole is greater than the sum of the parts. As with Mr. B., a definite synergy often occurs when the audiologic rehabilitation process for adults is managed multidimensionally and includes more than just targeting amplification.

Successful audiologic rehabilitation often can have a positive impact on an individual that goes beyond simply facilitating communication.

CASE 3   J. D.: AR FEATURING A SIGNIFICANT
■ OTHER

Introduction

J. D. is a 28-year-old male college student who, at his wife's insistence, made an appointment at a local audiology center for a complete evaluation. J. D. and his wife were married six months ago, and the stress of being newlyweds has been amplified considerably by communication difficulties on his part. J. D. had always felt that he had *some* difficulty hearing, but not as much as his wife seemed to describe. His wife felt that J. D. "just doesn't listen" and reported that "he tunes me out!"

J. D. was unaware of any history of hearing loss in his family but believed that he first noticed some difficulty hearing after working with a construction firm after graduation from high school. His wife admittedly hadn't had the opportunity to interact with too many people who had difficulty hearing and said that "my grandma and grandpa don't even wear hearing aids."

Informational Counseling

The policy for the audiology center is to invite the patient's significant other, if possible, to the evaluation. Having the significant other present during the evaluation and informational counseling session helps supplement case history and rehabilitative goal setting. The results of the evaluation and the communication implications were discussed in detail with both J. D. and his wife. It seemed to make perfect sense to J. D., but his wife was convinced that it was more of an "attention" problem than a "hearing" problem and that it seemed like a big expense to proceed with rehabilitation when all he would have to do is "listen."

Rehabilitation Assessment

COMMUNICATION STATUS: IMPAIRMENT AND ACTIVITY LIMITATIONS

AUDIOMETRY. The evaluation revealed a moderate, precipitous, high-frequency sensorineural hearing loss in both ears (see Figure 12.3). The loss was slightly greater at 4000 Hz in the right ear. His word recognition scores using phonetically balanced words (PB) were 88 percent in the right ear and 92 percent in the left ear. However, when high-frequency word lists were used (Gardner's High Frequency Words), his scores dropped dramatically to 68 percent in the right ear and 72 percent in the left ear.

A dynamic range (DR) assessment by frequency showed near-normal DR for the low frequencies (80 dB); reduced dynamic range for the mid frequencies (50 dB); and a very shallow DR (30 dB) for the frequencies above 2000 Hz.

COMMUNICATION ASSESSMENT. The *Self Assessment of Communication (SAC)* and the *Significant Other Assessment of Communication (SOAC)* (Schow & Nerbonne, 1982)

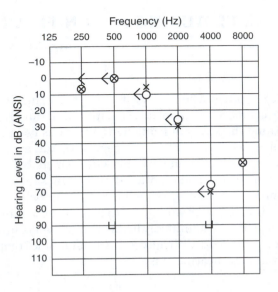

Speech Audiometry

	PTA	SRT	WRS PB Words	Level	WRS HF Words	Level
Right	12	15	88%	50 dB HL	68%	50 dB HL
Left	12	15	92%	50 dB HL	72%	50 dB HL

tools were used to help quantify J. D. and his wife's perception of the communication difficulty. Both of these assessment tools use the same ten questions to sample self-assessed difficulty in a variety of communication situations. The first five questions evaluate Activity Limitation (Disability) and include an open-ended communication situation item for the patient to identify a specific communication concern. Questions six through nine evaluate Participation Restriction (Handicap), and question ten applies to patients wearing amplification and asks them to estimate their hearing aid use in hours. The *SAC* and the *SOAC* are identical; however, the *patient* fills out the *SAC* and a "significant other" fills out the *SOAC*. Patients can be asked to complete the instrument prior to treatment (audiologic rehabilitation) and following treatment.

J. D.'s assessment of his communication difficulty revealed a total score of 33 percent, but his wife's assessment yielded a score of 80 percent, indicating that *her* perception of *his* communication difficulty was much greater (see Figure 12.4). When the individual items on the *SAC* and *SOAC* were compared, both J. D. and his wife indicated similar patterns for the "Various Communication Situations" section. For example, quiet one-to-one situations showed the least difficulty while group situations or difficult listening environments showed the most difficulty. However, in the "Social and Emotional" section, J. D. felt like his hearing loss "limited or hampered his personal or social life" only "occasionally," while his wife rated this item as "practically always." Similarly, the question asking "Do problems or dif-

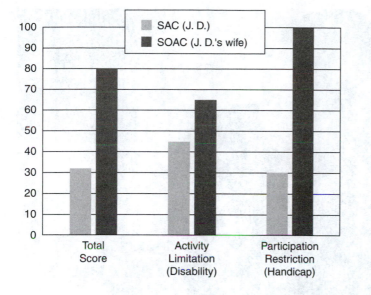

FIGURE 12.4

Summary of results for the initial administration of SAC and SOAC.

ficulty with your hearing upset you?" also showed a large difference, with J. D. reporting a 1 (Almost Never) and his wife reporting a 5 (Practically Always).

As shown in Figure 12.4, when the subcategories of Activity Limitation (Disability) and Participation Restriction (Handicap) were summarized, J. D.'s Activity Limitation (Disability) was computed at 45 percent and his wife's report revealed a score of 65 percent. For Participation Restriction (Handicap), J. D.'s score was 30 percent, while his wife estimated his Participation Restriction (Handicap) at 100 percent—again, a much different perception.

OVERALL PARTICIPATION VARIABLES. The demand on J. D.'s hearing is predictably high. He is a graduate student in biological sciences, and his classes are detailed in instruction and demanding. At home, it is important for him to be able to communicate with his wife and ease some of the stresses of being a newlywed.

RELATED PERSONAL FACTORS. Both J. D. and his wife indicated that he is a quiet person, somewhat introverted, but extremely intelligent. He is admittedly fascinated with technology and incorporates it in many aspects of his life, including computers, cellular phones, entertainment, and instruction.

ENVIRONMENTAL FACTORS. J. D. works part-time as a graduate assistant teaching an undergraduate biology laboratory course. The labs are taught in a large facility with poor acoustics and a substantial amount of noise for most of the class.

Rehabilitation Management

COUNSELING AND PSYCHOSOCIAL ISSUES. J. D. did not deny that he had a hearing problem, but at the same time didn't feel like the communication difficulties that he and his wife were experiencing were as bad as *she* indicated. Regardless, he was

Taking an ear impression for a new hearing aid.

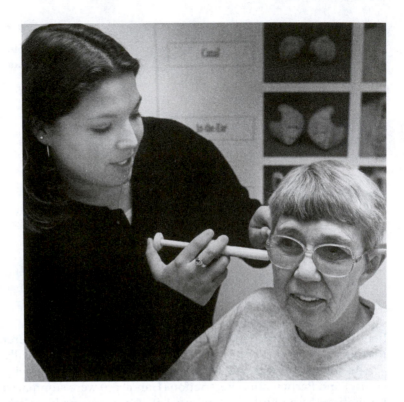

willing to do whatever was required to maximize his communication ability both at home and at school. As a way of setting rehabilitation goals, he was asked to pick two specific communication situations that he would like to improve. For the home environment, he wanted to be able to "hear his wife better, even if she is in another room." For his school environment, he wanted to be able to hear his students' questions even if they were in the back row.

The audiologist felt it was important at this point to provide some education and informational counseling to J. D.'s wife. It was clear that she continued to feel that it was nothing more than a "listening problem." As a way of helping her understand the difficulties associated with hearing loss, she was encouraged to experience hearing loss for one day. She was given two disposable foam ear plugs and instructed on how to insert them correctly. Her assignment was to place the earplugs first thing in the morning and wear them throughout the day. Additionally, she was asked to write down any difficulties or frustrations she experienced.

AUDIBILITY/IMPAIRMENT MANAGEMENT

AMPLIFICATION (MODIFYING AUDIBILITY). Since one of J. D.'s passions was technology, it was not difficult to talk about new technology in amplification. He was intrigued with the advances and eager to get started with a trial period. The goals that he had set were translated by the audiologist into focusing on maximizing the access to soft, speech-generated sounds while minimizing the impact of any type of competing nonspeech sound such as a running dishwasher (in the home environment) or a noisy laboratory (in his work environment). The audiologist felt that a binaural hearing aids with adaptive directional microphone technology along with aggressive nonspeech signal filtering would help J. D. to reach his goals. J. D. was given the option of either behind-the-ear (BTE) or in-the-ear (ITE) style hearing aids. While his wife felt that the BTE style was "ugly" and conspicuous, she ultimately yielded the decision to J. D., and he chose to stay with the BTE style.

The hearing aids were current state-of-the art and featured adaptive directional microphone technology that was coupled with a speech/nonspeech detector. The result allowed the hearing aids to not only reduce nonspeech generated noise, but to track and enhance sound that appeared to be speech. The intent was to provide J. D. with as much access to speech information as possible while reducing any potential competing noise.

The hearing aids were preprogrammed prior to his fitting appointment with his threshold and supra-threshold (uncomfortable levels) information, and an initial amplification target was set using the Desired Sensation Level (DSL) I/O fitting formula (Seewald, 1992). The hearing aids were equipped with multiple listening-situation memories. The first memory was set to adaptive processing, which allowed the hearing aid to manage the sound environment. The second memory was set to force the directional microphones to only receive from the front (the direction he would be facing). The third memory was optimized to use with his cellular phone.

When the appointment for the hearing aid fitting and orientation was set, he was encouraged to bring his wife. The hearing aids were placed in his ears and the actual fit of the hearing aids was inspected. The earmolds slipped in easily and seemed stable once in place. The BTE portion of the hearing aids fit nicely behind his ear and for the most part were covered by his hair. He reported that the hearing aids felt comfortable, and the circuits were then activated. He immediately had a look of disappointment because he expected that the hearing aids would sound louder. The audiologist explained to him that since his hearing loss was limited to just the high frequencies and that high frequencies carried more "clarity" information than "sound power" information, he would not get a large sensation of volume. Rather, he would just notice that sound was clearer and easier to understand. His wife mumbled something softly and he immediately responded appropriately.

Using both formal and informal measures, the hearing aids were set in such a way that soft sounds were audible but soft, average sounds (like the human voice) sounded appropriate, and loud sounds seemed loud, but not uncomfortable.

Speech mapping using probe-microphone measures was used as an objective way of evaluating not only *how* the hearing aids were providing him with amplification but *what* (in terms of speech or noise) type of signal the hearing aids were processing. The speech mapping indicated that not only did he have access to more of the clarity aspects of speech, but the hearing aids dynamically (using the directional microphones) followed the speech signal without having to move his head.

Finally, a formal functional assessment was performed under unaided and aided listening conditions using Gardner's high-frequency words. Unaided, binaural testing at 50 dB HL resulted in a score of 68 percent correct. Word recognition in the aided condition showed a score of 96 percent correct.

HEARING AID ORIENTATION. As a new user, it was important to cover the orientation topics (HIO BASICS) thoroughly, not only with J. D. but his wife as well.

Hearing expectations: Realistic (some situations will continue to be difficult and that the function of the hearing aids will be more "clarity" than power)

Instrument operation: On/off, telecoil, telephone use, memory button

Occlusion effect: User's voice with hearing aids in place

Batteries: Tabs, how long they will last, removal, replacement, dangers

Acoustic feedback: What causes it, when is it OK, not OK?

System troubleshooting: What to do when there are problems

Insertion/removal: Identifying left, right, insertion, and removal

Cleaning and maintenance: Wax/debris cleaning, hair spray, excessive heat, etc.

Summarize warranty, repairs, follow-up process, etc.

Both he and his wife were encouraged to write down situations where the hearing aids seem to be helping and situations that continue to be difficult. Additionally, a HIO BASICS DVD, produced at Idaho State University, was provided to them so that they could review the topics for clarification.

REMEDIATE COMMUNICATION ACTIVITY. Prior to proceeding with the first follow-up, his wife was asked to share her experience using the earplugs for a day. Initially (early in the morning), she felt that it wouldn't affect her at all, but as the day went on, she began to understand why J. D. seemed to ignore certain communication from her. By the end of the day, she was exhausted with having to strain to understand and constantly manipulate the situation (e.g., getting closer to the talker) to hear. Her experience simulating a hearing loss occurred at the same time J. D. was experiencing *better* access to sound through his new hearing aids. The communication difficulties, for a day, traded places.

Some minor adjustments were made to address some of the concerns that were written in both J. D.'s and his wife's journals, but overall, the hearing aids seemed to be giving him access to information that improved the clarity of speech and reduced the frustration for both of them.

The audiologist shared two types of communication strategy information: one for the talker and one for the receiver. For the receiver, the acronym CLEAR was used to represent five strategies: **C**ontrol the communication situation; **L**ook at the talker; **E**xpect realistic performance; **A**ssert yourself; and **R**epair communication breakdown. For the talker, the acronym SPEECH was used to represent six similar strategies: **S**potlight your face; **P**ause slightly between phrases; **E**mpathize with the person; **E**ase their listening by gaining their attention; **C**ontrol the listening situation; and **H**ave a plan for difficult listening situations.

ENVIRONMENTAL/COORDINATION: PARTICIPATION IMPROVEMENT. At J. D.'s one-month follow-up, the audiologist focused on improving specific situations that continued to be difficult. Additionally, the audiologist asked both J. D. and his wife to complete a *SAC* and *SOAC* form based on his experiences using amplification and the strategies offered in the audiologic rehabilitation session. One situation that continued to be difficult was his teaching environment. The background noise produced in the lab was a mix of nonspeech sounds and speech-generated noise. This made it difficult for the hearing aid circuitry to determine "what" speech to amplify and often resulted in J. D.'s turning off and removing his hearing aids. A number of environmental control suggestions were made. For example, it was suggested that the class be restructured so that instruction prior to the lab activity was done by having the entire class gather in the front of the lab. This increased the signal (students' questions and comments) as compared to the background noise. Then, the students would return to their lab tables and begin the activity. Another modification of the environment was to have the students signal J. D. when they needed to talk to him. J. D. would go to the student with the question, and because of the close proximity, the adaptive directional microphones on the hearing aids maximized the signal (student's voice) as compared to the background noise.

J. D. and his wife were asked to complete the *SAC* and *SOAC* forms again to estimate the residual communication difficulties following rehabilitation. The results are shown in Figure 12.5, and indicated that the use of amplification and the strategies offered in the rehabilitation process had resulted in benefits with an impact on both disability and handicap. The residual disability reported by J. D. was 20 percent (compared to an initial disability of 45 percent), resulting in a 25 percent benefit. His wife's assessment was more dramatic. The residual disability was 28

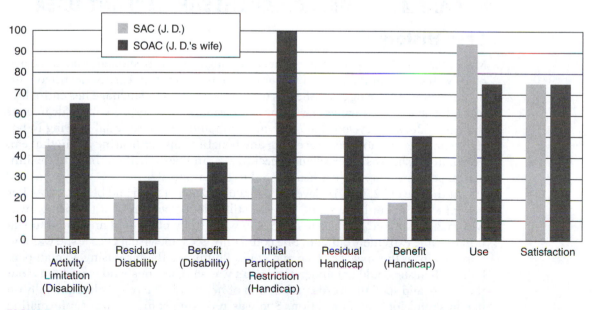

FIGURE 12.5

Summary of *SAC-SOAC* results (in percent), comparing results from the initial and follow-up administrations.

percent (compared to 65 percent initial disability) resulting in a 37 percent benefit. The residual handicap reported by J. D. was 12 percent (compared to an initial handicap of 30 percent) resulting in an 18 percent benefit. Again his wife's assessment showed greater benefit. For her the residual handicap was 50 percent (compared to 100 percent initial handicap), resulting in a 50 percent benefit. Both J. D. and his wife reported use and satisfaction scores of 75 percent or over.

Summary

Hearing impairment can result in communication difficulty and since "communication" implies both a sender and a receiver, it stands to reason that the hearing impairment *also* affects those people who interact with the hearing-impaired person. In the rehabilitative process, it is easy to focus on the individual with the hearing loss and forget about involving the significant other.

This case provides two examples of how the significant other can participate in the audiologic rehabilitation process. The first example is about *perception*. J. D. and his wife had very different feelings about his communication difficulties. This information helped the audiologist outline the rehabilitation process to include J. D.'s wife to a greater extent. The second example was using the rehabilitation process to work directly with the significant other. Having J. D.'s wife simulate a day with hearing loss helped her better understand the problem and move her from thinking it was just a "listening" problem.

■ CASE 4   MRS. D.: COCHLEAR IMPLANT USER

Case History

Mrs. D. was a 57-year-old woman whose hearing loss was first diagnosed at the age of 10 years after an infection of unknown origin. At that time, she was fitted with bilateral power hearing aids. She has used oral speech and language her entire life, was educated in the regular classroom, and went on to receive a college degree. At the age of 20, she developed another infection and lost all residual hearing in her right ear. She was no longer receiving any benefit from her hearing aid in that ear. Fortunately, she was an excellent speechreader and has relied on this and the limited benefit from her left ear hearing aid to communicate.

At the age of 52, Mrs. D. developed macular degeneration and began to lose her eyesight. For about three years, she was still able to speechread if the person was within 3 feet of her. By the age of 55, she was legally blind, and any communication became extremely difficult. She could only get some visual cues if she was 6 to 8 inches from the speaker's face and could illuminate the face using a small penlight. When she could not understand what was said, her husband would draw out the letters and spell the words in the palm of her hand. She relied almost totally on her husband for communication. She was receiving some auditory information from her power digital hearing aid in the left ear. Her audiologist referred her for a cochlear implant (CI) evaluation.

Assessment Information

Audiometric evaluation revealed a bilateral sensorineural hearing loss (Figure 12.6). Pure-tone thresholds indicated a severe loss at 250 Hz, rapidly dropping to a profound loss in the left ear and no measurable hearing at the limits of the audiometer in the right ear. Otoacoustic emissions (OAEs) were absent bilaterally. A Speech Awareness Threshold (SAT) was obtained at 90 dB HL in the left ear. Word recognition scores were not measurable bilaterally.

Aided thresholds were obtained at 45 dB HL at 250 Hz and 500 Hz, and 50 dB HL from 1000 Hz through 4000 Hz. Further aided evaluation was completed with

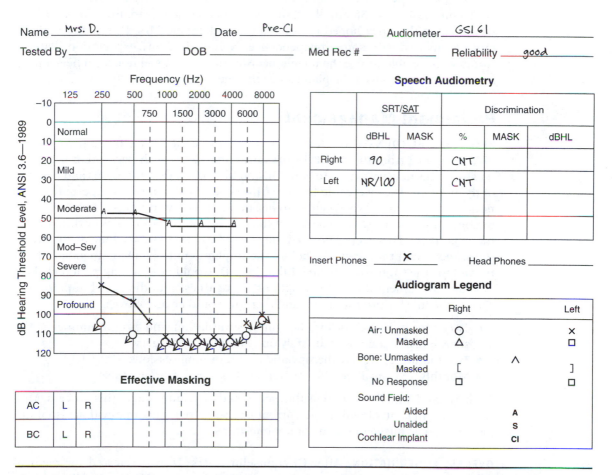

FIGURE 12.6

Case 4: Unaided and aided audiometric results for Mrs. D., preimplant.

Mrs. D. using the *Hearing in Noise Test* (*HINT;* Nilsson, Soli, & Sullivan, 1994) at a 55 dB HL presentation level in a quiet test condition. She was able to repeat 8 percent of the words on this test using twenty sentences in the auditory-only mode. On the *Consonant Nucleus Consonant Test* (*CNC;* Peterson & Lehiste, 1962), Mrs. D. correctly identified 26 percent of the phonemes and 0 percent of the words correctly. When presented the *CID Everyday Sentence List* (Davis & Silverman, 1970) via live voice with both auditory and visual cues, Mrs. D. was able to correctly identify 79 percent of the key words. This test was done 8 inches from the tester's face with the use of Mrs. D.'s penlight illuminating the speaker's face.

Paper and pencil questionnaires were given to Mrs. D. and her husband to ascertain their perceived handicap and expectations for a CI. Her score on the Screening version of the *Hearing Handicap Inventory for the Elderly* (*HHIE-S;* Ventry & Weinstein, 1983) was 38 out of 40, indicating severe handicap. Both Mr. and Mrs. D. indicated that they hoped the implant would enable Mrs. D. to communicate more easily and gain some independence. Neither had any expectation that she would ever be able to use the telephone. She stated that she hoped to hear music again, as she has played the piano since the age of 12.

Preimplant Management

PSYCHOSOCIAL/COUNSELING. Mrs. D. was determined to be a good audiologic candidate for a CI from the results of the pure-tone and speech-perception tests. Extensive counseling was given to both Mr. and Mrs. D. on the limitations and benefits of the implant. They were told that the CI was designed as an aid to speechreading, not a replacement for visual cues, so her blindness may still make it very difficult to communicate. They were also told that music appreciation is very difficult for many patients. They were informed they must have evaluations done medically by the surgeon and radiologically before the implant could be recommended. If approved for the CI, it was explained that Mrs. D. would need a long period of therapy and adjustment due to the length of her deafness and the visual impairment. Their schedule for programming and therapy would be as follows:

- Two consecutive days for the initial stimulation and programming of the speech processor, approximately one month after surgery
- Two months of weekly therapy and programming sessions
- Monthly sessions thereafter during the first year of implant use

Both Mr. and Mrs. D. assured us that she would be committed to this process. Mrs. D. was put in contact with three current CI users, including one with a visual impairment, who answered many of her questions.

OVERALL COORDINATION. After CI counseling, Mrs. D. was referred for medical evaluations that included a magnetic resonance imaging (MRI) test. All members of the CI team agreed Mrs. D. was a candidate for the CI. The decision was made to implant the right side since she was able to wear a hearing aid in her left ear. Mrs. D. was successfully implanted with a multichannel CI. The entire electrode was inserted surgically with no complications.

Postimplant Management

COCHLEAR IMPLANT INITIAL STIMULATION AND PROGRAMMING. Four weeks after surgery, Mrs. D. returned for electrical stimulation of her CI and follow-up therapy. Initial integrity testing indicated impedances within normal limits for all stimulation modes and demonstrated that all electrodes were functioning properly. During programming for the initial MAP, measurements of threshold and comfort values were attempted, but no reliable responses were obtained. Mrs. D. was very nervous and anxious during programming, which may have interfered with her concentration on obtaining accurate threshold and comfort levels across the electrode array. Therefore, initial threshold and comfort values were adjusted according to her detection to live voice and environmental noises. Upon initial activation of her speech processor, Mrs. D. stated tearfully that she heard things but nothing was clear. She said she knew it would take time to get adjusted. The proper workings and care of the processor were explained to Mrs. D. and her husband. She indicated that she would review the processor buttons with her magnifying glass to learn the orientation of buttons and see the indicator screen on the processor. They were together able to demonstrate how to use and care for the processor. She was instructed to continue using her hearing aid in the opposite ear.

The next day, measurements of Mrs. D.'s thresholds and comfort values were again attempted, with more reliable results. Her MAPs were modified and by the end of the session of programming, Mrs. D. was able to repeat back simple everyday sentences relying on auditory input alone.

During the following ten weeks programming consisted of trying different strategies and settings to optimize her MAPs. Continued monitoring of her threshold and comfort levels and subsequent MAP modifications were made throughout her therapy sessions. On the third week of programming she was fitted with an ear-level processor programmed similar to her best two body-worn processor MAPs. Throughout the process Mrs. D. was asked to keep a diary of her experiences. At home she is able write using a visual aid on her computer. She consistently wrote notes each day on her progress and brought them with her to the sessions.

AUDIOVISUAL TRAINING. Therapy sessions consisted of training Mrs. D. in a hierarchy of auditory skills including sound detection, word and sentence-length discrimination and identification, pattern discrimination and identification in phrases and sentences, and identification of overlearned speech (common expressions) using materials from Cochlear Corporation (1998). Drill work using consonant and vowel stimuli in auditory-only and auditory/visual modes was also used in each session. Her auditory-only scores with consonant-nucleus-consonant items (Peterson & Lehiste, 1962) improved from a preimplant score of 28 percent for phonemes and 0 percent for words to postimplant scores of 75 percent for phonemes and 54 percent for words within the first year of implant use. Through speech tracking (DeFilippo & Scott, 1978), Mrs. D. practiced using the CI and hearing aid in understanding running speech. The use of communication strategies was stressed and practiced during the tracking exercises. Her husband was trained to do tracking with her at home also. After one month of therapy, telephone use was introduced, using codes and overlearned speech. Telephone codes were developed to aid persons with severe to profound hearing loss to use the telephone with very limited hearing abilities (Castle, 1984). For example, the person with hearing loss asks yes-no questions and the other person responds with "yes–yes," "no," or "please repeat." The person with hearing loss can then listen for the number of syllables to know the answer. Mrs. D. found she could communicate with her mother and two sisters on the phone for the first time in ten years. After three months of use, she reported that she was using the telephone frequently with family and friends without the use of codes.

COUNSELING/OVERALL COORDINATION. Throughout the therapy sessions, Mrs. D. kept the ongoing diary of her experiences with the CI. She listed wearing times, environmental sounds heard, and communication situations. The diary served as a focal point of behavioral counseling. Specific problems were discussed, pointing out both the benefits and limitations of the CI, along with possible strategies she might use in each situation. The diary also served as a means of judging her perceived progress with the implant. Here are excerpts from her diary:

> *Six weeks postimplant.* Only a little more than a month has passed since the implant was turned on, but already I am hearing far, far better than before surgery! There is still a long row to hoe, and it is not easy, but to be able to converse so much more easily with people, even without lipreading, has made life more enjoyable—and easier for others, too. Music appreciation is still relatively primitive, but is improving. With the assistance of the hearing aid in the other ear, I have resumed piano lessons. And to learn about all the strange new sounds that the hearing aid cannot pick up is an adventure in itself.

> *Six months postimplant.* It is fascinating to listen to spoken words, to hear how they truly sound. In the past, words consisted of some sound supplemented by lipreading. Now I listen to the consonants in "quickly" and "temperature," for example, and <my husband> has a much easier time introducing names and terms we discuss with news reports. People have commented that my speech has improved, whatever that means! I've enjoyed playing Christmas carols, learning how they really sound. I've never heard cymbals before—that took some getting used to!

At her one-year evaluation, Mrs. D.'s audiogram was repeated using both her hearing aid and the CI. Her thresholds for narrow band noise were obtained from 30 to 35 dB HL from 250 through 6000 Hz. Her score on the *HINT* improved to 91 percent in quiet. At a 10 dB signal-to-noise ratio she was able to repeat 78 percent of the words on the *HINT*. She no longer uses the penlight to speechread and can carry on a conversation with most people with relative ease. She has become much more independent.

Examples of Overlearned Speech

How are you?	It is time for lunch.
What time is it?	Do you know him?
Do you know all of them?	Good morning.
I can see you now.	We have to do something.
I have been thinking.	We have to go now.
What would you do?	I have one more for you.

Summary

CIs offer an excellent opportunity for deafened adults to receive beneficial auditory information. Many CI benefits can be seen across patients, from those who have good open-set understanding even on the telephone to those who receive minimal auditory cues. Mrs. D. is representative of an average adult hearing-impaired CI patient. She is now able to communicate even with her visual impairment, can identify many more environmental sounds, and has telephone skills using the CI when talking with familiar individuals. Music, although not perfect, can be enjoyed.

Mrs. D.'s case also illustrates the importance of a full program of pre- and post-AR therapy and counseling with CI candidates and their families. Often, patients expect the CI to be a "bionic ear." Even after their expectations are tempered prior to surgery, they may be disappointed that the CI cannot provide "normal" hearing. Auditory training and communication strategy therapy help the patients learn to use the CI and deal with communication breakdowns. With appropriate training, the CI can improve the quality of life for an individual with severe-to-profound hearing impairment.

CASE 5   MRS. E.: NURSING HOME ■ HEARING AID USER

Case History

Mrs. E. was a 75-year-old resident of a local nursing home. She had been living in the facility for over two years and was quite alert mentally and able to move about the facility without any special assistance. Mrs. E. was using a behind-the-ear hearing aid in her right ear at the time she was first seen by an audiologist. It was later determined that she had been a longtime hearing aid user, having had four other instruments over a period of many years. Her present hearing aid was five years old and, according to Mrs. E., did not seem to be working as well as it once had.

Diagnostic Information

Initial efforts with Mrs. E. involved air conduction pure-tone testing and tympanometry in a quiet room within the nursing home. As seen in Figure 12.7, the client had a moderate hearing loss, which was bilaterally symmetrical. Type A tympanograms were traced bilaterally, suggesting the presence of a sensorineural disorder in each ear.

It is possible (and sometimes necessary) to gather basic, relevant audiometric information outside the traditional audiologic test booth if certain measures are taken to ensure the validity of the results obtained.

Audiologic Rehabilitation

Mrs. E. was concerned about the condition of her hearing aid, complaining that it did not seem to help her as much as it had in the past. She also appeared to be experiencing an excessive amount of acoustic feedback and reported having difficulty getting the earmold into her ear properly.

The hearing aid was analyzed electroacoustically by the audiologist, who found it to have a reduced gain and an abnormal amount of distortion. In discussing the

The repair and reconditioning of a hearing aid can be viable alternatives if the instrument is not too old and is still appropriate for the user's hearing loss.

feasibility of purchasing a new hearing aid, it became clear that Mrs. E. was not financially able to consider such a purchase. She was, therefore, advised to have her hearing aid serviced and reconditioned by the manufacturer. She was agreeable to this recommendation, and arrangements were made for this to occur.

In the course of working with Mrs. E., it became apparent that she needed a new earmold. In discussing this, Mrs. E. recalled that her current mold had also been used with her previous hearing aid. The mold was very discolored and did not appear to fit Mrs. E.'s ear canal and pinna adequately. The audiologist took an ear impression, which was sent to a laboratory for production of a new earmold.

In approximately two weeks, both the earmold and the hearing aid were returned. Mrs. E. was then fitted with the reconditioned aid, and her initial reaction was quite positive. She was instructed to use the aid as much as possible in the following days. A subsequent electroacoustic analysis of the instrument revealed an increase in gain and a significant improvement in the amount of distortion. Real-ear measures, taken at the nursing home with portable equipment, revealed satisfactory gain.

When she was seen again, Mrs. E. was still pleased with the help she was receiving from her hearing aid, but she indicated that she was still having difficulty inserting the earmold. Watching her attempt to do this herself made it apparent

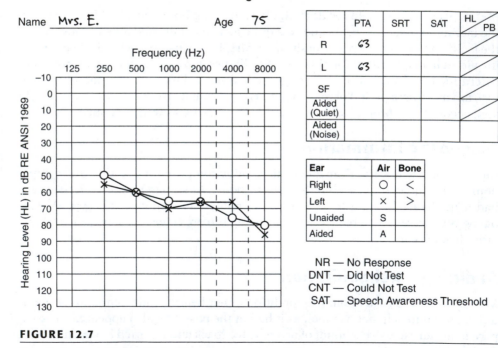

FIGURE 12.7

Case 5: Audiometric results for Mrs. E.

that Mrs. E. was not able to manipulate her hands sufficiently to allow her to insert the earmold without great effort. It was also apparent that she was not using an efficient method when inserting the mold. To assist her, Mrs. E. was given some basic instructions on how to best insert and remove the earmold. She was encouraged to practice the procedure and was visited by the audiologist several times during the next two weeks to review the procedure and to answer any questions she might have. During these visits it became apparent that Mrs. E.'s facility in placement of the earmold had improved.

More frequent monitoring of the status of some patients is important to facilitate success with audiologic rehabilitation.

Along with the work done with Mrs. E. to improve the way she inserted her earmold, several of the nursing home staff members working with Mrs. E. were also provided with information on how to put the earmold in properly. This allowed them to assist Mrs. E. in doing so each day. Both Mrs. E. and the staff also received helpful information on how to clean her earmold and basic instruction on the operation and use of her hearing aid.

Summary

Attempts to help Mrs. E. were successful. This is not always the case when working in a rehabilitative capacity with nursing home residents (Schow, 1982). Mrs. E.'s case illustrates one of the ways in which an audiologist can make a valuable contribution to a number of residents in a given nursing home. It is important first to identify those individuals within the facility for whom audiologic rehabilitation may be beneficial. Once this is done, the audiologist will generally work with each person individually, identifying those areas of AR that should be worked on. Individual needs must be considered, and the audiologist must be willing to devote the time necessary to accomplish the desired ends.

SUMMARY POINTS

- Hearing impairment can produce a variety of difficulties for an individual, and effective audiologic rehabilitation must address these particular needs.
- Information gathering, including discussions with the patient, the use of self-report scales, hearing tests, auditory–visual skills assessment, and other relevant sources of information, is an important component of audiologic rehabilitation.
- Successful intervention depends to a large extent on the degree of motivation possessed by the individual with hearing impairment.
- Today's hearing aids are complex instruments. Proper selection and fitting of these devices require extensive expertise and instrumentation in order to maximize their potential.
- The intervention process can be threatened if the person with hearing impairment has unrealistic hopes and expectations related to a component of audiologic rehabilitation (e.g., a cochlear implant) that are impossible to fulfill. Clinicians need to monitor this continuously with their patients, especially in the early stages of intervention.

■ Comprehensive and effective hearing aid fitting, particularly for first-time users, should include an extensive orientation to hearing aid use and exposure to factors that facilitate communication.

RECOMMENDED READING

Johnson, C. E., & Danhauer, J. L. (1999). *Guidebook for support programs in aural rehabilitation.* San Diego, CA: Singular Publishing Group.

Johnson, C. E., & Danhuer, J. L. (2002). *Handbook of outcomes measurement in audiology.* San Diego, CA: Singular Publishing Group.

REFERENCES

Castle, D. L. (1984). *Telephone training for the hearing-impaired persons.* Rochester, NY: NTID/RID.

Cochlear Corporation. (1998). *Rehabilitation manual.* Englewood, CO: Cochlear Corp.

Davis, H., & Silverman, R. (1970). *Hearing and deafness.* New York: Holt, Rinehart and Winston.

DeFilippo, C., & Scott, B. (1978). A method for training and evaluating the reception of ongoing speech. *Journal of the Acoustical Society of America, 63,* 1186–1192.

Gatehouse, S. (1999). Glasgow hearing aid benefit profile: Derivation and validation of a client-centered outcome measure for hearing aid services. *Journal of the American Academy, of Audiology, 10,* 80–103.

Goldstein, D., & Stephens, S. (1981). Audiological rehabilitation: Management model I. *Audiology, 20,* 432–452.

Nilsson, M. J., Soli, S. D., & Sullivan, J. A. (1994). Development of the *Hearing in Noise Test* for the measurement of speech reception in quiet and in noise. *Journal of the Acoustical Society of America, 95,* 1085–1099.

Peterson, G., & Lehiste, I. (1962). Revised CNC lists for auditory tests. *Journal of Speech and Hearing Disorders, 27,* 62–70.

Schow, R. L. (1982). Success of hearing aid fitting in nursing home residents. *Ear and Hearing, 3*(3),173–177.

Schow, R. L. (1989). Self assessment of hearing in rehabilitative audiology: Developments in the U.S.A. *British Journal of Audiology, 23,* 13–24.

Schow, R. L. & Nerbonne, M. (1982). Communication screening profile: Use with elderly clients. *Ear and Hearing, 3*(3), 133–147.

Seewald, R. (1992). The desired sensation level method for fitting children. *Hearing Journal, 45,* 36–46.

Seewald, R. (2000). An update of DSL [i/o]. *Hearing Journal, 53*(4), 10–16.

Ventry, I., & Weinstein, B. (1983). Identification of elderly people with hearing problems. *Journal of Speech Hear Research, 25,* 37–42.

World Health Organization (WHO). (2001). *International classification of functioning, disability, and health: ICF.* Geneva, Switzerland: Author.

■ AUTHOR INDEX

SUBJECT INDEX